Obesity

Causes, Mechanisms, Prevention, and Treatment

Obesity

Causes, Mechanisms, Prevention, and Treatment

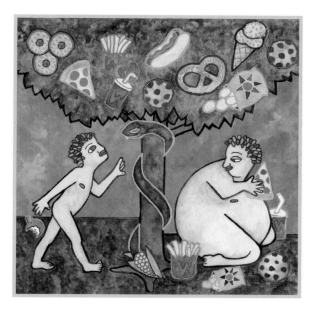

Edited by Elliott M. Blass

Sinauer Associates, Inc. • Publishers
Sunderland, MA 01375

About the Cover

The cover is by western Massachusetts artist Joanne Delphia (www.jdelphia.com). The theme of Adam and Eve, independently inspired artist and editor, captures the temptation of overeating. The snake, with a corn cob (the source of most energy-dense foods) instead of a rattle tail, masterminds each first taste. After taking a bite of the apple, Eve's determination is palpable as she strides towards the tree discarding the fruit, which does not stand a chance against temptation of the tree and advertising of the snake.

Obesity: Causes, Mechanisms, Prevention, and Treatment

Copyright 2008

For information address:
Sinauer Associates, Inc.
23 Plumtree Road
Sunderland, MA 01375 U.S.A.
FAX: 413-549-1118
Email: publish@sinauer.com
Internet: www.sinauer.com

Library of Congress Cataloging-in-Publication Data
Obesity: causes, mechanisms, prevention, and treatment / edited by Elliott M. Blass.
    p. ; cm.
  Includes bibliographical references and index.
   ISBN 978-0-87893-209-2 (hardcover) — ISBN 978-0-87893-037-1 (pbk.)
1. Obesity—Etiology. 2. Obesity—Psychological aspects. I. Blass,
Elliott M., 1940-
   [DNLM: 1. Obesity. 2. Diet. 3. Feeding Behavior. WD 210 O112193 2008]
   RC628.O245 2008
   616.3'98—dc22   2008010121

Printed in U.S.A.
4 3 2 1

CONTRIBUTING AUTHORS

CONTENTS

Chapter **6**

Development of Eating Behavior: Immediate and Long-Term Consequences   163
Julie Lumeng

Chapter 7

Chapter 8

Chapter 9

Built Environments and Obesity   281
Jeffery Sobal and Brian Wansink

Chapter 10

From Protocols to Populations: Establishing a Role for Energy Density of Food in the Obesity Epidemic   301
Marion M. Hetherington and Barbara J. Rolls

Chapter **11**

Proposed Modifications to the Food Stamp Program: Likely Effects and Their Policy Implications   319

Conner C. Mullally, Julian M. Alston, Daniel A. Sumner, Marilyn S. Townsend, and Stephen A. Vosti

Chapter **12**

Environmental Food Messages and Childhood Obesity   371

Shauna Harrison, Darcy A. Thompson, and Dina L. G. Borzekowski

Chapter **13**

A Framework for the Treatment of Obesity: Early Support   399

*Cecilia Bergh, Matthew Sabin, Julian Shield, Göran Hellers, Modjtaba
Zandian, Karolina Palmberg, Barbro Olofsson, Kerstin Lindeberg, Mikael
Björnström, and Per Södersten*

Epilogue   427

Elliott M. Blass

PREFACE

Elliott M. Blass

In late July 2007, the pharmaceutical giant Smith, Kline & French (SKF) received permission from the FDA to market the weight loss drug orlistat over the counter, under the brand name *alli*. At best, orlistat was a marginally effective weight loss agent, requiring large (120-milligram) doses three times daily. Moreover, because orlistat prevented absorption of about 30% of ingested fat, the effective dose caused almost all those who took it to experience mild to moderate gastric distress, excessive flatulence, bowel urgency, and in many cases, bowel incontinence. Orlistat as a prescription drug had an understandably poor track record. Alli, on the other hand, has been a smashing success; supplies have been exhausted, and newspapers and trade magazines have reported runaway sales. Given the dismal track record of orlistat and the startling price of $60 for a 2- to 4-week supply, one may well ask if there was an obesity epidemic threatening the land (think back to the recent run on the anti-anthrax drug Cipro, when the possible threat of anthrax release by terrorists gripped the nation), and if so, what can be done about it.

Addressing this vital public health issue has led to this text on obesity, its status as a public health entity, its causes, potential treatments, and possible means of prevention. In formulating this text while teaching an advanced undergraduate/graduate course, I realized that *obesity* is being directly addressed by a number of "unrelated" disciplines. The investigators who study obesity are unrelated in academic backgrounds and departments, which vary from epidemiology to gastrointestinal physiology to drug addiction, to exercise science, to agricultural policy, among others. They publish in very different journals with the understandable consequence that only very occasional references appear in literatures of sister disciplines also directly concerned with obesity sources and solutions. My students and I had to inform ourselves, and each other, of the issues confronting the individual fields and to integrate them as best we could. Clearly, a text was necessary, penned by experts in the various disciplines.

Accordingly, I had to ask myself and others a number of questions. First, are we an obese nation? Experts unanimously agree that the United States most definitely is, that the trajectory is not abating, and that the rest of the world is catching up.

Second, does this spreading trait constitute an illness? Are the obese sick? Given the rapidity of spread, are we in the throes of an obesity epidemic? Should we view obesity as one would look at smallpox, and seek a cure, or should we view obesity as graying, a physical trait that may not be welcomed by all who turn gray but would not be considered a health issue. The issue of defining a disease entity is more complex and, in this case especially, depends on medical costs and medical and social perceptions. The run on alli reminds us of the complexities and dangers of making available to an anxious public, without constraints of prescription, a drug that, in fact, can do harm. We have yet to reap the consequences of the FDA's having released this drug from its prescription restraint.

Epidemiological evidence shows clearly that the obese are considerably more likely than nonobese to develop adult-onset diabetes mellitus (type 2) and to be more vulnerable to cardiovascular compromises. Moreover, the obese uniquely bear severe personal burdens. As a group, they are underemployed and undereducated, more likely to be depressed and to harbor a poor self-image. Thus, independent of the direct physical consequences of the state, severe emotional sequellae have not yet been addressed in a comprehensive and systematic way. But ameliorating these sequellae has proven controversial. Some hold the view that dieting may actually be harmful and that the national concern about obesity has been foisted on the public by multibillion-dollar industries such as fashion, diet books and plans, and so on, that keep alive the contemporary idea that slim is beautiful. These views must be given serious consideration and will be evaluated, but in the end the data speak for themselves: *direct, identifiable, social and economic burdens have been engendered by a country whose eating habits are out of control.*

This text addresses what, if anything, can be done about these burdens. Can obesity, either as an individual state or as a national medical, social, and financial burden, be reversed? The odds are strongly against such a reversal in the near or even intermediate future. Can the trend be arrested and the tide held in check? Here the likelihood is greater. Obesity can be prevented through judicious eating habits and exercise. But this is not new to any reader of this text. What is new are discussions "under one roof" that are accessible to undergraduates, graduates, and professionals of disciplines concerned with obesity, about how things have come to this pass and how understanding the interplay of sources may help address how to deal with each source as part of a matrix of sources. The individual does not have to shoulder the problem alone. Like all epidemics, obesity directly or indirectly affects all of us and adjustments must be made in a broad and integrated manner. In this regard there is some room for optimism.

There are grounds for pessimism as well. The deck seems stacked in favor of obesity formation. We, especially the obese, are burdened by our inherited phylogentic tendency to find energy-dense foods palatable—as described by Smith (Chapter 1), Moran (3), Wise (4), Snyder and Bartoshuk (5), and Yeomans

(7)—and to eat even more of these energy-dense foods through conditioning, as described by Lumeng (Chapter 6) and Yeomans (7). When we encounter energy-dense, nutrition-poor foods in a safe environment, we ignore short-term satiety signals arising from stomach and gut, and we overeat. This putative phylogenetic indulgence may have provided a hedge against future food scarcities from resources that were patchily distributed in time and space. In today's energy-dense, supersized, underexercised environment, however, such capacity is a liability. This hypothesis is supported by the ease with which extra energy is rapidly, and almost without cost, converted to fat.

Our evolutionary history, therefore, has left short-term inhibitory signals vulnerable to override. Meals can be extended by food attractiveness, by palatability, by the eater's history with that food, and by environmental distractions such as watching TV or eating with a group of friends and relatives, as indicated by Smith (Chapter 1), Moran (3), Hetherington and Rolls (10), and Harrison et al. (12). Furthermore, the food-seeking and consumption behaviors of obese individuals are eerily akin to those of people who are addicted to drugs, including alcohol. In Chapter 4, Wise draws very compelling parallels between the two, leading me (in the Epilogue) to the inexorable conclusion of identical characteristics between overeating and established forms of addiction, with the exceptions of physiological dependence and the time of onset of withdrawal symptoms, although these resemblances have not been fully evaluated empirically.

We are vulnerable to portion size, to the proximity of serving bowls, to the sight, smells, and even sounds of foods, as reviewed by Sobal and Wansink (Chapter 9). From the perspective of obesity, we have been penalized by the astonishing progress in a contemporary agriculture and transport in which many steps in earlier processing have been eliminated and foods travel very rapidly from producers to widespread markets. The severe personal downside of these technical advances is that large agribusiness (Big Ag) has effectively squeezed out small farmers and, through savings of scale and select US Department of Agriculture (USDA) agricultural subsidies, prices have been lowered to make energy-dense foods very accessible. As argued by Mullaly et al. (Chapter 11), adjusting the Food Stamp Program in a serious way requires time, although changes will likely succeed in the intermediate and, especially, long terms as markets adjust to government policies.

Gaining a better understanding of these issues and others—such as the contributions of exercise to good health in general and fitness in particular, as documented by Filiault (Chapter 8)—help defray the pessimism expressed here. Through integration of the particular knowledge concerning the behavior of individuals, of neighborhoods, and of political systems, particular targets can be chosen to help effect change at these different organizational levels to yield healthier eating and exercise practices. Changes in feeding of our children (as described by Lumeng in Chapter 6 and Harrison et al. in Chapter 12), in exercise programs, and in agricultural practices—all aimed at reducing disease and improving fitness—are within our reach.

Such change will take some time, however, and effective programs for losing weight—and especially maintaining the new weight level—must be developed. Issues of compliance plague all branches of medicine, but none more than compliance in abstinence programs. In Chapter 13, Bergh et al. document the success that their program has had in working with getting anorexics to eat and gain weight. Their initial results in modifying eating patterns of obese individuals hold hope for success in helping dieters maintain a new weight level.

It remains for me to thank all of the authors for their contributions and for their acceptance of the unique challenge of participating in a deeply interdisciplinary undertaking and in making their chapters provoking to the expert and accessible to the novice. Their goodwill and cooperation have been a source of delight for me throughout the process.

Finally, I dedicate this book to my brother, Jacob Blass. The essence of all of our meals together has been the process itself, making all of them delicious, even when the food was not.

Bocé, France
August 2007

CAUSES OF OBESITY

Lack of exercise

Food addiction

Government policy

Portion size:
30 versus 1003 calories

USDA
A
GRADE

1 CRITICAL INTRODUCTION TO OBESITY

Gerard P. Smith

Introduction

There is an overwhelming mass of information about the development, pathophysiology, prevention, and treatment of obesity. The glut of information is matched by the variety of interested consumers: children, adolescents, adults, parents, students, teachers, lay and professional caregivers, investigators from many scientific and clinical disciplines, policy advisers, government officials, restaurateurs, caterers, and pharmaceutical, food product, and health care corporations.

How did something as obvious as an abnormally large amount of body fat become so hard to explain, and why are so many people interested in understanding it, preventing it, and treating it? How did eating properly and the avoidance of obesity become such a dominant topic in our cultural conversation? The answers are numerous, and all of them are incomplete.

To deal with the problem, the editor of this volume has thought "outside the box" in selecting his authors. The usual molecular and integrative biomedical types are here, but they are complemented by experts from disciplines concerned with developmental, psychological, sociological, and environmental aspects of obesity. Thus, the topics covered include the pitfalls of changing governmental policy, the impact of watching television, the promise of computer-assisted learning about how to eat better, the place of exercise in treatment and prevention, and the planning of community space and buildings—in addition to more traditional explanations in the vocabularies of molecular genetics, neuroendocrine physiology, learning, and social psychology. Critical thought and civility pervade the chapters. These authors are looking for answers, not villains. This is a book for intellectual adults, lay and professional; tabloid readers and media shouters will be disappointed.

Along with the wide range of topics and thoughtful essays, discussion of some fundamental information and issues will enable the reader to be a critical consumer of the various kinds of knowledge claims. This chapter aims to provide that foundation.

The Energy Equation

Investigation of the energetics of obesity was made possible by the demonstration in the late nineteenth and early twentieth centuries that homeothermic animals and humans obey the law of conservation of energy (Kinney, 2005; Kuhn, 1959). This demonstration was a decisive achievement. By refuting vitalist explanations of biological phenomena, it showed that biology is in the same fundamental framework of nature as physics and chemistry.

The energy equation of homeothermic animals and humans states that input of energy (intake of metabolizable food) minus expenditure of energy (heat, movement, and work) equals the storage of energy (primarily in white adipose tissue and heat; Kinney, 2005):

$$\text{In} - \text{Out} = \text{Storage} \tag{1.1}$$

This energy equation was the platform from which increasingly refined measurements of metabolism in lean and obese animals and people were launched. It was an attractive approach because it used the quantitative measurement of thermal and mechanical energy. Such measurements continue. They have given us a large amount of useful information, but they have not identified a reliable and significant cause of obesity within the metabolic transformations of nutrient or muscular energy.

Although measurements of metabolic transformations have not revealed a cause, all discussions of obesity—physiological, psychological, social, ecological, or environmental—are constrained by the absolute requirement of being consistent with what is known as the Working Energy Equation, which is good enough for most purposes:

$$\text{Food intake} - \text{Activity} = \text{Body weight} \tag{1.2}$$

This equation is not only a constraint; it also describes the fundamental problem of obesity as an abnormal amount of energy stored in adipose tissue. (*Abnormal* is defined statistically from measurements on populations of interest; see Chapter 2). Having defined obesity, the Working Energy Equation dictates that the intake of energy (food) must have exceeded energy expenditure in every obese person. The equation leads to the following conclusions:

$$\text{In} > \text{Out} = \text{Weight gain}$$

$$\text{In} = \text{Out} = \text{No change}$$

$$\text{In} < \text{Out} = \text{Weight loss}$$

Thus, obesity results from increased food intake (hyperphagia), decreased activity, or both.

Hypothalamic Obesity

In 1901 Alfred Fröhlich, a Viennese physician, described obesity in a 14-year-old boy. The obesity was characterized by marked increase of subcutaneous fat in the mammary region, on the abdomen, and around the genitals. Sexual development was retarded. The patient was seen in the clinic for increasing blindness (especially in the left eye), headaches, and vomiting (Bruch, 1939). These symptoms suggested a pituitary tumor without acromegaly. The tumor was removed in 1907. The obesity persisted after surgery, but the other symptoms improved.

Subsequent reports confirmed the clinical syndrome and showed that it was usually associated with tumors that damaged the hypothalamus. Whether the hyperphagia and obesity resulted from the neural or pituitary pathology produced by a tumor remained controversial until 1927, when P. E. Smith demonstrated that the neural damage was the critical lesion (Bray, 1993; G. P. Smith, 1997).

The production of a model of hypothalamic obesity in the rat by stereotaxic lesions in 1940 by Hetherington and Ranson (1940) opened up the systematic investigation of the relationship of obesity to hypothalamic structure and function. John Brobeck and his colleagues soon showed that rats with hypothalamic obesity ate more food, that they moved less than normal, and that the critical lesion involved the medial hypothalamus. Hypothalamic lesions made more laterally resulted in aphagia, not hyperphagia. On the basis of these results, Brobeck proposed that the lateral hypothalamus was a site for stimulating eating, that the medial hypothalamus was a site for stopping eating, and that eating was controlled by reciprocal inhibition between the lateral and medial mechanisms in the Sherringtonian manner (for details, see Smith, 1997). This hypothalamic representation of the controls of eating, now densely embroidered with specific peptides, amines, and short and long connections retains its importance (see Chapter 3).

Diet-Induced Obesity

Until 1976, the relevance of hypothalamic obesity to obese animals or people was not clear for three reasons: First, hypothalamic obesity was rare; almost all obese animals and humans lacked hypothalamic damage. Second, rodents and other animals were thought to be too machinelike in their eating behavior to be useful models of human obesity. Third, if eating too much caused human obesity, the hyperphagia was believed to be simply a "weakness of willpower"— a kind of character defect similar to the one leading to drinking too much and alcoholism. This explanation survives beneath the surface of current discussions of obesity in which hyperphagia is described as an addiction to palatable, energy-dense foods (discussed later in the chapter).

FIGURE 1.1   A rat with diet-induced obesity. (Courtesy of A. Sclafani.)

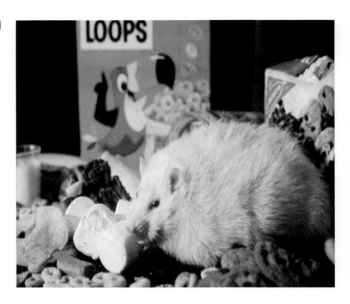

A more relevant model of obesity in the rat appeared in 1976, when Sclafani and Springer (1976) reported that lean rats became very obese if allowed constant access to a cafeteria diet that included a variety of foods that humans eat as snacks or desserts (Figure 1.1). This diet-induced obesity was soon shown to be an excellent model of human obesity. Hyperphagia caused it. The hyperphagia of the rat model had the following characteristics: First, it was expressed as increased meal size with little or no change in the number of meals. Second, the susceptibility of rats to diet-induced obesity varied within and between strains. Third, the obesity was reversed if the rats were switched to a less palatable diet. Fourth, although a number of diets could induce obesity, all of the obesity-inducing diets contained a mixture of calorically dense, sweet or fatty foods (Levin & Strack, 2008; Sclafani, 1989; West & York, 1998).

Diet became the link between diet-induced obesity and hypothalamic obesity. Diets that induced obesity in rats with intact brains also produced the largest increase of body weight in rats with mediobasal hypothalamic lesions.

Dynamic and Static Phases of Obesity

The two models—diet-induced obesity and hypothalamic obesity—also showed the same two phases of body weight gain (Brobeck et al., 1943). The phase of rapid weight gain was called the *dynamic phase*. It was followed by a phase in which weight gain slowed significantly or stopped—the *static phase*. In the static phase, meal size usually returned to normal.

When the body weight of rats in the static phase was reduced by limiting food intake, the dynamic phase of weight gain produced by ingesting abnormally large meals reappeared as soon as the rats were given free access to food. The reinstated dynamic phase continued until the lost body weight was regained and rats entered the second static phase. The body weight in this second static phase was very similar to the body weight in the first static phase. Rats selected for their susceptibility to diet-induced obesity are the exception; switched to a less palatable chow diet (standard commercial rat food), they remain obese (Levin & Dunn-Meynell, 2006).

The loss of body weight produced by food restriction reversed essentially all of the numerous endocrine and metabolic abnormalities but reinstated the hyperphagia. Thus, hyperphagia is most obvious during the dynamic phase of rapid body weight gain. In contrast, endocrine and metabolic abnormalities are largest during the static phase of body weight—an energy state in which hyperphagia disappears.

These two phases of obesity are familiar from the common experience in which obese people lose weight by dieting and then regain the lost weight when they stop following the diet. It is important to keep the dynamic and static phases in mind when reading the following chapters because most of our information about human obesity comes from people in the static phase. Note that the increased body weight in the static phase varies widely among individuals.

By contrast, relatively little information is available from intake studies on the development of obesity during the first dynamic phase or the reappearance of the dynamic phase, when people stop their dietary treatment and regain the body weight that was lost. This lack of data from the dynamic phase is unfortunate because the mechanisms causing hyperphagia are much more active and available for study during the dynamic phase than during the static phase.

Decreased activity can contribute to diet-induced obesity, but such decreases are not always detected. Decreased activity has recently been associated with a decrease in central orexin mechanisms (Novak et al., 2006).

Dietary Control of Meal Size

The observation that larger meals are responsible for the hyperphagia that produces obesity focused experimental attention on dietary control of meal size. Davis and his colleagues proposed that meal size was controlled by the central integration of orosensory stimulation of eating and postingestive inhibitory negative feedback (Davis et al., 1975; Davis & Levine, 1977).

The crucial evidence for this proposal came from comparing meal sizes during sham feeding and real feeding (Davis & Campbell, 1973; Young et al., 1974). First, meal size was always larger during sham feeding than during real feeding (Davis et al., 1999). Thus, the control of meal size always involved peripheral negative feedback control and was never produced by central ballistic con-

FIGURE 1.2 Dietary control of meal size by central integration of positive orosensory feedback and postingestive negative feedback. Conditioned negative feedback is due to prior association of orosensory stimulation and postingestive stimuli, particularly hypertonic stimuli. It operates in the first 6–8 minutes of the meal. Unconditioned negative feedback is produced by preabsorptive gastric and small-intestinal stimuli of food and digestive products mediated by peptides, such as cholecystokinin, and by the stimulation of vagal afferent fibers. It operates after 8 minutes of the meal.

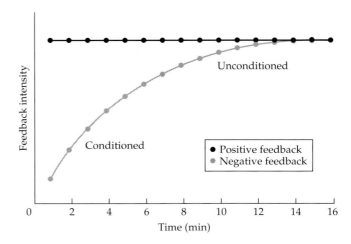

trol (i.e., control of meal size entirely by central mechanisms unaffected by peripheral feedback). Second, the concentration of orosensory stimuli determined the size of a sham-fed meal (Xenakis & Sclafani, 1982; Geary & Smith, 1985). Because a rat had to continue licking in order to maintain orosensory stimulation, orosensory control had the characteristics of positive feedback.

Thus, when meal size was under dietary control, it was mediated by the central processing, comparison, and integration of afferent peripheral feedback (Figure 1.2; Smith, 1996; Smith, 2000a; Smith, 2000b; Smith, 2005). The intensity of orosensory and postingestive feedback is produced by the dietary stimuli and their digestive products acting preabsorptively in the mouth, stomach, and small intestine. The preabsorptive site of action means that central integration of peripheral feedback for the control of meal size occurs before significant amounts of absorbed nutrients enter the energetics of metabolism and storage. The importance of preabsorptive stimuli in the dietary control of meal size emphasizes the neglected fact that the mucosa of the gut from the tip of the tongue to the end of the small intestine is a vast sensory sheet studded with receptors sensitive to the chemical and mechanical properties of ingested food and its digestive products.

Subsequent work revealed that orosensory positive feedback is mediated primarily by central dopaminergic and opioid mechanisms (see Chapters 4 and 7). In the case of dopamine, there is a positive feedback relationship between the concentration of sucrose orosensory stimulation and the concentration of dopamine in the microdialysate from the shell of the nucleus accumbens (Hajnal et al., 2004).

The potency of orosensory positive feedback to drive intake is usually due to conditioned effects produced by prior association of the orosensory stimuli and their postingestive effects (Sclafani, 2004). Dopaminergic-1 receptor mechanisms are critical for these conditioned effects (Azzara et al., 2001); opioid mechanisms appear less important.

Conditioned orosensory stimuli can also produce negative feedback effects. This relationship is due to prior association between the orosensory stimuli of a liquid diet and its hypertonic postingestive effects in the small intestine (Davis et al., 1999). Whereas these conditioned negative feedback effects of orosensory stimuli occur in the first 6 minutes of a liquid meal, the unconditioned postingestive negative feedback occurs later (see Figure 1.2). The conditioned negative feedback effects are extinguished by three consecutive sham-feeding tests and are acquired by two or three real-feeding tests (Davis, 1999). The intestinal hypertonic stimuli produce afferent vagal information to the hindbrain (Davis et al., 1995), probably through glutaminergic NMDA synaptic mechanisms (Hung et al., 2006).

Postingestive negative feedback is mediated by peptides and serotonin in peripheral and central sites. Vagal afferent mechanisms mediate the effects of peripheral stimuli to the hindbrain. The list of proven and candidate mechanisms continues to grow (see Chapter 3), and they are targets for drug development (see the Epilogue).

In contrast to the progress made on identifying peripheral positive and negative feedbacks and some of their mechanisms, almost no information is available concerning the central processing of afferent feedback information, the comparator function required to measure the relative central intensity of positive and negative feedback information, and the integration of the central information into motor commands to start, maintain, or stop eating. Some of these functions, however, have been localized anatomically (see the section on functional neurology later in this chapter).

Nondietary Controls of Meal Size

Dietary control of meal size is only one of many controls; meal size frequently increases or decreases on the same diet. For example, meal size varies as a function of food deprivation, social stimuli, prior experience, diurnal and sleep rhythms, level of estrogen, familiarity of location, ease of access, perceived caloric value, portion size, celebratory nature of the meal (e.g., Thanksgiving), instruction under laboratory conditions, and so on (see Chapter 9; Pliner & Rozin, 2000; Stroebele & de Castro, 2006; Walsh et al., 1989).

To deal with the many and diverse stimuli that increase or decrease meal size, investigators have proposed bipolar, categorical classifications of stimuli—for example, physiological versus psychological, internal versus external, short-term versus long-term, social versus individual, and homeostatic versus hedonic. Although useful for ordering certain sets of data and experimental results, none of these classifications is unambiguously defined or comprehensive, and all are in search of a neuroendocrine network that integrates the central effects of these stimuli into the rhythmic oromotor movements of eating that determine meal size.

Recent work on how meal size increases when rats regain weight after food deprivation has provided the first sketch of the neuroendocrine control of eating (see Chapter 3 for details). This is a clear example of eating serving a homeostatic function to restore energy balance. How much of the functional network of peptides involved in this metabolic control of eating also mediates the controls produced by other stimuli is an empirical question. To answer the question, the central networks for a representative number of classes of stimuli need to be identified and then compared. This is a formidable task. Each adequate stimulus could be mediated by a separate, specific network in what would be a pure parallel control system. If this is the answer, we will not know it for some time.

A Proposed Mechanism of Nondietary Controls: Central Modulation of Peripheral Feedback

An alternative means of nondietary control is based on the fact that whenever a stimulus increases or decreases meal size, the mechanisms of peripheral sensory feedback of the dietary control are also operating (Smith, 1996). Therefore, *all* stimuli that change meal size appear to act by changing the central potency of orosensory positive feedback, postingestive negative feedback, or both.[1] The advantages of this proposal are that it is comprehensive, it is unambiguous, it takes advantage of what we know about the differential mechanisms for orosensory and postingestive feedbacks (Smith & Geary, 2002), and it provides the first quantitative measurement of *all* stimuli using a common metric: curve-shift analysis of the potency of positive and negative peripheral feedbacks and their mechanisms (Smith, 1996). Quantitative measurement is essential; we need it to determine the relative potencies of different stimuli under representative conditions. That information, of course, will be crucial for guiding prevention and treatment. In contrast to the parallel control technique already described, this technique is available now.

The proposal is open to experimental test. Demonstration that a stimulus changes meal size without causing a measurable change in orosensory or postingestive feedback would refute the hypothesis.

Functional Neurology of the Controls of Meal Size

What kind of control system could mediate such a variety of adequate stimuli? Given that eating consists of rhythmic oral movements, the most relevant prece-

---

[1]Prior papers describing the dietary and nondietary controls referred to them as *direct* and *indirect* controls, respectively. This terminology emphasized that the two criteria for direct controls were direct preabsorptive stimulation of the orogastrointestinal mucosa and direct projection of afferent nerves from these sites to the hindbrain. Indirect controls were all of the controls that did not fulfill these criteria. Recent presentations have suggested that this terminology is confusing, so it has been changed here.

dent is the Sherringtonian analysis of the control of stepping or scratching (Sherrington, 1947). What are the major characteristics of Sherrington's control system? The adequate stimuli are many and varied, ranging from touch to vocal commands. The basic control is in the spinal cord, where the output of central pattern generators (CPGs) for the rhythmic movement is turned on and off in the chronic spinal dog by local afferent feedback stimuli from the surface of the body (Sherrington, 1947). The output of the CPG controls the spinal efferent nerves to the muscles that organize the movements of scratching or stepping. The spinal efferent neurons are an example of Sherrington's "final common path."

The spinal control of stepping or scratching is modulated by supraspinal controls that mediate the effects of all stimuli other than those impinging on the surface of the body (Stein et al., 1999). These supraspinal controls are mediated by nerve fibers that project into the spinal cord and that modulate the effect of the local spinal stimuli on the output of the CPG. Most, perhaps all, of these stimuli are conditioned.

The chronic decerebrate (CD) rat has served the neural analysis of eating in the same important way (Grill & Norgren, 1978a; Grill & Norgren, 1978b). In the CD rat, complete transection of the upper brainstem just behind the hypothalamus disconnects the caudal brainstem and spinal cord from the hypothalamus and forebrain (Figure 1.3). Experimental analysis of the CD rat revealed that (1) the peripheral afferent feedbacks from the oral, gastric, and small-intestinal mucosal surfaces project directly into the caudal brainstem; (2) the CPGs for licking, lapping, and chewing—the rhythmic oromotor movements of eating—are in the caudal brainstem; (3) the CD rat eats only in response to stimulation of

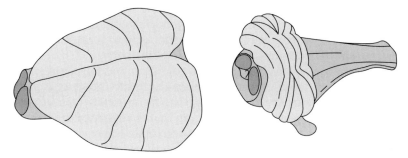

FIGURE 1.3   In this schematic of the chronic decerebrate rat, the disconnection of the large forebrain (visual left) from the smaller caudal brainstem capped by the cerebellum (visual right) is exaggerated to emphasize the functional importance of the connections between the forebrain and caudal brainstem for nondietary control of meal size and meal number. In contrast, the disconnected caudal brainstem has sufficient neural complexity to mediate the dietary controls of meal size.

the mucosal surface of the mouth by oral infusions of liquids; and (4) the caudal brainstem has sufficient neural complexity to process, compare, and integrate the afferent feedback information into a meal (Grill & Smith, 1988).

These properties of the caudal brainstem for eating can be considered the functional equivalent of the spinal cord for movement. Thus, the caudal brainstem is the spinal cord of eating (Smith, 2000b). This functional analogy has important implications for the neurological analysis of the controls of meal size.

Dietary control of meal size is the only control that operates in the CD rat. Nondietary controls that have been tested, such as deprivation and several conditioned stimuli, do not change meal size in the CD rat (Smith, 2000b). Thus, the fibers that connect the forebrain to the caudal brainstem must be intact for nondietary controls to work (see Figure 1.3; see Smith, 2000a; Smith, 2000b for specific examples). Given that the caudal brainstem's relationship to the rhythmic movements of eating is the same as the spinal cord's relationship to the rhythmic movements of scratching and stepping, it is reasonable to assume that the central neural networks for eating involve distributed and hierachical processing of various stimuli integrated into motor commands to turn on and off the CPG for licking or chewing, with the motor neurons for oromotor movements functioning as a final common path.

Since this functional neurology for the control of meal size was proposed, significant confirmation has come from experiments in preweaning rats (Smith, 2006) and adult rats (Berthoud et al., 2006; Morton et al., 2005; Schwartz, 2006; Williams & Schwartz, 2005). No failures to confirm have been reported. So far so good, but the neurology of the hypothesis needs more testing.

Although this functional neurology has been considered only as a control of meal size, it also provides insight into the control of meal number because the CD rat never initiates eating spontaneously (Grill & Norgren, 1978b). It eats only when liquid food is infused into its mouth. The conclusion is clear: normal initiation of eating prior to contact of food with the mouth requires some of the fibers connecting the forebrain and caudal brainstem to be intact. Again the situation parallels the spinal cat or dog; both begin to scratch or step only in response to stimuli from the sensory surface of the body.

Whatever the fate of this hypothesis, recognition that the control of eating is an example of the neurological control of rhythmic movement is heuristic because it is a neurology spacious enough to accommodate the numerous, varied physiological and psychological stimuli that change meal size. It also specifies for the *first* time the relationship between the dietary control of meal size by the food being eaten and all other stimuli that change meal size. The specific proposal is that *all* nondietary stimuli control meal size by modulating the central processing of the ongoing, orogastrointestinal feedback information produced by the ingested dietary stimuli. For these reasons, the analysis of the controls of eating should be pursued as a problem in behavioral neuroscience rather than solely as a problem in nutritional homeostasis (Smith, 2000a).

Prevention

The prevention of obesity includes treatment adjusted to age and psychosocial environment. The crucial question for prevention is, When do we intervene? This question reflects a developmental perspective, and Chapter 6 provides important answers, describing significant correlations between prenatal, infant, and childhood factors and adult body mass index (BMI). These factors include the mother's BMI and weight gain during pregnancy, diabetes in the mother, infant birth weight, childhood BMI at 2 and 4 years, and the onset of the loss of body fat and the "rebound" gain that occurs between 5 and 7 years of age. The last correlation has a temporal characteristic: the earlier the rebound gain, the larger the BMI! A deep biology must underlie these correlations, especially the last quantitative relationship, but it is a biology that no one knows.

Using psychophysics, Snyder and Bartoshuk have identified a new childhood risk factor for obesity: chronic otitis media. See Chapter 5 for details.

Taking all this into consideration, the answer of when to intervene is this: as soon as a significant risk factor is identified prenatally or postnatally. Other than good control of diabetes and of weight gain in the mother, and aggressive treatment of chronic otitis media, we do not know how best to intervene to undo the important specific correlations.

In addition to these specific interventions, general preventive measures of good eating habits and lifestyle changes, including age-appropriate exercise, need to be implemented as described in Chapter 14.

Treatment

The energy equation, (1.1), identifies the goals of the treatment of obesity. The abnormally large storage of fat is decreased by decreasing energy intake (food) or by increasing energy expenditure (exercise). Decreasing food intake is effective, but increasing exercise is not, except in a few fanatics. As discussed in Chapter 8, however, exercise reduces numerous pathological risk factors, probably increases compliance with diet treatment, and may well be a sign of high motivation for continuing treatment.

Two groups of investigators have reported promising therapeutic effects of exercise in obese rats. Levin has shown that exercise in rats with diet-induced obesity produces a long-lasting therapeutic effect (Levin & Dunn-Meynell, 2006; Patterson et al., 2008). Moran and Bi and their colleagues have shown a similar result in rats with diet-induced obesity and have used exercise to reverse the genetic obesity due to a null mutation of the cholecystokinin-1 receptor, the receptor that mediates the negative feedback effect of cholecystokinin released from the small intestine (see Chapter 3). The timing and type of exercise may be important for these effects.

Exercise does not affect only metabolism and physical performance. Exercise also has widespread effects on brain mechanisms (Dishman et al., 2006).

Decreasing food intake reduces body weight. Though true in a broad sense, this statement requires quantitative and temporal refinement. The reduction of intake must be large enough that the energy intake plus energy expenditure is less than the amount of energy stored. As predicted by the energy equation, decreased energy intake reduces adiposity and body weight in all forms of obesity—genetic, dietary, psychological, and so on. Diet, drugs, and surgery (Seaborg, 2007) are the main means of decreasing intake (see Chapters 9 through 13).

The temporal requirement is where diet therapy is weak. The energy equation has a temporal constraint: most people find maintaining dietary constraints for months or years too hard. Thus, the therapeutic limitation on diet therapy for obesity is failure of long-term compliance. In this respect obesity is similar to drug addiction, which is one of the reasons for recent interest in considering obesity an "addictive disease" (see Chapter 4). Of the established addictions, alcoholism may be the most relevant. The phenomenology of binges of ingestion, caloric and pharmacological effects, legal access, the cultural traditions of drinking alcoholic beverages prior to and with meals, and common peripheral (Kulkosky, 1998) and central (Schneider et al., 2007) mechanisms are reasons to consider alcoholism and obesity together.

The same is true of their treatments. The treatment of alcohol has two phases: detoxification and maintenance. The treatment of obesity is the same, if we consider the weight loss phase to be similar to detoxification.

The common problem of the maintenance phase in the treatment of alcoholism and obesity is relapse due to exposure to previously conditioned alcohol or food cues. The efficacy of naltrexone for decreasing relapse in alcohol-dependent individuals with the A118G polymorphism of the mu receptor gene (Oslin, et al., 2006) during the maintenance phase of alcohol treatment may be a model for the treatment of obese people during the maintenance phase of weight loss.

Leptin has also recently been used successfully to enhance compliance during the maintenance phase of weight loss in short-term trials by Rosenbaum and his colleagues (2005). These studies were based on the results in rats in which injection of leptin blocked the hyperphagia that occurs when rats are given free access to food after food deprivation or restriction.

Conclusion

Readers of this book will navigate through the varied perspectives more successfully by keeping the following points in mind.

Obesity is a phenotype produced by the interaction of the individual genome and environment. Like height or blood pressure, obesity is a quantitative trait; individuals with a BMI of 30 or 40 are both classified as obese, but they are in quite different metabolic states with different risks for associated diseases. Encountering the term *obesity*, the reader should bristle with specific questions: How obese? For how long has obesity been present? Is the obesity in its dynamic or stable phase? Is the obesity the result of relapse from treatment, or has the obese person never been treated? What kind of treatment has been used?

As this book shows, many aspects of obesity have been proposed as vulnerabilities or causes. Again certain questions should spring to mind: Is the aspect plausible, possible, or proven? Has the aspect been quantified? How big an effect does it produce on food intake? On meal size? Under what conditions?

Although vitalism was refuted more than a century ago (as noted earlier in the chapter), soft forms of it survive—for example, imputing personal powers (Nelkin & Lindee, 1995) or attributes, such as "thrift," to genes (Neel, 1962)[2] or explaining current problems by possible evolutionary scenarios.[3] Such vitalist ideas are an obstacle to clear thinking about potentially causal factors.

Hyperphagia expressed as larger-than-normal meals is the necessary and sufficient proximate cause in animal models of diet-induced obesity; decreased activity is also involved, but it is of secondary importance. The same is likely to be true in people as well, but meal size and exercise have not been measured directly in many relevant situations. Instead we have self-reports of uncertain quantitative validity. This scientific weakness should be remedied.

So far the search for successful prevention and treatment has assumed that all obese people share a common pathology that is susceptible to the identical pharmacological, dietary, or cognitive-behavioral treatment. This is the simplest case imaginable. It is probably time to pursue an alternative strategy that has proven effective in hypertension: using combinations of pharmacological agents based on characterization of the details of specific individual pathophysiology, such as the relative importance of increased angiotensin or aldosterone (Weber, 2007). The pharmacology takes place within a treatment program that emphasizes a healthful diet, appropriate exercise, and proactive surveillance and treatment of the risks of associated diseases, such as stroke and coronary artery disease.

Like hypertension, obesity is a warning, not a disease. This is an important point. There is no evidence that excess body fat is a disease in the traditional sense of a pathological abnormality.[4] A sufficient increase of body fat, like an increase in blood pressure, is of concern because it is associated with an increased

---

[2]A relevant example is positing thrifty genes as a "cause" of obesity. Neel proposed the thrifty gene hypothesis in 1962 to account for the common occurrence of diabetes and obesity in modern, developed countries and its absence in Yanomami and Xavante Indians of South America. He suggested that thrifty genes were selected for because they were adaptive in the cycles of feast and famine that the Indians (and other hunter-gatherers) experienced. The same genes were now maladaptive in us because of our easy access to energy-dense foods. Despite its wide acceptance, Neel concluded in 1998 that the idea was wrong and should be abandoned (Neel, 1999).

[3]The concept of thrifty genes has also been attacked on anthropological grounds. Speakmann (2007) has pointed out that thrifty genes involved in the intake and metabolism of food would not have been strongly selected for their survival value, because infection, not starvation, is the main cause of death during famines. Thus, it is no longer useful to appeal to the soft vitalism of thrifty genes to "explain" the increasing incidence of obesity in developed countries.

[4]The discovery that white adipose tissue is an active endocrine organ that secretes numerous molecules (adipokines) raises the possibility that increased secretion of one or more of them will cause a new pathology. Their role in type 2 diabetes and cardiovascular disease is under active investigation (Fischer-Posovszky, Wabitsch et al., 2007).

risk of traditional pathologies, such as diabetes, coronary heart disease, arthritis, and certain forms of cancer.

If obesity is a warning, why is it called a disease? The answers illuminate the medical-industrial-governmental complex of health care (Oliver, 2006). First, obesity is a disease because some physicians thought that it needed more attention from the scientific, medical, governmental, and insurance communities. It is a disease because it was lobbied for by the American Obesity Association and embraced by members of the Obesity Society (formerly the North American Association for the Study of Obesity).

This is part of the medicalization of conditions that put you at risk for traditional diseases. It's good because it is a sign that medicine is becoming more involved in prevention. There is potential for abuse, however, in that an arbitrary threshold for preventive treatment could be adjusted downward continuously under cover of the promised health benefits of early intervention. The result would be increases in the long-term cost to people and in the income of caregivers and drug companies.

Attaining disease status paved the way for a governmental decision to permit insurance companies and Medicare to pay for the treatment of obesity. All this stimulated pharmaceutical corporations to search for new drugs for weight loss and increased support by the NIH (National Institutes of Health) for relevant basic science for drug discovery. (Note that government-supported science is now responsible for the majority of drug development. Thus the drug corporations are free to spend most of their money on marketing and clinical trials. The fact that the public pays at both ends—drug discovery and drug consumption—is rarely mentioned; Angell, 2004; Relman, 2007.)

Thus, a disease is not just an idea whose sociocultural time has come, as Duffin (2005) has recently argued. Being designated a disease is a significant factor in the contemporary functioning of the medical-industrial-governmental complex of health care.

Reading this book brings to mind a remark by Georges Canguilhem (2000), the distinguished historian and philosopher of science: "An art of living—as medicine is in the full sense of the word—implies a science of life." We are far from a complete science of life, but to understand the ideas in this book and *their limits* is to press on toward a complete science of obesity.

Acknowledgments

I thank Professors James Gibbs, Anthony Sclafani, and Barry Levin, and the assiduous editor of this book for constructive criticism of earlier versions of this chapter. I am also grateful to Marcia Miller, medical librarian of the Payne Whitney Westchester Division of the New York-Presbyterian Hospital, for bibliographic assistance. Finally, I thank my chairman, Jack Barchas, for his continued support.

References Cited

Angell, M. (2004). *The Truth About the Drug Companies*. New York: Random House.

Azzara, A. V., Bodnar, R. J., Delamater, A.R., & Sclafani, A. (2001). D1 but not D2 dopamine receptor antagonism blocks the acquisition of a flavor preference conditioned by intragastric carbohydrate infusions. *Pharmacology, Biochemistry, and Behavior, 68*, 709–720.

Berthoud, H. R., Sutton, G. M., Townsend, R. L., Patterson, L. M., & Zheng, H. (2006). Brainstem mechanisms integrating gut-derived satiety signals and descending forebrain information in the control of meal size. *Physiology & Behavior, 89*, 517–524.

Bray, G. A. (1993). Commentary on classics of obesity 4. Hypothalamic obesity. *Obesity Research, 1*, 325–328.

Brobeck, J. R., Tepperman, J., & Long, C. N. H. (1943). Experimental hypothalamic hyperphagia in the rat. *Yale Journal of Biology and Medicine 15*, 831–853.

Bruch, H. (1939). The Fröhlich Syndrome: Report of the original case. *American Journal of Diseases of Children, 58*, 1281–1289.

Canguilhem, G. (2000). The identity of the two states. In F. Delaporte (Ed.), *A Vital Rationalist* (pp. 327–335). New York: Zone Books.

Davis, J. D. (1999). Some new developments in the understanding of oropharyngeal and postingestional controls of meal size. *Nutrition, 15*, 32–39.

Davis, J. D. & Campbell, C. S. (1973). Peripheral control of meal size in the rat. Effect of sham feeding on meal size and drinking rate. *Journal of Comparative and Physiological Psychology, 83*, 379–387.

Davis, J. D. & Levine, M. W. (1977). A model for the control of ingestion. *Psychological Review, 84*, 379–412.

Davis, J. D., Collins, B. J., & Levine, M. W. (1975). Peripheral control of drinking: gastrointestinal filling as a negative feedback signal, a theoretical and experimental analysis. *Journal of Comparative and Physiological Psychology, 89*, 985–1002.

Davis, J. D., Smith, G. P., & Kung, T. M. (1995). Abdominal vagotomy attenuates the inhibiting effect of mannitol on the ingestive behavior of rats. *Behavioral Neuroscience, 109*, 161–167.

Davis, J. D., Smith, G. P., Singh, B., & McCann, D. P. (1999). Increase in intake with sham feeding experience is concentration dependent. *American Journal of Physiology, 277*, R565–R571.

Dishman, R. K., Berthoud, H. R., Booth, F. W., Cotman, C. W., Edgerton, V. R., Fleshner, M. R. et al. (2006). Neurobiology of exercise. *Obesity, 14*, 345–356.

Duffin, J. (2005). *Lovers and Livers: Disease Concepts in History*. Toronto: University of Toronto Press.

Fischer-Posovszky, P., Wabitsch, M., & Hochberg, Z. (2007). Endocrinology of adipose tissue – an update. *Hormone and Metabolic Research, 39*, 314–321.

Geary, N. & Smith, G. P. (1985). Pimozide decreases the positive reinforcing effect of sham fed sucrose in the rat. *Pharmacology, Biochemistry, and Behavior, 22*, 787–790.

Grill, H. J. & Norgren, R. (1978a). Chronically decerebrate rats demonstrate satiation but not bait shyness. *Science, 201*, 267–269.

Grill, H. J. & Norgren, R. (1978b). Neurological tests and behavioral deficits in chronic thalamic and chronic decerebrate rats. *Brain Research, 143*, 299–312.

Grill, H. J. & Smith, G. P. (1988). Cholecystokinin decreases sucrose intake in chronic decerebrate rats. *American Journal of Physiology, 254*, R853–R856.

Hajnal, A., Smith, G. P., & Norgren, R. (2004). Oral sucrose stimulation increases accumbens dopamine in the rat. *American Journal of Physiology: Regulatory, Integrative and Comparative Physiology, 286*, R31–R37.

Hetherington, A. & Ranson, S. W. (1940). Hypothalamic lesions and adiposity in the rat. *Anatomical Record, 78*, 149–172.

Hung, C. Y., Covasa, M., Ritter, R. C., & Burns, G. A. (2006). Hindbrain administration of NMDA receptor antagonist AP-5 increases food intake in the rat. *American Journal of Physiology: Regulatory, Integrative and Comparative Physiology, 290*, R642–R651.

Kinney, J. M. (2005). Human energy metabolism. In M. E. Shils, M. Shike, A. C. Ross, B. Cabllero, & R. J. Cousins (Eds.), *Modern Nutrition in Health and Disease* (10th ed., pp. 10–16). Philadelphia: Lippincott Williams & Wilkins.

Kuhn, T. S. (1959). Energy conservation as an example of simultaneous discovery. In M. Clagett (Ed.), *Critical Problems in the History of Science* (pp. 321–356). Madison: The University of Wisconsin Press.

Kulkosky, P. J. (1998). Satiation of alcohol intake. In G. P. Smith (Ed.), *Satiation: From Gut to Brain* (pp. 263–286). New York: Oxford University Press.

Levin, B. E. & Dunn-Meynell, A. A. (2006). Differential effects of exercise on body weight gain and adiposity in obesity-prone and -resistant rats. *International Journal of Obesity* (Lond), *30*, 722–727.

Levin, B. E. & Strack, A. M. (2008). Diet-induced obesity in animal models and what they tell us about human obesity. In J. Harvey (Ed.), *The Neurobiology of Obesity* (pp. 164–195). Blue Ridge Summit, PA: University Press of America.

Morton, G. J., Blevins, J. E., Williams, D. L., Niswender, K. D., Gelling, R. W., Rhodes, C. J. et al. (2005). Leptin action in the forebrain regulates the hindbrain response to satiety signals. *Journal of Clinical Investigation, 115*, 703–710.

Neel, J. V. (1962). Diabetes mellitus: a "thrifty" genotype rendered detrimental by "progress"? *American Journal of Human Genetics, 14*, 353–362.

Neel, J. V. (1999). The "thrifty" genotype rendered detrimental by "progress"? *Nutrition Reviews* (5, Pt. 2), S2–S9.

Nelkin, D. & Lindee, M. S. (1995). The DNA mystique: the gene as a cultural icon. New York: W. H. Freeman.

Novak, C. M., Kotz, C. M., & Levine, J. A. (2006). Central orexin sensitivity, physical activity, and obesity in diet-induced obese and diet-resistant rats. *American Journal of Physiology: Endocrinology and Metabolism, 290*, E396–E403.

Oliver, J. E. (2006). The politics of pathology. *Perpspectives in Biology and Medicine, 49*, 611–627.

Oslin, D. W., Berrettini, W. H., & O'Brien, C. P. (2006). Targeting treatments for alcohol dependence: the pharmacogenetics of naltrexone. *Addiction Biology, 11*, 397–403.

Patterson C. M., Dunn-Meynell A. A., & Levin B. E. (2008). Three weeks of early onset exercise prolongs obesity-resistance in DIO rats after exercise cessation. *American Journal of Physiology: Regulatory, Integrative, and Comparative Physiology.*

Pliner, P. R. & Rozin, P. (2000). The psychology of the meal. In H. L. Meisselman (Ed.), *Dimensions of the Meal: the Science, Culture, and Art of eating* (pp. 19–46). Gaithersburg, MD: Aspen Publishers, Inc.

Relman, A. S. (2007). To lose trust, every day. *The New Republic*, 36–42.

Rosenbaum, M., Goldsmith, R., Bloomfield, D., Magnano, A., Weimer, L., Heymsfield, S. et al. (2005). Low-dose leptin reverses skeletal muscle, autonomic, and neuroendocrine adaptations to maintenance of reduced weight. *Journal of Clinical Investigation, 115*, 3579–3586.

Schneider, E. R., Rada, P., Darby, R. D., Leibowitz, S. F., & Hoebel, B. G. (2007). Orexigenic peptides and alcohol intake: differential effects of orexin, galanin, and ghrelin. *Alcoholism, Clinical and Experimental Research, 31*, 1858–1865.

Schwartz, G. J. (2006). Integrative capacity of the caudal brainstem in the control of food intake. *Philosophical Transactions of the Royal Society of London. Series B, Biological Sciences, 361*, 1275–1280.

Sclafani, A. (1989). Dietary-induced overeating. *Annals of the New York Academy of Sciences, 575*, 281–289.

Sclafani, A. (2004). Oral and postoral determinants of food reward. *Physiology & Behavior, 81*, 773–779.

Sclafani, A. & Springer, D. (1976). Dietary obesity in adult rats: similarities to hypothalamic and human obesity syndromes. *Physiology & Behavior, 17*, 461–471.

Seaborg, E. (2007). Bariatric surgery success in treating obesity & diabetes. *Endocrine News, 32*, 10–12.

Sherrington, C. (1947). *The Integrative Action of the Nervous System* (2nd ed.). New Haven, CT: Yale University Press.

Smith, G. P. (1996). The direct and indirect controls of meal size. *Neuroscience and biobehavioral reviews, 20*, 41–46.

Smith, G. P. (1997). Eating and the American Zeitgeist. *Appetite, 29*, 191–200.

Smith, G. P. (2000a). The controls of eating: a shift from nutritional homeostasis to behavioral neuroscience. *Nutrition, 16*, 814–820.

Smith, G. P. (2000b). The controls of eating: brain meanings of food stimuli. *Progress in Brain Research, 122*, 173–186.

Smith, G. P. (2005). Controls of food intake. In M. E. Shils, M. Shike, A. C. Ross, B. Cabllero, & R. J. Cousins (Eds.), *Modern Nutrition in Health and Disease* (10th ed., pp. 707–719). Philadelphia: Lippincott.

Smith, G. P. (2006). Ontogeny of ingestive behavior. *Developmental Psychobiology, 48,* 345–359.

Smith, G. P. & Geary, N. (2002). The behavioral neuroscience of eating. In K. L. Davis, D. Charney, J. T. Coyle, & C. Nemeroff (Eds.), *Neuropsychopharmacology: The Fifth Generation of Progress* (pp. 1665–1673). Philadelphia: Lippincott.

Speakmann, J. R. (2007). Gene environment interactions and the origin of modern obesity epidemic: a novel "nonadaptive drift" scenario (pp. 301–322). In T. C. Kirkham & S. J. Cooper, (Eds.), *Appetite and Body Weight*. New York: Academic Press.

Stein, P. S. G., Grillner, S. & Stuart, D. G. (1999). *Neurons, Networks, and Motor Behavior*. Cambridge, MA: MIT Press.

Stroebele, N. & de Castro, J. M. (2006). Influence of physiological and subjective arousal on food intake in humans. *Nutrition, 22,* 996–1004.

Walsh, B. T., Kissileff, H. R., Cassidy, S. M., & Dantzic, S. (1989). Eating behavior of women with bulimia. *Archives of General Psychiatry, 46,* 54–58.

Weber, M. A. (2007). New opportunities in cardiovascular patient management: a survey of clinical data on the combination of angiotensin-converting enzyme inhibitors and angiotensin receptor blockers. *American Journal of Cardiology, 100,* 45J-52J.

West, D. B. & York, B. (1998). Dietary fat, genetic predisposition, and obesity: lessons from animal models. *American Journal of Clinical Nutrition, 67,* 505S-512S.

Williams, D. L. & Schwartz, M. W. (2005). The melanocortin system as a central integrator of direct and indirect controls of food intake. *American Journal of Physiology: Regulatory, Integrative and Comparative Physiology, 289,* R2–R3.

Xenakis, S. & Sclafani, A. (1982). The dopaminergic mediation of a sweet reward in normal and VMH hyperphagic rats. *Pharmacology, Biochemistry, and Behavior 16,* 293–302.

Young, R. C., Gibbs, J., Antin, J., Holt, J., & Smith, G. P. (1974). Absence of satiety during sham feeding in the rat. *Journal of Comparative and Physiological Psychology, 87,* 795–800.

2 THE EPIDEMIOLOGY OF OBESITY: CAUSAL ROOTS—ROUTES OF CAUSE

Viktor E. Bovbjerg

> *Whoever would study medicine aright must learn of the follow-*
> *ing subjects . . . Lastly consider the life of the inhabitants them-*
> *selves; are they heavy drinkers and eaters and consequently*
> *unable to stand fatigue or, being fond of work and exercise, eat*
> *wisely but drink sparely?*
>
> —Hippocrates

Introduction

In 2008, it appears that the most important risk factor for obesity is to be human and alive in the first years of this new millennium. From an enormous volume of research reporting obesity incidence, prevalence, risk factors, and causes, one thing is clear: the epidemic of overweight and obesity is on the increase at every stage of the life span, in both women and men, among members of all racial and ethnic backgrounds, in all areas of the globe, and among rich and poor alike. Although population-level increases in obesity and overweight may have started earlier or later in some regions, may be distributed at any given time unevenly among populations, and may have had various contributing influences, it seems increasingly likely that overweight and obesity result from a world in which abundant and inexpensive food energy is available, and nei-ther work-related nor leisure-time physical activity is sufficient to balance the increase in caloric intake.

This chapter is a brief overview of the distribution and determinants—and consequences—of overweight and obesity. In 2008, this is well-trod ground, and the volume of such reviews, let alone primary sources and entire texts, is substantial. Rather than provide an exhaustive review (impossible at the cur-rent rate of publication on the topic of overweight and obesity), this chapter will briefly summarize the health effects of excess weight, highlight time trends in obesity, discuss the distribution of excess weight by place and person, and describe inherent challenges to uncritical use of such information to take action.

Health Effects of Excess Weight

It is clear that obesity, particularly central obesity, is associated with early mortality, contributes causally to a wide range of diseases, exacerbates existing conditions, complicates medical care, and is associated with psychological distress and decreased quality of life. The notion that obesity and overweight are associated with health consequences is not new. The elevated social status of those with relative corpulence was, until recent times, reflected in art, literature, and even medicine (Eknoyan, 2006). Only in the past century has excess weight as a health risk overcome in the public consciousness the perception of excess weight as a sign of wealth and status—although adiposity remains a sign of prosperity in settings where substantial undernourishment and famine are either still concerns or recent memories.

In times of famine, some excess weight is a boon, not only for humans but for many animal species. As human famine has receded across the globe, the benefits of excess weight have also receded, and the health risks associated with obesity have become clearer. The nutrition transition from a period of receding famine to one of degenerative diseases associated with changed food and activity environments (Figure 2.1), from famine to obesity-related chronic diseases, has spread around the world, with varied though predictable influences on public health (Popkin, 2005a).

Health threats associated with excess weight have been recognized and recorded since at least the time of Hippocrates. Formal observations connecting excess weight and health risks, however, are of a more recent origin. Much of our current conceptualization of obesity—including its relationship to fat cells, metabolism, and familial and genetic influences—dates back to the nineteenth century (Bray, 1990). In the late 1800s, actuarial data from insurance companies suggested a link between excess weight and mortality (Eknoyan, 2006), and pooled data collected between 1870 and 1899 from 34 insurance companies suggested that increases in both weight and girth were associated with earlier death (Kahn & Williamson, 1994). By the 1930s, insurance companies were adjusting premiums on the basis of body weight (Caballero, 2007). By midcentury, medical and nutrition science had made great strides in explaining obesity and its links to disease generally, and to metabolic disorders particularly (Goldner, 1957).

The profound effects of excess weight on both the development and management of disease can hardly be overstated. Overweight and obesity, in excess of 60% prevalence among US adults, is one of the few conditions that may shorten life expectancy, by as much as 5 years (Wyatt et al., 2006). As obesity and its related disorders become similarly prevalent in other countries, similar reductions in life expectancy, greater if resources are not available to treat them, may be looming. Excess weight contributes to an incredibly wide range of diseases (albeit in varying ways and with varying strengths of association), exacerbates preexisting conditions, and complicates medical care and disease management (Figure 2.2; Popkin et al., 2006; Pi-Sunyer, 1999). Childhood obesity, once seen primarily as a

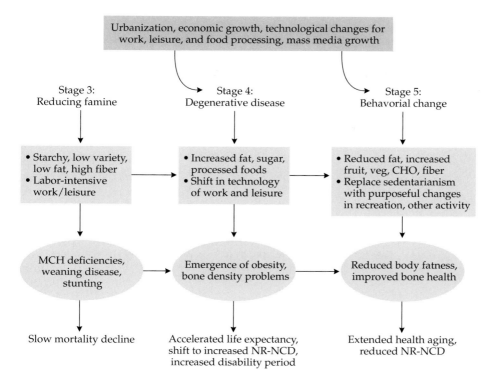

FIGURE 2.1   Stages in the nutrition transition (stages 1 and 2 not shown). (After Popkin & Gordon-Larsen, 2004.) NR-NCD=nutrition related non-communicable diseases, CHO=carbohydrate, MCH=maternal and child health.

cosmetic and social issue, is associated with adult risk of obesity and carries health consequences during both childhood and adulthood (Reilly et al., 2003).

The contributions of obesity to cardiovascular disease (including coronary heart disease, ventricular dysfunction, congestive heart failure, stroke, and cardiac arrhythmias) and type 2 diabetes are well documented (Ritchie & Connell, 2007); and they are more and more important as heart disease and diabetes become increasingly dominant global causes of early mortality and morbidity (Klein et al., 2004; Pearson, 2007; Krishnan et al., 2007). When obesity reaches countries with traditionally lower obesity rates, risk factors for cardiovascular disease and diabetes also rise (Nakamura et al., 2007). For example, obesity-related cardiovascular disease in the Asia-Pacific region, historically a region with generally low obesity rates, is on the rise (Asia Pacific Cohort Studies Collaboration, 2007).

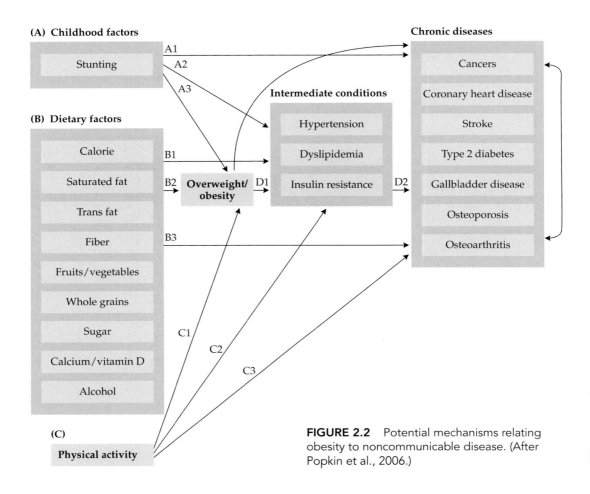

FIGURE 2.2 Potential mechanisms relating obesity to noncommunicable disease. (After Popkin et al., 2006.)

Figure 2.3, although stark, certainly underestimates the current burden of obesity: cardiovascular disease secondary to diabetes is not included, estimates of morbidity are not included, and obesity has risen rapidly in the Asia-Pacific region. A number of factors converge to increase the likelihood of obesity to spread worldwide. The World Health Organization expects diabetes-related deaths to rise by 50% in the next 10 years, in large part because of rises in obesity. In both cardiovascular disease and diabetes, the association of excess weight to health outcomes is complicated by the multiple pathways through which obesity may influence risk factors for disease (Menotti et al., 1993; Batty et al., 2007), and it seems likely that obesity influences cardiovascular disease and diabetes both through the well-known risk factors and by other means (Klein et al., 2004; He et al., 2007; Marini et al., 2007).

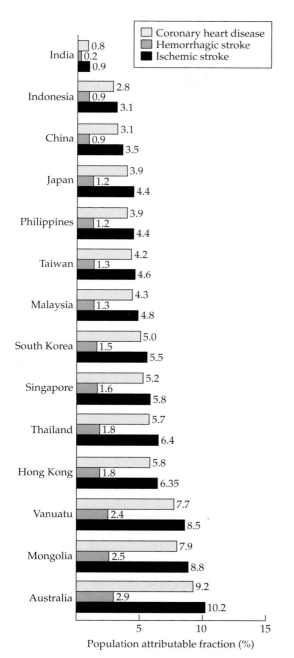

FIGURE 2.3   Proportion of cardiovascular disease deaths attributed to obesity in Asia-Pacific nations, 1993–2004. (After Asia Pacific Cohort Studies Collaboration, 2007.)

Prepregnancy weight and maternal obesity are also associated with similar conditions in pregnancy, including maternal preeclampsia and gestational diabetes (Stone et al., 2007; Frederick et al., 2006; Galtier-Dereure et al., 2000), as well as with perinatal complications (Mighty & Fahey, 2007; see also Chapter 6). As obesity becomes more common among youth and spreads in that population, we can expect the association between obesity and cardiovascular risk observed in young adults to become an even more dominant vector in early morbidity and mortality from heart disease and diabetes (Orio et al., 2007).

Excess weight contributes to disease risk beyond cardiovascular and metabolic disorders as well. After tobacco use, obesity may be the second leading cause of cancer worldwide (Calle & Thun, 2004). Several cancers are more common among those with excess weight (Ceschi et al., 2007), including liver (Larsson & Wolk, 2007), kidney (Bergström et al., 2001), breast (Harvie et al., 2003), ovarian (Olsen et al., 2007), colon and colorectal (Frezza et al., 2006; Dai et al., 2007), and prostate cancers (Presti, 2005). Relationships of obesity to cancer can be complex; for instance, central adiposity may be a stronger predictor of breast cancer among premenopausal than postmenopausal women (Harvie et al., 2003). Reflux disease—which, in addition to reducing quality of life, is associated with Barrett's esophagus (a change in esophageal tissue and a precursor to adenocarcinoma) and adenocarcinoma—is more likely among obese individuals (as is adenocarcinoma itself; Hampel et al., 2005). Obesity increases both the risk of pancreatitis and the risk of mortality from pancreatitis (Martinez et al., 2006). Compared with people below "normal" weight (body mass index $< 25\,\mathrm{kg/m^2}$), overweight individuals are at 40% increased risk, and obese individuals have nearly twice the risk (Beuther & Sutherland, 2007).

Excess weight spares few organ systems and affects certain behavioral functions as well. Obesity has been linked to sleep apnea, which in turn may lead to inflammatory responses, cardiovascular disease, and impaired safety behaviors (Miller & Cappuccio, 2007). Through changes in skin barrier function, sebum production, wound healing, and both micro- and macrocirculation, obesity is associated with a wide range of dermatologic conditions, including gout, acanthosis, keratosis, hyperandrogenism and hirsutism, lymphedema, cellulitis, infections, and psoriasis (Yosipovich et al., 2007). Obesity is the most important risk factor for chronic kidney disease (Kramer & Luke, 2007), and nonalcoholic fatty liver disease is substantially more common among those with excess weight, compared to others (Angulo, 2007). Obesity influences risk of osteoarthritis, perhaps through both mechanical and metabolic pathways (Eaton 2004; Powell et al., 2005). It has even been implicated in periodontal disease, through some of the same inflammatory mechanisms that increase cardiovascular disease risk (Pischon et al., 2007).

Though not cause to promote excess adiposity, obesity is associated with reduced risk of hip fracture in older adults (McTigue et al., 2006), and it slows further deterioration in patients reaching end-stage renal disease (Kramer & Luke, 2007). Although adiposity may help patients who have wasting diseases live longer once they reach end stage, any potential causal mechanism associating obesity to such outcomes must be balanced against the potential harm of excess weight in other areas of health.

Excess Weight, Medical Treatment, and Costs

Obesity also complicates medical treatment and disease management. Aside from causal links between obesity and cancer initiation or promotion, obesity has been associated with lower rates of cancer screening and increased complications of cancer treatment (Bordeaux et al., 2006). Cancer patients with obesity are more likely to experience problems following surgery, including wound complications (e.g., infection), lymphedema, second cancers, and chronic diseases that complicate cancer control (McTiernan, 2005). Obesity complicates labor and birth for both mother and child, and it increases the risk of birth defects, macrosomia (abnormally large size for gestational age), surgical deliveries (cesarean sections), prolonged labor, and postpartum anemia (Mighty & Fahey, 2007; Siega-Riz & Laraia, 2006).

Substantial adiposity influences the ability to provide quality medical care. For instance, obesity can lead to challenges in imaging (Uppot et al., 2007), greater complexity in anesthesia (Gaszynski, 2004), complications during surgery (Kurzer et al., 2006), and hampered postsurgical recovery (Yap et al., 2007). Treatment of obesity also carries risk. Most obviously, bariatric surgery—which has increased from 14,000 procedures in the United States in 1998 to 108,000 procedures in 2003 (Shinogle et al., 2005)—carries nontrivial risks of early mortality and morbidity, including chronic kidney failure (Byrne, 2001; Shinogle et al., 2005). Important results from two recent trials, however, suggest long-term weight loss and mortality benefit from such procedures (Adams et al., 2007; Sjöström et al., 2007).

The costs of obesity, though difficult to quantify accurately, are staggering by any measure (Figure 2.4). Each new review of obesity-related costs has shown a substantial increase over estimates from previous reviews (Colditz, 1992; Wolf & Colditz, 1998; Seidell, 1998). In 2004, the US expenditure for obesity-related conditions was estimated at more than $75 billion (Finkelstein et al., 2004). Figures from 15 member states in the European Union in roughly the same period estimated costs at €32.8 billion (Fry & Finley, 2005). Calculating indirect costs is a dicey affair, but one estimate using 1995 US figures suggested that indirect costs were nearly again as much as direct costs (Wolf & Colditz, 1998). Though precise estimates are even more difficult in other locations, a case study of the influence of changes in diet, physical activity, and obesity in China estimated that indirect costs were at least as important as direct medical costs, and that the productivity loss might range between roughly 3.5% and 9% of Chinese GNP (gross national product) during 2000 to 2005 (Popkin et al., 2006). Though estimates vary considerably, between $30 billion and $55 billion is spent each year on programs, equipment, and food aimed at weight loss—a remarkable expen-

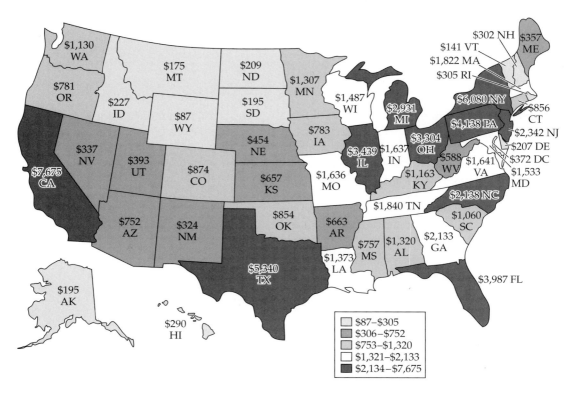

FIGURE 2.4 Estimated annual obesity-related medical expenditures, in millions of 2003 US dollars. (After Finkelstein et al., 2004.)

diture for an industry with such little documented long-term success and historically very little regulation (Tsai & Wadden, 2005; Ries, 1984; Begley, 1991). Of course, effective (and *cost*-effective) lifestyle, medical, and surgical treatments have the potential to *reduce* the medical, personal, and societal financial burden of disease.

The influence of obesity on employment and disability is substantial (Ells et al., 2006; Wolf & Colditz, 1998; Wyatt et al., 2006). Obesity predicts lower employment in both men and women, as well as greater work site disability in women (Tunceli et al., 2006); and it is associated with the awarding of disability pensions (Karnehed et al., 2007) and with restricted-activity days, bedridden days, and lost workdays (Wolf & Colditz, 1998). Overweight and obese employees use more sick leave and are at greater disability risk.

Obese employees are more likely to be injured, compared to other employees (Schmier et al., 2006). The "costs" of obesity are not limited to lost productivity and physical disability. Important psychological costs are borne by individuals with excess weight. Through poorly understood (and likely multiple) mechanisms, obesity is associated with increased prevalence of depression, suicidal ideation, and suicide attempts in the US population (Carpenter et al., 2000; Onyike et al., 2003). Similar associations between obesity and mental health have been observed in other cultures (Herva et al., 2006) and in youth (Sjöberg et al., 2005). Though cause-and-effect relationships between obesity and depression have not been well described—depression may not only lead to obesity but also be caused by it—evidence suggests that successful weight loss is associated with reduced depressive symptoms (Dixon et al., 2003). In addition, obese individuals may bear the costs of increased insurance premiums, diminished ability to be active, job discrimination, poorer education, and increased social stigma (Seidell, 1998).

In a previous age, when excess weight was restricted to the wealthy and prosperous, the burden of obesity-related disease in communities was low. The rise in overweight and obesity in the past few decades, however, and its distribution throughout the population, especially the poor, threatens to swamp our ability to treat the downstream sequelae of excess weight: diseases that are chronic, limit life, and reduce the quality of life. The rapid rise in obesity among developing nations, which may be simultaneously dealing with *under*nutrition and substantial threats from infectious disease, may widen the gap between disease burden and resources to meet the burden. The remainder of this chapter describes the current epidemic of obesity and overweight in the familiar epidemiological terms of person, place, and time—but in reverse order, to better emphasize the consistency in temporal and geographic trends.

Overview of the Current Epidemic

Reporting precise proportions for global prevalence of obesity and overweight is a futile exercise in a text. Prevalence is changing so rapidly and unevenly that reporting current rates is misleading. Many sources of up-to-date and comparable information on excess weight are available, and they will continue to be updated. For instance, the World Health Organization's Global Database on Body Mass Index (www.who.int/bmi), provides interactive and updated maps, tables, and graphs of national rates of obesity, overweight, and underweight by nationality. Even this database, however, is limited by the lack of reporting from some nations, and the lack of standardization in survey and measurement methods, BMI cutoffs, sampling frame, and year of sampling.

Nevertheless, it is clear from such databases, corroborated by independent samples, that the distribution of excess weight around the globe continues to show geographic patterns—but patterns that are rapidly changing with transitions in epidemiology, demographics, economic activity, and nutrition. Among the nations with the highest rates of overweight and obesity are the United States and the United Kingdom, with roughly two-thirds of the population classified as having excess weight by international standards. US figures—gleaned from the Behavioral Risk Factor Surveillance System (www.cdc.gov/brfss), the

National Health and Nutrition Examination Survey (www.cdc.gov/nchs/ nhanes.htm), or other sources—are similar (Wang & Beydoun, 2007; Baskin et al., 2005), suggesting that the two-thirds combined prevalence and one-third obesity prevalence currently cited are likely to be close to the mark.

Among developed North American and European nations, several (Poland, the Czech Republic, Germany, Spain, and several smaller central European nations) also reported overweight and obesity in greater than half their populations, and obesity rates of near 20%, similar to those reported by others (Fry & Finley, 2005). Rates comparable to those of the United States and the United Kingdom were also reported from the Middle East, in such disparate nations as Israel, Kuwait, Bahrain, and Saudi Arabia—in most cases representing substantial increases over estimates from as little as a decade earlier (Seidell, 2005). Most Scandinavian and central European countries, as well as several South American and northern African countries, have somewhat lower prevalence: under 50% but above 40% of their populations. Countries with the lowest rates of obesity and overweight—under 25% of the population—are primarily in the Asia-Pacific region but represent considerable variation in economic development; they include India, Japan, Pakistan, China, Korea, the Philippines, Indonesia, and Laos. Three African nations—Eritrea, Gambia, and Ghana—also report relatively low rates of excess weight. Obesity rates largely parallel combined rates, with the exception that the highest obesity rates include several island nations (e.g., Tonga, Nauru, French Polynesia), whose exceptionally high rates almost certainly reflect a confluence between strong genetic predisposition and rapid cultural shifts.

Though the previous few paragraphs seem to highlight differences in the prevalence of excess weight by regions and countries, the similarities of the epidemic curves are more important than the differences: the increase in overweight and obesity is not selective to certain regions, countries, or peoples, but rather the same phenomenon is occurring at different times in different settings. So a cross-sectional snapshot of obesity rates suggesting substantial differences among populations masks the more fundamental fact that nearly all populations have rising prevalence of obesity and overweight, and that the essential difference is the point in time at which the prevalence began to rise.

More illuminating than current prevalence rates, however, are trends in excess weight over time (*time*), the distribution of excess weight by environmental factors (*place*), and individual-level variables associated with excess weight (*person*). Each perspective tells part of the story of the current epidemic of excess weight, and each offers hope for intervention to stem the epidemic.

Time

The epidemic of overweight and obesity, which has been called "a new nutrition emergency" (Nishida & Mucavele, 2004), is largely a phenomenon of the past few decades, and to some extent a by-product of the technological and logistical advances that enabled food production of sufficient quality and quantity to reduce famine (Eknoyan, 2006). Other global forces, such as increased urbanization, as well as labor-saving technology at work and at home, have accelerated the imbalance between energy in and energy out. As these changes have occurred, excess weight has followed closely (Caballero, 2007; see also Chapter 8).

In 2008, it is apparent that calendar time is less relevant to the emergence of the epidemic of excess weight than is the timing of economic development. Globally, the rise in overweight and obesity has been enabled by changes in technology, agriculture, and transport. However, these changes have come at different times to different societies, so rising obesity prevalence has also emerged at different times (Popkin & Gordon-Larsen, 2004). In developed countries, however, the epidemic of obesity and overweight differs from that in developing nations, where increased prevalence of overweight and obesity may take place alongside ongoing undernourishment (Potera, 2004).

In the United States, the prevalence of obesity has risen dramatically since the 1970s. Data from the National Health and Nutrition Examination Survey (NHANES) document essentially a twofold increase in obesity in both women and men from the period 1971–1974 to 2003–2004, with mean body mass index (BMI) increasing from 24.4 to 27.6 in men, and from 25.3 to 28.2 in women (Wang & Beydoun, 2007). Similar trends were documented for central obesity and waist circumference, with average female waist circumference increasing from 77.1 cm (30.4 inches) in 1960–1962 to 94.3 cm (37.1 inches) in 1999–2000, and male waist circumference increasing from 89.1 to 99.0 cm (35 to 39 inches) during the same period (Wang & Beydoun, 2007). The increased prevalence has accelerated in recent years, with most of the doubling of adult obesity and tripling of adolescent overweight occurring since 1980 (Baskin et al., 2005).

Data from the Behavioral Risk Factor Surveillance System (BRFSS) suggested that in the short span of 1991 to 1998, adult obesity rose from 12% to 18%—a remarkable 50% increase. Just a year later, the estimate was nearly 20% (Mokdad et al., 2001). Recent NHANES data suggest that prevalence has continued to rise from 1999 to 2004 among children, adolescents, and adult men, though not among adult women. As is true in other cultures, US time trends in excess weight vary in complicated ways by socioeconomic status, race, gender, and age, though increases in prevalence have been similar across these variables. Though there were sometimes substantial cross-sectional differences in prevalence by gender, ethnicity, region, and socioeconomic status, all groups showed a dramatic rise in obesity during the period (Maskarinec et al., 2006; Truong & Sturm, 2005; Wang & Beydoun, 2007).

The Canadian experience is similar to that of the United States, suggesting that the same forces that have promoted excess weight in the United States are acting in Canada as well. Though first recognized as a health threat by the Canadian government in the 1950s, increases in weight for height have accelerated from the 1970s to the present, paralleling the US experience (Katzmarzyk, 2002a; Belanger-Ducharme & Tremblay, 2005). Average height has continued to increase, but average weight has increased disproportionately faster than height. From

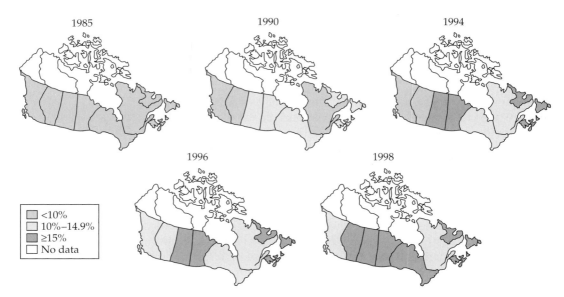

FIGURE 2.5   Prevalence of obesity among Canadian adults in 1985, 1990, 1994, 1996, and 1998. (After Katzmarzyk, 2002b.)

1953 to 1998, weight for height increased by roughly 5% for both men and women. Estimates of overweight increased from 40% in the early 1970s to 51% in the late 1990s. During a 13-year period, the prevalence of obesity in Canada nearly tripled in a series of five national surveys: 5.6% (1985), 9.2% (1990), 13.4% (1994), 12.7% (1996), and 14.8% (1998; Katzmarzyk, 2002b). Data from different population samples suggested that Canadian obesity rose from 10% in 1970 to 23% in 2004, with relatively few differences in rate *changes* between men and women, and occurring in all provinces (Luo et al., 2007; Katzmarzyk, 2002b), though the absolute prevalence of overweight and obesity varies by gender and region (Belanger-Ducharme & Tremblay, 2005; Katzmarzyk, 2002b) and lags US rates considerably (Figure 2.5).

Trends in other developed nations are similar to those in the United States and Canada. By 2002, obesity and overweight had increased among the (then) 15 member states of the European Union to the point that at least half of member nations exceeded 20% obesity prevalence (Fry & Finley, 2005). In the past two decades, obesity prevalence has tripled among European countries, with roughly one-half of adults and one-fifth of children classified as overweight (Watson, 2006). Though cross-national comparisons are difficult because of differences in timing and methodology, longitudinal surveys from the United Kingdom, the Netherlands, Sweden, Switzerland, and France suggest that the prevalence of childhood obesity has also risen steadily across the European Union, though absolute prevalence varies among countries (Livingstone, 2001).

Data from individual nations confirm these trends among both adults and children. Despite having relatively low absolute obesity prevalence, Sweden has seen adult obesity prevalence double—to 10%—in the past decade, and a parallel doubling has been observed in Swedish youth; among military conscripts, who are not in a position to underreport weight, prevalence of overweight doubled (to 16.3%), and obesity quadrupled (to 3.2%), during the period from 1971 to 1995 (Neovius et al., 2006). Population surveys from Denmark suggest that overweight and obesity there have been rising in parallel with the Swedish experience and that of other western European nations, with substantial increases over the past two decades (Due et al., 2007).

Because Scandinavian countries have kept both comprehensive population-level vital records and military conscription, Denmark has documented the rise in obesity using draft board records, from 5 per thousand in 1948 to 72 per thousand in 2004. In parallel, childhood obesity among children in Copenhagen increased 39-fold among 14- to 16-year-old girls and 115-fold in boys of the same ages between 1947 and 2003, with the greatest absolute increase after 1989. In 1947, the absolute prevalence at ages 6 to 8 was 0.2% in girls and 0.1% in boys; in 2003 the respective prevalences were 4.1% and 3.8%. Similar increases in both adults and children have been documented in the United Kingdom, with roughly twice the prevalence of obesity at the start of the millennium as there was two decades earlier (Rennie & Jebb, 2005). The advent of increased openness and subsequent changes in food availability in eastern Europe and the former Soviet states has probably hastened the rise of excess weight there as well. In Poland, during the decade following easing of political and trade restrictions, obesity increased among women (but not men) from 8.9% to 15.0% (Milewicz et al., 2005). During the period from 1994 to 2004, the Russian experience paralleled that of the United States, with overweight increasing slightly (from 34.3% to 36.1%) and obesity rising substantially (from 20.3% to 28.0%; Huffman & Rizov, 2007).

The developing nations of the world are where the *rate* increases in overweight and obesity are currently the greatest, however. Absolute prevalence among these countries in many cases is still below that of developed nations, but they are rapidly catching up, and the implications for life expectancy, chronic disease, and resource utilization are profound. Although many factors have influenced the rise in obesity among developing nations, the core influences are likely to be increased urbanization, changes in work and work technology, access to greater amounts of food, and more energy-dense food, which in turn collectively lead to caloric imbalance (Caballero, 2007).

As relative income increases in developing nations, the "nutrition transition"—marked at this stage by decreased physical activity and increased access to food in general, but particularly edible oils, caloric sweeteners, and animal foods—promotes obesity and the chronic diseases associated with it (Popkin,

2005a). Coupled with the ability to purchase more, increased economic development and improved logistics have expanded access to low-cost but calorically dense foods and beverages (Bray et al., 2004). Though the rise in obesity has followed similar patterns in developing countries—starting initially in upper income levels but expanding to encompass the entire population—the increases appear to occur more rapidly than those that occurred earlier in developed nations, and sometimes in a setting of ongoing undernourishment (Popkin & Gordon-Larsen, 2004; Campbell & Campbell, 2007; Potera, 2004).

In both northern and sub-Saharan Africa, as well as in the Middle East, overweight and obesity are on the rise. Among northern African nations, in which traditional culture has equated overweight (particularly in women) as a sign of social status and prosperity, overweight and obesity burgeoned in the last two decades of the twentieth century, as income increased and diets changed (Mokhtar et al., 2001). In Tunisia, female overweight increased from 28% to 50% between 1980 and 1997, and female obesity tripled within that time. Trends for Morocco are parallel. Trends are similar in sub-Saharan nations, where obesity has historically been unusual. However, the economic development and demographic shifts in, for instance, South Africa, Botswana, Namibia, and Zimbabwe, have been accompanied by rises in obesity (Walker et al., 2001). In Tanzania, a country historically thought of as grappling with undernutrition and wasting, obesity rose rapidly, from 3.6% in 1995 to 9.1% in 2004, with *no reduction in the prevalence of wasting* (Villamor et al., 2006).

Similar anecdotal observations have been made in other African nations, such as Gambia, where obesity appears no longer to be confined to wealthy families of tribal leaders, but is increasingly common as urbanization expands (Prentice & Webb, 2006). In South Africa, overweight and obesity, particularly among women and girls, has risen rapidly in the past few decades, in concert with the notion of "benign" or "healthy" obesity promoted from the 1960s to the late 1980s. Time trends in Middle Eastern countries parallel those of other nations in the region and have been driven by the same underlying societal changes. The increased prevalence of overweight and obesity in Egypt, for example, has paralleled the increasing availability, since the 1950s, of grains, oils, sugars, and meat, and the decline in legume consumption (Galal, 2002). In Turkey, the prevalence of adult obesity has increased slightly from 18.6% in 1990 to 21.9% in 2000 (Yumuk, 2005), coincident with ongoing economic development.

In Central and South America, a region with mixed economies and development, excess weight has been increasing during the last half century. Every country with longitudinal data on overweight and obesity (BMI $\geq$ 25) has reported substantially increased prevalence, to the point that the vast majority of nations are at least at 40% prevalence (Rueda-Clausen et al., 2007). Figure 2.6 demonstrates that, though there are differences by country, the increased prevalence of excess weight has been similar across the region.

The rapid demographic and nutrition transitions that have occurred or are occurring elsewhere have taken place in Central and South America as well, to

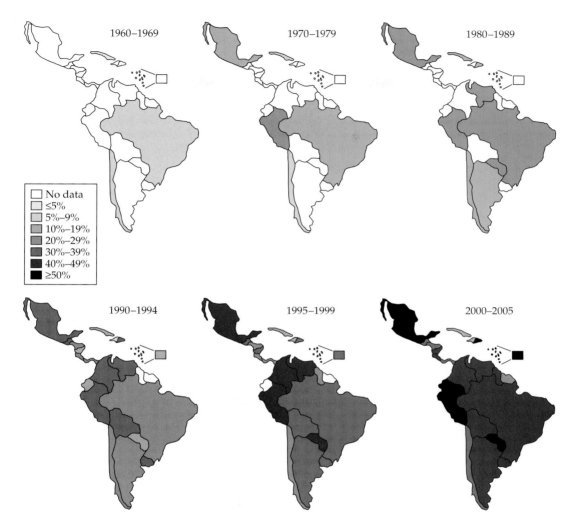

FIGURE 2.6 Changes in combined overweight and obesity prevalence among Central and South American countries, 1960–2005. (After Rueda-Clausen et al., 2007.)

similar effect. Countries that have substantially increased per capita income have seen the largest recent rises, particularly among the poor and urban citizens, while in the upper classes of some countries, obesity prevalence has declined somewhat from previously very high levels (Uauy et al., 2001). Because undernourishment and stunting have historically been challenges in many of these countries, ongoing food supplement programs may contribute to the epidemic of excess weight in the region, in addition to the well-documented changes in lifestyle, work habits, dietary intake, and residence.

Rises in obesity prevalence, as elsewhere, have been heterogeneous by demographic characteristics. In Brazil, for example, obesity has risen over time in both men and women, throughout rural and urban areas, and across income levels. However, absolute increases have been substantially greater among urban residents and among women—with the exception of upper-income urban women, who showed reduced prevalence from 12.8% to 9.2% in the decade from 1989 to 1997 (Filozof et al., 2001). In countries with longitudinal data on childhood obesity, several but not all—Chile, Bolivia, and Peru, but not Brazil—have reported increased prevalence (Filozof et al., 2001). Measurement of childhood obesity in the region is hampered, though, because of the long-standing focus on stunting and undernourishment rather than on excess weight.

The countries making up the Asia-Pacific region are highly heterogeneous in the prevalence of obesity, in the genetic and cultural histories of their peoples, in economic development, and in dietary and activity patterns. Across the region, however, the effects of the epidemiological, nutrition, and demographic transitions are clearly illustrated. Although many countries in the region continue to have low *absolute* prevalence of excess weight compared to other regions, the rate of increase in some instances far exceeds that of other regions. For instance, at the start of the twenty-first century, overweight and obesity prevalence was approximately 60% in Australia and only 19% in China. On the other hand, the prevalence of excess weight in Australia increased from approximately 50% in 1980 to roughly 60% in 2000, while prevalence in China rose from 3.7% to 19.0% during that same period—an increase of 414% (Asia Pacific Cohort Studies Collaboration, 2007). Given the trajectory of the increase, and the large absolute population of China, this change represents a serious and expanding threat. The threat is magnified by the likelihood that western BMI cutoffs are inappropriate for many Asian populations, and that lower cutoffs are needed to accurately convey the increased risk associated with greater BMI (Dudeja et al., 2001; James et al., 2002).

The economically developed nations of the Asia-Pacific region have experienced increases in excess weight, even in societies with traditionally little obesity and historically less influence from outside pressures. Among the economically developed island nations, combined overweight and obesity increased from 16.7% in the late 1970s to 24.0% in 2000 in Japan, and obesity from 0.8% to 2.0% between the late 1970s and mid 1990s; obesity increased from 11% in 1989 to 17% in 1997 in New Zealand; and obesity was roughly 21% in Australia in 2000, two and a half times the prevalence in 1980 (Asia Pacific Cohort Studies Collaboration, 2007; Seidell, 2005). In parallel with its substantial economic growth and change, overweight and obesity in Korea has increased rapidly in recent years. In surveys only 6 years apart, the obesity prevalence estimate for the population increased from under 15% to over 30% (Figure 2.7), with proportionally greater increases in men but greater absolute increases in women (Kim et al., 2005). This rapid rise corresponds with a decades-long shift in dietary pat-

(A)

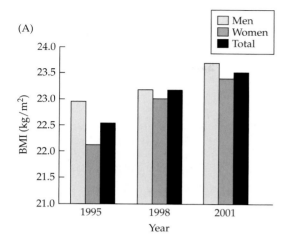

(B)

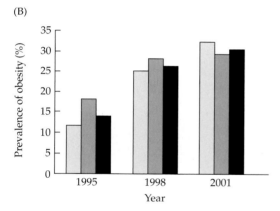

FIGURE 2.7   Mean BMI (A) and obesity prevalence (B) in Korea, 1995–2001. (After Kim et al., 2005.)

terns, with increased reliance on animal-based foods and oils, and with reduced reliance on cereals.

Excess weight is on the rise even in Asia-Pacific countries that are only now undergoing substantial shifts in economic and demographic development. In Vietnam, for instance, economic reforms initiated in 1986 have profoundly changed how and where people work and reside. In concert, overweight increased between 1992 and 2002 from 1.1% to 4.5% in men, and from 2.8% to 6.6% in women (Nguyen et al., 2007)—a huge proportional increase. Though the absolute rates are still low, the trend is clear, and it is consistent with other nations in the region: Vietnam, and nations with similar economic profiles, can expect substantial rises in excess weight unless interventions stem the increase.

India, too, has seen large proportional increases in excess weight as its population has become increasingly urbanized while it continues to focus on the ongoing challenge of undernutrition (Griffiths & Bentley, 2001; Chatterjee, 2002). Although the absolute rates of overweight in India remain lower than in many other countries, overweight and obesity are on the rise, particularly among the urban classes, which comprise the most rapidly growing population segments in Indian society.

China, currently the world's most populous nation, is also beginning to see rises in excess weight and related diseases as a result of the rapid demographic, economic, and nutrition trends of the past few decades. A review of trends in China has suggested that obesity increased from 3.3% to 5.6% in the decade 1992 to 2002, and that combined obesity and overweight rose from 16.1% to 23.2% during the same period (Wang, Mi, et al., 2007). As is now to be expected, these early rises in excess weight are greater among urban and well-off citizens, but they are likely to spread to the general population as buying power and distribution infrastructure expand.

The prevalence of overweight and obesity, far from being stemmed, is still on the rise globally. In a recent United Nations report, of 28 countries with longitudinal data, obesity was rising in 20 among men and in 19 among women (Nishida & Mucavele, 2004–05). In the few instances where prevalence seemed to be dropping, it was dropping from already high prevalence; while offering a glimmer of encouragement, these findings suggest that the road back from excess weight will be difficult and long.

Place

> *You will find, as a general rule, that the constitutions and the*
> *habits of a people follow the nature of the land where they live.*
> — Hippocrates

Nearly everyone has seen the maps, either cross-sectional or as a time series, depicting changes in overweight by region. The previous section showed the time course for excess weight by political jurisdictions for Canada and for Central and South America. Maps that show gradients of excess weight in the United States (Figure 2.8) are well known, and difficult to explain. As yet, no one has adequately explained what combination of genetics, culture, demography, environment, and behavior resulted in the southeastern states leading the way in obesity prevalence. Data-based speculation that the nature of modern rural living was to blame, or that economic and educational disadvantage drove the early southeastern rise, remain provocative but not definitive (Ramsey & Glenn, 2002). What is clear, from longitudinal data, is that prevalence has increased dramatically in all states across the United States; recent rates in the "thin" state of Colorado (in Figure 2.8) are comparable to those of Mississippi and Louisiana (dark gray) as recently as 1996. Large-scale geographic disparities do not "protect" some locations from the epidemic of excess weight. Similar patterns of rapid rises in excess weight can be seen around the globe.

Few generalizations are as tempting to make, but as difficult to support, as pat claims about geographic and environmental influences on obesity and over-

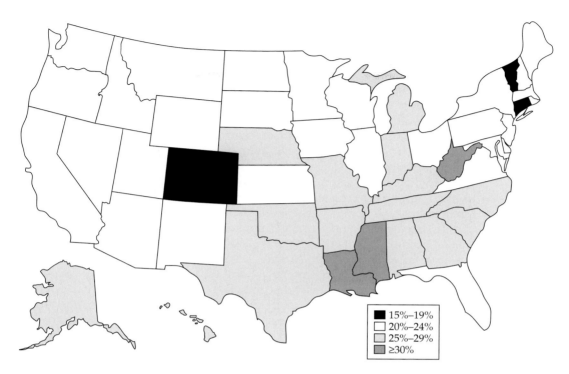

FIGURE 2.8   Obesity prevalence in the United States, 2005. (From Centers for Disease Control and Prevention.)

weight. Even a cursory review of the literature on the topic suggests that the relationships are complex, and differ depending on location, demography, and economics. These relationships are further clouded by the wide range in research methods used in this expanding field of public health. Nevertheless, some relationships between place and excess weight seem to be emerging, and the field is poised to make substantial contributions to our understanding of the epidemic.

At the same time, the rapid and global rise in excess weight suggests that the physical environment has a substantial influence on the development and maintenance of individual weight and on population levels of excess weight (Jeffery & Linde, 2005), and some have used the term *obesogenic environments* to describe environments that promote obesity at both the individual and population levels (Lake & Townshend, 2006). Precisely what elements of the environment promote excess caloric intake, encourage high-calorie food choices, or discourage or limit physical activity have yet to be firmly established. Research to date, however, suggests that there are many environmental determinants of weight gain—

and therefore many opportunities to take action. This section examines what is known, and what is not, about the ways in which environments promote overweight and obesity.

Many studies have examined whether the prevalence of excess weight is greater among urban than among rural residents. The answer likely depends on when during the nutrition transition the differences are assessed. In general, the epidemic of excess weight, at the population level, has seemed to start in urban populations and spread later to rural populations. In Tanzania, for instance, cross-sectional surveys found that residents in rural areas had significantly lower prevalence of obesity (and high blood pressure and cholesterol) than did their urban counterparts (Njelekela et al., 2003). In Malaysia, a country with rapid recent economic development, previous urban-versus-rural differences in obesity prevalence (and in dietary patterns) has been erased, with obesity prevalence among rural residents rivaling that of sedentary workers in Kuala Lumpur (Ismail et al., 2002). In Gambia, a similar pattern has emerged: obesity, once prevalent only in cities, has spread to the countryside with the advent of increased purchasing power and the availability of inexpensive but calorie-dense foods (e.g., oils; Prentice & Webb, 2006). In India, urban populations, with relatively greater wealth and access to less expensive calories, are experiencing increased obesity prevalence, but those living in the countryside continue to be more concerned with undernutrition (Chatterjee, 2002). In Iran, a similar pattern has been shown, with urban residents more likely to be overweight than their rural counterparts, against a backdrop of continuing concern with undernutrition (Rashidi et al., 2005). In Latin American countries, obesity is still more prevalent in urban settings, but differences have been shrinking as economic development has advanced. In Brazil, for instance, obesity was twice as prevalent in 1975 among urban residents compared to rural residents, but by 1997 obesity prevalence in the two populations was comparable. Similar narrowing of urban–rural differences have been observed for the Dominican Republic and Peru (Filozof et al., 2001).

Urban–rural differences can vary among subpopulations as countries develop economically. In Korea, obesity among younger women is more common in rural than in urban areas, but there is no urban–rural gradient among older women. In contrast, obesity among older men is more likely in urban than rural settings, but there is no urban–rural gradient among younger men (Chung et al., 2005). In Brazil, urban women of upper socioeconomic status have reduced prevalence of obesity compared to earlier assessments, but obesity among their rural counterparts has not appreciably abated (Filozof et al., 2001).

In a study of women in 36 developing countries (19 in sub-Saharan Africa, 8 in Central and South America and the Caribbean, 5 in Asia, and 4 in North Africa/Middle East), overweight was twice as common in urban than in rural areas, but with substantial variation among nations (Mendez et al., 2005). Among the developing nations with the highest gross national income, however, not only was overall prevalence of overweight greater, but the urban–rural differences were much less pronounced. Among the nations in the bottom third of gross national income, most showed a substantially greater proportion of urban overweight compared to rural overweight . The urban–rural difference was least in countries with both high income and high urbanization.

In economically developed countries, the historical advantage among rural residents is absent and in some instances reversed. A large population-based sample that crossed ten European nations found no differences by urban–rural status in overweight or obesity; adjusted odds ratios for risk of overweight by rural status ranged among the ten countries from 0.9 to 1.2 (Peytremann-Bridevaux et al., 2007). There were no urban–rural differences among strata of age, gender, education, or income. In Canada, a large national sample found that obesity was as prevalent in rural men (37%) and women (30%) as in their urban counterparts (34% and 28%, respectively; Reeder et al., 1997). In the Canadian west, obesity was more common in rural men (41%) and women (35%) than in their urban counterparts (34% and 25%, respectively).

In the United States, Behavioral Risk Factor Surveillance System data from 2000–2001 were used to compare obesity between urban and rural counties. Obesity was more common in rural counties (23.0%) compared to urban counties (20.5%), although both absolute prevalence and rates of increase from earlier estimates were similar (Jackson et al., 2005). Analysis of data from the National Survey of Children's Health (www.cdc.gov/nchs/about/major/slaits/nsch.htm) suggested that rural children were at 20% increased risk of being overweight compared to urban children (Lutfiyya et al., 2007). Taken as a whole, the large-scale ecological data suggest that there are geographic trends, both among and within countries, in the population-level rise of obesity—but that eventually, obesity and overweight spare no particular region or environment and require no particular type of neighborhood in which to flourish.

At both the local and the global level, it is clear that the food environment has changed considerably in the past few decades, in concert with the rise in obesity. Added fats and oils, caloric sweeteners, and refined grains are inexpensive, convenient, and appealing, and now available worldwide (Drewnowski, 2007). For instance, since 1970 food availability has increased by 15% in the United States, led by a sharp increase in the availability of carbohydrates (Jeffery & Linde, 2005).

The picture is complicated, however, by changes in food habits: during the same period, US consumption of red meat, butter, and whole milk dropped considerably, but that decrease was probably more than made up for calorically by steep rises in the intake of oils, cheeses, and corn sweeteners. Several obesity-promoting environmental changes in the United States and other developed nations have been noted, including the expansion of the availability (and purchase) of soft drinks, greater portion sizes in commercial food, and greater reliance on foods prepared away from home (Popkin, 2005a). In addition, government subsidies have promoted the production of ingredients used in low-cost, high-energy foods (e.g., high-fructose corn syrup).

In the developing world, food availability has shifted dietary patterns toward increased intake of edible oils, animal foods (e.g., meat, dairy), and caloric sweeteners (the same sweeteners that are so common in US soft drinks are available globally). For instance, food availability data from Egypt suggest that, between 1960 and 1997, the availability of cereals rose by 50%, while the availability of fats and oils rose by 300% (Galal, 2002), along with rises in animal-based foods, fruits, vegetables, and refined sugars but declines in legumes. Not only have available calories substantially increased, but those available are likely to result in less healthful diets—rises in fruit and vegetable consumption notwithstanding. The rapid and profound changes in the food environments among Pacific Islanders has led to rapid rises in overweight and obesity in the past four decades (Ulijaszek, 2005).

In parallel, and in both developed and developing nations, physical activity has declined because of decreased workplace activity—due to changes in employment patterns, as well as mechanization of work—increased labor-saving devices in home maintenance, and decreased reliance on human-powered transportation. The global changes in the food environment and physical activity patterns, and their subsequent influence on excess weight and disease, have been under way for decades, and they will influence our collective health for at least decades to come (Popkin, 2005b).

A growing body of evidence suggests that local environments—in addition to global, national, or regional environments—play an important role in the promotion and maintenance of obesity (Lopez & Hynes, 2006; Booth et al., 2005). A recent systematic review highlighted both the promise and the challenge of examining environmental influences on excess weight (Papas et al., 2007). Of 20 articles identified from three major online search engines, 17 (85%) reported statistically significant associations between an environmental variable and body mass index. The vast majority of studies reviewed focused on adults. Among studies of food availability, significant positive associations were reported between body weight and three factors: density of fast-food restaurants, density of grocery and convenience stores, and distance traveled to food shopping. In contrast, the presence of nearby supermarkets (versus grocery or convenience stores) was associated with lower BMI. In children, one study reported lower weights in metropolitan areas that had lower prices for fruits and vegetables, but two studies reported no associations between retail food outlets and childhood overweight.

Three of four studies suggested that urban sprawl was associated with increased BMI, while mixed land use was associated with reduced BMI in both studies in which it was examined. Increased BMI or overweight was also associated with living on roads having impediments to physical activity (e.g., high traffic density, limited sidewalks, low "walkability"). In two studies, BMI was higher in areas with limited access to physical activity facilities. It is clear, as the authors of the review noted, that one of the challenges in summarizing knowledge to date is the heterogeneity of measures used; 11 methods were used to characterize access to physical activity, 6 for access to food, and another 6 to define other environmental predictors (Papas et al., 2007). In addition, the studies were conducted in sometimes very different populations and at very different levels, from neighborhood to state.

The connections between environmental factors and overweight are difficult to tease apart from one another and from larger environmental influences on residence and behavior. For instance, proximity to supermarkets has been associated with body mass index in some settings (Laraia et al., 2004; Rose & Richards, 2004) and has been generally viewed as a marker for greater access to healthful foods (Popkin et al., 2005). In areas of Los Angeles, for instance, shopping at a grocery store in a "disadvantaged" area *or* traveling greater distances to shop at a supermarket was associated with greater BMI (Inagami et al., 2006), potentially revealing a complex environment–behavior interaction marked by substantial reliance on local, less healthfully stocked stores as either primary or supplemental sources of groceries. In four central and coastal California cities, however, obesity prevalence in women was greater among those living in neighborhoods with greater numbers of small grocery stores, but also among women living closer to chain supermarkets (Wang, Kim, et al., 2007).

Clearly, our typically individually targeted dietary interventions cannot succeed if the environment limits access to recommended foods. A recent study in New York City found that only 18% of stores in East Harlem, a relatively low income setting, stocked five foods typically recommended for diabetes control, compared to 58% of stores in the higher-income Upper East Side (Horowitz et al., 2004). It is not clear, however, whether this difference reflects reduced demand, cost-conscious choices, consumer preference, store policy, infrastructure or delivery limitations, or other factors.

Though associations between neighborhood factors and obesity have been mixed, there is growing evidence that physical activity is associated with aspects of the local environment—proximity, accessability, walkability, population density, and land-use mix (Popkin et al., 2005). The location of recreation facilities may influence obesity. In a large national sample, the risk of overweight was inversely related to the number of nearby recreation facilities (Gordon-Larsen et al., 2006). As Popkin and colleagues (2005) note, "this is a field in its infancy," and the cross-sectional design of this and many similar studies precludes drawing strong causal conclusions.

One major challenge in evaluating the role of the physical environment in promoting or preventing obesity is the issue of people selecting their environments. Even if it is true that elements of neighborhoods shape behavior associated with weight control—which they certainly do—it is equally true that people select neighborhoods to some extent on the basis of their preferred lifestyles. As part of a 13-county survey in the Atlanta, Georgia, region, 1455 people were asked a series of questions regarding their preferences for neighborhoods in which to live (Frank et al., 2007). Both the neighborhoods where respondents actually lived and their stated neighborhood preferences were categorized for walkability. Not surprisingly, walking was much more common in walkable neighborhoods among people who preferred such neighborhoods, and driving was more common in car-dependent neighborhoods. Among people who preferred and lived in car-dependent neighborhoods, 21.4% were obese, compared to 11.7% among those who lived in and preferred walkable neighborhoods. However, among those who lived in walkable neighborhoods but preferred car-dependent neighborhoods, obesity prevalence was 21.6%. In highly walkable neighborhoods, those who preferred to live in such neighborhoods were approximately five times as likely to walk as their neighbors who would have preferred more car-dependent neighborhoods.

Clearly, although the environment can shape behavior—particularly in settings where residents have little choice—it is also likely that people select environments that suit their preferred lifestyles. Many people have at least some choice in the nature of their residence. The willingness of citizens and their representatives to encourage or even demand health-promoting environments—through financial, social, or legal means—will in part determine the extent and rate of change. Along with improving the science of determining "what works" in environmental change, societies will also have to grapple with the limits of both collective action and individual choice.

It is worth considering one other definition of *environment* as it relates to excess weight: the social environment. Because excess weight is not gained in environmental or social isolation, weight gain by one individual may have the "collateral effect" of promoting obesity in others (Christakis, 2004), perhaps through shared behaviors or by the modification of norms for physical appearance. Modifying the immediate social environment and enlisting social support has long been a staple of change in dietary behavior (McCann & Bovbjerg, in press), and it makes intuitive sense that social networks might influence behaviors that promote excess weight as well.

In seven examinations administered during 3-year periods centered on 1973, 1981, 1985, 1989, 1992, 1997, and 1999, 5124 members of the Framingham Heart Study (www.nhlbi.nih.gov/about/framingham) listed first-degree relatives and close friends, along with their addresses (Christakis & Fowler, 2007). In every cross-sectional examination, risk of obesity was increased by having a direct connection to someone else in the network who was obese. The increased risk for a single degree of separation was 45%, for two degrees 20%, and for three degrees 10%, compared to randomly selected study participants (Figure 2.9). Mutual friendships put individuals at heightened risk of obesity: if two study participants were mutual friends and one of them became obese, the risk of the other participant's becoming obese rose by 171%. If a participant did not perceive friendship with another Framingham member, even though the second member did perceive such a friendship, there was no increased risk. Obesity was more likely in same-sex friends and siblings, with no association in mixed-sex friends or siblings. Married couples put each other at risk, too, while neigh-

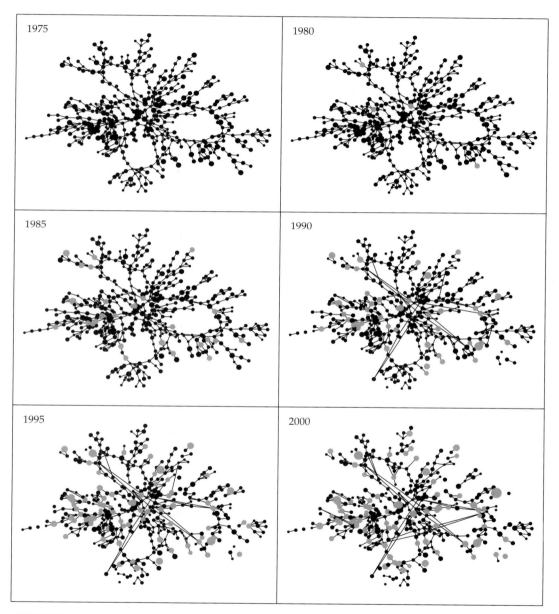

FIGURE 2.9 Increase in obesity within a social network, 1975–2000. Black circles, nonobese; grey circles, obese. (After Christakis & Fowler, 2007.)

bors did not. Though these findings are provocative, the relative contributions of social influences have not been entirely disentangled in this analysis from the influences of shared physical environments and genetics. It remains to be seen whether social networks contribute to the explanation of the obesity epidemic, over and above other environmental determinants, and more importantly, whether social networks will be an important element in reversing the prevalence of excess weight.

A wide range of other potential environmental influences on excess weight have been proposed but not yet thoroughly investigated, including intrauterine effects, unintended consequences of widespread pharmaceutical use, viruses that induce weight gain, and environmental pollutants (Cope & Allison, 2006). Some proposed influences are reasonably well documented, such as weight gain following the initiation of antidepressants (Fava, 2000), but are unlikely to account for much of the global increase in obesity and overweight. Potential infectious etiologies for obesity have been investigated in animal models (Dhurandhar, 2001), and they continue to capture popular attention (Borenstein, 2007), but their role in weight gain has not been demonstrated at either individual human or population levels. There is increasing interest in the intergenerational "transmission" of obesity (Benyshek, 2007), including the potential role of maternal malnutrition in obesity promotion among offspring (Varela-Silva et al., 2007), and the consistently reported preventive effect of breast-feeding (Owen et al., 2005; Arenz et al., 2004).

Environmental contaminants have been proposed as obesity promoters. For instance, exposure to bisphenol A from plastics, which has been shown to mimic estrogen in animal models, has been hypothesized as contributing to the worldwide obesity epidemic (Baillie-Hamilton, 2002), as well as causing a whole host of conditions from cancer to birth defects to pubertal acceleration (Howe & Borodinsky, 1998; Kuehn, 2007). Demonstration of such effects in humans, though, has been slow in coming, and there is considerable skepticism regarding the science underpinning claims against bisphenol A (Gray & Cohen, Harvard Center for Risk Analysis, 2004). Exposures to environmental contaminants are difficult to document, and their links to obesity will be very difficult to detect.

These are still early days in the exploration of the associations among environment, behavior, and excess weight. Caution is warranted in generalizing from current knowledge regarding the environment and obesity.

First, it is not clear that results obtained in one setting will generalize to others. For instance, in New York City, BMI was *inversely* related to mixed land use, density of bus and subway stops, and population density (Rundle et al., 2007). To what extent this inverse relationship is unique to New York or very similar settings is not yet known.

Second, we face the substantial methodological challenges common to an emerging field. The heterogeneity of environmental measures noted in systematic reviews (Papas et al., 2007) makes comparisons across settings and populations difficult. Measures surely will be refined as the field grows. In a study of urban sprawl and obesity, sprawl was (essentially) defined by subtracting the percentage of the population in high-density census tracts from the percentage in low-density tracts (Lopez, 2004). Although such an approach has the advantage of uncomplicated measurement and leads to some expected outcomes (e.g., New York City has the lowest sprawl index, 6.72), it can also lead to findings that need further explanation (e.g., Los Angeles' second lowest sprawl rating, at 10.61, and sprawl in Dothan, Alabama, rated at 100.00).

It is also unclear whether the important environmental variables consist of physical measurements (e.g., subway stop density, sidewalk presence), or whether these are elements of larger variables—the same way that individual items on a psychological scale are thought to be measuring part of a "latent" variable. Does the apparent paradox of suburban residents living in car-dependent neighborhoods having lower BMIs than urban residents with sidewalks everywhere (Lopez & Hynes, 2006) mean that we give up on sidewalks to promote activity *or* look for a more sophisticated understanding of the environment?

The now common cross-sectional and ecological study designs, useful though they are, must give way to more longitudinal multilevel studies. For instance, investigators have started examining the combined longitudinal roles of shared genes and shared environments on fast-food consumption, physical activity, and BMI changes (Nelson et al., 2006). Though many methodological challenges remain, our ability to use multiple sources of information and sophisticated mapping methods has enabled rapid gains in our ability to describe the associations among obesity, diet and activity, and the environment. It is now common, for instance, to see residences and recreational facilities mapped together to examine access to physical activity resources. Figure 2.10 shows study participants in relation to area recreation facilities. If something about the respondents is known, such figures can illustrate whether recreational facilities are poorly distributed among the population, or if access is limited in certain segments of the population or can help locate prime areas for future facility construction (Gordon-Larsen et al., 2006).

It is encouraging that investigators from formerly disparate fields, such as nutrition and urban planning, are collaborating to improve research methods (Popkin, 2005b; Handy et al., 2002), are identifying areas of commonality, and are seeking an understanding of issues that animate related disciplines interested in obesity—exemplified by the present compilation.

Third, though some evidence suggests that changing the food and built environment can lead to behavior change, to date we have limited evidence that the magnitude of those changes will be sufficient to result in changes in obesity and obesity-related disease prevalence (Sallis & Glanz, 2006). The surging growth of investigations on obesity and environment suggests that there will be increasingly sophisticated research methods, leading to more robust findings, which in turn will contribute to efforts to control excess weight.

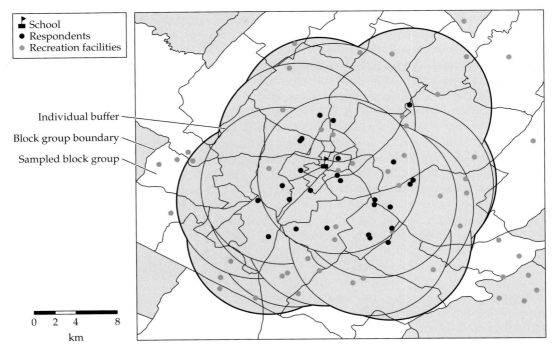

School
Respondents
Recreation facilities

Individual buffer
Block group boundary
Sampled block group

0   2   4   8
km

FIGURE 2.10   Spatial distribution of adolescent study respondents and nearby recreation facilities. (After Gordon-Larsen et al., 2006.)

Person

Although the global epidemic of excess weight is driven proximally by changes in society, technology, transportation and logistics, and income, the burden of excess weight—and its effects on health—falls unequally on individuals within societies. Most societies experience excess weight first among the wealthy—those with access to abundant and rich foods, and with little need for occupation-related physical activity. As the epidemic of excess weight has advanced, the burden typically has shifted to poorer groups, and evidence suggests that this shift is occurring more rapidly now than previously (Popkin & Gordon-Larsen, 2004). Within societies, the complex interaction of culture, income, environment, and genes profoundly influences who does and does not gain excess weight. The causal mechanisms behind weight gain and weight loss are the topics of other chapters, but it is worth reviewing the distribution of excess weight at the population level by socioeconomic status, sex, race or ethnicity, and age, and to take brief stock of the potential for genetic analysis to help unravel causal mechanisms in the epidemiology of excess weight.

SOCIOECONOMIC STATUS   The socioeconomic status of entire societies—that is, the wealth of a country or region—is clearly associated with excess weight. As countries become more wealthy, access to greater amounts of nutrient-dense food is coupled with reductions in work-related physical activity to promote obesity and overweight (Popkin & Gordon-Larsen, 2004). Typically, excess weight is observed initially in upper socioeconomic groups, but later in the epidemic in all groups. A recent systematic review of 333 published studies illustrates this pattern. Among women in high-income countries (those with high Human Development Index scores), the majority of associations were inverse; that is, higher socioeconomic status (SES) was associated with lower levels of excess weight (McLaren, 2007). Inverse relationships were noted in 72% of associations that examined excess weight and education, and in 68% of associations comparing excess weight to occupation.

In high-income countries, only 3% (23/731) of associations were positive—that is, suggesting greater excess weight at higher SES. In contrast, 43% of comparisons in medium-income countries and 94% of comparisons in low-income countries were positive, suggesting that higher SES is indeed predictive of excess weight in settings where inexpensive food may not be ubiquitous. Among men in both high- and medium-income countries, the most common finding was no association between SES and excess weight; in high-income countries, however, negative associations greatly exceeded positive associations, consistent with findings for women. In medium-income countries, by contrast, the second most common findings were positive associations, and every association in low-income countries was a positive association between SES and excess weight, though few studies focused on low-income countries.

China presents a clear example of how, during a period of development for urban upper classes, excess weight was not only much more common among those with higher incomes, but the rate of increase was greatest in upper-income groups as well (Figure 2.11; Wang, Mi, et al., 2007). Clearly the SES–excess weight gradient reverses in the progression from low- to high-income countries. Of course, prevalence of overweight at all levels of SES has generally risen over time. As countries that now have low incomes increase their per capita income, their SES–obesity patterns are likely to change, as well. Some evidence suggests that this is indeed happening, with the shift in obesity burden toward the poor occurring at the point when countries reach lower to middle GNP, approximately $2500 per capita in 2004 (Monteiro et al., 2004).

In the United States, the association between excess weight and SES is clear. At the start of the twenty-first century, obesity was more common among those in the Behavioral Risk Factor Surveillance System with less than high school educations (26%) than among those with high school education (22%), some college (20%), or at least a college degree (15%; Mokdad et al., 2001). A recent meta-analysis using data from the NHANES, BRFSS, Youth Risk Behavior Surveillance System (YRBSS; www.cdc.gov/HealthyYouth/yrbs), and National Longitudinal Survey of Adolescent Health (www.cpc.unc.edu/addhealth) revealed complex

FIGURE 2.11   Changes in combined overweight and obesity by socioeconomic status in China, 1989–1997. (After Wang, Mi, et al., 2007.)

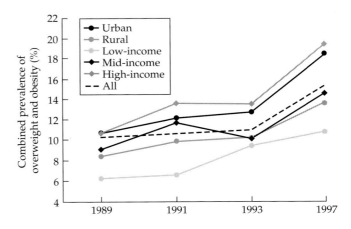

relationships between SES and obesity (Wang & Beydoun, 2007). In men, obesity prevalence rose in parallel from the early 1970s to 2000, with high-SES men less likely to be obese at any given time, but with all groups at substantially increased risk in 2000: high-SES men in 2000 had twice the prevalence of obesity compared to low-SES men in the early 1970s. Among women, SES differences were most pronounced in the early 1970s, with low-, medium-, and high-SES women converging on similar and much higher rates by 2000. In contrast, among those of African descent, obesity among low- and middle-SES men was similar until a sharp spike among low-SES men in the late 1990s, with middle- and high-SES men at lower prevalence. In African American women, rates among those with low SES were substantially elevated in the early 1970s compared to middle- and upper-SES groups, but all three SES groups had converged considerably by 2000. Among US children, the inverse relationship of higher SES to lower obesity prevalence holds among non-Hispanic Caucasians, but not among other races or ethnic groups (Baskin et al., 2005).

In countries in the middle of the income spectrum, the shift to increased burden among lower-SES groups is clear. In a series of surveys over 20 years in Brazil, for instance, obesity rose in both rural and urban men and women in all SES groups, but with a clear gradient of higher prevalence with higher SES in each time period until 1997 (Filozof et al., 2001). At that point, prevalence among upper-SES women dropped significantly from 1989 levels, while continuing to rise or remaining comparable among women in other SES groups, perhaps reflecting a combination of increased access to healthful foods and physical activity, social emphasis on body image, and greater knowledge of obesity-related illnesses. In Korea, which also has undergone substantial economic development in the past few decades, overweight is now more likely for both men and women in lower-education and lower-income groups compared to others (Kim et al., 2005).

In countries with relatively lower income levels, however, the positive association of SES to obesity is still common. In Tanzania, for instance, obesity is less common among lower-SES groups, in which undernutrition and wasting are still substantial concerns (Villamor et al., 2006). In South Africa, a nation in economic transition, there was a strong graded association between SES and weight among men, with BMI increasing consistently as years of education rose (Puoane et al., 2002). In women, however, the largest mean BMIs were seen among the least and most educated groups, and the authors speculated that this pattern might result from the combination of still-prevalent manual labor in low-SES groups and increased awareness of health and body image among higher-SES groups.

The mechanisms through which SES might influence obesity prevalence are many and difficult to untangle. SES is often associated with cultural norms and expectations, behavioral risk factors, environmental influences, and, in some settings, race or ethnicity (Ball & Crawford, 2005). SES and obesity may well be linked by such disparate mechanisms as limited access to physical activity resources (Gordon-Larsen et al., 2006), inadequate availability of healthful foods in low-SES neighborhoods (Horowitz et al., 2004), or the relatively low cost and ubiquity of high-energy foods (Drewnowski & Specter, 2004).

SEX   Overweight has been said to be more common in men, and obesity more common in women (Yumuk, 2005), but the variation in excess weight both over time and by setting suggests that this is a considerable overgeneralization. A quick review of the World Health Organization's Global Database on Body Mass Index, however, shows that country-level differences in female-to-male ratios of both overweight and obesity vary considerably. In the United States, Canada, and western European nations, male-to-female ratios in obesity have not consistently favored either gender, and they have hovered at about 1.0 in many nations; those for central and eastern Europe, the Baltic states, North Africa, and the Middle East have more often shown greater obesity prevalence in women relative to men (Seidell, 2005). Among 12 nations surveyed in the Asia-Pacific region, obesity was more prevalent among women than among men in 10 countries, and roughly equal in 2 others, and prevalence of overweight did not consistently favor either women or men (Asia Pacific Cohort Studies Collaboration, 2007).

In the United States, approximately two-thirds of both adult men and women were overweight in 2003–2004, though overweight is somewhat more likely in men than in women (Wang & Beydoun, 2007; Paeratakul et al., 2002). Between 30% and 40% were obese (BMI $\geq$ 30) or extremely obese (BMI $\geq$ 40), with both somewhat more prevalent among women. Mean BMI for men and women has reversed since the early 1970s, when it was 25.3 for men and 24.4 for women.

By the start of the twenty-first century, mean BMI was 27.6 for men and 28.2 for women, having crossed over in about 1990 (Wang & Beydoun, 2007).

Sex differences varied by race and ethnicity. Among Mexican Americans, overweight was more common compared to non-Hispanic Caucasians, and more equally prevalent in men and women, though both obesity and extreme obesity were more common in women. Among African Americans, women were more likely to be overweight, obese, and extremely obese, compared to men. Among Americans of Asian ancestry, obesity was substantially lower among women than men, and Asian American women had roughly one-half to one-third the prevalence of obesity, relative to other women. Regional and local influences make any generalization from national data problematic. In Texas, correlates of obesity in men and women differed from some national findings, suggesting, for instance, that obesity in women was not significantly different by ethnicity (Borders et al., 2006). Overall, however, the relatively greater burden of obesity among US women may have important implications for consequent burden of disease, disability, and decrements in quality of life (Muennig et al., 2006).

Gender differences in overweight and obesity are difficult to characterize globally, partly because of variation among nations, and partly because of the differences in sampling and measurement techniques adopted by various countries. For instance, in both Mongolia and China overweight was nearly as common in men as in women near the beginning of the twenty-first century, and obesity was more prevalent among women than men—but obesity in Chinese women was estimated at 3.4%, compared to 24.6% among Mongolian women (Asia Pacific Cohort Studies Collaboration, 2007). In the developing nations, greater obesity prevalence among women is commonly reported. In Ghana, recent nationwide surveys suggested that obesity prevalence was 2.8% in men, compared to 7.4% in women (Biritwum, 2005), but that there were powerful regional, residential, and ethnic differences as well. The greater prevalence of obesity among married persons in Ghana might reflect childbearing patterns (as well as age), and thus put women at greater risk for early excess weight in settings where food is in sufficient supply. Among Mediterranean and Middle Eastern countries, sex differences in obesity persist despite a wide range of economic, social, and political development: obesity is more common among women than men in Israel (Kaluski & Berry, 2005), Turkey (Yumuk, 2005), and Iran (Rashidi et al., 2005; Hajian-Tilaki & Heidari, 2007). As noted already, obesity rates in Europe as a whole do not show striking patterns of sex differences, but range from countries in which rates are nearly equal (obesity in 23% of men and 25% of women in England; Rennie & Jebb, 2005) to substantially greater among men (26% of men and 18% of women in Greece; Kapantais et al., 2006) or women (6.5% of men and 15% of women in Poland; Milewicz, 2005).

As in the United States, gender differences can depend on other factors. In China, both obesity and combined overweight and obesity were more prevalent among women of ages 45 to 59 and over 60 in 2002, but in the 18- to 44-year-old group, both obesity and combined obesity and overweight were more common in men (Wang, Mi, et al., 2007). In the youngest age group, obesity had risen in the previous decade by 224% among men but by "only" 97% among women. In South Korea, an economy that has boomed over the past couple of decades, obesity among older women does not depend on geography (and by extension, lifestyle), but obesity among younger women is now more common in rural areas, suggesting that young urban women are choosing to lead lifestyles different from those of their rural counterparts (Chung et al., 2005). Obesity rates have changed over time for men and women in Latin American countries as well. The rise in obesity, previously seen in both men and women at all ages, has been reversed among women with the highest incomes, and particularly among high-income urban women (Filozof et al., 2001), perhaps reflecting increased social pressure and body consciousness (combined with access to more healthful foods) among those women. Regardless of place or time, gender differences in overweight and obesity are likely to reflect a combination of underlying biology and a complex interaction of social norms, food availability, and socioeconomic status, which in turn leads to the substantial heterogeneity observed around the globe.

RACE/ETHNICITY   The concept of race is hotly debated and controversial, in part because it is often defined as a (usually unspecified) combination of genetics, geography, culture, and self-identity, and in part because of its association in some settings with subtle to extreme discrimination (Kaplan & Bennett, 2003). In most research, race is either self-identified or assigned by researchers, usually without clear criteria and often with poor agreement among methods of identification (Frost et al., 1992). Of 330 genetics research articles published between 2001 and 2003 that mentioned race or ethnicity, only 9.1% explained the criteria by which race or ethnicity was assigned (Sankar et al., 2007). Race and ethnicity, though conceptually separate, are often not treated as such in research, further complicating interpretation of results. Nevertheless, risk factors and disease are often distributed differentially by race or ethnicity, and in some settings this is true also of excess weight.

Overweight and obesity in the United States are reasonably well documented according to race and ethnicity. Americans of Asian heritage generally have the lowest mean BMI and lowest rates of both overweight and obesity, followed by non-Hispanic Caucasians, followed next by generally higher rates in African Americans, Hispanics, Native Americans, and Pacific Islanders (Wang & Beydoun, 2007). The eightieth percentile for BMI is higher in African Americans (32.2) than for Hispanics (30.2) and Caucasians (29.5; Truong & Sturm, 2005). BRFSS data from 2001 suggested that differences in obesity were relatively less pronounced in men—with the exception of Native American men at 41%, male obesity ranged from 19% to 22%—than in women, in which Asian Americans were lowest (9%), followed by Caucasians (21%), Hispanics (26%), Native Americans

(28%), and African Americans (34%; Wang & Beydoun, 2007). Even in fairly restricted environments, differences in obesity prevalence by heritage have been observed. Among residents of Hawaii, native Hawaiians and other Pacific Islanders have the highest prevalence of excess weight, and those of Asian descent have the lowest, with Caucasians exhibiting intermediate prevalence (Maskarinec et al., 2006; Davis et al., 2004).

Racial and ethnic differences vary by gender. Data from the 2003–2004 NHANES (based on measured weight and height) show a similar prevalence of obesity among men of European descent (31.1%) and Mexican descent (31.6%), and only slightly higher rates among men of African descent (34.0%). In contrast, prevalence among women of European descent (30.2%) was considerably lower than among women of Mexican descent (42.3%) or African descent (53.9%). Though obesity prevalence has risen in every NHANES examination from 1971 to the present, the pattern of similar rates by race and ethnicity in men, and disparate rates by race and ethnicity in women, has generally held throughout.

There are racial and ethnic differences in "transient" excess weight as well. Among pregnant women, one study reported that roughly one-third of Latinas and over one-half of African American women gained excess weight during pregnancy, putting them at increased risk of gestational diabetes (Kieffer et al., 2001). Differences in prevalence, as well as in potential biological, social, environmental, and economic mechanisms through which obesity confers risk, may help explain some differences in obesity-related disease risk by race and ethnicity in the United States (Cossrow & Falkner, 2004). In the United States particularly, it is very difficult to separate racial and ethnic differences in excess weight from SES-related differences (Zhang & Wang, 2004). More striking, however, than the differences in excess weight by race and ethnicity are the similarities in the extreme rise of excess weight across all racial and ethnic groups: though the processes might be somewhat different or occur with different timing, it is clear that the environmental forces promoting excess weight are operating across the entire US population.

Racial and ethnic differences in excess weight are less often reported outside the United States, partly because of the relative homogeneity of many smaller nations. Even in comparatively small nations, however, there can be important differences among groups. In the United Kingdom, BMI among those of Asian descent averaged 24.0 in 2003–2004, whereas BMI among those of Indian (24.0), Pakistani (27.6), and Bangladeshi (26.4) origin were similar but higher, and that of white (27.2) and black (28.5) English leaned toward the higher end of the spectrum (Diaz et al., 2007). Obesity rates varied considerably across the United Kingdom in 1999, with relatively low rates among those of Chinese or Bangladeshi origin, higher rates in those of Pakistani and Indian origin, and the highest rates among those of Caribbean heritage (Rennie & Jebb, 2005).

The ability of the environment to shape the relationship of ethnicity to overweight was demonstrated in a study of Afro-Caribbean women in which the prevalence of overweight rose from those in rural Cameroon (9.5%) to urban Cameroon (47.1%) to Jamaica (63.8%) to the United Kingdom (71.6%); the same pattern, however, was not observed in men (Jackson et al., 2007). Differences by ethnicity are observed in developing countries as well. In Ghana, obesity rates vary from 14.6% among those of Ga-Adangbe ethnicity to 0.9% among those of the Ghurma (Biritwum et al., 2005). As in the United States, however, ethnicity in Ghana is tied to other influences on obesity, in this case to residence by the Ga people in and around the capital Accra, with its attendant increase in income and food availability, and reduction in physical activity.

Among the various native peoples of South America, the same heterogeneity is apparent, in which differences between native peoples and others are related to geography and lifestyle. Among the Mapuche Indians of Chile, the prevalence of obesity was estimated at 34.4%, but mean BMI among urban Mapuche was higher than among their rural relatives (30.1 versus 27.5). Among native peoples living in mountainous areas of Peru, however, obesity prevalence was much lower—6.5%—reflecting differences in environmental pressures toward excess weight (Filozof et al., 2001). The association of excess weight to race and ethnicity varies globally, and it is likely that the associations depend heavily on social, environmental, and economic factors that may be specific to certain settings. Only a better understanding, both scientifically and conceptually, of what underlies race and ethnicity will allow these many effects to be disentangled.

AGE   In general, it has been a truism that overweight and obesity are more common at older ages than younger, for both men and women. Among adults, obesity has traditionally risen with age, though often at different rates for men and women. Figure 2.12, showing time trends in obesity by age group in the United Kingdom, is typical: at every measurement period, age is monotonically associated with increased prevalence of obesity; and virtually without exception, within each age group obesity prevalence rises with each successive survey (Rennie & Jebb, 2005). Because muscle mass declines beginning in middle age, older individuals have greater body fat than younger individuals with comparable BMIs. Though substantial methodological problems make it difficult to disentangle the effect of BMI and excess weight on health conditions and survival later in life, the health and quality-of-life benefits of weight control and healthful lifestyles are not debated. Curves similar to those in the United Kingdom are typical among developed countries, with body weight and BMI peaking at roughly 60 years of age and declining slightly thereafter (Elia, 2001).

In developing countries, however, the association of age with excess weight is not always monotonic. Among Chinese men in 2002, for instance, the prevalence of overweight was nearly rectangular by age, with prevalence among those 18 to 44 years old at 30.4%, those 45 to 59 years old at 33.55%, and those 60 or older at 30.1% (Wang, Mi, et al., 2007). In Korea, BMI is roughly equivalent among younger, middle-aged, and older men, and among rural women but not their urban counterparts (Chung et al., 2005). In Malaysia, a country undergo-

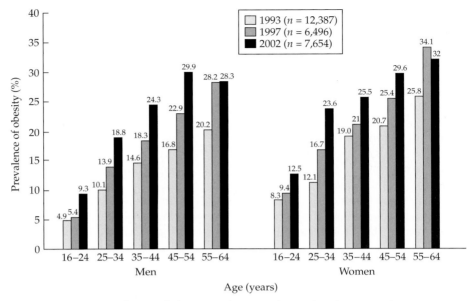

FIGURE 2.12   Prevalence of obesity in the United Kingdom by sex and age group, 1993–2002. (After Rennie & Jebb, 2005.)

ing rapid economic changes in recent decades, the increase in obesity in more recent cohorts can be seen in a cross-sectional survey of BMI in 1996 (Ismail et al., 2002). Figure 2.13 suggests that the increase in BMI was focused first in the younger generations, who are more likely to be affected by the rapid urbanization and changing dietary patterns of Malaysia. As these countries develop economically, and as the initial waves of the obesity epidemic become older, we can expect those countries to take on the familiar pattern of increasing BMI, overweight, and obesity with increasing age.

By far the most important development in the distribution of excess weight by age has been the downward shift in the age of onset of overweight and obesity. At one time confined to middle and older age, overweight and obesity are increasingly common among children and adolescents in both developed and developing countries (Kosti & Panagiotakos, 2006; Janssen et al., 2005). In addition to the immediate physical and psychological health challenges of excess weight in childhood, the early onset of excess weight represents a major long-term threat to longevity, health care expenditures, and quality of life. If the effects of obesity—formerly manifesting later in life—begin to appear in young adults who have been obese or overweight since youth, the financial and societal burden of treating chronic diseases for decades will overwhelm health care systems and social networks.

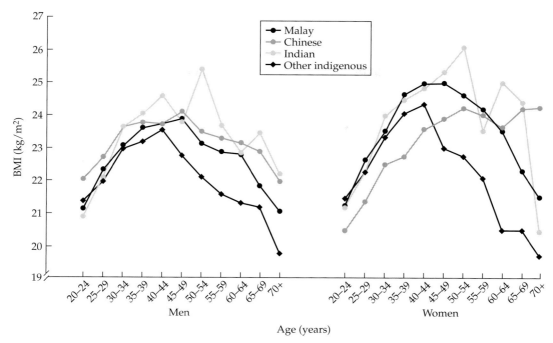

FIGURE 2.13   Mean BMI by age, Malaysia, 1996. (After Ismail et al., 2002.)

The US experience is similar to the experiences of other developed and, increasingly, developing nations. In the 1999–2004 NHANES survey, approximately 35% of children and adolescents between 6 and 19 years old exceeded the eighty-fifth percentile norm, and 17% exceeded the ninety-fifth percentile norm (corresponding to the unfortunate categories of "at risk for overweight" and "overweight," respectively); and the figures for 2- to 5-year-olds were 26% and 14%, respectively (Wang & Beydoun, 2007). The slopes of the increase in children of all ages are steep: NHANES estimates from 1963 to 1970 showed prevalences exceeding the ninety-fifth percentile in the mid single digits, and by 2003 to 2004, rates in the mid to upper teens. Prevalence was somewhat higher in boys than in girls in 2003–2004—a departure from the very similar (and much lower) rates observed in 1963–1970. Paralleling adult data, combined prevalence was lower among Caucasian children compared to African American and Hispanic children, with the lowest prevalence among those of Asian descent. Similar prevalences and rates of increase have been reported for Canada and the United Kingdom (Seidell, 2005).

In other European countries, childhood obesity has kept pace with that in North America and the United Kingdom. Though definitions of obesity vary by country and have changed over time, prevalence in northern European countries among 7- to 10-year-olds at the start of the twenty-first century ranged from 12% to 22%; whereas that in southern European countries was somewhat higher, ranging from 25% to 36% (Seidell, 2005; Tzotzas & Krassas, 2004). As part of the Health Behaviour in School-aged Children (www.hbsc.org) study (Janssen et al., 2005), a survey of nearly 140,000 children conducted in 34 countries demonstrated the generally high rates of overweight in North America, the United Kingdom, and southern Europe; moderate rates in most of western Europe; and lower rates in eastern Europe and Russia (Figure 2.14).

Prevalences of overweight, however, represented a substantial increase from that of earlier decades, even in countries with relatively low prevalence at the time of the survey. Overweight was associated with television viewing (in 22 of 34 countries) and sedentary behavior (in 29 of 34), suggesting that some of the environmental changes acting on adults were influencing excess weight in children as well. Similar patterns have been observed in non-Western developed nations. In Japan, the prevalence of obesity in girls rose from 7.1% in the late 1970s to 10.2% in the late 1990s, and in boys from 6.1% to 11.1% (Matsushita et al., 2004).

In developing nations, increases in childhood obesity, often concentrated in urban areas, may come in the face of ongoing concerns about undernutrition, particularly in rural settings. In some settings, heavy children remain an outward symbol of health and high socioeconomic status. A recent systematic review of published literature on childhood obesity in developing nations suggests that childhood obesity rates vary widely around the world (Kelishadi, 2007). Though there is substantial heterogeneity among countries—in part because of real differences along geopolitical lines and in part because of variation in methods—childhood obesity is particularly high in the countries of the Mediterranean, Balkans, North Africa, and Middle East, with rates comparable to those in the United States or United Kingdom. In South America, prevalence of excess weight in childhood is somewhat lower and more uniform across countries but has risen rapidly.

Although prevalence of overweight and obesity remain relatively low in the most populous countries of Asia—notably India and China—excess weight among children in those countries as well is rising in concert with demographic, nutritional, and lifestyle changes. In China, increased urbanization and income are likely to have the same effects on childhood overweight as they have in other developed nations. In urban China, childhood obesity increased from 1.5% in 1989 to 12.6% one decade later, and overweight increased from 14.6% to 28.9% (Luo & Hu, 2002). Other estimates place the prevalence of overweight (using current definitions) among Beijing 6- to 12-year-olds at 14.2% in girls and 27.7% in boys (Iwata et al., 2003), and increased prevalence has been observed in other urban areas of China (Hui & Bell, 2003). Social and environmental forces, notably the popularity and status associated with consuming Western diets and the relative de-emphasis on physical activity, will continue to promote weight gain among Chinese youth.

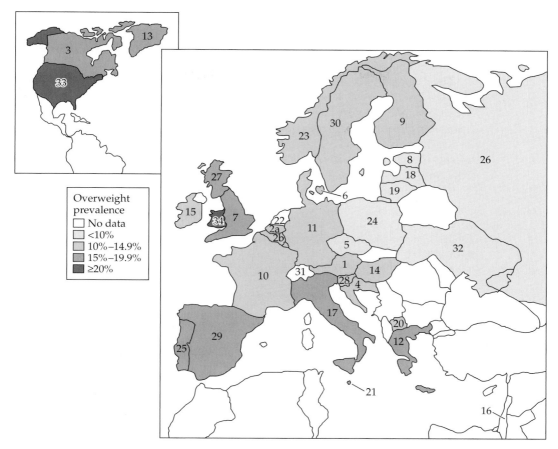

FIGURE 2.14   Prevalence of overweight among 10- to 16-year-olds, 2001–2002. 1, Austria; 2a, Flemish Belgium; 2b, French Belgium; 3, Canada; 4, Croatia; 5, Czech Republic; 6, Denmark; 7, England; 8, Estonia; 9, Finland; 10, France; 11, Germany; 12, Greece; 13, Greenland; 14, Hungary; 15, Ireland; 16, Israel; 17, Italy; 18, Latvia; 19, Lithuania; 20, Macedonia; 21, Malta; 22, Netherlands; 23, Norway; 24, Poland; 25, Portugal; 26, Russia; 27, Scotland; 28, Slovenia; 29, Spain; 30, Sweden; 31, Switzerland; 32, Ukraine; 33, United States; 34, Wales. (After Janssen et al., 2005.)

Similarly, rates of excess weight among children in India remain low overall, but they are growing among the more affluent urban populations. In a sample of 431 affluent Bengalee 6- to 9-year-old schoolgirls, 17.63% were overweight and 5.10% were obese—both higher rates than the national prevalence (Bose et al., 2007). These findings of increased prevalence of excess weight among urban and upper-class children have been replicated in both boys and girls in other Indian settings (Sidhu et al., 2006), and one study across SES groups suggested that excess weight in childhood is more likely among upper-SES children (Chhatwal et al., 2004), though this pattern can be expected to change, just as excess weight in adults has spread beyond its origins among upper-SES groups.

The global environment has changed as much for children as it has for adults. The decline in physical activity and increase in consumption of energy-dense foods brought about by changes in relative wealth, technology and logistics, distribution systems, urbanization and mechanization of work, and lifestyle choices is affecting children as well as adults (Dehghan et al., 2005). It seems likely that efforts to stem the rise in excess weight among children will have to target environments and behavior specific to children, but such measures can't be expected to work well outside a context of population-wide efforts to reduce overweight and obesity.

GENES   As yet, the specific roles of genetics in the worldwide obesity epidemic have not been identified. The rise of obesity is clearly an interaction of environment, behavior, and genetics (Yang et al., 2007). Without the availability of excess calories, excess weight at the population level is impossible—and indeed was not for most of human history. Behavioral changes in diet and physical activity must precede large-scale changes in relative weight. And without a genetic predisposition to store excess calories as fat (or other tissue), changes in neither environment nor behavior would result in excess weight.

Given the similar descriptive epidemiology of obesity and overweight around the globe, it is likely that humans in general are genetically disposed to store excess calories as fat. The thrifty gene hypothesis suggests that natural selection promoting fat deposition during times of plenty occurred in human populations that historically experienced cycles of undernutrition (i.e., nearly all), and may account for the global "reaction" of excess weight to the modern environment characterized by ample calories and reduced physical activity (Bell et al., 2005). Increases in human height, which has a high degree of heritability, are clearly the result of gene–environment interaction, in which the genetic makeup has remained nearly identical in the past century but the nutrition environment has changed. Similarly, changes in overweight and obesity, which also have considerable heritability, are taking place in a changed nutrition and physical activity environment (Farooqi & O'Rahilly, 2006).

The substantial heritability of obesity has been well documented, and even similarities between spouses have been ascribed to assortative mating (the tendency to seek and select mates with important similarities) as much as to shared environments (Sackett et al., 1975; Stunkard et al., 1986; Stunkard et al., 1990). Weight gain and loss appear also to have substantial heritability: twin studies have reported substantial variation between pairs in weight gain among intentionally overfed pairs, but high correlations in weight gain within pairs, followed by high correlations in spontaneous weight loss after the resumption of usual diets (Bell et al., 2005). Heritability estimates for BMI range considerably, from 16% to 85% (Yang et al., 2007), suggesting both that heritability may vary among different samples and that research techniques are not yet as precise as could be hoped, or that the genetic dispositions are pretty much overwhelmed in situations that afford energy-dense foods tailored to mass palatability. Similarly, the genetic contribution to obesity has been difficult to quantify, despite the huge advances in research methods that enable both genomewide and candidate gene investigations (Yang et al., 2007).

The several forms of monogenic obesity have been well described and their genetic basis explored. Though these forms of obesity are very severe and often start in childhood, they are also quite rare and constitute an extremely small proportion of obesity cases (Yang et al., 2007; Farooqi & O'Rahilly, 2006). The most common form of syndromic obesity occurs in one in 25,000 births (Mutch & Clement, 2006). Most obesity is polygenic, with each of many genes making a relatively small contribution to the collectively substantial influence of inheritance on body weight and fat distribution (Lyon & Hirschhorn, 2005). In both genomewide and candidate gene approaches, many potential obesity-related genes have been identified. A recent systematic review reported that genomewide studies have identified genes linked to BMI on every chromosomal region except Y, but only a few reports have been replicated. Similarly, of the over 400 positive associations to obesity observed in more than 120 candidate genes, only 22 have been supported in five or more studies (Yang et al., 2007). For example, a meta-analysis reviewing studies of polymorphisms in three genes involved in leptin regulation found no associations with obesity, either overall or after stratification by ethnicity (Paracchini et al., 2005).

This failure to replicate has been a major challenge to advancing the field, and it may be the result of some combination of statistical false positives, underpowered studies resulting in false negatives, the relatively small effects of single genes in polygenic disorders, the genetic heterogeneity of human populations underlying study samples, dissimilar obesity definitions and ascertainment methods, and gene–environment and gene–diet interactions that are complex and poorly understood (Mutch & Clement, 2006; Yang et al., 2007; Bell et al., 2005; Lyon & Hirschhorn, 2005). More sophisticated approaches to characterizing the genetic contribution to obesity, such as explorations of gene–environment, gene–diet, and gene–activity interactions, have shown initial promise but are far from clinical application (Yang et al., 2007). If gene–diet interactions, for instance, can identify people likely to be responsive to one or another lifestyle intervention, such interventions might be more effectively targeted (Uusitupa, 2005). Though we are in the early days of research in this area, understanding the genetic contribution to obesity seems likely to play an important role in its control.

Summary

This brief overview of the distribution of obesity and overweight suffers from three important challenges. First, descriptive epidemiology is inherently retrospective. At best, descriptions of the prevalence of disease and its predictors are done in near real time. Given the lag in collecting and aggregating data, and then reporting results, such efforts can provide a clear picture of the path followed to reach the current state of the world. In a retrospective look at the obesity epidemic, the path behind seems clear enough. The path ahead, however, is much less obvious; trying to describe and predict a rapidly changing epidemic is perilous. Using the past to speculate on the future is problematic, as epidemics spread to new populations and new regions, and as efforts are undertaken to stem the epidemic.

Obesity is no different; in 20 years, the worst fears about global obesity-related reductions in both life expectancy and quality of life may have been realized. Although concerted global effort may yet identify and implement multimodal, cost-effective interventions to prevent and reverse obesity, it is still not clear whether knowing the causes of this epidemic will lead to its control. Because many cultural and economic causes of obesity are well ingrained in our societies, obesity control may have to come from fiscal and public health pressures that can no longer be resisted and interventions not yet envisioned (Kumanyika, 2007). Understanding the current state of the epidemic may suggest fruitful avenues for amelioration, however. It *is* clear now, and has been for some time, that if unchecked, the current epidemic of overweight and obesity will take a substantial toll on human life expectancy and quality of life.

Second, the social and medical construct of "obesity" has changed over time. Obesity has been transformed from a symbol of health and wealth to an indicator of health risk. Central adiposity, which may have once been a means to survive through lean times, is now a chronic health threat. In clinical and research settings as well, the definition of obesity has varied over time and among investigators. In 2003, the World Health Organization (WHO) defined overweight as a body mass index (BMI) of over 25 kg/m^2, and obesity as a BMI of greater than 30 kg/m^2, and more refined categories (underweight, preobese, class I obesity, etc.) have been promoted (Seidell, 2005), but not as widely adopted. As the WHO notes, however, common cutoffs for weight categories are not necessarily based on thresholds for excess risk of any particular disease. Rather, many conditions have a dose–response relationship to excess weight that can be complex and vary from condition to condition (Caballero, 2007).

For childhood obesity, BMI and BMI cutoffs are more problematic. BMI cutoffs for children, despite efforts by the International Obesity Taskforce and others, tend to be based on norms (e.g., eighty-fifth percentile for overweight and ninety-fifth for obesity) rather than on any objective association of BMI to disease risk (Chinn, 2006; Wang, Mi, et al., 2007). This approach not only defines obesity and overweight entirely in the context of the population used to create norms, but it makes cross-cultural and transnational comparisons difficult because norms are often created from national samples. BMI itself is an imperfect assessment tool. The relationship of BMI to body fat varies among ethnic groups (Deurenberg & Yap, 1999; Charbonneau-Roberts et al., 2005), and it is weaker among older adults (McTigue et al., 2006). Calculating BMI from self-reported weights and heights leads to substantial underestimates of overweight and obesity because those at the highest BMI tend to underreport weight; obesity prevalence has been underreported by 25% to 30% in some national samples (Visscher et al., 2006). Waist-to-hip ratios, and more recently waist circumference alone, have been promoted as better measures of the central adiposity that seems to convey the greatest health risks (Klein et al., 2007). Such measures are logistically more difficult to assess in large population samples, and a recent meta-analysis reported that BMI, waist circumference, and waist-to-hip ratio were nearly identical in their association to diabetes risk (Vazquez et al., 2007). Other methods to assess adiposity—such as the measurement of bioelectrical impedance, body density, or body water, as well as dual-energy X-ray absorptiometry—are useful in clinical research settings but not practical at the population level (Chumlea & Guo, 2000).

Such variation in the definition of obesity, and the means used to estimate its changing prevalence and to identify risk factors, clouds our ability to describe trends over time and across populations, and to identify potential foci for intervention. Debate over the best ways to measure overweight and obesity, though valuable, does not diminish the need to take action; despite the variation in the definitions of overweight and obesity, it is clear from *any* measure of obesity that the epidemic is widespread and accelerating.

Third, the volume of academic writing on the subject of obesity can no longer be summarized in detail. If learned publications on obesity were preventive or curative by themselves, the epidemic would now be a historical footnote. Of the 40,688 publications listed by the National Library of Medicine as having the words *obese* or *obesity* in the title (suggesting that the authors themselves wished to focus on the topic) as of August 2007, 19,770 (48.6%) were published in the past decade, and 12,933 (31.8%) within the past 5 years (Figure 2.15). The volume of work represents admirable effort on the part of academics to explain and control obesity, but the sheer quantity of information makes it impossible to summarize objectively. Fortunately, there have been substantial attempts to summarize findings through systematic reviews and meta-analyses (despite their drawbacks), and recently many journal issues and texts have been devoted to summarizing the history of the current obesity epidemic, and speculating on its possible course and control. The literature, whether from the genetic, psychological, nutritional, environmental, medical, or epidemiological perspective, has converged on the notion that obesity is a multicausal phenomenon, not likely the result of a single influence, nor likely to be resolved by a single approach.

These challenges to our scientific method should not obscure the central facts: that overweight and obesity have been rising and continue to rise around the

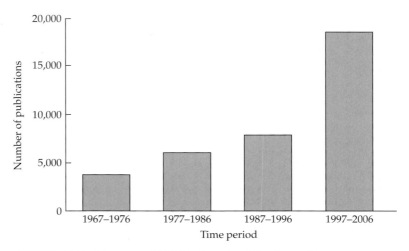

FIGURE 2.15   Number of NLM-indexed publications with *obese* or *obesity* in the title.

globe in every population at every age, and that they cause or are contributing factors to early mortality, a wide range of diseases, psychological distress and diminished quality of life, and substantial direct and indirect costs both to individuals and society. Science is never perfect or final; a central challenge to public health is deciding when enough information exists to take action (Weed, 1996).

The most recent (2005) information from the WHO states that approximately 1.6 billion adults were overweight, of which 400 million were obese, with projections for 2015 of 2.3 billion and 700 million, respectively. A compelling argument can be made that action should be and is being taken to stem the epidemic of obesity, but the form of those efforts is still under debate (Schwartz & Brownell, 2005). As the epidemic of diet- and activity-related disorders spreads across the globe, it is becoming clear that an individual approach to diet change will not by itself stem the tide of overweight and obesity. Criticism of individual-level dietary change interventions (Mann et al., 2007) is hardly novel (Wooley & Garner, 1991; Goodrick & Foreyt, 1991). Only recently, however, has it become more common to point out that individual-level dietary change faces an uphill struggle when attempted in *obesogenic environments* and societies (Caballero, 2007). Clearly, approaches that take into account the traditional triad of person, behavior, and environment provide the greatest promise of success (Glanz, 2002; Caballero, 2007). Applied scientists (such as epidemiologists) have the obligation to provide the best available evidence to communities, organizations, corporations, clinicians, and policy makers, on which they in turn can recommend and initiate action, and evaluate the relative success of their efforts.

Acknowledgments

The writing of this chapter was supported in part by a grant from the National Institute of Diabetes and Digestive and Kidney Diseases (R18 DK062942).

References Cited

Adams, T. D., Gress, R. E., Smith, S. C., Halverson, R. C., Simper, S. C., Rosamond, et al. (2007). Long-term mortality after gastric bypass surgery. *New England Journal of Medicine, 357*, 753–761.

Angulo, P. (2007). Obesity and nonalcoholic fatty liver disease. *Nutrition Reviews, 65*, S57–S63.

Arenz, S., Rückerl, R., Koletzko, B., & von Kries, R. (2004). Breast-feeding and childhood obesity—a systematic review. *International Journal of Obesity and Related Metabolic Disorders, 28*, 1247–1256.

Asia Pacific Cohort Studies Collaboration (2007). The burden of overweight and obesity in the Asia-Pacific region. *Obesity Reviews, 8*, 191–196.

Baillie-Hamilton, P. F. (2002). Chemical toxins: A hypothesis to explain the global obesity epidemic. *Journal of Alternative and Complementary Medicine, 8*, 185–192.

Ball, K., & Crawford, D. (2005). The role of socio-cultural factors in the obesity epidemic. In D. Crawford & R. W. Jeffery (Eds.), *Obesity prevention and public health*. Oxford: Oxford University Press.

Baskin, M. L., Ard, J., Franklin, F., & Allison, D. B. (2005). Prevalence of obesity in the United States *Obesity Reviews, 6*, 5–7.

Batty, G. D., Kivimaki, M., Smith, G. D., Marmot, M. G., & Shipley, M. J. (2007). Obesity and overweight in relation to mortality in men with and without type 2 diabetes/impaired glucose tolerance: the original Whitehall study. *Diabetes Care, 30*, 2388–2391.

Begley, C. E. (1991). Government should strengthen regulation in the weight loss industry. *Journal of the American Dietetic Association, 91*, 1255–1257.

Bélanger-Ducharme, F., & Tremblay, A. (2005). Prevalence of obesity in Canada. *Obesity Reviews, 6*, 183–186.

Bell, C. G., Walley, A. J., & Froguel, P. (2005). The genetics of human obesity. *Nature Reviews Genetics, 6*, 221–234.

Benyshek, D. C. (2007). The developmental origins of obesity and related health disorders—prenatal and perinatal factors. *Collegium Antropologicum, 31*, 11–17.

Bergström, A., Hsieh, C. C., Lindblad, P., Lu, C. M., Cook, N. R., & Wolk, A. (2001). Obesity and renal cell cancer—a quantitative review. *British Journal of Cancer, 85*, 984–990.

Beuther, D. A., & Sutherland, E. R. (2007). Overweight, obesity, and incident asthma: a meta-analysis of prospective epidemiologic studies. *American Journal of Respiratory and Critical Care Medicine, 175*, 661–666.

Biritwum, R., Gyapong, J., & Mensah, G. (2005). The epidemiology of obesity in Ghana. *Ghana Medical Journal, 39*, 82–85.

Booth, K. M., Pinkston, M. M., & Poston, W. S. (2005). Obesity and the built environment. *Journal of the American Dietetic Association, 105*(5, Suppl. 1), S110–S117.

Bordeaux, B. C., Bolen, S., & Brotman, D. J. (2006). Beyond cardiovascular risk: the impact of obesity on cancer death. *Cleveland Clinic Journal of Medicine, 73*, 945–950.

Borders, T. F., Rohrer, J. E., & Cardarelli, K. M. (2006). Gender-specific disparities in obesity. *Journal of Community Health, 31*, 57–68.

Borenstein, S. (2007, August 20). Study Finds Virus Contributes to Obesity. *ABC News*. Retrieved October 19, 2007 from http://abcnews.go.com/Health/wirestory?id=3503014

Bose, K., Bisai, S., Mukhopadhyay, A., & Bhadra, M. (2007). Overweight and obesity among affluent Bengalee schoolgirls of Lake Town, Kolkata, India. *Maternal & Child Nutrition, 3*, 141–145.

Bray, G. A. (1990). Obesity: Historical development of scientific and cultural ideas. *International journal of obesity, 14*, 909–926.

Bray, G. A., Nielsen, S. J., & Popkin, B. M. (2004). Consumption of high-fructose corn syrup in beverages may play a role in the epidemic of obesity. *American Journal of Clinical Nutrition, 79*, 537–543.

Byrne, T. K. (2001). Complications of surgery for obesity. *Surgical Clinics of North America, 81*, 1181–1193.

Caballero, B. (2007). The global epidemic of obesity: An overview. *Epidemiologic Reviews, 29*, 1–5.

Calle, E. E., & Thun, M. J. (2004). Obesity and cancer. *Oncogene, 23*, 6365–6378.

Campbell, T., & Campbell, A. (2007). Emerging disease burdens and the poor in cities of the developing world. *Journal of Urban Health, 84*(Suppl. 3), i54–i64.

Carpenter, K. M., Hasin, D. S., Allison, D. B., & Faith, M. S. (2000). Relationships between obesity and DSM-IV major depressive disorder, suicide ideation, and suicide attempts: results from a general population study. *American Journal of Public Health, 90*, 251–257.

Ceschi, M., Gutzwiller, F., Moch, H., Eichholzer, M., & Probst-Hensch, N. M. (2007). Epidemiology and pathophysiology of obesity as cause of cancer. *Swiss Medical Weekly, 137*, 50–56.

Charbonneau-Roberts, G., Saudny-Unterberger, H., Kuhnlein, H. V., & Egeland, G. M. (2005). Body mass index may overestimate the prevalence of overweight and obesity among the Inuit. *International Journal of Circumpolar Health, 64*, 163–169.

Chatterjee, P. (2002). India sees parallel rise in malnutrition and obesity. *Lancet, 360*, 1948.

Chhatwal, J., Verma, M., & Riar, S. K. (2004). Obesity among pre-adolescent and adolescents of a developing country (India). *Asia Pacific Journal of Clinical Nutrition, 13*, 231–235.

Chinn, S. (2006). Definitions of childhood obesity: current practice. *European Journal of Clinical Nutrition, 60*, 1189–94.

Christakis, N. A. (2004). Social networks and collateral health effects. *BMJ, 329*, 184–185.

Christakis, N. A., & Fowler, J. H. (2007). The spread of obesity in a large social network over 32 years. *New England Journal of Medicine, 357*, 370–379.

Chumlea, W. M., & Guo, S. S. (2000). Assessment and prevalence of obesity: application of new methods to a major problem. *Endocrine, 13*, 135–142.

Chung, S. J., Han, Y. S., Lee, S. I., & Kang, S. H. (2005). Urban and rural differences in the prevalence of gender and age specific obesity and related health behaviors in Korea. *Journal of Korean Medical Science, 20*, 713–720.

Colditz, G. A. (1992). Economic costs of obesity. *American Journal of Clinical Nutrition, 55*(Suppl. 2), 503S–507S.

Cope, M. B., & Allison, D. B. (2006). Obesity: person and population. *Obesity, 14*(Suppl. 4), 156S–159S.

Cossrow, N., & Falkner, B. (2004). Race/ethnic issues in obesity and obesity-related comorbidities. *Journal of Clinical Endocrinology and Metabolism, 89*, 2590–2594.

Dai, Z., Xu, Y. C., & Niu, L. (2007). Obesity and colorectal cancer risk: A meta-analysis of cohort studies. *World Journal of Gastroenterology, 13*, 4199–4206.

Davis, J., Busch, J., Hammatt, Z., Novotny, R., Harrigan, R., Grandinetti, A., et al. (2004). The relationship between ethnicity and obesity in Asian and Pacific Islander populations: a literature review. *Ethnicity & Disease, 14*, 111–118.

Dehghan, M., Akhtar-Danesh, N., & Merchant, A. T. (2005). Childhood obesity, prevalence and prevention. *Nutrition Journal, 4*, 24.

Deurenberg, P., & Yap, M. (1999). The assessment of obesity: methods for measuring body fat and global prevalence of obesity. *Baillière's Best Practice & Research: Clinical Endocrinology & Metabolism, 13*, 1–11.

Dhurandhar, N. V. (2001). Infectobesity: obesity of infectious origin. *Journal of Nutrition, 131*, 2794S–2797S.

Diaz, V. A., Mainous, A. G., Baker, R., Carnemolla, M., & Majeed, A. (2007). How does ethnicity affect the association between obesity and diabetes? *Diabetic Medicine, 11*, 1199–1204.

Dixon, J. B., Dixon, M. E., & O'Brien, P. E. (2003). Depression in association with severe obesity: changes with weight loss. *Archives of Internal Medicine, 163*, 2058–2065.

Drewnowski, A. (2007). The real contribution of added sugars and fats to obesity. *Epidemiologic Reviews, 29*, 160–171.

Drewnowski, A., & Specter, S. E. (2004). Poverty and obesity: the role of energy density and energy costs. *American Journal of Clinical Nutrition, 79*, 6–16.

Dudeja, V., Misra, A., Pandey, R. M., Devina, G., Kumar, G., & Vikram, N. K. (2001). BMI does not accurately predict over-weight in Asian Indians in northern India. *British Journal of Nutrition, 86,* 105–112.

Due, P., Heitmann, B. L., & Sørensen, T. I. (2007). Prevalence of obesity in Denmark. *Obesity Reviews, 8,* 187–189.

Eaton, C. B. (2004). Obesity as a risk factor for osteoarthritis: mechanical versus metabolic. *Medicine and Health, Rhode Island, 87,* 201–204.

Eknoyan, G. (2006). A history of obesity, or how what was good became ugly and then bad. *Advances in Chronic Kidney Disease, 13,* 421–427.

Elia, M. (2001). Obesity in the elderly. *Obesity Research, 9*(Suppl. 4), 244S–248S.

Ells, L. J., Lang, R., Shield, J. P., Wilkinson, J. R., Lidstone, J. S., Coulton, S., et al. (2006). Obesity and disability—a short review. *Obesity Reviews, 7,* 341–345.

Farooqi, S., & O'Rahilly, S. (2006). Genetics of obesity in humans. *Endocrine Reviews, 27,* 710–718.

Fava, M. (2000). Weight gain and antidepressants. *Journal of Clinical Psychiatry, 61*(Suppl. 11), 37–41.

Filozof, C., Gonzalez, C., Sereday, M., Mazza, C., & Braguinsky, J. (2001). Obesity prevalence and trends in Latin-American countries. *Obesity Reviews, 2,* 99–106.

Finkelstein, E. A., Fiebelkorn, I. C., & Wang, G. (2004). State-level estimates of annual medical expenditures attributable to obesity. *Obesity Research, 12,* 18–24.

Frank, L. D., Saelens, B. E., Powell, K. E., & Chapman, J. E. (2007). Stepping towards causation: Do built environments or neighborhood and travel preferences explain physical activity, driving, and obesity. *Social Science and Medicine, 65,* 1898–1914.

Frederick, I. O., Rudra, C. B., Miller, R. S., Foster, J. C., & Williams, M. A. (2006). Adult weight change, weight cycling, and prepregnancy obesity in relation to risk of preeclampsia. *Epidemiology, 17,* 428–434.

Frezza, E. E., Wachtel, M. S., & Chiriva-Internati, M. (2006). Influence of obesity on the risk of developing colon cancer. *Gut, 55,* 285–291.

Frost, F., Taylor, V., & Fries, E. (1992). Racial misclassification of Native Americans in a surveillance, epidemiology, and end results cancer registry. *Journal of the National Cancer Institute, 84,* 957–962.

Fry, J., & Finley, W. (2005). The prevalence and costs of obesity in the EU. *Proceedings of the Nutrition Society, 64,* 359–362.

Galal, O. M. (2002). The nutrition transition in Egypt: obesity, undernutrition and the food consumption context. *Public Health Nutrition, 5,* 141–148.

Galtier-Dereure, F., Boegner, C., & Bringer, J. (2000). Obesity and pregnancy: complications and cost. *American Journal of Clinical Nutrition, 71*(Suppl. 5), 1242S–1248S.

Gaszynski, T. (2004). Anesthetic complications of gross obesity. *Current Opinion in Anaesthesiology, 17,* 271–276.

Glanz, K. (2002). Perspectives on group, organization, and community interventions. In K. Glanz, B. K. Rimer, & F. M. Lewis (Eds.), *Health behavior and health education,* (3rd ed.). San Francisco: Wiley.

Goldner, M. G. (1957). Symposium on obesity: Introduction, with a few historical remarks on obesity. *Metabolism, 6,* 404–406.

Goodrick, G. K., & Foreyt, J. P. (1991). Why treatments for obesity don't last. *Journal of the American Dietetic Association, 91,* 1243–1247.

Gordon-Larsen, P., Nelson, M. C., Page, P., & Popkin, B. M. (2006). Inequality in the built environment underlies key health disparities in physical activity and obesity. *Pediatrics, 117,* 417–424.

Gray, G. & Cohen, J.; Harvard Center for Risk Analysis. (2004, August). Weight of the evidence: Evaluation of low-dose reproductive and developmental effects of bisphenol A. *Risk in Perspective, 12* (3).

Griffiths, P. L., & Bentley, M. E. (2001). The nutrition transition is underway in India. *Journal of Nutrition, 131,* 2692–2700.

Hajian-Tilaki, K. O., & Heidari, B. (2007). Prevalence of obesity, central obesity and the associated factors in urban population aged 20–70 years, in the north of Iran: a population-based study and regression approach. *Obesity Reviews, 8,* 3–10.

Hampel, H., Abraham, N. S., & El-Serag, H. B. (2005). Meta-analysis: obesity and the risk for gastroesophageal reflux disease and its complications. *Annals of Internal Medicine, 143,* 199–211.

Handy, S. L., Boarnet, M. G., Ewing, R., & Killingsworth, R. E. (2002). How the built environment affects physical activity:

views from urban planning. *American Journal of Preventive Medicine, 23*(Suppl. 2), 64–73.

Harvie, M., Hooper, L., & Howell, A. H. (2003). Central obesity and breast cancer risk: a systematic review. *Obesity Reviews, 4*, 157–173.

He, Y., Jiang, B., Wang, J., Feng, K., Chang, Q., Zhu, S., et al. (2007). BMI versus the metabolic syndrome in relation to cardiovascular risk in elderly Chinese individuals. *Diabetes Care, 30*, 2128–2134.

Herva, A., Laitinen, J., Miettunen, J., Veijola, J., Karvonen, J. T., Läksy, K., et al. (2006). Obesity and depression: results from the longitudinal Northern Finland 1966 Birth Cohort Study. *International Journal of Obesity, 30*, 520–527.

Horowitz, C. R., Colson, K. A., Hebert, P. L., & Lancaster, K. (2004). Barriers to buying healthy foods for people with diabetes: evidence of environmental disparities. *American Journal of Public Health, 94*, 1549–1554.

Howe, S. R., & Borodinsky, L. (1998). Potential exposure to bisphenol A from food-contact use of polycarbonate resins. *Food Additives and Contaminants, 15*, 370–375.

Huffman, S. K., & Rizov, M. (2007). Determinants of obesity in transition economies: The case of Russia. *Economics and Human Biology, 5*, 379–391.

Hui, L., & Bell, A. C. (2003). Overweight and obesity in children from Shenzhen, Peoples Republic of China. *Health Place, 9*, 371–376.

Inagami, S., Cohen, D. A., Finch, B. K., & Asch, S. M. (2006). You are where you shop: grocery store locations, weight, and neighborhoods. *American Journal of Preventive Medicine, 31*, 10–17.

Ismail, M. N., Chee, S. S., Nawawi, H., Yusoff, K., Lim, T. O., & James, W. P. (2002). Obesity in Malaysia. *Obesity Reviews, 3*, 203–208.

Iwata, F., Hara, M., Okada, T., Harada, K., & Li, S. (2003). Body fat ratios in urban Chinese children. *Pediatrics International, 45*, 190–192.

Jackson, J. E., Doescher, M. P., Jerant, A. F., & Hart, L. G. (2005). A national study of obesity prevalence and trends by type of rural county. *Journal of Rural Health, 21*, 140–148.

Jackson, M., Walker, S., Cruickshank, J. K., Sharma, S., Cade, J., Mbanya, J. C., et al.

(2007). Diet and overweight and obesity in populations of African origin: Cameroon, Jamaica and the UK. *Public Health Nutrition, 10*, 122–130.

James, W. P. T., Chunming, C., & Inoue, S. (2002). Appropriate Asian body mass indices? *Obesity Reviews, 3*, 139.

Janssen, I., Katzmarzyk P. T., Boyce, W. F., Vereecken, C., Mulvihill, C., Roberts, C., et al.; Health Behaviour in School-Aged Children Obesity Working Group. (2005). Comparison of overweight and obesity prevalence in school-aged youth from 34 countries and their relationships with physical activity and dietary patterns. *Obesity Reviews, 6*, 123–132.

Jeffery, R. W., & Linde, J. A. (2005). Evolving environmental factors in the obesity epidemic. In D. Crawford & R. W. Jeffery (Eds.), *Obesity prevention and public health.* Oxford: Oxford University Press.

Kahn, H. S., & Williamson, D. F. (1994). Abdominal obesity and mortality risk among men in nineteenth-century North America. *International Journal of Obesity and Related Metabolic Disorders, 18*, 686–691.

Kaluski, D. N., & Berry, E. M. (2005). Prevalence of obesity in Israel. *Obesity Reviews, 6*, 115–116.

Kapantais, E., Tzotzas, T., Ioannidis, I., Mortoglou, A., Bakatselos, S., Kaklamanou, M., et al. (2006). First national epidemiological survey on the prevalence of obesity and abdominal fat distribution in Greek adults. *Annals of Nutrition and Metabolism, 50*, 330–338.

Kaplan, J. B., & Bennett, T. (2003). Use of Race and Ethnicity in Biomedical Publication. *Journal of the American Medical Association, 289*, 2709–2716.

Karnehed, N., Rasmussen, F., & Kark, M. (2007). Obesity in young adulthood and later disability pension: a population-based cohort study of 366,929 Swedish men. *Scandinavian journal of public health, 35*, 48–54.

Katzmarzyk, P. T. (2002a). The Canadian obesity epidemic: an historical perspective. *Obesity Research, 10*, 666–674.

Katzmarzyk, P. T. (2002b). The Canadian obesity epidemic, 1985–1998. *Canadian Medical Association Journal, 166*, 1039–1040.

Katzmarzyk, P. T., Pérusse, L., Rao, D. C., & Bouchard, C. (2000). Familial risk of overweight and obesity in the Canadian population using the WHO/NIH criteria. *Obesity Research, 8,* 194–197.

Kelishadi, R. (2007). Childhood overweight, obesity, and the metabolic syndrome in developing countries. *Epidemiologic Reviews, 29,* 62–76.

Kieffer, E. C., Carman, W. J., Gillespie, B. W., Nolan, G. H., Worley, S. E., & Guzman, J. R. (2001). Obesity and gestational diabetes among African-American women and Latinas in Detroit: implications for disparities in women's health. *Journal of the American Medical Women's Association, 56,* 181–187, 196.

Kim, D. M., Ahn, C. W., & Nam, S. Y. (2005). Prevalence of obesity in Korea. *Obesity Reviews, 6,* 117–121.

Klein, S., Allison, D. B., Heymsfield, S. B., Kelley, D. E., Leibel, R. L., Nonas, C., et al. (2007). Waist Circumference and Cardiometabolic Risk: a Consensus Statement from Shaping America's Health: Association for Weight Management and Obesity Prevention; NAASO, the Obesity Society; the American Society for Nutrition; and the American Diabetes Association. *Obesity, 15,* 1061–1067.

Klein, S., Burke, L. E., Bray, G. A., Blair, S., Allison, D. B., Pi-Sunyer, X., et al.; American Heart Association Council on Nutrition, Physical Activity, and Metabolism. (2004). Clinical implications of obesity with specific focus on cardiovascular disease: a statement for professionals from the American Heart Association Council on Nutrition, Physical Activity, and Metabolism: endorsed by the American College of Cardiology Foundation. *Circulation, 110,* 2952–2967.

Kosti, R. I., & Panagiotakos, D. B. (2006). The epidemic of obesity in children and adolescents in the world. *Central European Journal of Public Health, 14,* 151–159.

Kramer, H., & Luke, A. (2007). Obesity and kidney disease: a big dilemma. *Current Opinion in Nephrology and Hypertension, 16,* 237–241.

Krishnan, S., Rosenberg, L., Djoussé, L., Cupples, L. A., & Palmer, J. R. (2007). Overall and central obesity and risk of type 2 diabetes in U.S. black women. *Obesity, 15,* 1860–1866.

Kuehn, B. M. (2007). Expert Panels Weigh Bisphenol-A Risks. *Journal of the American Medical Association, 298,* 1499–1503.

Kumanyika, S. K. (2007). The obesity epidemic: Looking in the mirror. *American Journal of Epidemiology, 166,* 243–245.

Kurzer, E., Leveillee, R., & Bird, V. (2006). Obesity as a risk factor for complications during laparoscopic surgery for renal cancer: multivariate analysis. *Journal of Endourology, 20,* 794–799.

Lake, A., & Townshend, T. (2006). Obesogenic environments: Exploring the built and food environments. *Journal of the Royal Society of Health, 126,* 262–267.

Laraia, B. A., Siega-Riz, A. M., Kaufman, J. S., & Jones, S. J. (2004). Proximity of supermarkets is positively associated with diet quality index for pregnancy. *Preventive Medicine, 39,* 869–875.

Larsson, S. C., & Wolk, A. (2007). Overweight, obesity and risk of liver cancer: a meta-analysis of cohort studies. *British Journal of Cancer, 97,* 1005–1008.

Livingstone, M. B. (2001). Childhood obesity in Europe: a growing concern. *Public Health Nutrition, 4,* 109–116.

Lopez, R. (2004). Urban sprawl and risk for being overweight or obese. *American Journal of Public Health, 94,* 1574–1579.

Lopez, R. P., & Hynes, H. P. (2006). Obesity, physical activity, and the urban environment: Public health research needs. *Environmental Health, 5,* 25.

Luo, J., & Hu, F. B. (2002). Time trends of obesity in pre-school children in China from 1989 to 1997. *International Journal of Obesity and Related Metabolic Disorders, 26,* 553–558.

Luo, W., Morrison, H., de Groh, M., Waters, C., DesMeules, M., Jones-McLean, E., et al. (2007). The burden of adult obesity in Canada. *Chronic Diseases in Canada, 27,* 135–144.

Lutfiyya, M. N., Lipsky, M. S., Wisdom-Behounek, J., & Inpanbutr-Martinkus, M. (2007). Is rural residency a risk factor for overweight and obesity for U.S. Children? *Obesity, 15,* 2348–2356.

Lyon, H. N., & Hirschhorn, J. N. (2005). Genetics of common forms of obesity: A brief overview. *American Journal of Clinical Nutrition, 82*(Suppl.), 215S–217S.

Mann, T., Tomiyama, A. J., Westling, E., Lew, A. M., Samuels, B., & Chatman, J. (2007). Medicare's search for effective obesity treatments: diets are not the answer. *American Psychologist, 62,* 220–233.

Marini, M. A., Succurro, E., Frontoni, S., Hribal, M. L., Andreozzi, F., Lauro, R., et al. (2007). Metabolically healthy but obese women have an intermediate cardiovascular risk profile between healthy nonobese women and obese insulin-resistant women. *Diabetes Care, 30*, 2145–2147.

Martínez, J., Johnson, C. D., Sánchez-Payá, J., de Madaria, E., Robles-Díaz, G., & Pérez-Mateo, M. (2006). Obesity is a definitive risk factor of severity and mortality in acute pancreatitis: an updated meta-analysis. *Pancreatology, 6*, 206–209.

Maskarinec, G., Takata, Y., Pagano, I., Carlin, L., Goodman, M. T., Le Marchand, L., et al. (2006). Trends and dietary determinants of overweight and obesity in a multiethnic population. *Obesity, 14*, 717–726.

Matsushita, Y., Yoshiike, N., Kaneda, F., Yoshita, K., & Takimoto, H. (2004). Trends in childhood obesity in Japan over the last 25 years from the national nutrition survey. *Obesity Research, 12*, 205–214.

McCann, B. S., & Bovbjerg, V. E. (in press). Promoting dietary change. In S. A. Shumaker, J. K. Ockene, & K. Riekert (Eds.), *The handbook of health behavior change* (3rd ed.). New York: Springer.

McLaren, L. (2007). Socioeconomic status and obesity. *Epidemiologic Reviews, 29*, 29–48.

McTiernan, A. (2005). Obesity and cancer: the risks, science, and potential management strategies. *Oncology, 19*, 871–881.

McTigue, K. M., Hess, R., & Ziouras, J. (2006). Obesity in older adults: a systematic review of the evidence for diagnosis and treatment. *Obesity, 14*, 1485–1497.

Mendez, M. A., Monteiro, C. A., & Popkin, B. M. (2005). Overweight exceeds underweight among women in most developing countries. *American Journal of Clinical Nutrition, 81*, 714–721.

Menotti, A., Descovich, G. C., Lanti, M., Spagnolo, A., Dormi, A., & Seccareccia, F. (1993). Indexes of obesity and all-causes mortality in Italian epidemiological data. *Preventive Medicine, 22*, 293–303.

Mighty, H. E., & Fahey, A. J. (2007). Obesity and pregnancy complications. *Current Diabetes Reports, 7*, 289–294.

Milewicz, A., Jedrzejuk, D., Lwow, F., Bialynicka, A. S., Lopatynski, J., Mardarowicz, G., et al. (2005). Prevalence of obesity in Poland. *Obesity Reviews, 6*, 113–114.

Miller, M. A., & Cappuccio, F. P. (2007). Inflammation, sleep, obesity and cardio-vascular disease. *Current Vascular Pharmacology, 5*, 93–102.

Mokdad, A. H., Bowman, B. A., Ford, E. S., Vinicor, F., Marks, J. S., & Koplan, J. P. (2001). The continuing epidemics of obesity and diabetes in the United States. *Journal of the American Medical Association, 286*, 1195–1200.

Mokhtar, N., Elati, J., Chabir, R., Bour, A., Elkari, K., Schlossman, N. P., et al. (2001). Diet culture and obesity in northern Africa. *Journal of Nutrition, 131*, 887S–892S.

Monteiro, C. A., Moura, E. C., Conde, W. L., & Popkin, B. M. (2004). Socioeconomic status and obesity in adult populations of developing countries: a review. *Bulletin of the World Health Organization, 82*, 940–946.

Muennig, P., Lubetkin, E., Jia, H., & Franks, P. (2006). Gender and the burden of disease attributable to obesity. *American Journal of Public Health, 96*, 1662–1668.

Mutch, D. M., & Clement, K. (2006). Unraveling the genetics of human obesity. *PLoS Genetics, 2*, e188.

Nakamura, K., Okamura, T., Hayakawa, T., Hozawa, A., Kadowaki, T., Murakami, Y., et al.; for the NIPPON DATA80, 90 Research Group. (2007). The proportion of individuals with obesity-induced hypertension among total hypertensives in a general Japanese population: NIPPON DATA80, 90. *European Journal of Epidemiology, 30*, 663–668.

Nelson, M. C., Gordon-Larsen, P., North, K. E., & Adair, L. S. (2006). Body mass index gain, fast food, and physical activity: effects of shared environments over time. *Obesity, 14*, 701–709.

Neovius, M., Janson, A., & Rössner, S. (2006). Prevalence of obesity in Sweden. *Obesity Reviews, 7*, 1–3.

Nguyen, M. D., Beresford, S. A., & Drewnowski, A. (2007). Trends in overweight by socio-economic status in Vietnam: 1992 to 2002. *Public Health Nutrition, 10*, 115–121.

Nishida, C., & Mucavele, P. (2004–2005). Monitoring the rapidly emerging public health problem of overweight and obesity: the WHO Global Database on Body Mass Index. *SCN News, 29*, 5–12.

Njelekela, M., Sato, T., Nara, Y., Miki, T., Kuga, S., Noguchi, T., et al. (2003). Nutritional variation and cardiovascular risk factors in Tanzania—rural-urban difference. *South African Medical Journal, 93,* 295–299.

Olsen, C. M., Green, A. C., Whiteman, D. C., Sadeghi, S., Kolahdooz, F., & Webb, P. M. (2007). Obesity and the risk of epithelial ovarian cancer: a systematic review and meta-analysis. *European Journal of Cancer, 43,* 690–709.

Onyike, C. U., Crum, R. M., Lee, H. B., Lyketsos, C. G., & Eaton, W. W. (2003). Is obesity associated with major depression? Results from the Third National Health and Nutrition Examination Survey. *American Journal of Epidemiology, 158,* 1139–1147.

Orio, F., Jr., Palomba, S., Cascella, T., Savastano, S., Lombardi, G., & Colao, A. (2007). Cardiovascular complications of obesity in adolescents. *Journal of Endocrinological Investigation, 30,* 70–80.

Owen, C. G., Martin, R. M., Whincup, P. H., Smith, G. D., & Cook, D. G. (2005). Effect of infant feeding on the risk of obesity across the life course: a quantitative review of published evidence. *Pediatrics, 115,* 1367–1377.

Paeratakul, S., Lovejoy, J. C., Ryan, D. H., & Bray, G. A. (2002). The relation of gender, race and socioeconomic status to obesity and obesity comorbidities in a sample of US adults. *International Journal of Obesity and Related Metabolic Disorders, 26,* 1205–1210.

Papas, M. A., Alberg, A. J., Ewing, R., Helzlsouer, K. J., Gary, T. L., & Klassen, A. C. (2007). The built environment and obesity. *Epidemiologic Reviews, 29,* 129–143.

Paracchini, V., Pedotti, P., & Taioli, E. (2005). Genetics of leptin and obesity: a HuGE review. *American Journal of Epidemiology, 162,* 101–114.

Pearson, W. S. (2007). Ten-year comparison of estimates of overweight and obesity, diagnosed diabetes and use of office-based physician services for treatment of diabetes in the United States. *Preventive Medicine, 45,* 353–357.

Peytremann-Bridevaux, I., Faeh, D., & Santos-Eggimann, B. (2007). Prevalence of overweight and obesity in rural and urban settings of 10 European countries. *Preventive Medicine, 44,* 442–446.

Pischon, N., Heng, N., Bernimoulin, J. P., Kleber, B. M., Willich, S. N., & Pischon, T. (2007). Obesity, inflammation, and peri-odontal disease. *Journal of Dental Research, 86,* 400–409.

Pi-Sunyer, F. X. (1999). Comorbidities of overweight and obesity: Current evidence and research issues. *Medicine and Science in Sports and Exercise, 31*(Suppl. 11), S602–S608.

Popkin, B. M. (2005a). The implications of the nutrition transition for obesity in the developing world. In D. Crawford & R. W. Jeffery (Eds.), *Obesity prevention and public health.* Oxford: Oxford University Press.

Popkin, B. M. (2005b). Using research on the obesity pandemic as a guide to a unified vision of nutrition. *Public Health Nutrition, 8,* 724–729.

Popkin, B. M., Duffey, K., & Gordon-Larsen, P. (2005). Environmental influences on food choice, physical activity and energy balance. *Physiology and Behavior, 86,* 603–613.

Popkin, B. M., & Gordon-Larsen, P. (2004). The nutrition transition: worldwide obesity dynamics and their determinants. *International Journal of Obesity and Related Metabolic Disorders, 28*(Suppl. 3), S2–S9.

Popkin, B. M., Kim, S., Rusev, E. R., Du, S., & Zizza, C. (2006). Measuring the full economic costs of diet, physical activity and obesity-related chronic diseases. *Obesity Reviews, 7,* 271–293.

Potera, C. (2004). The opposite of obesity: undernutrition overwhelms the world's children. *Environmental Health Perspectives, 112,* A802.

Powell, A., Teichtahl, A. J., Wluka, A. E., & Cicuttini, F. M. (2005). Obesity: a preventable risk factor for large joint osteoarthritis which may act through biomechanical factors. *British Journal of Sports Medicine, 39,* 4–5.

Prentice, A., & Webb, F. (2006). Obesity amidst poverty. *International Journal of Epidemiology, 35,* 24–30.

Presti, J. C. (2005). Obesity and prostate cancer. *Current Opinion in Urology, 15,* 13–16.

Puoane, T., Steyn, K., Bradshaw, D., Laubscher, R., Fourie, J., Lambert, V., et al. (2002). Obesity in South Africa: the South African demographic and health survey. *Obesity Research, 10,* 1038–1048.

Ramsey, P. W., & Glenn, L. L. (2002). Obesity and health status in rural, urban, and suburban southern women. *Southern Medical Journal, 95,* 666–671.

Rashidi, A., Mohammadpour-Ahranjani, B., Vafa, M. R., & Karandish, M. (2005).

Prevalence of obesity in Iran. *Obesity Reviews, 6*, 191–192.

Reeder, B. A., Chen, Y., Macdonald, S. M., Angel, A., & Sweet, L. (1997). Regional and rural-urban differences in obesity in Canada. Canadian Heart Health Surveys Research Group. *Canadian Medical Association Journal, 157*(Suppl. 1), S10–S16.

Reilly, J. J., Methven, E., McDowell, Z. C., Hacking, B., Alexander, D., Stewart, L., et al. (2003). Health consequences of obesity. *Archives of Disease in Childhood, 88*, 748–752.

Rennie, K. L., & Jebb, S. A. (2005). Prevalence of obesity in Great Britain. *Obesity Reviews, 6*, 11–12.

Ries, G. (1984). Diet industry flourishes without regulation. *Iowa Medicine, 74*, 77–78, 80.

Ritchie, S. A., & Connell, J. M. (2007). The link between abdominal obesity, metabolic syndrome and cardiovascular disease. *Nutrition, Metabolism, and Cardiovascular Diseases, 17*, 319–326.

Rose, D., & Richards, R. (2004). Food store access and household fruit and vegetable use among participants in the US Food Stamp Program. *Public Health Nutrition, 7*, 1081–1088.

Rueda-Clausen, C. F., Silva, F. A., & López-Jaramillo, P. (2007). Epidemic of overweight and obesity in Latin America and the Caribbean. *International Journal of Cardiology*. Retrieved September 20, 2007 from http://www.sciencedirect.com/science?_ob=ArticleURL&_udi=B6T16-4NGB9WF-2&_user=709071&_rdoc=1&_fmt=&_orig=search&_sort=d&view=c&_acct=C000039638&_version=1&_urlVersion=0&_userid=709071&md5=773b3612769f19087e4ee34adb940a9d

Rundle, A., Roux, A. V., Free, L. M., Miller, D., Neckerman, K. M., & Weiss C. C. (2007). The urban built environment and obesity in New York City: a multilevel analysis. *American Journal of Health Promotion, 21*(Suppl. 4), 326–334.

Sackett, D. L., Anderson, G. D., Milner, R., Feinleib, M., & Kannel, W. B. (1975). Concordance for coronary risk factors among spouses. *Circulation, 52*, 589–595.

Sallis, J. F., & Glanz, K. (2006). The role of built environments in physical activity, eating, and obesity in childhood. *Future of Children, 16*, 89–108.

Sankar, P., Cho, M. K., & Mountain, J. (2007). Race and ethnicity in genetic research. *American Journal of Medical Genetics Part A, 143*, 961–970.

Schmier, J. K., Jones, M. L., & Halpern, M. T. (2006). Cost of obesity in the workplace. *Scandinavian Journal of Work, Environment & Health, 32*, 5–11.

Schwartz, M. B., & Brownell, K. D. (2005). The need for courageous action to prevent obesity. In D. Crawford & R. W. Jeffery (Eds.), *Obesity prevention and public health*. Oxford: Oxford University Press.

Seidell, J. C. (1998). Societal and personal costs of obesity. *Experimental and Clinical Endocrinology & Diabetes, 106*(Suppl. 2), 7–9.

Seidell, J. C. (2005). The epidemiology of obesity: A global perspective. In D. Crawford & R. W. Jeffery (Eds.), *Obesity prevention and public health*. Oxford: Oxford University Press.

Shinogle, J. A., Owings, M. F., & Kozak, L. J. (2005). Gastric bypass as treatment for obesity: trends, characteristics, and complications. *Obesity Research, 13*, 2202–2209.

Sidhu, S., Kaur, N., & Kaur, R. (2006). Overweight and obesity in affluent school children of Punjab. *Annals of Human Biology, 33*, 255–259.

Siega-Riz, A. M., & Laraia, B. (2006). The implications of maternal overweight and obesity on the course of pregnancy and birth outcomes. *Maternal and Child Health Journal, 10*(Suppl. 5), S153–S156.

Sjöberg, R. L., Nilsson, K. W., & Leppert, J. (2005). Obesity, shame, and depression in school-aged children: a population-based study. *Pediatrics, 116*, e389–e392.

Sjöström, L., Narbro, K., Sjöström, C. D., Karason, K., Larsson, B., Wedel, H., et al. (2007). Effects of bariatric surgery on mortality in Swedish obese subjects. *New England Journal of Medicine, 357*, 741–752.

Sobal, J., & Stunkard, A. J. (1989). Socioeconomic status and obesity: a review of the literature. *Psychological Bulletin, 105*, 260–275.

Spanier, P. A., Marshall, S. J., & Faulkner, G. E. (2006). Tackling the obesity pandemic: a call for sedentary behaviour research. *Canadian Journal of Public Health, 97*, 255–257.

Stone, C. D., Diallo, O., Shyken, J., & Leet, T. (2007). The combined effect of maternal smoking and obesity on the risk of preeclampsia. *Journal of Perinatal Medicine, 35*, 28–31.

Stunkard, A. J., Harris, J. R., Pedersen, N. L., & McClearn, G. E. (1990). The body-mass index of twins who have been reared apart. *New England Journal of Medicine, 322,* 1483–1487.

Stunkard, A. J., Sørensen, T. I., Hanis, C., Teasdale, T. W., Chakraborty, R., Schull, W. J., et al. (1986). An adoption study of human obesity. *New England Journal of Medicine, 314,* 193–198.

Truong, K. D., & Sturm, R. (2005). Weight gain trends across sociodemographic groups in the United States. *American Journal of Public Health, 95,* 1602–1606.

Tsai, A. G., & Wadden, T. A. (2005). Systematic review: an evaluation of major commercial weight loss programs in the United States. *Annals of Internal Medicine, 142,* 56–66.

Tunceli, K., Li, K., & Williams, L. K. (2006). Long-term effects of obesity on employment and work limitations among U.S. Adults, 1986 to 1999. *Obesity, 14,* 1637–1646.

Tzotzas, T., & Krassas, G. E. (2004). Prevalence and trends of obesity in children and adults of South Europe. *Pediatric Endocrinology Reviews, 1*(Suppl. 3), 448–454.

Uauy, R., Albala, C., & Kain, J. (2001). Obesity trends in Latin America: transiting from under- to overweight. *Journal of Nutrition, 131,* 893S–899S.

Ulijaszek, S. (2005). Modernisation, migration and nutritional health of Pacific Island populations. *Environmental Sciences, 12,* 167–176.

Uppot, R. N., Sahani, D. V., Hahn, P. F., Gervais, D., & Mueller, P. R. (2007). Impact of obesity on medical imaging and image-guided intervention. *American Journal of Roentgenology, 188,* 433–440.

Uusitupa, M. (2005). Gene-diet interaction in relation to the prevention of obesity and type 2 diabetes: evidence from the Finnish Diabetes Prevention Study. *Nutrition, Metabolism, and Cardiovascular Diseases, 15,* 225–233.

Varela-Silva, M. I., Frisancho, A. R., Bogin, B., Chatkoff, D., Smith, P. K., Dickinson, F., et al. (2007). Behavioral, environmental, metabolic and intergenerational components of early life undernutrition leading to later obesity in developing nations and in minority groups in the U.S.A. *Collegium Antropologicum, 31,* 39–46.

Vazquez, G., Duval, S., Jacobs, D. R., Jr., & Silventoinen, K. (2007). Comparison of body mass index, waist circumference, and waist/hip ratio in predicting incident diabetes: a meta-analysis. *Epidemiologic Reviews, 29,* 115–128.

Villamor, E., Msamanga, G., Urassa, W., Petraro, P., Spiegelman, D., Hunter, D. J., et al. (2006). Trends in obesity, underweight, and wasting among women attending prenatal clinics in urban Tanzania, 1995–2004. *American Journal of Clinical Nutrition, 83,* 1387–1394.

Visscher, T. L., Viet, A. L., Kroesbergen, I. H., & Seidell, J. C. (2006). Underreporting of BMI in adults and its effect on obesity prevalence estimations in the period 1998 to 2001. *Obesity, 14,* 2054–2063.

Walker, A. R., Adam, F., & Walker, B. F. (2001). World pandemic of obesity: the situation in Southern African populations. *Public Health, 115,* 368–372.

Walley, A. J., Blakemore, A. I., & Froguel, P. (2006). Genetics of obesity and the prediction of risk for health [Special issue]. *Human Molecular Genetics, 15*(2), R124–R130.

Wang, M. C., Kim, S., Gonzalez, A. A., MacLeod, K. E., & Winkleby, M. A. (2007). Socioeconomic and food-related physical characteristics of the neighbourhood environment are associated with body mass index. *Journal of Epidemiology and Community Health, 61,* 491–498.

Wang, Y., & Beydoun, M. A. (2007). The obesity epidemic in the United States—gender, age, socioeconomic, racial/ethnic, and geographic characteristics: a systematic review and meta-regression analysis. *Epidemiologic Reviews, 29,* 6–28.

Wang, Y., Mi, J., Shan, X. Y., Wang, Q. J., & Ge, K. Y. (2007). Is China facing an obesity epidemic and the consequences? The trends in obesity and chronic disease in China. *International journal of obesity, 31,* 177–188.

Watson, R. (2006). European nations draw up strategy to fight obesity. *BMJ, 333,* 1088.

Weed, D. L. (1996). Epistemology and ethics in epidemiology. In S. S. Coughlin & T. L. Beauchamp (Eds.), *Ethics and epidemiology* (pp. 76–94). New York: Oxford University Press.

Wolf, A. M., & Colditz, G. A. (1998). Current estimates of the economic cost of obesity in the United States. *Obesity Research, 6,* 97–106.

Wooley, S. C., & Garner, D. M. (1991). Obesity treatment: the high cost of false hope. *Journal of the American Dietetic Association, 91,* 1248–1251.

Wyatt, S. B., Winters, K. P., & Dubbert, P. M. (2006). Overweight and obesity: prevalence, consequences, and causes of a growing public health problem. *American Journal of the Medical Sciences, 331,* 166–174.

Yang, W., Kelly, T., & He, J. (2007). Genetic epidemiology of obesity. *Epidemiologic Reviews, 29,* 49–61.

Yap, C. H., Mohajeri, M., & Yii, M. (2007). Obesity and early complications after cardiac surgery. *Medical Journal of Australia, 186,* 350–354.

Yosipovitch, G., DeVore, A., & Dawn, A. (2007). Obesity and the skin: skin physiology and skin manifestations of obesity. *Journal of the American Academy of Dermatology, 56,* 901–916.

Yumuk, V. D. (2005). Prevalence of obesity in Turkey. *Obesity Reviews, 6,* 9–10.

Zhang, Q., & Wang, Y. (2004). Trends in the association between obesity and socioeconomic status in U.S. adults: 1971 to 2000. *Obesity Research, 12,* 1622–1632.

3 METABOLIC INFLUENCES ON THE CONTROLS OF MEAL SIZE

Timothy H. Moran

Introduction

Multiple neural, hormonal, and metabolic systems interact to influence what and how much we eat. Both stimulatory and inhibitory mechanisms for feeding exist. The recent increase in the prevalence of obesity points to the primacy of systems that stimulate food intake, protract meals, or both. In the face of caloric abundance and a reduced need for regular physical exertion, mean body weights are elevated in Western societies, and the prevalence of disorders secondary to excess weight gain is increasing at an alarming rate. Recent work in the basic sciences of energy balance has revealed multiple interactions among systems that monitor energy stores and assess the nutrient and hedonic value of what we consume. This chapter focuses on the relationships between two such regulatory systems in the controls of meal size. These systems mediate responses to (1) signals that arise during and following the consumption of nutrients, and (2) signals related to metabolic state, especially the degree of stored or available energy. The interactions between these two systems play a major role in determining how intake in meals is modulated and, in that way, contribute to the maintenance of energy balance. Identifying and understanding the circumstances that disengage these processes, thereby leading to and culminating in obesity, will yield considerable information about the etiology of obesity and may provide novel directions toward its mitigation.

Meals as Ingestive Units

Humans and most rodents and primates spontaneously feed in distinct bouts (meals) separated by periods of noneating and other activities. Meal size is highly variable both within and among individuals in all animals studied (Collier, 1985). In fact, alteration in meal size is the major determinant of overall daily food intake, which is the average meal size multiplied by the number of meals consumed. Manipulating meal costs increases variability in meal number and size to stabilize overall intake (Collier, 1985). However, in standard laboratory settings in which a single commercially prepared food is continuously available, patterns of food intake become fairly regular, thereby allowing the study of factors that contribute to meal initiation, maintenance, and termination. This situation represents a classic trade-off between experimental control and measurement on the one hand, and variability in food availability under natural conditions on the other. Although this chapter focuses on factors that terminate meals, a brief review of determinants of meal initiation and maintenance will provide a context for that discussion.

The factors that trigger feeding are poorly understood. A number of conditioned stimuli related to the characteristics of the nutrients themselves or to the settings associated with meal initiation have been identified (Weingarten, 1984) that may be involved in sustaining overeating. In contrast, remarkably few unconditioned stimuli for meal initiation have received serious attention. Metabolic signals tied to decreased glucose or fatty acid use are sufficient for meal initiation (Scharrer & Langhans, 1986), but whether these signals act under normal physiological circumstances has not yet been demonstrated.

Ghrelin, one of the gastric peptides, may stimulate feeding. It was first identified in 1999 as the endogenous ligand for the growth hormone stimulating receptor (GHSR; Kojima et al., 1999). Unexpectedly, peripheral and central ghrelin administration were found to potently stimulate food intake and decrease energy expenditure in rodents (Nakazato et al., 2001; Tschop et al., 2000). Such a role for the endogenous peptide is supported by data demonstrating reduced food intake in response to ghrelin antagonist administration (Asakawa et al., 2003) and by the decreased body weight and fat mass in knockout mice, lacking ghrelin receptors, that ate a high-fat diet (Sun et al., 2004).

Ghrelin is secreted by endocrine cells within the stomach and circulates in plasma. Fasting increases circulating ghrelin (Gualillo et al., 2002); indeed, in humans circulating ghrelin levels increase and decline before and following meals, respectively (Cummings et al., 2001). Meal-induced declines in plasma ghrelin appear to depend on postgastric nutrient factors (Williams et al., 2003), although the specific site and mechanism underlying these declines remain to be determined. Ghrelin decreases the time to meal initiation and increases the overall number of meals consumed (Faulconbridge et al., 2003). The pattern of ghrelin release around meals and the ability of exogenous ghrelin to increase meal number suggest that premeal ghrelin elevations may provide a signal for meal initiation.

Taste is an important determinant of meal size: it either extends or curtails contact with a nutrient source. Palatable (good-tasting) substances are consumed more rapidly, for longer periods of time, and in greater amounts than unpalatable foods. A number of experimental paradigms have been developed to isolate taste influences on ingestion; sham feeding is the most widely used. In this paradigm, a fistula is created, generally in the stomach, that can be opened or left closed according to test condition. With the fistula open, ingested liquids drain outside the body, thereby minimizing postingestive feedback. For example, when a gastric fistula is open, ingested nutrients contact mouth, esophagus, and stomach but do not collect in the stomach or pass into the upper intestine, thereby eliminating signals that normally arise from gastric distension or intestinal nutrient contact and absorption. In Pavlov's (1910) original demonstration that dogs eating with open esophageal fistulas continued to eat for hours, the act of tasting and swallowing was not sufficient to induce satiety. This finding is especially noteworthy because when dehydrated dogs sham-drink water, the amount sham-drunk is exactly the amount drunk normally and is appropriate to the deficit, although the animals return after a while to drink the same amount again (Thrasher et al., 1980). Thus for drinking, an act that uses the same neuromusculature as consuming a liquid diet, the oropharyngeal monitoring mechanisms are sufficient for accurate regulation.

Although oropharyngeal metering or other mechanisms that track the passage of food from mouth to stomach cannot alone account for meal termination, orosensory stimuli contribute substantially to the ingestive process, as revealed by the sham-feeding paradigm. Increasing the concentration of saccharide solutions or oil emulsions, for example, increases intake linearly over an extensive range of concentrations (Grill & Kaplan, 1992; Mook, 1963; Weingarten & Watson, 1982). Palatability, therefore, can help sustain ingestion once it is initiated. Conversely, unpalatable foods or liquids curtail the ingestive process. The neural systems underlying the effects of palatability and their interactions with systems that mediate meal termination are discussed in other chapters.

Analyses of sham-feeding patterns have also demonstrated how other pregastric factors may induce satiety. Sham feeding does eventually stop, of course, as a reflection of the individual or joint contribution(s) of a number of processes. These could include oral metering (Mook, 1990), habituation (Swithers & Hall, 1994), and sensory-specific satiety (decreasing pleasantness of a specific food as more is ingested; Rolls, 1986). The amount sham-fed also depends on the animal's experience with the sham-feeding paradigm. Although the initial sham-feeding bout lasts about twice as long as bouts with the fistula closed, intake significantly increases with repeated testing. These data have been interpreted to demonstrate the presence of a conditioned inhibition on food intake that is due to an association of the oral stimulation with postingestive negative feedback. Only with continued experience with sham feeding is this conditioned inhibition on intake gradually overcome (Davis, 1990; Weingarten & Kulikovsky, 1989).

Data such as these demonstrate interactions among the various influences on food intake. Palatability sustains intake and, in the absence of negative feedback, or with the waning of associative controls on the basis of experience, the effects of palatability can be the primary determinants of intake. This becomes an important issue in considerations of the current obesity epidemic. Calorically dense, highly palatable foods are readily available, increasing the positive drives on ingestion. If the amount of food consumed represents the outcome of the balance of positive and negative feedback, increasing the positive side of the equation will increase overall intake. In this regard, the set point around which body weight is regulated may be specific to different diets (Tremblay, 2004). As diet palatability increases, so, too, does the set point around which weight will be regulated.

Controls of Meal Termination

Factors determining meal termination are well documented. During normal ingestion, consumed nutrients contact multiple mechano- and chemosensitive receptors in the stomach and the intestine that inform the brain of gut volume and contents. The potential range of feedback mechanisms that could operate during a meal is determined by the distribution of ingested nutrients through the gastrointestinal tract. The main determinants of this distribution are the controls of gastric emptying and intestinal motility that either confine or distribute the ingested nutrients. Gastric emptying is differentially controlled during and following a meal (Kaplan et al., 1992; Moran et al., 1999). During a meal, gastric emptying is rapid; it occurs at a constant rate for the duration of the meal and is not affected by nutrient concentration (Kaplan et al., 1992). Similar patterns of emptying are obtained whether the meal is ingested or infused into the stomach at a rate that matches meal ingestion (Kaplan et al., 1997). After a meal, gastric emptying is slower and is determined primarily by the caloric concentration of the gastric contents.

These differential controls are depicted in the data from nonhuman primates shown in Figure 3.1. Examinations of gastric contents at various times while the stomach is being filled at a constant rate indicate that a constant proportion of infused volume empties over this period; emptying is rapid and linear, and it is primarily a product of the total gastric volume. When the filling period ends, the overall rate of emptying slows but continues to be linear; the rate is constant and not affected by volume. Such data demonstrate that a significant portion of ingested nutrients enters the duodenum, contacts duodenal receptors, and is available for absorption during a meal. Thus, both the stomach and a significant proportion of the upper intestine provide potential sites for feedback signal generation during a meal that could be important for meal termination.

Gut neural signaling

Nutrients within the gut elicit both neural and chemical signals that provide feedback information about the quantity and quality of what has been ingested. Vagal afferent fibers with cell bodies in the nodose ganglion relay information from various digestive organs and project centrally to the nucleus of the solitary tract (NST) within the dorsal hindbrain. The NST distribution of vagal afferent terminations approximates a viscerotopic representation of the alimentary canal (Altschuler et al. 1989). In rats, afferents constitute the majority of vagal fibers, accounting for greater than 75% of those projecting from subdiaphragmatic organs (Prechtl & Powley, 1990). Thus, the potential for simultaneous feedback from multiple gastrointestinal sites is significant.

Vagal afferents are often categorized by their anatomical terminations or response properties. The terminations of vagal afferents often reflect the organ

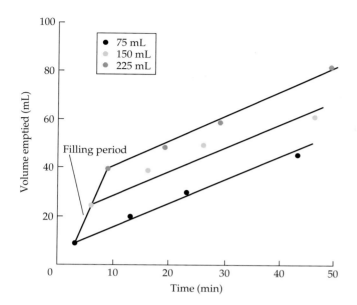

FIGURE 3.1   Patterns of gastric emptying during and following gastric infusions mimicking ingestion rates. During the filling period, emptying represents a constant fraction of the increasing gastric volume. When filling stops, the rate of emptying slows and is independent of volume. (After Moran et al., 1999, with permission.)

from which they arise. Within the gastric and intestinal musculature, two distinct mechanosensitive vagal afferent terminations have been identified: intramuscular arrays and intraganglionic laminar endings. Intramusculature arrays (IMAs) are found in both the longitudinal and circular muscle layers of the gastrointestinal tract and consist of an array of free endings lying in parallel with the muscle fibers (Berthoud & Powley, 1992). IMAs have been proposed to serve as stretch receptors responding to passive stretch (Phillips & Powley, 2000). The other primary termination, intraganglionic laminar endings (IGLEs), are localized to the myenteric plexus and consist of a series of arborizing endings within the myenteric ganglia (Rodrigo et al., 1975). IGLEs are widely distributed throughout the esophagus, stomach, and intestine; and these endings may be tension receptors responding to local muscle contraction (Phillips & Powley, 2000).

The location of IGLEs suggests that they may respond to local chemical stimulation arising from myenteric neurons or paracrine release from gastrointestinal secretory cells (Berthoud et al., 1997; Schwartz, 2000). Polymorphic individual vagal afferent fibers are known to have collateral terminations consisting of both IMAs and IGLEs. Thus, single fibers may respond to and integrate information from multiple stimulation modalities (Berthoud & Powley, 1992). Therefore, the degree to which a fiber responds to a mechanical stimulation such as intraluminal volume or stretch may be modified by nutrient-induced transmitter or peptide release, as will be discussed in greater detail shortly.

Vagal afferents arising from the gastrointestinal tract are often categorized according to their response properties. Thus, fibers can be mechanosensitive (responding to intraluminal volume changes), chemosensitive (responding to the chemical nature of the intraluminal contents), or both. Two functional mechanosensitive fibers have been identified that together provide information about both changes in and absolute intraluminal volume. Rapidly adapting fibers increase their response rate as volume increases. When a new volume is reached, the firing rate rapidly decreases back to baseline levels (Schwartz et al., 1993). Slowly adapting gastric mechanoreceptive fibers increase their response rate with increasing gastric volume, remain active while load volume is retained, and show an *off response* in which electrophysiological activity briefly drops below baseline levels when the load volume is removed (Andrews et al., 1980).

Individual afferents are differentially tuned to reflect differences in their dynamic range (Schwartz et al., 1993). Some afferents reach their maximal activity at small intraluminal volumes; others do not begin to respond until a significant load volume is present. Gastric mechanoreceptive vagal afferents do not respond directly to the chemical character of the gastric load. Response rate is similarly increased by nutrient and non-nutrient load volumes that are confined to the stomach by a pyloric noose (Mathis et al., 1998). Thus, information transmitted via the vagal afferent innervation from the stomach appears to be specific to the volume of gastric contents. A role for such gastric volume–related feedback signaling in the controls of food intake is suggested from data demonstrating the ability of gastric distension to inhibit food intake (Geliebter et al., 1988; Phillips & Powley, 1996) and the attenuation of such inhibition in response to vagotomy (Phillips & Powley, 1998).

Vagal afferent terminations have also been identified within the duodenal mucosa (Berthoud et al., 1995). Although fine afferent fibers have been localized within the intestinal villi, the terminations do not appear to penetrate the duodenal lumen, leading to the view that any direct nutrient stimulation would follow rather than precede absorption. Alternatively, nutrient absorption could stimulate local chemical release and activate vagal afferents secondary to such release. Duodenal vagal afferents are activated by both intraluminal load volume and nutrient character. Duodenal slowly adapting mechanoreceptive fibers have been identified. As with gastric mechanoreceptive fibers, activity increases with increases in load volume. Duodenal vagal afferents also respond directly to nutrient character. For example, both intestinal casein (Eastwood et al., 1998) and lipid infusions (Randich et al., 2000) have been shown to result in increases in vagal afferent activity beyond those produced by similar non-nutrient loads.

Elimination of aspects of vagal afferent feedback can significantly alter the way that rats pattern their food intake. Surgical vagal deafferentation results in alterations in meal patterns in rats maintained on a liquid diet, in that such rats consume larger, less frequent meals than do sham-operated controls (Schwartz et al., 1999). Meal frequency is reduced in response to these meal size increases such that overall food intake is unchanged. Similar alterations in meal size have been reported in response to capsaicin-induced chemical vagal deafferentation. These rats consume larger meals of a novel diet (Chavez et al., 1997) or of calorically dilute sucrose (Kelly et al., 2000). Although such data demonstrate a role for vagal afferent feedback in the controls of meal size, the particular signal(s) being blocked have yet to be identified.

Within-meal gut peptide signaling

A number of peptides are released from the gastrointestinal tract in response to nutrient ingestion. Many of these restrict feeding. The best characterized of these inhibitors is the brain–gut peptide cholecystokinin (CCK), which has been demonstrated to inhibit feeding in a variety of species, including human and nonhuman primates (Moran & McHugh, 1982; Pi-Sunyer et al., 1982). Exogenously administered CCK reduces meal size and results in earlier appearance of a behavioral sequence that indicates satiety (Antin et al., 1975). A specific role for CCK in controlling the size of individual meals was first suggested by experiments examining the feeding effects of repeated meal-contingent CCK administration. CCK given in conjunction with meal initiation consistently reduced meal size, which was compensated for by an increase in the number of meals consumed, thereby stabilizing daily food intake (West et al., 1984). Such an action in meal termination is consistent with the dynamics of nutrient-induced CCK release. Plasma CCK rises rapidly following meal initiation, peaking within 10 to 15 minutes and gradually returning to baseline levels (Liddle et al., 1985), and it is rapidly broken down (Koulischer et al., 1982).

The satiety actions of CCK reflect its interactions with multiple receptor sites. Substantial populations of CCK1 receptors, the subtype through which CCK satiety actions are mediated, are found on vagal afferent fibers and on circular muscle cells within the pyloric sphincter. CCK receptors are expressed in the cell bodies of vagal afferents within the nodose ganglion (Broberger et al., 2001) and are transported along subdiaphragmatic vagal afferent fibers to terminations within gastrointestinal organs (Moran et al., 1990). CCK increases vagal afferent activity. As Figure 3.2 shows, CCK induces activity in vagal mechanosensitive afferent fibers, and these increases are similar in magnitude to those induced by intragastric loads (Schwartz et al., 1993) or intraduodenal loads (Schwartz et al., 1995). Combinations of load volumes and CCK administration result in levels of activity beyond those produced by either stimulus alone. Importantly, CCK increases responsiveness to load volumes even after the direct response to CCK has disappeared. Thus, gastric load volumes result in greater vagal afferent activity following than preceding activation by CCK. The ability of CCK to activate and sensitize mechanosensitive vagal afferents is likely the result of individual afferent fibers expressing multiple terminations, as discussed earlier. This capacity allows for signal integration at the level of the peripheral afferent fiber.

CCK is involved in mediating vagal chemosensitive responses to intraluminal nutrients. CCK activates both mechanosensitive (Schwartz et al., 1995) and nonmechanosensitive (Eastwood et al., 1998) duodenal vagal afferents, and such activation appears to be a role of the endogenous peptide. CCK antagonists block the increase in vagal afferent activity produced by intraduodenal casein (Eastwood et al., 1998) and fatty acids (Cox et al., 2004).

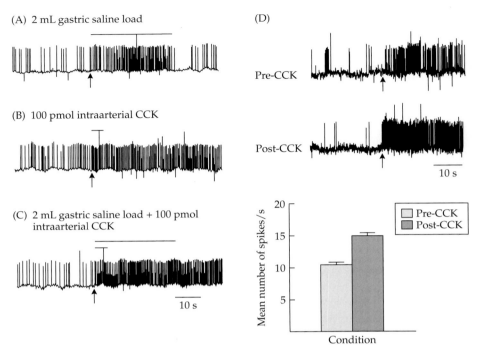

FIGURE 3.2 Electrophysiological responses of gastric vagal afferents to gastric volume (A), intraarterial CCK (B), gastric volume + intraarterial CCK (C), and gastric volume before and after CCK exposure (D). Gastric vagal afferent fibers respond to both load and CCK. CCK both activates and sensitizes gastric mechanosensitive vagal afferent fibers. (A–C from Schwartz et al., 1993, used with permission.)

Surgical or chemical disruption of subdiaphragmatic vagal afferent innervation compromises CCK inhibition of food intake (Moran et al., 1997; Ritter & Ladenheim, 1985; Smith et al., 1981), as manifested in a rightward shift in the CCK satiety dose–response function (Figure 3.3). Low doses of CCK that inhibit food intake in intact rats are ineffective for reducing intake following vagal afferent lesions. Higher doses inhibit intake but do so much more modestly than in control animals. CCK also interacts with receptors localized to the circular muscle layer of the pyloric sphincter (Smith et al., 1984). CCK receptor activation at this site results in pyloric contraction (Margolis et al., 1989) and in the inhibition of nutrient flow from stomach to duodenum (Moran et al., 1991). In contrast with the vagotomy findings, surgical removal of the pyloric sphincter does not prevent low doses of CCK from inhibiting intake but, as Figure 3.3 shows, truncates the dose–effect curve such that the additional suppression that normally accompanies higher CCK doses is eliminated (Moran et al., 1988). CCK satiety, therefore, is mediated by multiple mechanisms and is, in part, secondary to its local gastrointestinal actions.

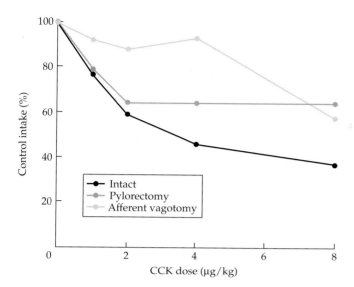

Control intake (%)

CCK dose (μg/kg)

- Intact
- Pylorectomy
- Afferent vagotomy

FIGURE 3.3 Contributions to CCK's satiety actions. In intact rats, peripheral CCK administration results in dose-related reductions in meal size. With disconnection of the afferent vagus (vagotomy), the ability of low doses of CCK to inhibit food intake is eliminated. With surgical removal of the pyloric sphincter (pylorectomy), the actions of low doses are intact but the dose–response curve is truncated.

Endogenous CCK likely contributes to satiety during normal feeding. CCK antagonists with specificity for the CCK1 receptor increase food intake (Moran et al., 1993; Reidelberger & O'Rourke, 1989). In nonhuman primates, the effect is related to dose, with a maximum increase of about 40% in daily 4-hour feeding sessions. Enhanced intake is almost completely accounted for by the increased size of the first meal (Moran et al., 1993). Alterations in meal patterns are also evident in mice or rats lacking CCK1 receptors, including the Otsuka Long Evans Tokushima Fatty (OLETF) CCK1 receptor knockout rat (Takiguchi et al., 1997). OLETF rats are hyperphagic and obese, consuming roughly 35% more calories than do control rats of similar age. This increase in overall intake results from an 80% increase in meal size that is not sufficiently compensated for by decreases in meal frequency (Moran et al., 1998). CCK1 receptor knockout mice also increase meal size, although not to the same degree as in OLETF rats, and CCK1 receptor knockout mice adjust meal frequency to compensate for the larger meals so that total food intake remains stable (Bi et al., 2004).

Satiety actions for the pancreatic peptides glucagon and amylin have also been demonstrated. Eating rapidly increases pancreatic glucagon secretion (Langhans et al., 1984), as does sham feeding, suggesting cephalic influences on glucagon release (Nilsson & Uvnas-Wallensten, 1977). Glucagon is quickly cleared from the circulation by the liver (Langhans et al., 1984), which appears to be the site of glucagon's satiety action (Geary, et al., 1993): direct hepatic-portal vein infusions of glucagon at meal onset elicit dose-related reductions in meal size (Geary & Smith, 1982a). Furthermore, hepatic vagotomy prevents exogenously administered glucagons from inhibiting food intake (Geary & Smith, 1983). Glucagon's actions appear to be specific to meal termination because meal-contingent glucagon administration reliably reduces meal size without affecting subsequent meal initiation (Le Sauter & Geary, 1991). Furthermore, hepatic-portal infusions of glucagon antibody reliably increase meal size, suggesting a role for endogenous glucagons in the control of meal size (Le Sauter et al., 1991). Glucagon's satiety action is not direct and requires the presence of other forms of ingestive consequences. Although glucagon alone does not affect sham feeding (even at very high doses; Geary & Smith, 1982b), it potently augments sham-feeding suppression produced by CCK (Le Sauter & Geary, 1987).

Amylin inhibits feeding in a dose-dependent and behaviorally specific manner following either peripheral or central administration (Lutz, et al., 1995). Amylin is obligatorily co-secreted with insulin by pancreatic beta cells (Cooper, 1994). Amylin levels rise rapidly with meal onset and remain high during and following meals. Amylin's site of action is within the area postrema, a hindbrain structure lacking a complete blood–brain barrier. Amylin receptors are densely expressed within the area postrema, and area postrema lesions block feeding inhibition by peripherally administered amylin (Lutz et al., 1998). Amylin also inhibits sham feeding, but higher doses are required than for inhibition of real feeding. Thus, amylin-induced signals may normally combine with others to inhibit feeding (Asarian et al., 1998). Feeding is increased in response to peripheral (Reidelberger et al., 2004) or central administration of amylin antagonists (Mollet et al., 2004; Rushing et al., 2001), with maximal increases in 3-hour tests as high as 171%.

Modulation of neural activity within the dorsal hindbrain is the signature central change caused by peptides that contribute to meal termination, regardless of signaling origin—that is, direct peptide action at hindbrain sites or activation subsequent to vagal afferent activation. For example, both CCK (Fraser & Davison, 1992) and amylin (Rowland & Richmond, 1999) activate neurons in the NST (the site of vagal afferent termination) and within the area postrema, as demonstrated by the induction of the immediate early gene c-*fos* (Figure 3.4), a commonly used surrogate for neuronal activation.

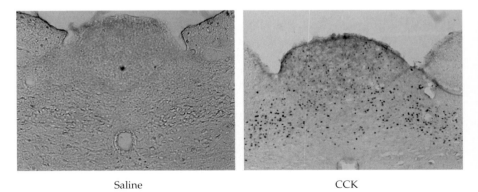

Saline   CCK

FIGURE 3.4 NST and area postrema c-*fos* responses to peripheral CCK administration. CCK activates NST and area postrema neurons.

Considerable integration of within-meal feedback signaling occurs within the dorsal hindbrain. Experiments in which oral, gastric, and intestinal sites have been exposed to nutrients either individually or in combination have revealed both negative and positive interactions. For example, gastric nutrient exposure reduces the degree of NST c-*fos* activation induced by oral exposure during sham feeding and, as Figure 3.5 shows, combined gastric and duodenal exposure results in greater activation than does either exposure alone (Emond et al., 2001). Such signal integration at this hindbrain site is consistent

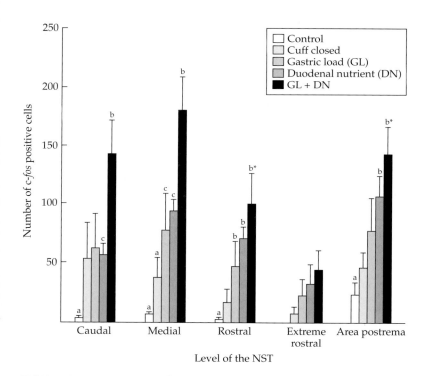

FIGURE 3.5   Integration of gastrointestinal inputs in the dorsal hindbrain. Levels of c-*fos* positive cells differ in response to individual gastric, individual duodenal, and combined gastric and duodenal stimulation at different levels of the NST. "Cuff closed" is a control condition for isolating gastric nutrients in which the pyloric cuff was closed but the stomach was not filled. Bars with different letters are different from one another within a level of the NST; * indicates significant difference from corresponding cuff closed condition. Individual gastric and duodenal stimulation activates the medial and rostral NST, but combined stimulation resulted in greater activation. (After Emond et al., 2001, with permission.)

with the sufficiency of the hindbrain for mediating many aspects of within-meal feedback signaling.

The evidence comes from experiments in decerebrate rats in which the neural axis at the level of the mesodiencephalic junction is complete transected. This preparation allows the study of the capacities of the caudal hindbrain in isolation from descending forebrain influences. Although decerebrate rats will not spontaneously consume food, they are capable of metering their intake if nutrients are infused into their mouths by either swallowing or allowing the food to drip out. Using such oral feeding procedures, Grill and colleagues have demonstrated the sufficiency of the hindbrain for mediating sophisticated within-meal feedback controls. For example, decerebrate rats reduce their intake appropriately to nutrient preloads or peripheral CCK administration (Grill et al., 1997; Grill & Kaplan, 2001; Grill & Smith, 1988).

Across-meal gut peptide signaling

A number of additional gut peptides inhibit food intake following peripheral administration but do so with characteristics different from those already discussed. Typically their nutrient-stimulated release is slower and/or longer-lasting than that of peptides that act within a meal, and, consistent with this pattern of release, they affect feeding beyond the proximal meal. Examples include glucagon-like peptide-1 (GLP-1) and peptide YY_{3-36}, whose actions are not limited to terminating the individual meal that produced their release.

GLP-1 is released by ileal endocrine L cells upon ingestion of nutrients. It functions as a gut hormone that helps regulate blood glucose and feeding behavior in mammals (Drucker et al., 1987). Circulating levels of GLP-1 rise within minutes of food ingestion and remain elevated for over 3 hours (Verdich et al., 2001). Carbohydrates (Ritzel et al., 1997) and long-chain unsaturated fatty acids (Rocca & Brubaker, 1995) are particularly good secretagogues. The rapid rise in plasma GLP-1 following meal initiation makes it unlikely that this is a local response to nutrients in the ileum. Duodenal nutrients probably stimulate endocrine and neural mediators that activate GLP-1 secretion (Roberge & Brubaker, 1993; Roberge et al., 1996). Consistent with this view, pharmacological or surgical vagotomy significantly attenuates meal-stimulated increases in GLP-1.

Exogenous GLP-1 reduces blood glucose in both normal and diabetic subjects (Nathan et al., 1992) by stimulating insulin secretion and synthesis in response to elevations in blood glucose (Fehmann & Habener, 1992), and by suppressing glucagon secretion (Komatsu et al., 1989). GLP-1 also plays a part in what is termed the *ileal brake*—the inhibition of gastric emptying and intestinal motility that is stimulated by the presence of undigested nutrients in the lower intestine (Giralt & Vergara, 1999; Lavin et al., 1998). In human subjects, prolonged peripheral GLP-1 infusions reduce food intake in lean, obese, and type 2 diabetic subjects (Gutzwiller, Drewe et al., 1999; Gutzwiller, Goke et al., 1999; Naslund et al., 1999; Naslund et al., 1998). However, peripheral bolus injections of GLP-1 into rats have little (Rodriquez de Fonseca et al., 2000) or no (Turton et al., 1996) effect on food intake.

The short half-life of peripheral GLP-1 provides a potential explanation for the relative inability of exogenous GLP-1 to influence feeding in rats. In vivo studies in rats demonstrated that dipeptidyl peptidase IV (DPP-IV), an enzyme present in the capillaries surrounding intestinal cells that catabolizes GLP-1, cleaved 50% of a bolus GLP-1 infusion within 2 minutes (Kieffer et al., 1995). GLP-1 analogues that are resistant to degradation have been shown to reduce food intake and body weight in lean and obese rats (Larsen et al., 2001), and recent data have demonstrated the ability of such compounds to produce dose-related suppressions of food intake in nonhuman primates (Scott & Moran, 2007).

The mechanisms underlying the feeding-inhibitory actions of intestinally derived GLP-1 are not yet fully understood. In human studies, exogenous GLP-1 infusions result in significant reductions in the size of a test meal comparable to those found with CCK (Gutzwiller et al., 2004), suggesting a similar mediation. The possibility of such vagal mediation is further suggested from data demonstrating that GLP-1 receptors are expressed in vagal afferent cell bodies in the nodose ganglion (Nakagawa et al., 2004), that vagal afferent denervation abolishes the actions of central and peripheral GLP-1 on gastric emptying (Imeryuz et al., 1997), and that surgical vagotomy attenuates the feeding-inhibitory actions of peripheral GLP-1 in the rat (Abbott et al., 2005).

In a second proposed mode of action, peripheral GP-1 exerts its effects via specific carriers or endothelial leaks that allow the peptide access to central binding sites. Evidence supporting this idea comes from data demonstrating that when radiolabeled GLP-1 is injected peripherally, it can be identified in the area postrema and other circumventricular organs (Orskov et al., 1996). These data suggest that peripheral GLP-1 gains access to the brain and may bind to brainstem sites from which efferent projections are directed to major hypothalamic nuclei involved in energy homeostasis (Shapiro & Miselis, 1985). Consistent with such mediation are data showing the ability of centrally administered GLP-1 to reduce food intake (Tang-Christensen et al., 1996).

Although the site of action for central GLP-1 to inhibit feeding appears to be the within the dorsal hindbrain (Kinzig et al., 2002), GLP-1 administration does activate hypothalamic sites involved in energy balance (as will be discussed shortly), and activation of these sites appears to be necessary for GLP-1–induced feeding suppression to occur (Tang-Christensen et al., 1998). Involvement of hypothalamic sites may underlie the ability of GLP-1 to affect feeding across multiple meals. Although effects of GLP-1 on hypothalamic gene expression have not yet been identified, such actions seem likely because repeated administration of GLP-1 analogues can result in long-term reduction in food intake and reductions in body weight without apparent subsequent compensation (Larsen et al., 2001).

Peptide YY_{3-36}, a cleavage product of peptide YY (PYY), shares a number of similarities with GLP-1. It is also secreted from L cells located primarily in the distal intestine (Grandt et al., 1994) and plays a part in the ileal brake (Lin et al., 1996; Pironi et al., 1993). PYY_{3-36} and PYY are both released into the circulation during and following a meal (Grandt et al., 1994). Although little is known about the specific dynamics of PYY_{3-36} in circulation, it is likely released and degraded along with PYY. The temporal pattern of PYY release differs from that of other gastrointestinal peptides in that PYY levels gradually rise following meal initiation, reaching a peak at about 60 minutes, which is then maintained for a number of hours following the meal (Onaga et al., 2002). This release pattern suggests a more protracted influence beyond the meal that triggered its release.

PYY_{3-36} suppresses eating in both rodents and humans (Batterham et al., 2002). Although the original findings of a feeding-inhibitory action of exogenous PYY_{3-36} in rodents were controversial (Tschop et al., 2004), they have now been confirmed by multiple investigators; and recent work employing sustained infusions of PYY_{3-36} aimed at mimicking prandial and postprandial PYY release has demonstrated significant feeding-inhibitory actions across multiple meals in rodents (Chelikani et al., 2005), nonhuman primates (Moran et al., 2004), and humans (Batterham et al., 2003).

The site(s) and mechanisms of action through which peripheral PYY_{3-36} inhibits food intake remain under investigation. Both direct central and vagus-mediated mechanisms have been proposed. Peripheral PYY_{3-36} administration has been shown to reduce arcuate neuropeptide Y (NPY) and increase arcuate pro-opiomelanocortin (POMC) mRNA expression (Challis et al., 2003) and the localization of presynaptic Y2 receptors (the receptor subtype through which the anorexigenic actions of PYY_{3-36} are probably mediated) to arcuate NPY neurons has led to the hypothesis that circulating PYY_{3-36} could have direct access to this neuronal population. In support of this view are data demonstrating that mice in whom the Y2 receptor is knocked out do not respond to PYY_{3-36} and that direct arcuate PYY_{3-36} injection inhibits food intake (Batterham et al., 2002). Importantly, PYY has been demonstrated to cross the blood–brain barrier, providing a potential mechanism for arcuate access of circulating PYY_{3-36} (Nonaka et al., 2003). Recent data suggest a vagal mediation. It has recently been demonstrated (Koda et al., 2005) that the vagus contains Y2 receptors and that intravenous administration of PYY_{3-36} activates gastric vagal afferent fibers. Furthermore, multiple reports have now shown that vagotomy blocks the ability of PYY_{3-36} to inhibit food intake and to activate arcuate NPY neurons (Koda et al., 2005), suggesting a peripheral site of action but leaving open a role for hypothalamic mediation of the feeding-inhibitory effects.

Figure 3.6 illustrates how gut peptides influence feeding. Feedback depends on vagal afferent transmission of multiple gut peptides that are involved in both meal termination and across-meal signaling. Other peptides exploit direct hindbrain access to sites that receive ascending neural inputs. Finally, direct access to hypothalamic sites and actions, dependent on modulating hypothalamic signaling, has also been suggested.

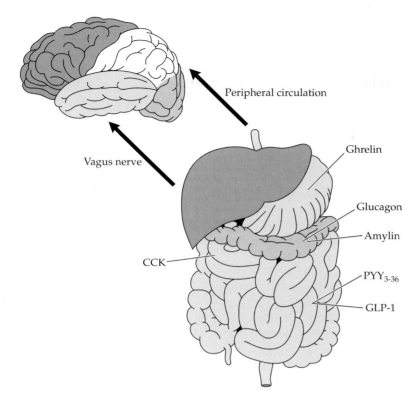

Peripheral circulation

Ghrelin

Vagus nerve

Glucagon

Amylin

CCK

PYY_{3-36}

GLP-1

FIGURE 3.6 Peptide feedback from the gut to the brain.

Mediation of Metabolic Signals

A role for signals related to metabolic state or to the availability of energy stores in the control of food intake has long been postulated. Depletion/repletion models tied to carbohydrate availability (Mayer, 1953) and to the extent of fat stores (Kennedy, 1953) dominated the early years of feeding research. Early studies of mouse genetic obesity models suggested the importance of circulating factors in signaling metabolic status. Having identified two different forms of genetic obesity in mice (*ob/ob* and *db/db*), Coleman (1973) studied food intake and body weight gains in these obese mice under conditions in which their blood supply was shared with the other obese or normal-weight mice in parabiotic pairs. The *ob/ob* mice reduced their food intake and lost body weight whether paired with normal or with *db/db* mice. The food intake and body weight of *db/db* mice was not affected by these manipulations. This overall pattern of results led to the conclusions that *ob/ob* mice lacked a circulating factor whose absence resulted in hyperphagia and obesity, and that *db/db* mice produced that factor but lacked the ability to respond to it appropriately.

Some 20 years later, the positional cloning of leptin as the protein product of the *ob* gene (Zhang et al., 1994) and the subsequent identification of the leptin receptor as the protein product of the *db* gene (Chua et al., 1996; Tartaglia et al., 1995) provided the basis for understanding Coleman's observations. Leptin was the circulating factor that was lacking in the *ob/ob* mouse. When exogenously administered, leptin normalized food intake and body weight in *ob/ob* mice. It also reduced eating and body weight in normal mice and rats (Campfield et al., 1995). Leptin is produced in white adipose tissue and circulates in proportion to the adipose mass, increasing in plasma as animals and humans become obese (Maffei et al., 1995) and decreasing in times of food deprivation and weight loss (Scarpace et al., 1998). Thus, leptin is a circulating factor that signals the extent of the body's fat stores.

Consistent with Coleman's predictions, *db/db* mice lack the leptin receptor. Leptin receptors are members of the cytokine receptor superfamily. Multiple leptin receptor isoforms arise from differential splicing of the receptor protein. The predominant, short form (Ob-Ra), is widely expressed in multiple tissues, including the choroid plexus and brain microvasculature (Bjorbaek et al., 1998). These brain binding sites have been proposed to function as part of a saturable transport system allowing circulating leptin to enter the brain (Bjorbaek et al., 1997). The long form of the leptin receptor (Ob-Rb), is highly expressed in neurons, with maximal expression in hypothalamic nuclei that have identified roles in energy balance. Thus, dense concentrations of Ob-Rb are found within the arcuate, paraventricular, and dorsomedial hypothalamic nuclei, as well as within the lateral hypothalamus (Elmquist et al., 1998).

Although leptin is viewed as the major adiposity factor important for the long-term control of energy balance, similar actions have been proposed for insulin. Insulin is also secreted in proportion to the body mass (Bagdade et al., 1967), mechanisms for insulin's transport into the brain have been demonstrated (Baura et al., 1993), and, as discussed in the next section, insulin interacts with the same hypothalamic circuits as leptin to affect overall energy balance (Niswender et al., 2004).

Hypothalamic systems involved in feeding control

The identification of leptin and its sites of action in the brain allowed rapid advances in our understanding of the hypothalamic influences on food intake and shifted the focus from nuclei-specific influences to the identification of orexigenic and anorexigenic peptide systems that respond to circulating signals reflecting overall metabolic state. A major site for leptin's actions in feeding control is the hypothalamic arcuate nucleus, which, as Figure 3.7 shows, contains

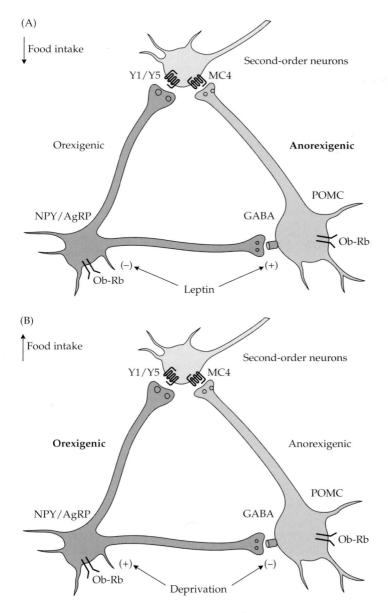

FIGURE 3.7   Arcuate nucleus peptide signaling in response to leptin and food deprivation. (A) Leptin increases POMC and decreases NPY/AgRP signaling to shift the balance to anorexigenic signaling and decreased food intake. (B) Food deprivation decreases POMC and increases NPY/AgRP signaling to shift the balance toward orexigenic signaling and increased food intake. GABA, γ-aminobutyric acid; MC4, melanocortin-4 receptor; Y1/Y5, NPY receptors.

two distinct neuronal populations, each of which express leptin and insulin receptors (Elias et al., 1999; Schwartz et al., 1996).

The first is a population of neurons that express the pro-peptide POMC (Figure 3.7). A precursor peptide, POMC is processed into multiple peptides, including α-melanocyte-stimulating hormone (α-MSH). α-MSH is an anorexigenic peptide that reduces food intake following exogenous administration (Giraudo, 1998). Leptin activates POMC-containing neurons both by direct depolarization (Cowley et al., 2001) and by increasing POMC mRNA expression. Leptin also interacts with a second population of arcuate neurons that contain the orexigenic peptides neuropeptide Y (NPY) and the endogenous melanocortin antagonist agouti-related peptide (AgRP). Leptin hyperpolarizes these neurons, reducing their activity (Cowley et al., 2001) and reducing NPY and AgRP mRNA expression (Korner et al., 2001). Leptin inhibition of these neurons also results in a reduction of their GABAergic inhibitory input onto the POMC-containing neurons (Cowley et al., 2001).

Thus, elevated leptin levels at times of metabolic excess directly activate an arcuate anorexigenic pathway and reduce activity in arcuate orexigenic pathways (see Figure 3.7A). Low leptin levels, occurring at times of nutrient deficit, have the opposite effect. Inhibitory influences on NPY/AgRP neurons are reduced, resulting in increased NPY/AgRP mRNA expression and increased inhibitory GABAergic input to POMC-containing neurons. The result is an overall increase in orexigenic signaling (see Figure 3.7B).

Exogenous administration of the peptide products of NPY, AgRP, and POMC gene expression results in changes in food intake. Intracerebroventricular or direct hypothalamic injection of NPY potently stimulates feeding in a variety of paradigms (Clark et al., 1984; Morley et al., 1985; Stanley et al., 1986), and repeated or chronic NPY administration results in obesity (Stanley et al., 1986; Zarjevski et al., 1993). Expression of NPY mRNA and release of the peptide increase in response to food deprivation (Kalra et al., 1991) or exercise (Lewis et al., 1993), and decrease in response to overconsumption of a highly palatable high-energy diet (Widdowson et al., 1997). The orexigenic effects of NPY are mediated through interactions with both the Y1 and Y5 receptor subtypes. Both receptor subtypes are expressed in hypothalamic areas involved in feeding control (Parker, 1999), and compounds with specific activity at these receptors affect food intake (Daniels et al., 2001). Chronic NPY infusions result in sustained increases in food intake and obesity in both Y1 and Y5 knockout mice, further suggesting redundancies in these receptor networks (Raposinho et al., 2004).

Melanocortins are the additional class of arcuate peptides that mediate the energy balance effects of leptin and insulin. Melanocortins can have both feeding-stimulatory and feeding-inhibitory actions. As noted already, POMC, with hypothalamic expression limited to the arcuate nucleus, is the precursor for a number of peptides, including the anorexigenic melanocortin agonist peptide α-MSH. Central administration of α-MSH or synthetic melanocortin agonists potently inhibits food intake (Benoit et al., 2000; Fan et al., 1997). POMC mRNA expression also decreases with food deprivation (Kim et al., 2000) and increases with overfeeding (Hagan et al., 1999), suggesting a regulatory role for this peptide in feeding control. Important roles for melanocortin signaling in energy balance have been demonstrated with POMC knockouts (Yaswen et al., 1999) or melanocortin receptor knockouts (Huszar et al., 1997). Such interruptions in melanocortin signaling result in obese phenotypes, and mutations in POMC and the melanocortin-4 receptor are also linked to some forms of monogenic human obesity (Huszar et al., 1997).

A unique aspect of melanocortin signaling is the existence of an endogenous melanocortin antagonist, agouti-related protein (AgRP). AgRP is co-localized with NPY in the arcuate nucleus, and its expression is up-regulated by fasting and down-regulated by leptin and insulin (Hahn et al., 1998). AgRP or synthetic melanocortin antagonists increase food intake when centrally administered, and their effects are long-lasting (Fan et al., 1997). Melanocortin signaling is thought to represent the balance between α-MSH and AgRP signaling at melanocortin-4 receptors, with increased food intake in the presence of increased AgRP release and decreased food intake in the presence of increased α-MSH release.

Arcuate NPY/AgRP- and POMC-containing neurons have primary projections to both the paraventricular nucleus (PVN; Baker & Herkenham, 1995; Elmquist, 2001) and the lateral hypothalamus (LH; Elias et al., 1999)—two nuclei involved in autonomic regulation. The arcuate-to-PVN projection appears to play a major role in anorexigenic signaling. Lesions of the PVN result in hyperphagia and obesity (Choi et al., 1999), and the PVN contains multiple neuronal cell types that express NPY and melanocortin receptors. These neurons also express other peptides that themselves can inhibit food intake when exogenously administered; such intake-inhibiting peptides include corticotropin-releasing hormone (CRH; Sawchenko & Swanson, 1982), oxytocin (Rogers et al., 1980), and gastrin-releasing peptide (GRP; Lynn et al., 1997).

In contrast to the feeding-inhibitory action of PVN stimulation, the other major hypothalamic projection site for arcuate neurons, the LH, seems to play a role in stimulating or maintaining food intake. LH lesions result in aphagia and profound weight loss (Teitelbaum & Epstein, 1962), and LH electrical or chemical stimulation increases food intake in sated animals (Mendelson, 1969). The LH is the site for neurons containing two additional peptides that have been implicated in feeding control: orexin (Chen et al., 1999) and melanin-concentrating hormone (MCH; Qu et al., 1996). Both of these peptides are orexigenic and have been proposed to be downstream mediators of reduced leptin signaling (Rossi et al., 1997; Sweet et al., 1999).

Orexin-containing neurons are found in the perifornical area of the hypothalamus and project widely throughout the hypothalamus and to extrahypothalamic sites (Peyron et al., 1998). Prepro-orexin expression is increased in response to deprivation (Lopez et al., 2000), and administration of an orexin A antagonist has been demonstrated to inhibit food intake, suggesting a role for endogenous orexin A in food intake control (Haynes et al., 2000). MCH-expressing neurons in the lateral hypothalamus are distinct from neurons that express hypocretin/orexin, although, like orexin neurons, they are innervated by arcuate nucleus NPY/AgRP- and POMC-containing fibers (Broberger et al., 1998). NPY has been demonstrated to activate orexin and MCH neurons (Niimi et al., 2001), and leptin has been demonstrated to inhibit orexin and MCH mRNA expression (Kokkotou et al., 2001; Niimi et al., 2001). MCH expression is increased in obesity, and MCH levels are modulated by fasting (Qu et al., 1996).

As well as responding to circulating hormones such as leptin and insulin, hypothalamic neurons respond directly to changes in the levels of circulating nutrients. Hypothalamic neurons have long been known to alter their activity in response to changes in glucose concentration (Oomura et al., 1969), and there are now reasons to think that hypothalamic neurons also respond to local changes in the availability of fatty acids. Intraventricular administration of oleic acid inhibits food intake and reduces hepatic glucose production (Obici et al., 2002). Results with compounds that inhibit fatty acid synthesis are also consistent with the idea of neuronal nutrient signaling. Administration of the fatty acid synthase inhibitor C75 results in decreases in food intake and body weight (Loftus et al., 2000), by altering patterns of hypothalamic gene expression, reducing NPY and AgRP signaling, and increasing POMC expression relative to levels found in animals whose intake was restricted to that consumed by the C75 treated animals. (Kim et al., 2002; Tu et al., 2005).

Although the hypothalamus has been the main focus of study for anorexigenic and orexigenic peptides, a number of these peptides also have effects on food intake when they are delivered to the dorsal hindbrain. For example, administration of NPY (Corp et al., 1990), ghrelin (Faulconbridge et al., 2005; Kinzig et al., 2006), or a melanocortin antagonist (Grill et al., 1998) into the fourth cerebroventrical potently increases food intake, but administration of leptin (Grill et al., 2002), a melanocortin agonist (Grill et al., 1998), CART (Aja et al., 2001), or urocortin (Grill et al., 2000) at this site inhibits food intake. These hindbrain actions suggest that the central feeding regulatory system is a distributed system (Grill, 2006).

Interactions between gut peptide and hypothalamic signaling

As detailed in the preceding discussion, some of the effects of gut peptides have been proposed to depend on alterations in hypothalamic signaling, whether through direct contact or secondary to activation of ascending neural pathways. There is also evidence for interactions between hypothalamic peptide signaling and the processing of ascending within-meal satiety signals. A number of the clearest demonstrations of interactions involve the adiposity signal leptin. As noted already, leptin circulates in direct relation to the degree of adiposity, serving as a feedback signal for the overall regulation of energy balance. Both peripheral and central leptin administration reduce food intake, and various experiments have demonstrated that leptin's effects on feeding are specific to reducing meal size without changing meal frequency (Eckel et al., 1998; Flynn et al., 1998; Kahler et al., 1998).

How does a signal that is critically involved in regulating hypothalamic energy balance pathways produce reductions in the size of individual meals? There are multiple possibilities for such an action. Leptin may reduce meal size through direct actions on taste sensitivity. Leptin specifically reduces chorda tympani and glossopharyngeal sensitivity to sweet stimuli without altering responses to other tastants (Kawai et al., 2000). This result appears to be a direct effect at the level of the taste bud, since leptin hyperpolarizes the taste cell. Leptin may also decrease meal size by altering the reinforcing effects of ingestion. Leptin has been shown to reduce the rewarding efficacy of electrical brain stimulation (Fulton, 2000), and leptin receptors have been localized to mesolimbic dopaminergic cell bodies that play a role in reinforcement (Figlewicz, 2003). Actions such as these may lead to earlier meal termination because the ability of the ingested nutrients to maintain feeding may be reduced.

Leptin's ability to limit meal size also depends on its ability to modulate the actions of within-meal feedback signaling. Leptin has been demonstrated to enhance the feeding-inhibitory actions of a variety of gastrointestinal feedback stimuli, including gastric distension (Emond et al., 2001) and several gastrointestinal peptides (Emond et al., 1999; Ladenheim et al., 2005; Williams et al., 2006). The best-studied example of such enhancement is the interaction between leptin and CCK (Barrachina et al., 1997; Emond et al., 1999).

As Figure 3.8 shows, central administration of leptin, at a dose that is subthreshold for inhibiting feeding when administered alone, enhances the satiat-

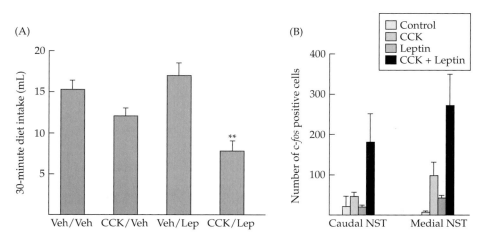

FIGURE 3.8   Leptin enhances satiety responses (A) and NST c-*fos* responses to peripheral CCK (B). CCK, cholecystokinin; Lep, leptin; Veh, vehicle. (After Emond et al., 1999, with permission.)

ing potential of peripheral CCK. This action of leptin appears to depend on its ability to enhance the degree of NST neural activation produced by these peripheral manipulations. That is, leptin enhances the dorsal hindbrain representation of ascending vagal afferent feedback signals arising from CCK, as demonstrated by the increase in the number of c-*fos* positive neurons in the leptin/CCK condition compared to the level induced by CCK alone. Reducing leptin levels through food deprivation has the opposite result: the satiating potency of CCK is reduced (Billington et al., 1983; McMinn et al., 2000). This effect may be mediated through enhanced NPY signaling, since NPY administration has the opposite effect of leptin on both the behavioral and neural activation potency of CCK: NPY administration attenuates the ability of CCK to reduce food intake and to induce c-*fos* in the NST (McMinn et al., 2000).

Such actions of leptin or its downstream signaling appear to depend on altered responsiveness of individual NST neurons to ascending vagal afferent signaling (Schwartz & Moran, 2002). As Figure 3.9A shows, central leptin enhances the degree of electrophysiological activity in single NST neurons to a gastric load volume. Central NPY administration has the opposite effect (Figure 3.9B). Following NPY administration, the degree of electrophysiological activation produced by a given intragastric volume is significantly reduced (Schwartz & Moran, 2002).

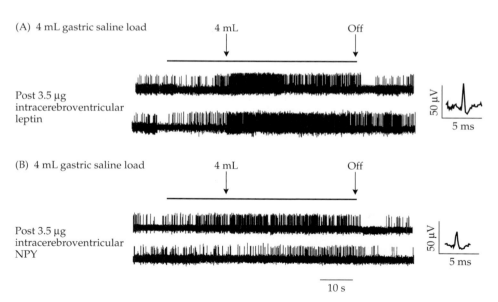

FIGURE 3.9 Electrophysiological responses of single NST neurons to gastric loads. Leptin increases (A) and NPY decreases (B) NST neuronal gastric load responses. (After Schwartz & Moran, 2002. Copyright 2002, The Endocrine Society.)

Such effects of leptin or NPY could depend on direct local hindbrain actions of these peptides. The dorsal hindbrain contains both leptin and NPY receptors (Grill et al., 2002; Harfstrand et al., 1986; Mercer et al., 1998), and, as noted earlier, hindbrain injections of these peptides alter feeding in the predicted directions (Corp et al., 1990; Grill et al., 2002). In addition, administration of leptin to the fourth cerebroventrical, which should access hindbrain but not forebrain sites, does enhance the feeding-inhibitory response to gastric distension (Huo et al., 2007).

Alternatively, the modulation of hindbrain responsiveness to within-meal signals could depend on activation of a descending pathway from the hypothalamus to the dorsal hindbrain. Recent data support such an additional possibility. Adenoviral replacement of functional leptin receptors limited to the arcuate nucleus of Koletsky rats (which lack all forms of the leptin receptor at all sites), was sufficient to normalize behavioral and hindbrain neural activational responses to CCK (Morton et al., 2005). In the absence of these leptin receptors, Koletsky rats are relatively insensitive to the satiety actions of CCK, and CCK produces only a mild degree of NST activation. Arcuate replacement of leptin receptors significantly increases the potency of CCK for both inhibiting feeding and activating NST neurons. These data demonstrate that forebrain signaling induced by leptin is sufficient to limit meal size by regulating hindbrain responses to within-meal satiety signaling.

A number of neuropeptide systems are candidates for mediating such hypothalamic modulation of hindbrain responsiveness. A role for PVN oxytocin-containing neurons in mediating leptin's modulation of responses to CCK has been suggested (Blevins et al., 2003; Blevins et al., 2004). Oxytocin-containing neurons are localized to the parvocellular subdivision of the PVN (Sawchenko et al., 1984). These neurons project to the NST, and the PVN is the source for NST oxytocin-containing fibers (Rinaman, 1998; Sawchenko & Swanson, 1982). Leptin increases c-*fos* expression in PVN oxytocin-containing neurons, and regions of the NST activated by CCK are densely innervated by oxytocin-containing fibers (Blevins et al., 2004). Ventricular administration of an oxytocin antagonist attenuates the effect of leptin on food intake and results in a significant decrease in the potentiating effect of leptin on CCK activation of NST neuronal c-*fos* expression (Blevins et al., 2003). Furthermore, fourth-ventricular administration of an oxytocin antagonist increases food intake. Oxytocin has long been known to affect gastrointestinal function (Rogers & Hermann, 1987), and local hindbrain administration of oxytocin has been shown to activate gastric-related NST and dorsal motor nucleus (DMX) neurons (McCann & Rogers, 1990). Whether oxytocin modulates the NST electrophysiological response to gastric distension or other satiety signals has not yet been directly assessed.

GRP-expressing neurons localized to the magnocellular layer of the PVN are another potential candidate. These neurons project to the dorsal vagal complex (Costello et al., 1991; Lynn et al., 1997). Fourth-ventricular administration of GRP inhibits intake (Ladenheim & Ritter, 1988), and fourth-ventricular administration of a GRP antagonist increases intake (Flynn, 1993), demonstrating a role for endogenous hindbrain GRP in feeding modulation. Electrophysiological studies have shown that NST neurons responsive to gastric distension also respond to local application of GRP, and that activation of NST neurons induced by electrical stimulation of the PVN can be modulated by local administration of GRP antagonists (Zhang et al., 2002). It is not known whether local application of GRP has the ability to modulate responses to gastric distension, or whether GRP can affect the activity of CCK-responsive NST neurons.

Finally, a discrete population of parvocellular PVN neurons expresses corticotropin-releasing hormone (CRH; Sawchenko et al., 1984), and PVN CRH neurons project to the NST (Rogers et al., 1980). Intracerebroventricular (ICV) administration of CRH can be shown to inhibit food intake and activate c-*fos* expression within the caudal brainstem (Imaki et al., 1993; Levine et al., 1983), and ICV administration of CRH antagonists blocks the anorexic actions of both leptin (Uehara et al., 1998) and a melanocortin agonist (Lu et al., 2003), suggesting that there is also a role for CRH signaling in these pathways. Roles for the orexigenic peptide systems in the lateral hypothalamus for mediating the meal size effects of leptin and NPY have yet to be evaluated. However, given the multiplicity of hypothalamic and hindbrain interactions, such contributions seem likely.

Summary

The body contains multiple systems for regulating overall energy balance. These systems derive from and control different aspects of ingestive behavior and its consequences. Signals arising from the gastrointestinal tract in response to nutrient ingestion, and the salience of these signals for affecting ongoing and subsequent intake, depend on signals from multiple other sources, including, but not limited to, metabolic status. As discussed in other chapters, multiple controls affect food intake, and the overall contributions of those detailed here depend on factors that go beyond physiological status. Given the multiplicity of systems that both ensure adequate energy intake and limit intake to appropriate amounts, it might be surprising that we now have such marked increases in obesity. Where have things gone awry? There are a number of potential explanations.

One explanation for the apparent ineffectiveness of negative feedback systems with the development of obesity is the onset of leptin resistance. As leptin levels increase in response to increased adiposity (Rodriquez de Fonseca et al., 2000), negative feedback to reduce food intake and body weight should also increase. However, the incidence of human obesity continues to increase, providing an argument against the potency of such signals within the current feeding environment. Developed insensitivity to leptin has been postulated to explain the lack of responsiveness of obese animals and humans to the negative feedback signal of prolonged elevations of plasma leptin levels (Halaas et al., 1997).

Leptin insensitivity is a multistage process with initially reduced feeding-inhibitory responses to peripheral, but not central, leptin administration and eventual loss of response to central leptin with further obesity. Thus, a down-regulation of leptin transport may precede a down-regulation of central leptin receptors against a background of high circulating leptin levels (Banks et al., 1999; El-Haschimi et al., 2000). Additional reductions in intracellular signaling in response to leptin's interaction with its receptor have also been demonstrated (Dunn et al., 2005). Similar mechanisms for insulin insensitivity have been proposed (Kaiyala et al., 2000).

Another possibility may be specific to the current availability of dietary fat. As discussed earlier, fatty foods have both denser caloric content and increased palatability. The increased palatability alone could account for increased intake because the balance between excitatory and inhibitory influences over ingestion would be altered. Dietary fat also affects aspects of both gastrointestinal and adiposity signaling. Consumption of a high-fat diet over time has been demonstrated to down-regulate receptor systems responding to peptide signaling. Thus, high-fat diet reduces the ability of CCK to activate hindbrain regions critical to the controls of meal size (Covasa et al., 2000), thereby reducing the satiating potency of CCK and shifting the dose–response curve to the right (Covasa & Ritter, 1998). High-fat diet also contributes to leptin resistance. Circulating triglycerides, which are elevated on a high-fat diet, reduce leptin transport across the blood–brain barrier (Banks et al., 2004), and thus reduce the feedback signaling from adiposity stores, adding to leptin insensitivity.

Though these mechanisms may underlie the propensity for increased food intake in the current environment, why would the system develop in this way? One possibility is that the feeding control systems are simply biased in the direction of maintaining adequate nutrient stores and, in the face of current levels of caloric excess, are not able to sufficiently down-regulate. This view points to the mismatch between our current environmental circumstances and those that molded evolutionary selection (Speakman, 2004). In an environment of relative caloric scarcity, a tendency to overconsume at times of nutrient availability and thus increase energy stores would impart a competitive advantage protecting against times of relative scarcity. In an environment of caloric excess, such a trait would be detrimental, leading to overconsumption and obesity.

An alternative perspective (Seeley & Woods, 2003) on this issue is that, in fact, the feedback systems are working very well. Even with the increases in the prevalence of obesity over the past 30 years, average weight has changed by less than a pound per year. Given that a pound represents a caloric excess of about 4000 kilocalories and that the average male consumes upwards of 900,000 kilocalories per year, this excess translates to an error rate of less than 0.5%. What the obesity epidemic might be like without such exquisite control mechanisms is a sobering thought.

References Cited

Abbott, C. R., Monteiro, M., Small, C. J., Sajedi, A., Smith, K. L., Parkinson, J. R., et al. (2005). The inhibitory effects of peripheral administration of peptide YY(3-36) and glucagon-like peptide-1 on food intake are attenuated by ablation of the vagal-brainstem-hypothalamic pathway. *Brain Research, 1044*, 127–131.

Aja, S., Sahandy, S., Ladenheim, E. E., Schwartz, G. J., & Moran, T. H. (2001). Intracerebroventricular CART peptide reduces food intake and alters motor behavior at a hindbrain site. *American Journal of Physiology – Regulatory, Integrative and Comparative Physiology, 281*, R1862–1867.

Altschuler, S. M., Bao, X. M., Bieger, D., Hopkins, D. A., & Miselis, R. R. (1989). Viscerotopic representation of the upper alimentary tract in the rat: sensory ganglia and nuclei of the solitary and spinal trigeminal tracts. *Journal of Comparative Neurology, 283*, 248–268.

Andrews, P. L., Grundy, D., & Scratcherd, T. (1980). Vagal afferent discharge from mechanoreceptors in different regions of the ferret stomach. *Journal of Physiology, 298*, 513–524.

Antin, J., Gibbs, J., Holt, J., Young, R. C., & Smith, G. P. (1975). Cholecystokinin elicits the complete behavioral sequence of satiety in rats. *Journal of Comparative and Physiological Psychology, 89*, 784–790.

Asakawa, A., Inui, A., Kaga, T., Katsuura, G., Fujimiya, M., Fujino, M. A., et al. (2003). Antagonism of ghrelin receptor reduces food intake and body weight gain in mice. *Gut, 52*, 947–952.

Asarian, L., Eckel, L. A., & Geary, N. (1998). Behaviorally specific inhibition of sham feeding by amylin. *Peptides, 19*, 1711–1718.

Bagdade, J. D., Porte, D., Jr., & Bierman, E. L. (1967). Diabetic lipemia. A form of acquired fat-induced lipemia. *New England Journal of Medicine, 276*, 427–433.

Baker, R. A., & Herkenham, M. (1995). Arcuate nucleus neurons that project to the hypothalamic paraventricular nucleus: neuropeptidergic identity and consequences of adrenalectomy on mRNA levels in the rat. *Journal of Comparative Neurology, 358*, 518–530.

Banks, W. A., Coon, A. B., Robinson, S. M., Moinuddin, A., Shultz, J. M., Nakaoke, R., et al. (2004). Triglycerides induce leptin resistance at the blood-brain barrier. *Diabetes, 53*, 1253–1260.

Banks, W. A., DiPalma, C. R., & Farrell, C. L. (1999). Impaired transport of leptin across the blood-brain barrier in obesity. *Peptides, 20*, 1341–1345.

Barrachina, M. D., Martinez, V., Wang, L., Wei, J. Y., & Tache, Y. (1997). Synergistic interaction between leptin and cholecystokinin to reduce short-term food intake in lean mice. *Proceedings of the National Academy of Sciences, USA, 94*, 10455–10460.

Batterham, R. L., Cohen, M. A., Ellis, S. M., Le Roux, C. W., Withers, D. J., Frost, G. S., et al. (2003). Inhibition of food intake in obese subjects by peptide YY(3-36). *New England Journal of Medicine, 349*, 941–948.

Batterham, R. L., Cowley, M. A., Small, C. J., Herzog, H., Cohen, M. A., Dakin, C. L., et al. (2002). Gut hormone PYY(3-36) physiologically inhibits food intake. *Nature, 418*, 650–654.

Baura, G. D., Foster, D. M., Porte, D., Jr., Kahn, S. E., Bergman, R. N., Cobelli, C., et al. (1993). Saturable transport of insulin from plasma into the central nervous system of dogs in vivo. A mechanism for regulated insulin delivery to the brain. *Journal of Clinical Investigation, 92*, 1824–1830.

Benoit, S., Schwartz, M., Baskin, D., Woods, S. C., & Seeley, R. J. (2000). CNS melanocortin system involvement in the regulation of food intake. *Hormones and Behavior, 37*, 299–305.

Berthoud, H. R., Kressel, M., Raybould, H. E., & Neuhuber, W. L. (1995). Vagal sensors in the rat duodenal mucosa: distribution and structure as revealed by in vivo DiI-tracing. *Anatomy and Embryology, 191*, 203–212.

Berthoud, H. R., Patterson, L. M., Neumann, F., & Neuhuber, W. L. (1997). Distribution and structure of vagal afferent intraganglionic laminar endings (IGLEs) in the rat gastrointestinal tract. *Anatomy and Embryology, 195*, 183–191.

Berthoud, H. R., & Powley, T. L. (1992). Vagal afferent innervation of the rat fundic stomach: morphological characterization of the gastric tension receptor. *Journal of Comparative Neurology, 319,* 261–276.

Bi, S., Scott, K. A., Kopin, A. S., & Moran, T. H. (2004). Differential roles for cholecystokinin a receptors in energy balance in rats and mice. *Endocrinology, 145,* 3873–3880.

Billington, C. J., Levine, A. S., & Morley, J. E. (1983). Are peptides truly satiety agents? A method of testing for neurohumoral satiety effects. *American Journal of Physiology, 245,* R920–926.

Bjorbaek, C., Elmquist, J. K., Michl, P., Ahima, R. S., van Bueren, A., McCall, A. L., et al. (1998). Expression of leptin receptor isoforms in rat brain microvessels. *Endocrinology, 139,* 3485–3491.

Bjorbaek, C., Uotani, S., da Silva, B., & Flier, J. S. (1997). Divergent signaling capacities of the long and short isoforms of the leptin receptor. *Journal of Biological Chemistry, 272,* 32686–32695.

Blevins, J. E., Eakin, T. J., Murphy, J. A., Schwartz, M. W., & Baskin, D. G. (2003). Oxytocin innervation of caudal brainstem nuclei activated by cholecystokinin. *Brain Research, 993,* 30–41.

Blevins, J. E., Schwartz, M. W., & Baskin, D. G. (2004). Evidence that paraventricular nucleus oxytocin neurons link hypothalamic leptin action to caudal brain stem nuclei controlling meal size. *American Journal of Physiology – Regulatory, Integrative and Comparative Physiology, 287,* R87–96.

Broberger, C., De Lecea, L., Sutcliffe, J. G., & Hokfelt, T. (1998). Hypocretin/orexin- and melanin-concentrating hormone-expressing cells form distinct populations in the rodent lateral hypothalamus: relationship to the neuropeptide Y and agouti gene-related protein systems. *Journal of Comparative Neurology, 402,* 460–474.

Broberger, C., Holmberg, K., Shi, T. J., Dockray, G., & Hokfelt, T. (2001). Expression and regulation of cholecystokinin and cholecystokinin receptors in rat nodose and dorsal root ganglia. *Brain Research, 903,* 128–140.

Campfield, L. A., Smith, F. J., Guisez, Y., Devos, R., & Burn, P. (1995). Recombinant mouse OB protein: evidence for a peripheral signal linking adiposity and central neural networks. *Science, 269,* 546–549.

Challis, B. G., Pinnock, S. B., Coll, A. P., Carter, R. N., Dickson, S. L., & O'Rahilly, S. (2003). Acute effects of PYY(3-36) on food intake and hypothalamic neuropeptide expression in the mouse. *Biochemical and Biophysical Research Communications, 311,* 915–919.

Chavez, M., Kelly, L., York, D. A., & Berthoud, H. R. (1997). Chemical lesion of visceral afferents causes transient overconsumption of unfamiliar high-fat diets in rats. *American Journal of Physiology, 272,* R1657–1663.

Chelikani, P. K., Haver, A. C., & Reidelberger, R. D. (2005). Intravenous infusion of peptide YY(3-36) potently inhibits food intake in rats. *Endocrinology, 146,* 879–888.

Chen, C. T., Dun, S. L., Kwok, E. H., Dun, N. J., & Chang, J. K. (1999). Orexin A-like immunoreactivity in the rat brain. *Neuroscience Letters, 260,* 161–164.

Choi, S., Sparks, R., Clay, M., & Dallman, M. F. (1999). Rats with hypothalamic obesity are insensitive to central leptin injections. *Endocrinology, 140,* 4426–4433.

Chua, S. C., Jr., Chung, W. K., Wu-Peng, X. S., Zhang, Y., Liu, S. M., Tartaglia, L., et al. (1996). Phenotypes of mouse diabetes and rat fatty due to mutations in the OB (leptin) receptor. *Science, 271,* 994–996.

Clark, J. T., Kalra, P. S., Crowley, W. R., & Kalra, S. P. (1984). Neuropeptide Y and human pancreatic polypeptide stimulate feeding behavior in rats. *Endocrinology, 115,* 427–429.

Coleman, D. L. (1973). Effects of parabiosis of obese with diabetes and normal mice. *Diabetologia, 9,* 294–298.

Collier, G. (1985). Satiety: an ecological perspective. *Brain Research Bulletin, 14,* 693–700.

Cooper, G. J. (1994). Amylin compared with calcitonin gene-related peptide: structure, biology, and relevance to metabolic disease. *Endocrine Reviews, 15,* 163–201.

Corp, E. S., Melville, L. D., Greenberg, D., Gibbs, J., & Smith, G. P. (1990). Effect of fourth ventricular neuropeptide Y and peptide YY on ingestive and other behaviors. *American Journal of Physiology, 259,* R317–323.

Costello, J. F., Brown, M. R., & Gray, T. S. (1991). Bombesin immunoreactive neurons in the hypothalamic paraventricular nucleus innervate the dorsal vagal complex in the rat. *Brain Research, 542,* 77–82.

Covasa, M., Grahn, J., & Ritter, R. C. (2000). High fat maintenance diet attenuates hindbrain neuronal response to CCK. *Regulatory Peptides, 86,* 83–88.

Covasa, M., & Ritter, R. C. (1998). Rats maintained on high-fat diets exhibit reduced satiety in response to CCK and bombesin. *Peptides, 19,* 1407–1415.

Cowley, M. A., Smart, J. L., Rubinstein, M., Cerdan, M. G., Diano, S., Horvath, T. L., et al. (2001). Leptin activates anorexigenic POMC neurons through a neural network in the arcuate nucleus. *Nature, 411,* 480–484.

Cox, J. E., Kelm, G. R., Meller, S. T., & Randich, A. (2004). Suppression of food intake by GI fatty acid infusions: roles of celiac vagal afferents and cholecystokinin. *Physiology & Behavior, 82,* 27–33.

Cummings, D. E., Purnell, J. Q., Frayo, R. S., Schmidova, K., Wisse, B. E., & Weigle, D. S. (2001). A preprandial rise in plasma ghrelin levels suggests a role in meal initiation in humans. *Diabetes, 50,* 1714–1719.

Daniels, A. J., Chance, W. T., Grizzle, M. K., Heyer, D., & Matthews, J. E. (2001). Food intake inhibition and reduction in body weight gain in rats treated with GI264879A, a non-selective NPY-Y1 receptor antagonist. *Peptides, 22,* 483–491.

Davis, J. D., & Smith, G. P. (1990). Learning to sham feed: Behavioral adjustments to loss of physiological postingestive stimuli. *American Journal of Physiology, 259,* R1228–R1235.

Drucker, D. J., Philippe, J., Mojsov, S., Chick, W. L., & Habener, J. F. (1987). Glucagon-like peptide I stimulates insulin gene expression and increases cyclic AMP levels in a rat islet cell line. *Proceedings of the National Academy of Sciences, USA, 84,* 3434–3438.

Dunn, S. L., Bjornholm, H., Bates, S. H., Chen, Z., Seifert, M., & Myers, M. G., Jr. (2005). Feedback inhibition of leptin receptor/Jak 2 signaling via Tyr1138 of the leptin receptor suppressor of cytokine signaling 3. *Molecular Endocrinology 19,* 925–938.

Eastwood, C., Maubach, K., Kirkup, A. J., & Grundy, D. (1998). The role of endogenous cholecystokinin in the sensory transduction of luminal nutrient signals in the rat jejunum. *Neuroscience Letters, 254,* 145–148.

Eckel, L. A., Langhans, W., Kahler, A., Campfield, L. A., Smith, F. J., & Geary, N. (1998). Chronic administration of OB protein decreases food intake by selectively reducing meal size in female rats. *American Journal of Physiology, 275*(1, Pt. 2), R186–193.

El-Haschimi, K., Pierroz, D. D., Hileman, S. M., Bjorbaek, C., & Flier, J. S. (2000). Two defects contribute to hypothalamic leptin resistance in mice with diet-induced obesity. *Journal of Clinical Investigation, 105,* 1827–1832.

Elias, C. F., Aschkenasi, C., Lee, C., Kelly, J., Ahima, R. S., Bjorbaek, C., et al. (1999). Leptin differentially regulates NPY and POMC neurons projecting to the lateral hypothalamic area. *Neuron, 23,* 775–786.

Elmquist, J. K. (2001). Hypothalamic pathways underlying the endocrine, autonomic, and behavioral effects of leptin. *Physiology & Behavior, 74*(4–5), 703–708.

Elmquist, J. K., Bjorbaek, C., Ahima, R. S., Flier, J. S., & Saper, C. B. (1998). Distributions of leptin receptor mRNA isoforms in the rat brain. *Journal of Comparative Neurology, 395,* 535–547.

Emond, M., Ladenheim, E. E., Schwartz, G. J., & Moran, T. H. (2001). Leptin amplifies the feeding inhibition and neural activation arising from a gastric nutrient preload. *Physiology & Behavior, 72,* 123–128.

Emond, M., Schwartz, G. J., Ladenheim, E. E., & Moran, T. H. (1999). Central leptin modulates behavioral and neural responsivity to CCK. *American Journal of Physiology, 276*(5, Pt. 2), R1545–1549.

Emond, M., Schwartz, G. J., & Moran, T. H. (2001). Meal-related stimuli differentially induce c-Fos activation in the nucleus of the solitary tract. *American Journal of Physiology – Regulatory, Integrative and Comparative Physiology, 280,* R1315–1321.

Fan, W., Boston, B. A., Kesterson, R. A., Hruby, V. J., & Cone, R. D. (1997). Role of melanocortinergic neurons in feeding and the agouti obesity syndrome. *Nature, 385,* 165–168.

Faulconbridge, L. F., Cummings, D. E., Kaplan, J. M., & Grill, H. J. (2003). Hyperphagic effects of brainstem ghrelin administration. *Diabetes, 52,* 2260–2265.

Faulconbridge, L. F., Grill, H. J., & Kaplan, J. M. (2005). Distinct forebrain and caudal brainstem contributions to the neuropeptide Y mediation of ghrelin hyperphagia. *Diabetes, 54,* 1985–1993.

Fehmann, H. C., & Habener, J. F. (1992). Insulinotropic hormone glucagon-like peptide-I(7–37) stimulation of proinsulin gene expression and proinsulin biosynthesis in insulinoma beta TC-1 cells. *Endocrinology, 130*, 159–166.

Figlewicz, D. P., Evans, S. B., Murphy, J., Hoen, M., & Baskin, D. G. (2003). Expression of receptors for insulin and leptin in the ventral tegmental area/substantia nigra (VTA/SN) of the rat. *Brain Research, 964*, 107–115.

Flynn, F. W. (1993). Fourth ventricular injection of selective bombesin receptor antagonists facilitates feeding in rats. *American Journal of Physiology, 264*(1, Pt. 2), R218–221.

Flynn, M. C., Scott, T. R., Pritchard, T. C., & Plata-Salaman, C. R. (1998). Mode of action of OB protein (leptin) on feeding. *American Journal of Physiology, 275*(1, Pt. 2), R174–179.

Fraser, K. A., & Davison, J. S. (1992). Cholecystokinin-induced c-fos expression in the rat brain stem is influenced by vagal nerve integrity. *Experimental Physiology, 77*, 225–228.

Fulton, S., Woodside, B., & Shizgal, P. (2000). Modulation of brain reward circuitry by leptin. *Science, 287*, 125–128.

Geary, N., Le Sauter, J., & Noh, U. (1993). Glucagon acts in the liver to control spontaneous meal size in rats. *American Journal of Physiology, 264*(1, Pt. 2), R116–122.

Geary, N., & Smith, G. P. (1982a). Pancreatic glucagon and postprandial satiety in the rat. *Physiology & Behavior, 28*, 313–322.

Geary, N., & Smith, G. P. (1982b). Pancreatic glucagon fails to inhibit sham feeding in the rat. *Peptides, 3*, 163–166.

Geary, N., & Smith, G. P. (1983). Selective hepatic vagotomy blocks pancreatic glucagon's satiety effect. *Physiology & Behavior, 31*, 391–394.

Geliebter, A., Westreich, S., & Gage, D. (1988). Gastric distention by balloon and test-meal intake in obese and lean subjects. *American Journal of Clinical Nutrition, 48*, 592–594.

Giralt, M., & Vergara, P. (1999). Glucagonlike peptide-1 (GLP-1) participation in ileal brake induced by intraluminal peptones in rat. *Digestive Diseases and Sciences, 44*, 322–329.

Giraudo, S., Billington, C. J., & Levine, A. S. (1998). Feeding effects of hypothalamic injeciton of melanocortin 4 ligands. *Brain Research, 809*, 302–306.

Grandt, D., Schimiczek, M., Struk, K., Shively, J., Eysselein, V. E., Goebell, H., et al. (1994). Characterization of two forms of peptide YY, PYY(1-36) and PYY(3-36), in the rabbit. *Peptides, 15*, 815–820.

Grill, H. J. (2006). Distributed neural control of energy balance: contributions from hindbrain and hypothalamus. *Obesity, 14*(Suppl. 5), 216S–221S.

Grill, H. J., Donahey, J. C., King, L., & Kaplan, J. M. (1997). Contribution of caudal brainstem to d-fenfluramine anorexia. *Psychopharmacology, 130*, 375–381.

Grill, H. J., Ginsberg, A. B., Seeley, R. J., & Kaplan, J. M. (1998). Brainstem application of melanocortin receptor ligands produces long-lasting effects on feeding and body weight. *Journal of Neuroscience, 18*, 10128–10135.

Grill, H. J., & Kaplan, J. M. (1992). Sham feeding in intact and chronic decerebrate rats. *American Journal of Physiology, 262*(6, Pt. 2), R1070–1074.

Grill, H. J., & Kaplan, J. M. (2001). Interoceptive and integrative contributions of forebrain and brainstem to energy balance control. *International Journal of Obesity and Related Metabolic Disorders, 25*(Suppl. 5), S73–77.

Grill, H. J., Markison, S., Ginsberg, A., & Kaplan, J. M. (2000). Long-term effects on feeding and body weight after stimulation of forebrain or hindbrain CRH receptors with urocortin. *Brain Research, 867*, 19–28.

Grill, H. J., Schwartz, M. W., Kaplan, J. M., Foxhall, J. S., Breininger, J., & Baskin, D. G. (2002). Evidence that the caudal brainstem is a target for the inhibitory effect of leptin on food intake. *Endocrinology, 143*, 239–246.

Grill, H. J., & Smith, G. P. (1988). Cholecystokinin decreases sucrose intake in chronic decerebrate rats. *American Journal of Physiology, 254*(6, Pt. 2), R853–856.

Gualillo, O., Caminos, J. E., Nogueiras, R., Seoane, L. M., Arvat, E., Ghigo, E., et al. (2002). Effect of food restriction on ghrelin in normal-cycling female rats and in pregnancy. *Obesity Research, 10*, 682–687.

Gutzwiller, J. P., Degen, L., Heuss, L., & Beglinger, C. (2004). Glucagon-like peptide

1 (GLP-1) and eating. *Physiology & Behavior, 82,* 17–19.

Gutzwiller, J. P., Drewe, J., Goke, B., Schmidt, H., Rohrer, B., Lareida, J., et al. (1999). Glucagon-like peptide-1 promotes satiety and reduces food intake in patients with diabetes mellitus type 2. *American Journal of Physiology, 276*(5, Pt. 2), R1541–1544.

Gutzwiller, J. P., Goke, B., Drewe, J., Hildebrand, P., Ketterer, S., Handschin, D., et al. (1999). Glucagon-like peptide-1: a potent regulator of food intake in humans. *Gut, 44,* 81–86.

Hagan, M. M., Rushing, P. A., Schwartz, M. W., Yagaloff, K. A., Burn, P., Woods, S. C., et al. (1999). Role of the CNS melanocortin system in the response to overfeeding. *Journal of Neuroscience, 19,* 2362–2367.

Hahn, T. M., Breininger, J. F., Baskin, D. G., & Schwartz, M. W. (1998). Coexpression of Agrp and NPY in fasting-activated hypothalamic neurons. *Nature Neuroscience, 1,* 271–272.

Halaas, J. L., Gajiwala, K. S., Mafei, M., Cohen, S. L., Chait, B. T., Rabinopwitz, D., Lallone, R. L., Burley S. K. & Friedman, J. M. (1995). Weight reducing effects of the plasma protein encoded by the obese gene. *Science, 269,* 543–546.

Harfstrand, A., Fuxe, K., Agnati, L. F., Benfenati, F., & Goldstein, M. (1986). Receptor autoradiographical evidence for high densities of 125I-neuropeptide Y binding sites in the nucleus tractus solitarius of the normal male rat. *ACTA Physiologica Scandinavica, 128,* 195–200.

Haynes, A. C., Jackson, B., Chapman, H., Tadayyon, M., Johns, A., Porter, R. A. & Arch, J. R. (2000) A selective orexin-1 antagonist reduces food consumption in male and female rats. *Regulatory Peptides, 96,* 45–51.

Huo, L., Maeng, L., Bjorbaek, C., & Grill, H. J. (2007). Leptin and the control of food intake: neurons in the nucleus of the solitary tract are activated by both gastric distension and leptin. *Endocrinology, 148,* 2189–2197.

Huszar, D., Lynch, C. A., Fairchild-Huntress, V., Dunmore, J. H., Fang, Q., Berkemeier, L. R., et al. (1997). Targeted disruption of the melanocortin-4 receptor results in obesity in mice. *Cell, 88,* 131–141.

Imaki, T., Shibasaki, T., Hotta, M., & Demura, H. (1993). Intracerebroventricular administration of corticotropin-releasing factor induces c-fos mRNA expression in brain regions related to stress responses: comparison with pattern of c-fos mRNA induction after stress. *Brain Research, 616,* 114–125.

Imeryuz, N., Yegen, B. C., Bozkurt, A., Coskun, T., Villanueva-Penacarrillo, M. L., & Ulusoy, N. B. (1997). Glucagon-like peptide-1 inhibits gastric emptying via vagal afferent-mediated central mechanisms. *American Journal of Physiology, 273,* G920–927.

Kahler, A., Geary, N., Eckel, L. A., Campfield, L. A., Smith, F. J., & Langhans, W. (1998). Chronic administration of OB protein decreases food intake by selectively reducing meal size in male rats. *American Journal of Physiology, 275,* R180–185.

Kaiyala, K. J., Prigeon, R. L., Kahn, S. E., Woods, S. C., & Schwartz, M. W. (2000). Obesity induced by a high-fat diet is associated with reduced brain insulin transport in dogs. *Diabetes, 49,* 1525–1533.

Kalra, S. P., Dube, M. G., Sahu, A., Phelps, C. P., & Kalra, P. S. (1991). Neuropeptide Y secretion increases in the paraventricular nucleus in association with increased appetite for food. *Proceedings of the National Academy of Sciences, USA, 88,* 10931–10935.

Kaplan, J. M., Siemers, W., & Grill, H. J. (1997). Effect of oral versus gastric delivery on gastric emptying of corn oil emulsions. *American Journal of Physiology, 273*(4, Pt. 2), R1263–1270.

Kaplan, J. M., Spector, A. C., & Grill, H. J. (1992). Dynamics of gastric emptying during and after stomach fill. *American Journal of Physiology, 263*(4, Pt. 2), R813–819.

Kawai, K., Sugimoto, K., Nakashima, K., Miura, H., & Ninomiya, Y. (2000). Leptin as a modulator of sweet taste sensitivities in mice. *Proceedings of the National Academy of Sciences, USA, 97,* 11044–11049.

Kelly, L., Morales, S., Smith, B. K., & Berthoud, H. R. (2000). Capsaicin-treated rats permanently overingest low- but not high-concentration sucrose solutions. *American Journal of Physiology – Regulatory, Integrative and Comparative Physiology, 279,* R1805–1812.

Kennedy, G. C. (1953). The role of depot fat in the hypothalamic control of food intake in the rat. *Proceedings of the Royal Society of London B, 140,* 578–596.

Kieffer, T. J., McIntosh, C. H., & Pederson, R. A. (1995). Degradation of glucose-dependent insulinotropic polypeptide and truncated glucagon-like peptide 1 in vitro and in vivo by dipeptidyl peptidase IV. *Endocrinology, 136*, 3585–3596.

Kim, E. K., Miller, I., Landree, L. E., Borisy-Rudin, F. F., Brown, P., Tihan, T., et al. (2002). Expression of FAS within hypothalamic neurons: a model for decreased food intake after C75 treatment. *American Journal of Physiology – Endocrinology and Metabolism, 283*, E867–879.

Kim, E. M., O'Hare, E., Grace, M. K., Welch, C. C., Billington, C. J., & Levine, A. S. (2000). ARC POMC mRNA and PVN alpha-MSH are lower in obese relative to lean zucker rats. *Brain Research, 862*(1–2), 11–16.

Kinzig, K. P., D'Alessio, D. A., & Seeley, R. J. (2002). The diverse roles of specific GLP-1 receptors in the control of food intake and the response to visceral illness. *Journal of Neuroscience, 22*, 10470–10476.

Kinzig, K. P., Scott, K. A., Hyun, J., Bi, S., & Moran, T. H. (2006). Lateral ventricular ghrelin and fourth ventricular ghrelin induce similar increases in food intake and patterns of hypothalamic gene expression. *American Journal of Physiology – Regulatory, Integrative and Comparative Physiology, 290*, R1565–1569.

Koda, S., Date, Y., Murakami, N., Shimbara, T., Hanada, T., Toshinai, K., et al. (2005). The Role of the Vagal Nerve in Peripheral PYY(3-36)–Induced Feeding Reduction in Rats. *Endocrinology, 146*, 2369–2375.

Kojima, M., Hosoda, H., Date, Y., Nakazato, M., Matsuo, H., & Kangawa, K. (1999). Ghrelin is a growth-hormone-releasing acylated peptide from stomach. *Nature, 402*, 656–660.

Kokkotou, E. G., Tritos, N. A., Mastaitis, J. W., Slieker, L., & Maratos-Flier, E. (2001). Melanin-concentrating hormone receptor is a target of leptin action in the mouse brain. *Endocrinology, 142*, 680–686.

Komatsu, R., Matsuyama, T., Namba, M., Watanabe, N., Itoh, H., Kono, N., et al. (1989). Glucagonostatic and insulinotropic action of glucagonlike peptide I-(7-36)-amide. *Diabetes, 38*, 902–905.

Korner, J., Savontaus, E., Chua, S. C., Jr., Leibel, R. L., & Wardlaw, S. L. (2001). Leptin regulation of Agrp and Npy mRNA in the rat hypothalamus. *Journal of Neuroendocrinology, 13*, 959–966.

Koulischer, D., Moroder, L., & Deschodt-Lanckman, M. (1982). Degradation of cholecystokinin octapeptide, related fragments and analogs by human and rat plasma in vitro. *Regulatory Peptides, 4*, 127–139.

Ladenheim, E. E., Emond, M., & Moran, T. H. (2005). Leptin enhances feeding suppression and neural activation produced by systemically administered bombesin. *American Journal of Physiology – Regulatory, Integrative and Comparative Physiology, 289*, R473–R477.

Ladenheim, E. E., & Ritter, R. C. (1988). Low-dose fourth ventricular bombesin selectively suppresses food intake. *American Journal of Physiology, 255*(6, Pt. 2), R988–993.

Langhans, W., Pantel, K., Muller-Schell, W., Eggenberger, E., & Scharrer, E. (1984). Hepatic handling of pancreatic glucagon and glucose during meals in rats. *American Journal of Physiology, 247*(5, Pt. 2), R827–832.

Larsen, P. J., Fledelius, C., Knudsen, L. B., & Tang-Christensen, M. (2001). Systemic administration of the long-acting GLP-1 derivative NN2211 induces lasting and reversible weight loss in both normal and obese rats. *Diabetes, 50*, 2530–2539.

Lavin, J. H., Wittert, G. A., Andrews, J., Yeap, B., Wishart, J. M., Morris, H. A., et al. (1998). Interaction of insulin, glucagon-like peptide 1, gastric inhibitory polypeptide, and appetite in response to intraduodenal carbohydrate. *American Journal of Clinical Nutrition, 68*, 591–598.

Le Sauter, J., & Geary, N. (1987). Pancreatic glucagon and cholecystokinin synergistically inhibit sham feeding in rats. *American Journal of Physiology, 253*(5, Pt. 2), R719–725.

Le Sauter, J., & Geary, N. (1991). Hepatic portal glucagon infusion decreases spontaneous meal size in rats. *American Journal of Physiology, 261*(1, Pt. 2), R154–161.

Le Sauter, J., Noh, U., & Geary, N. (1991). Hepatic portal infusion of glucagon antibodies increases spontaneous meal size in rats. *American Journal of Physiology, 261*(1, Pt. 2), R162–165.

Levine, A. S., Rogers, B., Kneip, J., Grace, M., & Morley, J. E. (1983). Effect of centrally administered corticotropin releasing factor

(CRF) on multiple feeding paradigms. *Neuropharmacology, 22,* 337–339.

Lewis, D. E., Shellard, L., Koeslag, D. G., Boer, D. E., McCarthy, H. D., McKibbin, P. E., et al. (1993). Intense exercise and food restriction cause similar hypothalamic neuropeptide Y increases in rats. *American Journal of Physiology, 264*(2, Pt. 1), E279–284.

Liddle, R. A., Goldfine, I. D., Rosen, M. S., Taplitz, R. A., & Williams, J. A. (1985). Cholecystokinin bioactivity in human plasma. Molecular forms, responses to feeding, and relationship to gallbladder contraction. *Journal of Clinical Investigation, 75,* 1144–1152.

Lin, H. C., Zhao, X. T., Wang, L., & Wong, H. (1996). Fat-induced ileal brake in the dog depends on peptide YY. *Gastroenterology, 110,* 1491–1495.

Loftus, T. M., Jaworsky, D. E., Frehywot, G. L., Townsend, C. A., Ronnett, G. V., Lane, M. D., et al. (2000). Reduced food intake and body weight in mice treated with fatty acid synthase inhibitors. *Science, 288,* 2379–2381.

Lopez, M., Seoane, L., Garcia, M. C., Lago, F., Casanueva, F. F., Senaris, R., et al. (2000). Leptin regulation of prepro-orexin and orexin receptor mRNA levels in the hypothalamus. *Biochemical and Biophysical Research Communications, 269,* 41–45.

Lu, X. Y., Barsh, G. S., Akil, H., & Watson, S. J. (2003). Interaction between alpha-melanocyte-stimulating hormone and corticotropin-releasing hormone in the regulation of feeding and hypothalamo-pituitary-adrenal responses. *Journal Neuroscience, 23,* 7863–7872.

Lutz, T. A., Geary, N., Szabady, M. M., Del Prete, E., & Scharrer, E. (1995). Amylin decreases meal size in rats. *Physiology & Behavior, 58,* 1197–1202.

Lutz, T. A., Senn, M., Althaus, J., Del Prete, E., Ehrensperger, F., & Scharrer, E. (1998). Lesion of the area postrema/nucleus of the solitary tract (AP/NTS) attenuates the anorectic effects of amylin and calcitonin gene-related peptide (CGRP) in rats. *Peptides, 19,* 309–317.

Lynn, R. B., Bechtold, L. S., & Miselis, R. R. (1997). Ultrastructure of bombesin-like immunoreactive nerve terminals in the nucleus of the solitary tract and the dorsal motor nucleus. *Journal of the Autonomic Nervous System, 62,* 174–182.

Maffei, M., Halaas, J., Ravussin, E., Pratley, R. E., Lee, G. H., Zhang, Y., et al. (1995). Leptin levels in human and rodent: measurement of plasma leptin and ob RNA in obese and weight-reduced subjects. *Nature Medicine, 1,* 1155–1161.

Margolis, R. L., Moran, T. H., & McHugh, P. R. (1989). In vitro response of rat gastrointestinal segments to cholecystokinin and bombesin. *Peptides, 10,* 157–161.

Mathis, C., Moran, T. H., & Schwartz, G. J. (1998). Load-sensitive rat gastric vagal afferents encode volume but not gastric nutrients. *American Journal of Physiology, 274*(2, Pt. 2), R280–286.

Mayer, J. (1953). Glucostatic mechanism of regulation of food intake. *New England Journal of Medicine, 249,* 13–16.

McCann, M. J., & Rogers, R. C. (1990). Oxytocin excites gastric-related neurones in rat dorsal vagal complex. *Journal of Physiology, 428,* 95–108.

McMinn, J. E., Sindelar, D. K., Havel, P. J., & Schwartz, M. W. (2000). Leptin deficiency induced by fasting impairs the satiety response to cholecystokinin. *Endocrinology, 141,* 4442–4448.

Mendelson, J. (1969). Lateral hypothalamic stimulation: inhibition of aversive effects by feeding, drinking, and gnawing. *Science, 166,* 1431–1433.

Mercer, J. G., Moar, K. M., & Hoggard, N. (1998). Localization of leptin receptor (Ob-R) messenger ribonucleic acid in the rodent hindbrain. *Endocrinology, 139,* 29–34.

Mollet, A., Gilg, S., Riediger, T., & Lutz, T. A. (2004). Infusion of the amylin antagonist AC 187 into the area postrema increases food intake in rats. *Physiology & Behavior, 81,* 149–155.

Mook, D. G. (1963). Oral and postingestional determinants of intake of various solutions in rats with esophageal fistulas. *Journal of Comparative and Physiological Psychology, 56,* 645–659.

Mook, D. G. (1990). Satiety, specifications and stop rules: Feeding as a voluntary act. In A. N. Epstein & A. R. Morrison (Eds.), *Progress in Psychobiology and Physiological Psychology* (Vol. 14, pp. 1–65). New York: Academic Press.

Moran, T. H., Ameglio, P. J., Peyton, H. J., Schwartz, G. J., & McHugh, P. R. (1993). Blockade of type A, but not type B, CCK receptors postpones satiety in rhesus monkeys. *American Journal of Physiology, 265*(3, Pt. 2), R620–624.

Moran, T. H., Baldessarini, A. R., Salorio, C. F., Lowery, T., & Schwartz, G. J. (1997). Vagal afferent and efferent contributions to the inhibition of food intake by cholecystokinin. *American Journal of Physiology, 272*(4, Pt. 2), R1245–1251.

Moran, T. H., Crosby, R. J., & McHugh, P. R. (1991). Effects of pylorectomy on cholecystokinin-induced inhibition of liquid gastric emptying. *American Journal of Physiology, 261*(3, Pt. 2), R531–535.

Moran, T. H., Katz, L. F., Plata-Salaman, C. R., & Schwartz, G. J. (1998). Disordered food intake and obesity in rats lacking cholecystokinin A receptors. *American Journal of Physiology, 274*(3, Pt. 2), R618–625.

Moran, T. H., Knipp, S., & Schwartz, G. J. (1999). Gastric and duodenal features of meals mediate controls of liquid gastric emptying during fill in rhesus monkeys. *American Journal of Physiology, 277*(5, Pt. 2), R1282–1290.

Moran, T. H., & McHugh, P. R. (1982). Cholecystokinin suppresses food intake by inhibiting gastric emptying. *American Journal of Physiology, 242*, R491–497.

Moran, T. H., Norgren, R., Crosby, R. J., & McHugh, P. R. (1990). Central and peripheral vagal transport of cholecystokinin binding sites occurs in afferent fibers. *Brain Research, 526*, 95–102.

Moran, T. H., Shnayder, L., Hostetler, A. M., & McHugh, P. R. (1988). Pylorectomy reduces the satiety action of cholecystokinin. *American Journal of Physiology, 255*(6, Pt. 2), R1059–1063.

Moran, T. H., Smedh, U., Kinzig, K. P., Scott, K. A., Knipp, S., & Ladenheim, E. E. (2004). Peptide YY(3-36) inhibits gastric emptying and produces acute reductions in food intake in rhesus monkeys. *American Journal of Physiology – Regulatory, Integrative and Comparative Physiology, 288*, R384–R388.

Morley, J. E., Levine, A. S., Grace, M., & Kneip, J. (1985). Peptide YY (PYY), a potent orexigenic agent. *Brain Research, 341*, 200–203.

Morton, G. J., Blevins, J. E., Williams, D. L., Niswender, K. D., Gelling, R. W., Rhodes, C. J., et al. (2005). Leptin action in the forebrain regulates the hindbrain response to satiety signals. *Journal of Clinical Investigation, 115*, 703–710.

Nakagawa, A., Satake, H., Nakabayashi, H., Nishizawa, M., Furuya, K., Nakano, S., et al. (2004). Receptor gene expression of glucagon-like peptide-1, but not glucose-dependent insulinotropic polypeptide, in rat nodose ganglion cells. *Autonomic Neuroscience, 110*, 36–43.

Nakazato, M., Murakami, N., Date, Y., Kojima, M., Matsuo, H., Kangawa, K., et al. (2001). A role for ghrelin in the central regulation of feeding. *Nature, 409*, 194–198.

Naslund, E., Barkeling, B., King, N., Gutniak, M., Blundell, J. E., Holst, J. J., et al. (1999). Energy intake and appetite are suppressed by glucagon-like peptide-1 (GLP-1) in obese men. *International Journal of Obesity and Related Metabolic Disorders, 23*, 304–311.

Naslund, E., Gutniak, M., Skogar, S., Rossner, S., & Hellstrom, P. M. (1998). Glucagon-like peptide 1 increases the period of postprandial satiety and slows gastric emptying in obese men. *American Journal of Clinical Nutrition, 68*, 525–530.

Nathan, D. M., Schreiber, E., Fogel, H., Mojsov, S., & Habener, J. F. (1992). Insulinotropic action of glucagonlike peptide-I-(7–37) in diabetic and nondiabetic subjects. *Diabetes Care, 15*, 270–276.

Niimi, M., Sato, M., & Taminato, T. (2001). Neuropeptide Y in central control of feeding and interactions with orexin and leptin. *Endocrine, 14*, 269–273.

Nilsson, G., & Uvnas-Wallensten, K. (1977). Effect of teasing and sham feeding on plasma glucagon concentration in dogs. *Acta Physiologica Scandinavica, 100*, 298–302.

Niswender, K. D., Baskin, D. G., & Schwartz, M. W. (2004). Insulin and its evolving partnership with leptin in the hypothalamic control of energy homeostasis. *Trends in Endocrinology and Metabolism, 15*, 362–369.

Nonaka, N., Shioda, S., Niehoff, M. L., & Banks, W. A. (2003). Characterization of blood-brain barrier permeability to PYY(3-36) in the mouse. *Journal of Pharmacology and Experimental Therapeutics, 306*, 948–953.

Obici, S., Feng, Z., Morgan, K., Stein, D., Karkanias, G., & Rossetti, L. (2002). Central administration of oleic acid inhibits glucose production and food intake. *Diabetes, 51*, 271–275.

Onaga, T., Zabielski, R., & Kato, S. (2002). Multiple regulation of peptide YY secretion in the digestive tract. *Peptides, 23*, 279–290.

Oomura, Y., Ono, T., Ooyama, H., & Wayner, M. J. (1969). Glucose and osmosensitive neurones of the rat hypothalamus. *Nature, 222*, 282–284.

Orskov, C., Poulsen, S. S., Moller, M., & Holst, J. J. (1996). Glucagon-like peptide I receptors in the subfornical organ and the area postrema are accessible to circulating glucagon-like peptide I. *Diabetes, 45*, 832–835.

Parker, R. & Herzog, H. (1999). Regional distribution of Y receptor subtype mRNA in rat brain. *European Journal of Neuroscience, 11*, 1431–1448.

Pavlov, I. P. (1910). *The work of the digestive glands* (2nd ed.). London: Charles Griffin.

Peyron, C., Tighe, D. K., van den Pol, A. N., de Lecea, L., Heller, H. C., Sutcliffe, J. G., et al. (1998). Neurons containing hypocretin (orexin) project to multiple neuronal systems. *Journal of Neuroscience, 18*, 9996–10015.

Phillips, R. J., & Powley, T. L. (1996). Gastric volume rather than nutrient content inhibits food intake. *American Journal of Physiology, 271*(3, Pt. 2), R766–769.

Phillips, R. J., & Powley, T. L. (1998). Gastric volume detection after selective vagotomies in rats. *American Journal of Physiology, 274*(6, Pt. 2), R1626–1638.

Phillips, R. J., & Powley, T. L. (2000). Tension and stretch receptors in gastrointestinal smooth muscle: re-evaluating vagal mechanoreceptor electrophysiology. *Brain Research, 34*, 1–26.

Pironi, L., Stanghellini, V., Miglioli, M., Corinaldesi, R., De Giorgio, R., Ruggeri, E., et al. (1993). Fat-induced ileal brake in humans: a dose-dependent phenomenon correlated to the plasma levels of peptide YY. *Gastroenterology, 105*, 733–739.

Pi-Sunyer, X., Kissileff, H. R., Thornton, J., & Smith, G. P. (1982). C-terminal octapeptide of cholecystokinin decreases food intake in obese men. *Physiology & Behavior, 29*, 627–630.

Prechtl, J. C., & Powley, T. L. (1990). The fiber composition of the abdominal vagus of the rat. *Anatomy and Embryology, 181*, 101–115.

Qu, D., Ludwig, D. S., Gammeltoft, S., Piper, M., Pelleymounter, M. A., Cullen, M. J., et al. (1996). A role for melanin-concentrating hormone in the central regulation of feeding behaviour. *Nature, 380*, 243–247.

Randich, A., Tyler, W. J., Cox, J. E., Meller, S. T., Kelm, G. R., & Bharaj, S. S. (2000). Responses of celiac and cervical vagal afferents to infusions of lipids in the jejunum or ileum of the rat. *American Journal of Physiology – Regulatory, Integrative and Comparative Physiology, 278*, R34–43.

Raposinho, P. D., Pedrazzini, T., White, R. B., Palmiter, R. D., & Aubert, M. L. (2004). Chronic neuropeptide Y infusion into the lateral ventricle induces sustained feeding and obesity in mice lacking either Npy1r or Npy5r expression. *Endocrinology, 145*, 304–310.

Reidelberger, R. D., Haver, A. C., Arnelo, U., Smith, D. D., Schaffert, C. S., & Permert, J. (2004). Amylin receptor blockade stimulates food intake in rats. *American Journal of Physiology – Regulatory, Integrative and Comparative Physiology, 287*, R568–574.

Reidelberger, R. D., & O'Rourke, M. F. (1989). Potent cholecystokinin antagonist L 364718 stimulates food intake in rats. *American Journal of Physiology, 257*(6, Pt. 2), R1512–1518.

Rinaman, L. (1998). Oxytocinergic inputs to the nucleus of the solitary tract and dorsal motor nucleus of the vagus in neonatal rats. *Journal of Comparative Neurology, 399*, 101–109.

Ritter, R. C., & Ladenheim, E. E. (1985). Capsaicin pretreatment attenuates suppression of food intake by cholecystokinin. *American Journal of Physiology, 248*(4, Pt. 2), R501–504.

Ritzel, U., Fromme, A., Ottleben, M., Leonhardt, U., & Ramadori, G. (1997). Release of glucagon-like peptide-1 (GLP-1) by carbohydrates in the perfused rat ileum. *Acta Diabetologica, 34*, 18–21.

Roberge, J. N., & Brubaker, P. L. (1993). Regulation of intestinal proglucagon-derived peptide secretion by glucose-dependent insulinotropic peptide in a novel enteroendocrine loop. *Endocrinology, 133*, 233–240.

Roberge, J. N., Gronau, K. A., & Brubaker, P. L. (1996). Gastrin-releasing peptide is a novel mediator of proximal nutrient-induced proglucagon-derived peptide secretion from the distal gut. *Endocrinology, 137*, 2383–2388.

Rocca, A. S., & Brubaker, P. L. (1995). Stereospecific effects of fatty acids on proglucagon-derived peptide secretion in fetal rat intestinal cultures. *Endocrinology, 136*, 5593–5599.

Rodrigo, J., Hernandez, J., Vidal, M. A., & Pedrosa, J. A. (1975). Vegetative innervation of the esophagus. II. Intraganglionic laminar endings. *Acta Anat (Basel), 92*, 79–100.

Rodriquez de Fonseca, F., Navarro, M., Alvarez, E., Roncero, I., Chowen, J. A., Maestre, O., et al. (2000). Peripheral versus central effects of glucagon-like peptide-1 receptor agonists on satiety and body weight loss in Zucker obese rats. *Metabolism, 49*, 709–717.

Rogers, R. C., & Hermann, G. E. (1987). Oxytocin, oxytocin antagonist, TRH, and hypothalamic paraventricular nucleus stimulation effects on gastric motility. *Peptides, 8*, 505–513.

Rogers, R. C., Kita, H., Butcher, L. L., & Novin, D. (1980). Afferent projections to the dorsal motor nucleus of the vagus. *Brain Research Bulletin, 5*, 365–373.

Rolls, B. J. (1986). Sensory-specific satiety. *Nutrition Reviews, 44*, 93–101.

Rossi, M., Choi, S. J., O'Shea, D., Miyoshi, T., Ghatei, M. A., & Bloom, S. R. (1997). Melanin-concentrating hormone acutely stimulates feeding, but chronic administration has no effect on body weight. *Endocrinology, 138*, 351–355.

Rowland, N. E., & Richmond, R. M. (1999). Area postrema and the anorectic actions of dexfenfluramine and amylin. *Brain Research, 820*(1–2), 86–91.

Rushing, P. A., Hagan, M. M., Seeley, R. J., Lutz, T. A., D'Alessio, D. A., Air, E. L., et al. (2001). Inhibition of central amylin signaling increases food intake and body adiposity in rats. *Endocrinology, 142*, 5035.

Sawchenko, P. E., & Swanson, L. W. (1982). Immunohistochemical identification of neurons in the paraventricular nucleus of the hypothalamus that project to the medulla or to the spinal cord in the rat. *Journal of Comparative Neurology, 205*, 260–272.

Sawchenko, P. E., Swanson, L. W., & Vale, W. W. (1984). Corticotropin-releasing factor: co-expression within distinct subsets of oxytocin-, vasopressin-, and neurotensin-immunoreactive neurons in the hypothalamus of the male rat. *Journal of Neuroscience, 4*, 1118–1129.

Scarpace, P. J., Nicolson, M., & Matheny, M. (1998). UCP2, UCP3 and leptin gene expression: modulation by food restriction and leptin. *Journal of Endocrinology, 159*, 349–357.

Scharrer, E., Langhans, W. (1986). Control of food itnake by fatty acid oxidation. *American Journal of Physiology, 250*, R1003–R1006.

Schwartz, G. J. (2000). The role of gastrointestinal vagal afferents in the control of food intake: current prospects. *Nutrition, 16*, 866–873.

Schwartz, G. J., McHugh, P. R., & Moran, T. H. (1993). Gastric loads and cholecystokinin synergistically stimulate rat gastric vagal afferents. *American Journal of Physiology, 265*(4, Pt. 2), R872–876.

Schwartz, G. J., & Moran, T. H. (2002). Leptin and neuropeptide Y have opposing modulatory effects on nucleus of the solitary tract neurophysiological responses to gastric loads: implications for the control of food intake. *Endocrinology, 143*, 3779–3784.

Schwartz, G. J., Salorio, C. F., Skoglund, C., & Moran, T. H. (1999). Gut vagal afferent lesions increase meal size but do not block gastric preload-induced feeding suppression. *American Journal of Physiology, 276*(6, Pt. 2), R1623–1629.

Schwartz, G. J., Tougas, G., & Moran, T. H. (1995). Integration of vagal afferent responses to duodenal loads and exogenous CCK in rats. *Peptides, 16*, 707–711.

Schwartz, M. W., Seeley, R. J., Campfield, L. A., Burn, P., & Baskin, D. G. (1996). Identification of targets of leptin action in rat hypothalamus. *Journal of Clinical Investigation, 98*, 1101–1106.

Scott, K. A., & Moran, T. H. (2007). The GLP-1 agonist exendin-4 reduces food intake in non-human primates through changes in meal size. *American Journal of Physiology – Regulatory, Integrative and Comparative Physiology, 293*, R983–R987.

Seeley, R. J., & Woods, S. C. (2003). Monitoring of stored and available fuel by the CNS: implications for obesity. *Nature Reviews – Neuroscience, 4*, 901–909.

Shapiro, R. E., & Miselis, R. R. (1985). The central neural connections of the area postrema of the rat. *Journal of Comparative Neurology, 234*, 344–364.

Smith, G. P., Jerome, C., Cushin, B. J., Eterno, R., & Simansky, K. J. (1981). Abdominal vagotomy blocks the satiety effect of cholecystokinin in the rat. *Science, 213*, 1036–1037.

Smith, G. T., Moran, T. H., Coyle, J. T., Kuhar, M. J., O'Donahue, T. L., & McHugh, P. R. (1984). Anatomic localization of cholecystokinin receptors to the pyloric sphincter. *American Journal of Physiology, 246*(1, Pt. 2), R127–130.

Speakman, J. R. (2004). Obesity: the integrated roles of environment and genetics. *Journal of Nutrition, 134*(Suppl. 8), 2090S–2105S.

Stanley, B. G., Kyrkouli, S. E., Lampert, S., & Leibowitz, S. F. (1986). Neuropeptide Y chronically injected into the hypothalamus: a powerful neurochemical inducer of hyperphagia and obesity. *Peptides, 7,* 1189–1192.

Sun, Y., Wang, P., Zheng, H., & Smith, R. G. (2004). Ghrelin stimulation of growth hormone release and appetite is mediated through the growth hormone secretagogue receptor. *Proceedings of the National Academy of Sciences, USA, 101,* 4679–4684.

Sweet, D. C., Levine, A. S., Billington, C. J., & Kotz, C. M. (1999). Feeding response to central orexins. *Brain Research, 821,* 535–538.

Swithers, S. E., & Hall, W. G. (1994). Does oral experience terminate ingestion? *Appetite, 23,* 113–138.

Takiguchi, S., Takata, Y., Funakoshi, A., Miyasaka, K., Kataoka, K., Fujimura, Y., et al. (1997). Disrupted cholecystokinin type-A receptor (CCKAR) gene in OLETF rats. *Gene, 197*(1–2), 169–175.

Tang-Christensen, M., Larsen, P. J., Goke, R., Fink-Jensen, A., Jessop, D. S., Moller, M., et al. (1996). Central administration of GLP-1 (7-36) amide inhibits food and water intake in rats. *American Journal of Physiology, 271*(4, Pt. 2), R848–856.

Tang-Christensen, M., Vrang, N., & Larsen, P. J. (1998). Glucagon-like peptide 1(7-36) amide's central inhibition of feeding and peripheral inhibition of drinking are abolished by neonatal monosodium glutamate treatment. *Diabetes, 47,* 530–537.

Tartaglia, L. A., Dembski, M., Weng, X., Deng, N., Culpepper, J., Devos, R., et al. (1995). Identification and expression cloning of a leptin receptor, OB-R. *Cell, 83,* 1263–1271.

Teitelbaum, P., & Epstein, A. N. (1962). The lateral hypothalamic syndrome: recovery of feeding and drinking after lateral hypothalamic lesions. *Psychological Review, 69,* 74–90.

Thrasher, T. N., Brown, C. J., Keil, L. C., & Ramsay, D. J. (1980). Thirst and vasopressin release in the dog: an osmoreceptor or sodium receptor mechanism? *American Journal of Physiology, 238,* R333–339.

Tremblay, A. (2004). Dietary fat and body weight set point. *Nutrition Reviews, 62,* S75-77.

Tschop, M., Castaneda, T. R., Joost, H. G., Thone-Reineke, C., Ortmann, S., Klaus, S., et al. (2004). Physiology: does gut hormone PYY(3-36) decrease food intake in rodents? *Nature, 430,* 1–4.

Tschop, M., Smiley, D. L., & Heiman, M. L. (2000). Ghrelin induces adiposity in rodents. *Nature, 407,* 908–913.

Tu, Y., Thupari, J. N., Kim, E. K., Pinn, M. L., Moran, T. H., Ronnett, G. V., et al. (2005). C75 alters central and peripheral gene expression to reduce food intake and increase energy expenditure. *Endocrinology, 146,* 486–493.

Turton, M. D., O'Shea, D., Gunn, I., Beak, S. A., Edwards, C. M., Meeran, K., et al. (1996). A role for glucagon-like peptide-1 in the central regulation of feeding. *Nature, 379,* 69–72.

Uehara, Y., Shimizu, H., Ohtani, K., Sato, N., & Mori, M. (1998). Hypothalamic corticotropin-releasing hormone is a mediator of the anorexigenic effect of leptin. *Diabetes, 47,* 890–893.

Verdich, C., Toubro, S., Buemann, B., Lysgard Madsen, J., Juul Holst, J., & Astrup, A. (2001). The role of postprandial releases of insulin and incretin hormones in meal-induced satiety—effect of obesity and weight reduction. *International Journal of Obesity and Related Metabolic Disorders, 25,* 1206–1214.

Weingarten, H. P. (1984) Meal initiation controlled by learned cues: basic behavioral properties. *Appetite, 5,* 147–158.

Weingarten, H. P., & Kulikovsky, O. T. (1989). Taste-to-postingestive consequence conditioning: is the rise in sham feeding with repeated experience a learning phenomenon? *Physiology & Behavior, 45,* 471–476.

Weingarten, H. P., & Watson, S. D. (1982). Sham feeding as a procedure for assessing the influence of diet palatability on food intake. *Physiology & Behavior, 28,* 401–407.

West, D. B., Fey, D., & Woods, S. C. (1984). Cholecystokinin persistently suppresses meal size but not food intake in free-feeding rats. *American Journal of Physiology, 246*(5, Pt. 2), R776–787.

Widdowson, P. S., Upton, R., Henderson, L., Buckingham, R., Wilson, S., & Williams, G. (1997). Reciprocal regional changes in brain NPY receptor density during dietary restriction and dietary-induced obesity in the rat. *Brain Research, 774*(1–2), 1–10.Williams, D. L., Baskin, D. G., & Schwartz, M. W. (2006). Leptin regulation of the anorexic response to glucagon-like peptide-1 receptor stimulation. *Diabetes, 55*, 3387–3393.

Williams, D. L., Cummings, D. E., Grill, H. J., & Kaplan, J. M. (2003). Meal-related ghrelin suppression requires postgastric feedback. *Endocrinology, 144*, 2765–2767.

Yaswen, L., Diehl, N., Brennan, M. B., & Hochgeschwender, U. (1999). Obesity in the mouse model of pro-opiomelanocortin deficiency responds to peripheral melanocortin. *Nature Medicine, 5*, 1066–1070.

Zarjevski, N., Cusin, I., Vettor, R., Rohner-Jeanrenaud, F., & Jeanrenaud, B. (1993). Chronic intracerebroventricular neuropeptide-Y administration to normal rats mimics hormonal and metabolic changes of obesity. *Endocrinology, 133*, 1753–1758.

Zhang, X., Sun, X., Renehan, W., & Fogel, R. (2002). GRP mediates an inhibitory response of gut-related vagal motor neurons to PVN stimulation. *Peptides, 23*, 1649–1661.

Zhang, Y., Proenca, R., Maffei, M., Barone, M., Leopold, L., & Friedman, J. M. (1994). Positional cloning of the mouse obese gene and its human homologue. *Nature, 372*, 425–432.

4 OBESITY AND ADDICTION

Roy A. Wise

Introduction

Obesity and drug addiction result from homologous behaviors—behaviors with common biological roots. For the most part, the brain mechanisms of food and drug intake are the same as those of food and drug seeking. It is difficult to imagine how it could be otherwise. What evolutionary pressure could select in advance for a dedicated mechanism of addiction, a uniquely human and relatively recent phenomenon? Rather than independent brain mechanisms, the brain mechanisms of drug addiction evolved in the management and integration of vital motivated behaviors—sexual and ingestive behavior among them. Thus, our knowledge of compulsive drug intake and consequent addiction offers a heuristic model of compulsive food intake and consequent obesity. This chapter provides an overview of the increasing evidence for considering compulsive overeating of refined, high-energy foods as something akin to the compulsive ingestion of addictive drugs.

It should not be surprising that our animal ancestors first came into contact with addictive substances when foraging for food. By the end of the Jurassic period, several lines of plants had evolved the ability to synthesize poisonous alkaloids, some of which are addictive (Siegel, 1989). Such alkaloids are known as *secondary* plant compounds because they play no role in the primary metabolism of the plant. Rather, they enhance plant survival by protecting the plant from overgrazing by insects and other herbivores (Fraenkel, 1959; Freeland & Janzen, 1974). The early classes of bitter addictive substances—nicotine, opium, cocaine, and caffeine—are examples of such secondary plant alkaloids.

Although addiction has been imposed on lower animals in laboratory settings, animals do not become truly addicted in the wild. Birds, elephants, and other species do self-intoxicate by ingesting fermenting fruits, grains, and saps (Siegel, 1989), but their access to alcohol is too brief for them to develop alcohol dependence. Even when animals are given continual access to alcohol in the laboratory, it has proven remarkably difficult to establish alcohol dependence (Lester & Freed, 1973; Mello, 1973; Cicero, 1980). The key to establishing alcohol dependence is the maintenance of around-the-clock intoxication (Falk et al., 1972), but laboratory animals are more likely to drink alcohol if it is given intermittently (Wise, 1973).

Other than alcohol, few, if any, natural substances are truly addictive when ingested orally. Although mildly intoxicating levels of caffeine can be ingested by chewing the seeds, bark, or leaves of some 60 plants, only by steeping the plants in hot water do we extract concentrations that might be considered seriously addictive (Juliano & Griffiths, 2004). Intoxicating levels of cocaine were ingested for thousands of years by Incas who chewed the coca leaf (Paly et al., 1980). However, the levels of the drug that reach the blood after oral ingestion are low and slowly absorbed (Van Dyke et al., 1978) compared to those reached by the most dangerous routes of administration: smoking (Paly et al., 1982) and intravenous injection (Byck et al., 1980). Human ingenuity is required even to obtain intoxicating concentrations; the leaf is chewed along with an alkaline substance—*tocra* or *llipta*—that extracts significant concentrations of cocaine from the chewed leaf and hydrolyzes it. Although laboratory animals will self-administer laboratory solutions of opiates and cocaine by the oral route (Macenski & Meisch, 1994), they do not take them to the compulsive degree that is seen in humans with intravenous injections or smoking.

Indeed, many animal species have developed a love–hate relationship with plants containing addictive substances. As poisonous alkaloids evolved in plants, herbivores that avoided or limited their intake survived to reproduce. Many modern species learn with a single exposure to avoid new tastes and smells that are followed by nausea (Palmerino et al., 1980) or drug intoxication (Cappell & LeBlanc, 1975; Wise et al., 1976). This form of learning is remarkably robust; animals learn to avoid new foods that have made them sick even when the sickness develops many hours after ingestion of the food (Garcia et al., 1966). Animals are said to be particularly "prepared" to learn the association between novel tastes and illness (Seligman, 1970; Shettleworth, 1972). Thus, animals in the wild are unlikely to experience intoxication more than once from any given substance.

Human achievements were required to set the stage for addiction. The harnessing of fire made addiction to smoked opium and tobacco (and more recently heroin, cocaine, and methamphetamine) possible. The invention of cork, bottle, and distillation made alcohol available year-round and thus made alcoholism possible. The invention of the hypodermic syringe led to the primary method of addicting laboratory animals. And, of course, humans invented a number of our most troublesome addictive substances, including heroin, amphetamines, and barbiturates. Thus, addiction to drugs originated with the human species, the species that developed means for introducing drugs with sufficient speed and concentration to the long-established brain mechanisms of reward and motivation—mechanisms that had served foraging, the unique tendency of animals to seek out nourishment and mates rather than waiting, like plants, for food and fertilization to come to them.

Needs, Drives, and Reinforcement

Obesity is ultimately the result of overconsumption, of taking in more energy than is expended. We have many hypotheses to explain what makes us overeat: we eat in response to energy depletion or hormonal imbalance, because of stress, for pleasure, out of habit, and as an integral part of social interactions. Regardless of the origins we assign it, obesity ultimately results from eating unneeded nutritive substances, just as addiction results from ingesting unneeded addictive substances.[1] These are not surface resemblances. Rather, common mechanisms, common behavioral properties, and common dependency characteristics characterize both drug addiction and the overfeeding that results in obesity.

Despite the obvious fact that most humans in industrialized societies take in more energy than they burn, early behaviorists looked to biological need states for an explanation of our motivations to find and ingest food (Hull, 1943). Hunger was seen as a drive caused by energy depletion and was operationally defined as a function of time since the last meal. The motivations to drink, to find shelter from heat or cold, and to avoid pain were also seen as drives based on physiological needs. To make it fit the dominant model of the day, the motivation for sexual interaction was also discussed as satisfying a need: the "need" of the species for reproduction.

The formal theory that feeding is under the direct control of need states was quickly falsified. It was most directly contradicted by the finding that rats learn to work for non-nutritive saccharin as well as for nutritive sucrose (Sheffield & Roby, 1950). This fact gave rise to discussions of eating for the "pleasures of sensation" (Pfaffmann, 1960). The eagerness with which animals will work for direct electrical stimulation of so-called pleasure centers in the brain (Olds, 1958) was also seen as an example of working for pure sensation. The examples of social affiliation, play, manipulation, and novelty seeking (Harlow, 1953; Fiske & Maddi, 1961) each contributed further to the notion that many things are done for their intrinsic rewards and not merely because they satisfy biological needs. The study of animals in social settings revealed another source of cause for feeding: social imitation. Social animals often eat simply in response to the sight or sound of another animal eating (Santos et al., 2001; Galef, 2002; Ferrari et al., 2005).

Though it is obvious that evolution has favored animals that meet their bodily needs, it has not necessarily favored species that respond *only* or *very precisely* to their immediate needs. If our ancestors delayed eating until they really needed fuel, they would not have survived periods of prolonged danger or drought. Human sexual activity, another naturally motivated behavior, offers a clear example of how behavior can evolve away from biological necessity and toward

---

[1]One line of theory suggests that addictions result from the self-medication of preexisting conditions like depression or from the need to alleviate withdrawal distress resulting from prior recreational drug use. This is an interesting, if not universally accepted, view of addiction. An argument can be made for a parallel in obesity: eating to alleviate anxiety, stress, or other needs (Peters et al., 2007).

purely sensory rewards. In most other species, periods of fertility are marked by sensory cues that determine when copulation occurs, and copulation is restricted to times when procreation is possible. In humans, on the other hand, the sensory correlates of ovulation have been largely lost, presumably through natural selection (Diamond, 1997). Humans are unique in their lack of sensory awareness of ovulation, and they often continue to copulate during menstruation and after menopause—when conception is not possible. Indeed, humans have invented contraception and found ways to avoid or reduce the probability of conception even at times when the female is ovulating. For many humans, unique in the animal kingdom, sexual interaction has become an end in itself, no longer tied, as in lower animals, to the reproduction that accounts for its evolutionary success.

Similarly, the mechanisms of feeding are not limited to need reduction. Indeed, the phenomenon of obesity refutes the notion that we eat only in response to energy depletion. Fat is our vehicle for storing energy in advance of metabolic need. Such storage may have served our ancestors well during periods of drought and danger, but it serves us badly now, when energy-rich foods are abundant, inexpensive, and aggressively marketed. Although intake tends to precede need, the need to take in *at least* as much energy as we expend clearly explains our inherited tendency to graze when we encounter food. Among the mechanisms that encourage our inclination to eat beyond what we need is the mechanism of reinforcement and habit formation.

What makes a given reward rewarding? The answer is neither simple nor obvious. Water reward—a simpler case than food—illustrates this point. Unlike most foods, water is a simple substance, making its primary reinforcing property easier to identify. The reinforcing consequence of drinking water is the cooling of the oral cavity, as suggested by the fact that humans tend to prefer cool water over warm (Gold et al., 1973). More telling, however, is the fact that thirsty rats, in the absence of water, will compulsively lick a cool airstream (Mendelson & Chillag, 1970). Moreover, thirsty rats will even lick at a warm airstream, as long as the air is dry and warm and causes oral cooling through the evaporation of saliva (Freed & Mendelson, 1974). Not only does licking a warm, dry airstream fail to satisfy the need to hydrate; it actually dehydrates the animal further. Thus the tendency to cool the oral cavity when we are dehydrated is a tendency to respond for a sensory pleasure that is usually, *but not necessarily*, correlated with the satisfaction of a pending need. This tendency is usually sufficient to ensure that we take in more fluid than we need. In the case of drinking, surplus is simply voided by urination (Blass & Hall, 1976); unlike excess food, excess fluid is not stored.

In the case of food, the nature of reinforcement is more complicated. Most foods are complex mixtures of nutritive and non-nutritive substances. Most foods, therefore, help satisfy several nutritional needs at once, and they can be reinforcing for a variety of reasons. Some foods are intrinsically reinforcing because of their taste. Humans have what appear to be inborn preferences for sweet (Steiner, 1979) and salty (Denton, 1982) foods, but of course we have to learn through experience to identify the objects in our environment that have these qualities. Other foods can be reinforcing because they contain a needed vitamin or mineral (Garcia et al., 1967; Rozin & Rodgers, 1967). Thus there is no universal source of food reinforcement or satisfaction. Some people compulsively eat sweet foods; others compulsively eat fatty or salty foods. Initial tasting of specific foods often results from imitation of conspecifics (Galef, 2002) or even members of another species (Santos et al., 2001). However, whether or not we return to a given food—and how often and aggressively we do so—depends largely on the habit-forming property of the foods we sample, the property of *reinforcement*.

The most familiar form of reinforcement—termed *instrumental* or *operant* reinforcement—is the reinforcement we typically use to train our pets and children. Reinforcers are the rewards that we are willing to approach and work for. They include the things we consciously like (White, 1989) but also extend to things we don't necessarily recognize as liked—things that influence our behavior without being perceived as having influence (Aharon et al., 2001; Berridge & Winkielman, 2003). Under some circumstances, aversive events can be reinforcing (Kelleher & Morse, 1968). An instrumental reinforcer is defined as an object or event that, when its occurrence is contingent upon a given behavior, increases the probability of recurrence of that behavior. Through repeated reinforcement, initially random or imitative acts can rapidly evolve into habits, and certain food habits can escalate and result in obesity. This is the form of reinforcement common to addictive drugs (Johanson, 1978; Collins et al., 1984; Wise, 1987). As a reinforcing food or drug is repeatedly tried, the probability that it will be tried again steadily increases. Successive reinforcements change investigatory intake to "recreational" intake, and further repetition changes recreational intake to compulsive intake (Everitt & Robbins, 2005).

The things we come to crave are, for the most part, things we have experienced and found reinforcing in the past.[2] Although we appear to respond innately to the taste of sweet (Steiner, 1974) and salty (Denton, 1982) substances, we learn which foods to approach for these tastes only through our individual reinforcement histories. Why would a monkey, for example, crave a banana before learning that the yellow skin surrounds a sweet and edible white flesh? Humans (Harper & Sanders, 1975; de Castro, 1990), monkeys (Visalberghi & Addessi, 2000; Santos et al., 2001), pigs (Hsia & Wood-Gush, 1984), chicks (Strobel et al., 1970), blackbirds (Mason & Reidinger, 1981), and laboratory rats (Galef, 2002) are all known to sample foods that they see others eating, but it is a stretch to suggest that they truly crave specific foods before experiencing them.

---

[2]Humans, uniquely, can come to crave things that they have only heard or read about. Sexual cravings or cravings for caviar, for example, can develop in humans prior to significant experience with either. Word of mouth can similarly establish initial drug cravings. Although imitation can account for initial sexual or feeding incidents, it is reinforcement—perhaps only a single powerful reinforcement—that dramatically elevates cravings and establishes response habits that usually become increasingly compulsive.

Even when a sexually naive male is attracted to a receptive female by pheromones or other innate releasing stimuli, the initial attraction is much less powerful than the attraction exerted by the same cues after the male has had previous successful sexual experience (Whalen, 1966). The conditioned stimuli that come to trigger true cravings are termed *incentive motivational stimuli* in the specialist literature, and they come to exert increasing control over feeding, drug self-administration, and other forms of motivated behavior (Bindra, 1978).

Brain reinforcement mechanisms

Much of what we know about the brain mechanisms of acquired cravings and reinforcement comes from studies of the reinforcing effects of direct electrical stimulation of the brain. Focal brain stimulation all along the medial forebrain bundle is strongly rewarding in a broad variety of species; goldfish, guinea pigs, bottlenose dolphins, cats, dogs, goats, and monkeys have each been trained to make arbitrary responses for such stimulation (Olds, 1962). Human neurological and psychiatric patients have also shown willingness to stimulate this and related regions of their own brains, reporting that such stimulation is pleasurable (Monroe & Heath, 1954; Sem-Jacobsen, 1959; Heath, 1963).

The effects of stimulation of medial forebrain bundle sites are quite profound; rats will press a lever several thousand times per hour for such stimulation (Olds et al., 1960) and will cross a strongly electrified grid for the opportunity to do so (Olds, 1958). Remarkably, except for periods of eating and exhaustion, they will work hour after hour for weeks for such stimulation (Valenstein & Beer, 1964), appearing never to satiate (Olds & Olds, 1963). Most specialists concur that a subset of fibers within the medial forebrain bundle forms a critical part of the substrate through which most drug and naturally occurring reinforcers exert their influence over behavior. Electrolytic or neurotoxic lesions of the medial forebrain bundle at the level of the lateral hypothalamus render animals aphagic (unable to eat), adipsic (unable to regulate water intake properly), and seemingly lacking in positive affect (Teitelbaum & Epstein, 1962; Ungerstedt, 1971).

Pharmacological studies have pinpointed the mesocorticolimbic dopamine system as a major link in the brain's reward circuitry (Wise & Rompré, 1989). The fibers of this system ascend the medial forebrain bundle, are small and unmyelinated, and are relatively insensitive to direct stimulation (Gallistel et al., 1981); thus, few dopamine fibers are directly activated by the stimulating currents typically used (Yeomans et al., 1988). Other medial forebrain bundle fibers are activated directly, however; and they, in turn, activate the dopamine system (You et al., 2001; Hernandez et al., 2006). Lateral hypothalamic stimulation preferentially activates large myelinated fibers that descend the medial forebrain bundle (Bielajew & Shizgal, 1986) and are thought to activate the dopamine system directly (Wise, 1982) or, via the pedunculopontine tegmental and laterodorsal tegmental nuclei, transsynaptically (Yeomans et al., 2001).

Whether direct or indirect, rewarding lateral hypothalamic stimulation activates the dopamine fibers, causing dopamine release in the nucleus accumbens and other forebrain sites (Gratton et al., 1988; You et al., 2001; Hernandez et al., 2006). Drugs such as amphetamine, heroin, and cocaine, given intravenously, also elevate extracellular dopamine (Figure 4.1); self-administered doses tend

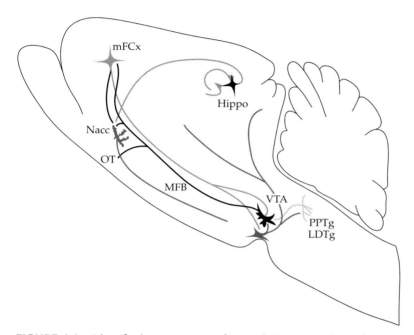

FIGURE 4.1   Identified components of reward circuitry in the rat brain. Food reward activates cells in the ventral tegmental area (VTA) probably via taste input from the cranial nerves. Nicotine activates dopaminergic neurons either directly or by causing local release of the excitatory neurotransmitter glutamate (which is found in fibers originating in the medial prefrontal cortex (mFCx) among other sources. Heroin activates the dopamine system by attenuating the inhibitory effects of GABAergic cells that are also found in the VTA. Amphetamine causes dopamine release from nerve terminals in nucleus accumbens (Nacc), olfactory tubercle (OT), and mFCx; cocaine causes dopamine accumulation in these structures by blocking the normal inactivation process. The medial forebrain bundle (MFB) carries the dopamine fibers to their terminal fields in Nacc, OT, and mFCx, where the rewarding effects of these substances and of MFB electrical stimulation are triggered. The MFB also carries glutamatergic fibers from the mFCx and GABA fibers from Nacc, plus about 50 other fiber pathways, most with unrelated functions, back to and beyond the VTA. The schematic shows single lines to represent this sampling of reward-relevant circuitry, but each line represents hundreds of fibers of a particular projection. Thus, the drawing is a very oversimplified introduction to the known portions of the circuitry.

to do so by 300% to 500% (Wise, Leone, et al., 1995; Wise, Newton, et al., 1995; Ranaldi et al., 1999). Blocking the receptors that normally respond to the released dopamine blocks the rewarding effects of medial forebrain bundle brain stimulation (Fouriezos & Wise, 1976; Franklin, 1978; Gallistel et al., 1982), as well as of intravenous amphetamine (Yokel & Wise, 1975) and cocaine (de Wit & Wise, 1977; Ettenberg et al., 1982); it does so by devaluing these rewards rather than by impairing the response capability of the animal (Wise & Rompré, 1989).

Animals treated with low doses of dopamine antagonists respond to electrical stimulation as if the stimulating current were weaker than normal (Fouriezos & Wise, 1976; Fouriezos et al., 1978; Franklin, 1978; Gallistel & Karras, 1984). This tendency is reflected in a rightward shift of the function relating response rate to stimulation frequency or intensity; although normal response rates can be obtained, stronger-than-normal stimulation is required to produce normal responding in animals with blocked dopamine receptors (Franklin, 1978; Gallistel & Karras, 1984; Gallistel & Freyd, 1987; Rompré & Wise, 1989).

In rats pretreated with low and moderate doses of dopamine antagonists, normal rates of responding are seen in the first few minutes of testing, and normal renewal of responding can be triggered by reward-predicting stimuli; however, once the animals have sampled the reward in this condition, they slow or cease responding (Fouriezos & Wise, 1976; Fouriezos et al., 1978; Franklin & McCoy, 1979). Similarly, animals treated with dopamine antagonists respond to amphetamine or cocaine as if the dose were less than what is actually given (Yokel & Wise, 1975; de Wit & Wise, 1977). Here, when treated with low doses of dopamine antagonists, they compensate by taking more amphetamine or cocaine; when high doses of dopamine antagonists are given, the animals respond at high initial rates but then cease responding completely (Yokel & Wise, 1975; de Wit and Wise, 1977).

Natural rewards like food (Hernandez & Hoebel, 1988; Bassareo & Di Chiara, 1999) and sex (Fiorino et al., 1997) also increase extracellular dopamine levels, although they tend to do so to a lesser degree (Figure 4.2)—increases of 150% to 200% of normal (Hernandez & Hoebel, 1988; Fiorino et al., 1997; Bassareo & Di Chiara, 1999)—than is seen with the previously mentioned drugs. As with brain stimulation and drug reward, animals treated with dopamine antagonists treat food reward as if it had been devalued. They approach food and begin to eat it or work for it normally, but eating or responding is not sustained at a normal level as the animals gain experience with the taste of the food under the condition of dopamine receptor blockade (Wise et al., 1978; Geary & Smith, 1985; Schneider et al., 1986; Wise & Raptis, 1986). Animals that are trained when hungry but tested when satiated (Morgan, 1974) cease responding progressively in the same pattern (Wise et al., 1978). Rats drinking sucrose under dopamine blockade respond at normal rates but require higher concentrations of sucrose to do so (Bailey et al., 1986; Schneider et al., 1990).

Several additional chemical messengers are involved in both drug reward and natural rewards. These are the neurotransmitters of various systems that

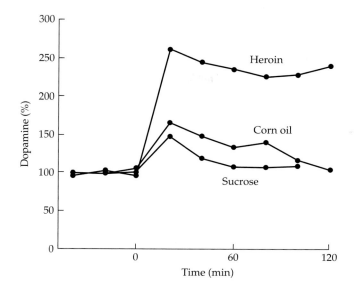

FIGURE 4.2   Relative effects of self-administered oral sucrose, oral corn oil, and intravenous heroin rewards on nucleus accumbens dopamine levels. Based on data of Hajnal et al. (2004), Liang et al. (2006) and Wise et al. (1995).

synapse on dopamine neurons or receive synapses from dopamine neurons. Most addictive drugs (alcohol is the notable exception) are known to act at one or more of the receptors or transporters for the other neurotransmitters. These include receptors for two classes of neurotransmitters known to modulate food intake: the endogenous opioid and cannabinoid neurotransmitters. Pharmacological blockade of opioid receptors attenuates feeding not only in mammals (Holtzman, 1974; Jalowiec et al., 1981; Wise & Raptis, 1986; Kavaliers & Hirst, 1987), but also in such primitive animals as slugs and snails (Kavaliers & Hirst, 1987), and even the single-celled amoeba (Josefsson and Johansson, 1979). Thus, endogenous opioids have been involved in the control of feeding throughout our evolutionary history.

Administration of opioids directly into the ventral tegmental area, where endogenous opioids synapse, stimulates feeding (Jenck et al., 1986; Mucha & Iversen, 1986; Wise et al., 1986; Noel & Wise, 1993, 1995); both mu (μ) and delta (δ) opioids are effective in this region, and they are effective in proportion to their differential abilities to activate the dopamine system (Devine et al., 1993) and to serve as rewards in their own right (Devine & Wise, 1994). The administration of opioids into the dopamine terminal fields of the striatum, particularly into the shell portion of the nucleus accumbens, also facilitates feeding (Mucha & Iversen, 1986; Evans & Vaccarino, 1990; Bakshi & Kelley, 1993; Zhang & Kelley, 2000). Nucleus accumbens opioids appear to increase preferentially the consumption of sweet and high-fat foods (Zhang & Kelley, 2002; Will et al., 2006), and they enhance the orofacial responses typically associated with the taste of sucrose (Pecina & Berridge, 2005). Morphine (Olds, 1982) and the endogenous opioid methionine enkephalin (Goeders et al., 1984) have rewarding actions in this same region.

Similarly, intravenous (Tanda et al., 2000) and intracranial (Zangen et al., 2006) injections of Δ^9-tetrahydrocannabinol (the active ingredient in marijuana and hashish) and intravenous injections of the endogenous cannabinoid anandamide (Justinova et al., 2005) are rewarding. Cannabinoids have long been known for their ability to facilitate feeding, particularly the eating of sweet foods (Hollister, 1971; Abel, 1975; Gross et al., 1983; Foltin et al., 1986). Endogenous cannabinoids are found in many places in the brain; among their actions is the ability to elevate brain dopamine levels (Chen et al., 1991; Tanda et al., 1997). Two reward sites in the brain have been identified for cannabinoids: the ventral tegmental area and the nucleus accumbens (Zangen et al., 2006). Antagonists for endogenous cannabinoids attenuate the rewarding effects not only of marijuana and hashish (Tanda et al., 2000; Zangen et al., 2006), but also of food (Thornton-Jones et al., 2005) and nicotine (Cohen et al., 2002). Cannabinoids and endogenous opioids appear to have a shared mechanism of action, since blocking ventral tegmental opioid receptors blocks the effect of cannabinoids on dopamine levels (Tanda et al., 1997). Clinical trials are in progress to determine if cannabinoid receptor antagonists might be useful for dieters or smokers (Curioni & Andre, 2006; Lopez-Moreno et al., 2006; Tucci et al., 2006).

As mentioned earlier, brain dopamine is important for the habit-forming effects of brain stimulation reward and of several addictive drugs. It is also important for the habit-forming effects of food. Animals pretreated with dopamine antagonists behave as if the food were somehow devalued, as if it were unrewarding or less rewarding than usual (Wise et al., 1978; Ettenberg & Camp, 1986; Wise & Raptis, 1986; Bailey et al., 1986; Schneider et al., 1990). Such animals fail to learn new instrumental responses for food (Wise & Schwartz, 1981); if already trained, they show extinction of food-rewarded habits (Wise et al., 1978; Beninger, 1982; Ettenberg & Camp, 1986). Thus the brain circuitry of food reward involves dopamine, the neurotransmitter most broadly implicated in drug and brain stimulation reward, as well as the endogenous opioid endomorphin (Zangen et al., 2002) and the endogenous cannabinoid anandamide (Justinova et al., 2005).

Interestingly, brain dopamine appears to be more involved in responsiveness to food-associated cues (Schultz et al., 1993) and the approach behaviors that these cues control (Bakshi & Kelley, 1991; Salamone et al., 1994), than to the sensory properties of food itself (Berridge et al., 1989). Thus, although opioid and cannabinoid antagonists attenuate free feeding, dopamine antagonists attenuate lever pressing for food long before they block the consumption of the earned food (Wise et al., 1978; Salamone et al., 1994).

Another indication that the mechanisms of feeding and addiction overlap is that natural motivational states interact with drug reward. Food restriction enhances the rewarding effects not only of food, but also of lateral hypothalamic brain stimulation (Blundell & Herberg, 1968; Carr & Wolinsky, 1993) and of cocaine, amphetamine, heroin, and nicotine (Carroll, 1999). Conversely, the satiety factor leptin attenuates not only the hunger for food but also the ability of food restriction to enhance motivation for brain stimulation and cocaine rewards (Fulton et al., 2000; Shalev, Yap, et al., 2001). Thus, hunger mechanisms modulate the impact of addictive drugs.

Finally, recent animal studies reveal that excessive intermittent binge eating can lead to an opiate-type dependence syndrome. Rats given intermittent access to 25% glucose solutions come to drink large amounts in the first hour of each exposure. After a week of exposure on a once-a-day schedule, challenge with the opioid antagonist naloxone precipitates opiate-type withdrawal symptoms: tooth chattering and heightened reactivity in a test of fear (Colantuoni et al., 2002). Inasmuch as these animals never received exogenous opiates, their dependence syndrome appears to result from excessive release of endogenous opioids: endogenous opioid neurotransmitter release caused by the binge feeding of glucose.

Taken together, these several lines of evidence implicate brain mechanisms of food reward and food intake in aspects of drug reward and drug intake. Brain dopamine plays a major role in both food-seeking and drug-seeking behaviors, and endogenous opioid and cannabinoid systems appear to play important roles in sweet palatability and sweet and fat intake. In addition, recent studies have begun to link peptide modulators of food intake such as leptin (Fulton et al., 2000), hypocretin (orexin; Boutrel et al., 2005; Harris et al., 2005), and melanin-concentrating hormone (Duncan et al., 2006) to aspects of drug reward and intake.

Genetic predispositions

Genetic variation contributes to differences in the vulnerability to both addiction and obesity. Estimates of the heritability of obesity tend to be in the range of 50% to 70% (Baessler et al., 2005; Walley et al., 2006); for risk of addiction, these estimates tend to be in the similar range of 40% to 60% (Uhl et al., 2002). Such global estimates can be misleading, however, because they imply that heredity and environment are additive when they are really interactive (see Hebb, 1980, pp. 72–74). Heritability estimates are valid only for the species tested and the environment in which the tests were made; because they are interactive, the same genotype will not necessarily carry the same importance in a different ecological niche. Obviously heritability estimates from a country where a drug like alcohol is illegal will not generalize to a country where it is freely available (Johnson et al., 1998). Indeed, estimates of the heritability of body mass in sheep can vary significantly depending merely on what time of year the estimates are made (Reale et al., 1999). Although statements of the percentage of variance controlled by genetics can be misleading when generalized across substances, routes of administration, and availability, genotypic variation clearly contributes importantly to the variability of both obesity and addiction.

Early studies on the genetics of vulnerability to addiction and obesity have tended to focus on monogenetic sources such as mutations in the genes for specific receptors, neurotransmitters, gut peptides, or enzymes (Volkow et al., 1993; Montague et al., 1997; Krude et al., 1998; Vaisse et al., 2000; Martinez et al., 2004; Martinez et al., 2005). However, polygenetic risk factors are probably more important for the explosive rise in addiction and obesity in recent decades (Crabbe, 2002; Walley et al., 2006); indeed, single-gene mutations have been suggested to explain less than 5% of human obesity (Walley et al., 2006).[3] Identification of polygenetic influences on behavioral traits is expensive and progresses slowly (Crabbe & Belknap, 1992), but it is interesting that the C57BL and 129 mice, with high and low sensitivity to sweet taste, respectively (Bachmanov et al., 2001), are among those with the highest and lowest acceptance of alcohol and other addictive drugs (Belknap, Crabbe, & Young, 1993; Belknap, Crabbe, Riggan, et al., 1993).

Environmental factors in craving

Although genetic factors are important, genetic drift and natural selection have not had time to contribute much to the rapid increase in human obesity over the last few decades. Genetic risk for addiction has surely been with us for centuries, and probably millennia. The number of overweight young people in the United States has roughly tripled since 1980; the human genome has probably changed very little during this period. What has changed dramatically in recent years is the availability of calorie-enriched processed foods and exposure to food symbols and advertising. Just as modern farming and chemical processing in the undeveloped world have made addictive drugs more available, so have modern farming and chemical processing in the developed world (for an overview, see Pollan, 2006) made energy-dense foods inexpensive and widely available. Unlike most addictive drugs, addictive foods can be marketed openly and aggressively.

Food availability has increased in both obvious and subtle ways over the last half century. First, expendable income has increased since World War II and the Depression years. Snacks and luxury foods have become affordable not only because they have become less expensive, but also because the more basic needs of much of the population are now more easily met. Second, meals—particularly commercially prepared meals—have become larger. Meal portions in restaurants have generally increased, despite attempts, such as accompanying large plates with small portions in the "nouvelle cuisine" of the 1980s, to restrict them. Indeed, fast-food restaurants have not only offered very energy-rich meals at low prices but have encouraged the "supersizing" of portions. As the adult population becomes increasingly obese, social facilitation of feeding encourages larger meals (de Castro, 1990). Where "balanced" diets are still offered in school cafeterias, unbalanced alternatives are also increasingly offered, if not at the meal

---

[3]Again, this figure should not be generalized very far beyond the population on which it was based.

counter then in candy, snack, and drink machines that are now widely found in schools, hospitals, and other public places.

Along with snack and drink machines and fast-food restaurants has come a proliferation of snack, drink, and fast-food advertising. Though we have curtailed tobacco and alcohol advertising on the assumption that it increases the use of unhealthful substances, advertising for unhealthful foods has increased in pace with the obesity epidemic. Advertising is certainly an environmental factor relevant to both addiction, where it has been discouraged, and obesity, where it goes unchecked. As discussed in the next section, the advertising itself is a stimulus to eat, and the increase of advertising is, in a way, a contribution to increased food availability.

Animal Models of Relapse: Priming, Stress, and Cues

Animal models have been used to study the conditions under which drug-seeking habits become reinstated after periods of abstinence. In these models, animals are first trained to press a lever to receive intravenous injections of a drug such as cocaine or heroin. Abstinence is then imposed and the lever-pressing habit is nearly extinguished by allowing the animals to continue pressing the lever for nonrewarding physiological saline injections. The animals continue, for a few weeks, to press the lever despite the absence of drug; however, their response rate eventually drops to pretraining levels. When spontaneous lever pressing has become very infrequent, the animals are challenged with conditions associated with relapse in human addicts.

Three classes of challenge cause animals to resume drug seeking (lever pressing) despite the continued absence of reward (Shaham et al., 2003). First, an unearned injection of the training drug (de Wit & Stewart, 1981, 1983) or a related drug (Wise et al., 1990) causes renewed responding; such "priming injections" are among the most effective provocations for reinstatement of the drug-seeking response habit. Second, stressors such as mild foot shock or food deprivation can also be very effective (Shaham & Stewart, 1995; Erb et al., 1996). Finally, stimuli that have been associated with drug injections in the past—drug-predictive stimuli—can also reinstate drug-seeking behaviors in this model (Meil & See, 1996).

This model has also been used to study the reinstatement of habits trained under food reward, and parallel findings have been obtained. Foot shock or the stress caused by the adrenergic antagonist yohimbine reinstates lever pressing in rats previously trained to work for sucrose reward (Ghitza et al., 2006), much as it does in rats previously trained to work for cocaine (Lee et al., 2004), alcohol (Le et al., 2005), or methamphetamine reward (Shepard et al., 2004). Thus, just as findings from the reinstatement model are consistent with the widely held view that stress precipitates relapse to addiction (Sinha et al., 1999), so too are they consistent with the widely held view that stress can precipitate relapse to eating highly palatable foods (Herman & Polivy, 1975; Crowther et al., 2001;

Dallman et al., 2003). For an understanding of the recent escalation in obesity, however, the more important implications of the reinstatement model may come from studies of priming- and cue-induced reinstatement.

The administration of a small unearned reward is termed *priming*; like the priming of a dry pump, priming gets things flowing. Priming has long been used to trigger prompt reinitiation of intracranial self-stimulation (Deutsch et al., 1964) or drug self-administration (Pickens & Harris, 1968) at the start of a new testing session. Animals that have learned to self-administer electrical stimulation of the brain (Annau et al., 1974) or intravenous drugs (Pickens & Harris, 1968) occasionally stop responding because of exhaustion during a prolonged session; here, too, priming appears to remind the animal of the reward and turn its attention back to the response lever.

Priming exerts similar power over self-imposed abstinence in humans.[4] Thus, 12-step programs stress total abstinence (Nowinski et al., 1992): a single drink or a single cigarette puts the abstinent addict at risk for obsessive thoughts and actual relapse. In the animal model, priming (de Wit & Stewart, 1981, 1983; Wise et al., 1990) is usually much more effective than stress or reward-predictive cues (Shaham et al., 2003) in reinstating a no-longer-rewarded (but clearly not forgotten) response habit. It can take weeks of additional extinction training to reverse the effects of a single priming injection of cocaine given to an animal that has undergone extinction training (Wang et al., 2005).

The implications for obesity are profound because dieting by total abstinence requires hospitalization and intubation. We cannot totally abstain from eating. At best we can abstain for a limited period or from a subset of specified problem foods, and even that is difficult because most or our commercially available foods are laced with effective priming stimuli, like sugar and salt. Foods offered at social occasions are even more problematic. The temptation to join the party— to have just one small piece of cake or chocolate—increases the risk of relapse to old and unhealthy eating habits. No matter how hard it is for the dieter or the addict to avoid the first bite or the first drink, it is much more difficult to avoid the second. The effects of eating salted peanuts and potato chips are good examples of the priming effects of taste stimuli.

Cue-induced relapse is a less obvious but perhaps more pervasive phenomenon among those attempting to control their food intake. The efforts of the advertising industry are predicated on the assumption that food-associated stimuli (symbols) provoke food-seeking behaviors. Two kinds of cues can induce relapse to food or drug seeking. The first, known as a *discriminative* stimulus or an *occasion setter*, is a stimulus that signals *availability* of the reward. In many experiments, the discriminative stimulus is a start signal such as illumination

---

[4]Self-imposed abstinence, like addiction itself, is a uniquely human phenomenon. In the cases of self-administration of intravenous cocaine, amphetamine, or heroin, self-imposed abstinence by well-trained laboratory animals is rarely, if ever, seen—unless there is a problem with the intravenous catheter.

of the house lights or insertion of a response lever into the animal's cage; in others, it is the testing context itself. At home it is the smell of food cooking. It is a stimulus that says the reward will soon be available.

The second kind of cue is a conditioned or *secondary* reinforcer—a stimulus that we work for because of its association with an unconditioned reinforcer. It appears only after we make a particular required response. For humans, the best example is money—something we work for because of its arbitrary and learned value. For the laboratory rat it might be a light that is earned by every lever press and is presented along with a primary reinforcer that is earned, say, by every tenth lever press. The two cues differ necessarily only in that one is a priming stimulus, telling the animal that it is time to make the learned response, whereas the other is a reinforcing stimulus, signaling that the animal has made the correct response and the reward is coming or that the animal has made a part of the correct response and is thus on the right track.

Each of these types of cues has the potential to reinstate extinguished responding in the animal model. Each serves as a reminder of the reward, and each increases the probability that the animal will repeat or continue the acts that have led to the reward in the past (Grimm et al., 2001). The pictures of foods, the smells of food cooking, the jingle of the ice cream truck, and the signs and symbols of the fast-food restaurant are among the discriminative stimuli of modern society; the taste of artificial sweeteners is the conditioned reinforcer that sustains our interest in diet drinks.

A recently discovered phenomenon of cue-induced reinstatement of drug seeking—*incubation of craving*—may also have important implications for understanding food cravings and food-seeking behaviors. Here a period of abstinence was imposed between training animals to self-administer intravenous cocaine and extinguishing the response prior to subsequent reinstatement testing. The longer the period of abstinence was, the stronger the responding was during the extinction period (Grimm et al., 2001). The craving for the unobtainable drug appeared to incubate—to grow spontaneously stronger—as the traditional physiological abstinence symptoms were growing weaker. Only after 3 months of abstinence does the strength of responding in extinction begin to weaken in cocaine-trained animals. Similar time-dependent increases in craving for heroin (Shalev, Morales, et al., 2001) and sucrose (Grimm et al., 2002) have been found, although the times of peak craving are shorter in these cases. The obvious implication for dieters is that however hard it is to initiate a diet, it will be even harder, perhaps for quite some time, to maintain it.

Cue-induced craving is known in the specialist literature as *incentive motivation*, the kind of craving or motivation that is provoked not by inner need or hormonal states, but rather by an external stimulus (Bindra, 1974). Sexual motivation in the male, for example, can be triggered by the various cues of receptivity given by the females of different species, such as the release of a pheromone or the reddened vulva of the receptive baboon. These are unconditioned stimuli that best illustrate the concept of incentive motivation: arousal and focused attention elicited by the incentive itself. The notion of incentive motivation is traditionally invoked, however, to explain situations in which the primary incentives themselves are not present and behavior is controlled by *conditioned* incentives—*predictors* of reward—rather than by the rewards themselves. These are the environmental cues that tell us we are getting closer to the reward—cues that keep us going toward the anticipated reward when it is not yet within our reach.

Studies of drug self-administration and intracranial self-stimulation in animals illustrate the importance of incentive motivation (Wise, 2002). In such studies, the primary incentive is never itself available to the senses. The animal cannot see, smell, touch, taste, or hear the drug or the stimulation before it is perceived internally. The stimulation or injection is not a distal object in the environment. In these studies, there is no unconditioned incentive to be approached. The animals learn to approach only conditioned incentives—for example, the lever, the part of a maze where the lever can be found, the side of the apparatus where the stimulation or drug has been given in the past. The lever-pressing and approach responses can be very compulsive, but they are conditioned responses and are directed toward conditioned stimuli. Even though these behaviors are controlled entirely by conditioned environmental stimuli, the approach and ingestive responses established by such stimuli can be extremely compulsive. Responses to such conditioned stimuli can remain strong for long periods, particularly if they are occasionally reinforced by association with their unconditioned reward (Jenkins & Stanley, 1950).

Though we tend to think of our own behavior as involving approach to the reward itself, our commonsense assumptions are misleading. How do we identify something as a "primary" food reward? How do we know, from their distal sense impressions, the difference between foods and nonfoods? To be sure, we have unconditioned aversions to certain nonfood smells. But visual distal food stimuli—the sight of the reward—are conditioned stimuli. The monkey has to learn to associate the yellow skin of the banana with the white flesh inside; it also has to learn to associate the white flesh with the sweet taste. Thus the craving elicited by the sight of a banana (Tinklepaugh, 1928) is a learned craving, much as is the craving of an animal for the lever that delivers intravenous drugs. Similarly, the craving for a chocolate bar triggered by the sight of the candy wrapper in a vending machine is a conditioned craving, a craving instigated by the reward-associated cue—the wrapper that says the candy is available—rather than by the sense impression of the unconditioned reward itself. Such stimuli can be very effective in reinstating temporarily extinguished reward-seeking behaviors.

Treatment

The addiction field has had limited success with treatment and prevention. It should not be surprising that many attempts have been made to manage addiction with medications. In the case of heroin addiction, opiate agonists (Dole &

Nyswander, 1965) and opiate antagonists (Zaks et al., 1971) have each been tried. Methadone is an opiate agonist—a drug that, like heroin and morphine, has its primary pharmacological action through its ability to activate mu-type opioid receptors (Selley et al., 1998). It alleviates opiate withdrawal symptoms by its opiate-like action, but it is less addictive than morphine, which, in turn, is less addictive than heroin. The relative addictive potency of the three drugs appears to be largely due to differences in the speed of action and clearance (Oldendorf et al., 1972). Methadone enters and leaves the brain more slowly than morphine, which, in turn, is slower than heroin. Presumably for this reason, methadone produces neither the rapid "high" nor the rapid withdrawal distress that is seen with morphine and heroin. Addicts treated with methadone remain addicted, but they are more successful in all other aspects of life than are those who maintain their addiction with heroin or morphine (Vocci et al., 2005).

The opiate antagonist naltrexone is also used with abstinent opiate addicts. Naltrexone precipitates opiate withdrawal symptoms in opiate users, making opiate use very aversive. It is used as a preventive against relapse, and its major limitation is one of compliance (Greenstein et al., 1997). It is also used in the treatment of alcoholism (Oslin et al., 2006) and nicotine dependence (Schnoll & Lerman, 2006). Similarly, the cannabinoid antagonist rimonabant, which blocks the rewarding effects of cannabinoids (Tanda et al., 2000) such as marijuana and hashish (Huestis et al., 2001), is under study as an addiction medication (Le Foll and Goldberg, 2005). It appears to have potential usefulness in the treatment of nicotine addiction (Tucci et al., 2006), nicotine-induced relapse to alcoholism (Lopez-Moreno et al., 2006), and obesity (Despres et al., 2005; Van Gaal et al., 2005).

Note, however, that two drugs with strong abuse liability, amphetamine and cocaine, are among the most effective appetite suppressants. Thus, not all drugs that effectively treat addiction will effectively treat obesity, and not all drugs that are effective against obesity will be free from abuse liability. Most drugs have the problematic characteristic of acting in more than one brain circuit, often having opposing actions at different brain sites. Morphine, for example, has stimulant and reward properties in the ventral tegmental area and sedative and dependence-producing properties in the brainstem (Wise & Bozarth, 1987). Amphetamine appears to be another case in point, suppressing appetite in some ways but enhancing it in others (Colle & Wise, 1988). Amphetamines have long been used as dietary aids (Craddock, 1976), but various amphetamines have serious abuse liability (Greenhill, 2006).

Prevention

Although efforts to reduce drug addiction have had limited success, important insights about the reduction of obesity can be extrapolated from the addiction literature. These have less to do with the traditional defining property of addiction—physiological dependence—and more to do with the role of conditioned stimuli in craving and habit.

A first lesson is that some rewards are more seductive than others. Heroin is more seductive than morphine; morphine, more than methadone (Dole & Nyswander, 1965). Similarly, some foods appear to be much more seductive than others. Humans often binge on chocolate, fat-saturated potato and corn chips, and sugar-coated, butter-rich pastries; we tend to enjoy nuts and berries more than vegetables. The advice of dietitians to shift our diet back in the direction of high fiber and away from refined sugars and flours is consistent with the advice we give addicts to restrict their diet to slow-acting methadone and away from fast-acting heroin. One reason for preferring unrefined, high-fiber foods is that they, like methadone, go through the system more slowly and produce less compulsive intake.

A second lesson—out of sight, out of mind—comes from the effectiveness of cues in triggering craving. In cue-induced relapse studies, the primary cue that triggers reinstatement of lever pressing is the insertion of the response lever into the test box. The sight of the lever and the noise of lever insertion are the stimuli that arouse and attract the animal and reinstate the old response habit. It is very difficult not to see the response knobs and buttons on the frequently present office vending machines that dispense high-sugar, high-fat or high-salt, high-fat foods as the equivalent, for the human, of the laboratory animal's response lever. Similarly, it is hard not to see the large, familiar, gaudy, fast-food icons or the signature cans and wrappers of our favorite snacks and drinks as the equivalent, for the human, of the onset of the laboratory animal's reward-associated house lights. Both the visible display of candy, chips, and soft drink containers and the advertising symbols that represent these products are likely sources of cue-induced cravings for at least some people. It seems almost certain that removing machines offering unhealthful snacks and drinks from our schools, hospitals, and other public places would be a positive step toward slowing the obesity epidemic.

A final lesson from efforts in drug prevention is that the most effective stimulus for relapse is a priming stimulus—a "taste" of the drug in question. Although we cannot avoid the priming effects of food altogether, we can try to avoid sampling the specific foods that are problematic for us individually. The addiction models teach us that it is easier to avoid problem foods than to eat limited portions of them.

Summary

Addiction reflects the compulsive ingestion of various drugs—most notably heroin, cocaine, methamphetamine, nicotine, and alcohol—to the point of lost health, lost jobs, lost families, lost shelter, and other serious negative consequences. Obesity reflects the arguably compulsive intake of various foods—most notably high-fat, high-sugar foods—leading to the loss of health, job, and sometimes family. The drugs that are the most addictive are drugs that elevate brain dopamine to three to five times normal levels. The most addictive foods (sweets and fats) also elevate brain dopamine levels, though to a somewhat lesser degree. However, through the sensory detection of sweet taste and fat flavor, they can elevate dopamine levels very rapidly.

Homeostatic controls that usually limit intake are to some extent ineffective in regulating the rapid intake of sweet, fatty foods, because postingestive satiating effects of food intake can take tens of minutes to come into play (Davis et al., 1969). The excess energy of calorically dense meals is stored as fat, which accumulates gradually, but irrevocably, to result in obesity. Dopaminergic systems are crucial for the rewarding effects of both natural (food, sex) and unnatural (brain stimulation, addictive drugs) pleasures of life. The brain circuitry of drug motivation and the brain circuitry of food motivation are, for the most part, common circuitries; thus, the lessons of addiction and the lessons of obesity are, for the most part, common lessons. We have much to learn about the mechanisms, treatment, and prevention of each; and cross-fertilization between the addiction and obesity literatures is likely to be valuable to both.

References Cited

Abel, E. L. (1975). Cannabis: effects on hunger and thirst. *Behavioral biology, 15,* 255–281.

Aharon, I., Etcoff, N., Ariely, D., Chabris, C. F., O'Connor, E., & Breiter, H. C. (2001). Beautiful faces have variable reward value: fMRI and behavioral evidence. *Neuron, 32,* 537–551.

Annau, Z., Heffner, R., & Koob, G. F. (1974). Electrical self-stimulation of single and multiple loci: Long term observations. *Physiology & Behavior, 13,* 281–290.

Bachmanov, A. A., Tordoff, M. G., & Beauchamp, G. K. (2001). Sweetener preference of C57BL/6ByJ and 129P3/J mice. *Chemical Senses, 26,* 905–913.

Baessler, A., Hasinoff, M. J., Fischer, M., Reinhard, W., Sonnenberg, G. E., Olivier, M., Erdmann, J., et al. (2005). Genetic linkage and association of the growth hormone secretagogue receptor (ghrelin receptor) gene in human obesity. *Diabetes, 54,* 259–267.

Bailey, C. S., Hsiao, S., & King, J. E. (1986). Hedonic reactivity to sucrose in rats: Modification by pimozide. *Physiology & Behavior, 38,* 447–452.

Bakshi, V. P., & Kelley, A. E. (1991). Dopaminergic regulation of feeding behavior: I. Differential effects of haloperidol microinfusion into three striatal subregions. *Psychobiology, 19,* 223–232.

Bakshi, V. P., & Kelley, A. E. (1993). Striatal regulation of morphine-induced hyperphagia: an anatomical mapping study. *Psychopharmacology, 111,* 207–214.

Bassareo, V., & Di Chiara, G. (1999). Differential responsiveness of dopamine transmission to food-stimuli in nucleus accumbens shell/core compartments. *Neuroscience, 89,* 637–641.

Belknap, J. K., Crabbe, J. C., Riggan, J., & O'Toole, L. A. (1993). Voluntary consumption of morphine in 15 inbred mouse strains. *Psychopharmacology, 112,* 352–358.

Belknap, J. K., Crabbe, J. C., & Young, E. R. (1993). Voluntary consumption of ethanol in 15 inbred mouse strains. *Psychopharmacology, 112,* 503–510.

Beninger, R. J. (1982). A comparison of the effects of pimozide and nonreinforcement on discriminated operant responding in rats. *Pharmacology, Biochemistry, and Behavior, 16,* 667–669.

Berridge, K. C., & Winkielman, P. (2003). What is an unconscious emotion? (The case for unconscious "liking"). *Cognition and Emotion, 17,* 181–211.

Berridge, K. D., Venier, I. L., & Robinson, T. E. (1989). Taste reactivity analysis of 6-hydroxydopamine-induced aphagia: Implications for arousal and anhedonia hypotheses of dopamine function. *Behavioral Neuroscience, 103,* 36–45.

Bielajew, C., & Shizgal, P. (1986). Evidence implicating descending fibers in self-stimulation of the medial forebrain bundle. *Journal of Neuroscience, 6,* 919–929.

Bindra, D. (1974). A motivational view of learning, performance, and behavior modification. *Psychological Review, 81,* 199–213.

Bindra, D. (1978). How adaptive behavior is produced: A perceptual-motivational alternative to response-reinforcement. *Behavioral and Brain Sciences, 1,* 41–91.

Blass, E. M., & Hall, W. G. (1976). Drinking termination: interactions among hydrational, orogastric and behavioral controls in rats. *Journal of Comparative and Physiological Psychology, 83,* 356–374.

Blundell, J. E., & Herberg, L. J. (1968). Relative effects of nutritional deficit and deprivation period on rate of electrical self-stimulation of lateral hypothalamus. *Nature, 219,* 627–628.

Boutrel, B., Kenny, P. J., Specio, S. E., Martin-Fardon, R., Markou, A., Koob, G. F., et al. (2005). Role for hypocretin in mediating stress-induced reinstatement of cocaine-seeking behavior. *Proceedings of the National Academy of Sciences, USA, 102,* 19168–19173.

Byck, R., Van Dyke, C., Jatlow, P., & Barash, P. (1980). Clinical pharmacology of cocaine. In F. R. Jeri (Ed.), *Cocaine 1980* (pp. 250–256). Lima, Peru: Pacific Press.

Cappell, H., & LeBlanc, A. E. (1975). Conditioned aversion by psychoactive drugs: Does it have significance for understanding drug dependence. *Addictive behaviors, 1,* 55–64.

Carr, K. C., & Wolinsky, T. D. (1993). Chronic food restriction and weight loss produce opioid facilitation of perifornical hypothalamic self-stimulation. *Brain Research, 607,* 141–148.

Carroll, M. E. (1999). Interactions between food and addiction. In R. J. M. Niesink, R. M. A. Jaspers, L. M. W. Kornet, & J. M. van Ree (Eds.), *Drugs of abuse and addiction: Neurobehavioral toxicology* (pp. 286–311). Boca Raton, FL: CRC Press.

Chen, J. P., Paredes, W., Lowinson, J. H., & Gardner, E. L. (1991). Strain-specific facilitation of dopamine efflux by delta 9-tetrahydrocannabinol in the nucleus accumbens of rat: an in vivo microdialysis study. *Neuroscience Letters, 129,* 136–180.

Cicero, T. J. (1980). Animal models of alcoholism. In K. Eriksson, J. D. Sinclair, & K. Kiianmaa (Eds.), *Animal Models in Alcohol Research* (pp. 99–118). New York: Academic Press.

Cohen, C., Perrault, G., Voltz, C., Steinberg, R., & Soubrie, P. (2002). SR141716, a central cannabinoid (CB(1)) receptor antagonist, blocks the motivational and dopamine-releasing effects of nicotine in rats. *Behavioural pharmacology, 13,* 451–463.

Colantuoni, C., Rada, P., McCarthy, J., Patten, C., Avena, N. M., Chadeayne, A., et al. (2002). Evidence that intermittent, excessive sugar intake causes endogenous opioid dependence. *Obesity Research, 10,* 478–488.

Colle, L. M., & Wise, R. A. (1988). Concurrent facilitory and inhibitory effects of amphetamine on stimulation-induced eating. *Brain Research, 459,* 356–360.

Collins, R. J., Weeks, J. R., Cooper, M. M., Good, P. I., & Russell, R. R. (1984). Prediction of abuse liability of drugs using IV self-administration by rats. *Psychopharmacology, 82,* 6–13.

Crabbe, J. C. (2002). Alcohol and genetics: new models. *American Journal of Medical Genetics, 114,* 969–974.

Crabbe, J., & Belknap, H. (1992). Genetic approaches to drug dependence. *Trends in Pharmaceutical Science, 13,* 212–219.

Craddock, D. (1976). Anorectic drugs: use in general practice. *Drugs, 11,* 378–393.

Crowther, J. H., Sanftner, J., Bonifazi, D. Z., & Shepherd, K. L. (2001). The role of daily hassles in binge eating. *International Journal of Eating Disorders, 29,* 449–454.

Curioni, C., & Andre, C. (2006). Rimonabant for overweight or obesity. *Cochrane Database of Systematic Reviews, 4,* Article CD006162. Retrieved July, 2007, from http://www.ncbi.nlm.nih.gov/sites/entrez?Db=pubmed&Cmd=ShowDetailView&TermToSearch=17054276&ordinalpos=1&itool=EntrezSystem2.PEntrez.Pubmed.Pubmed_ResultsPanel.Pubmed_RVDocSum

Dallman, M. F., Pecoraro, N., Akana, S. F., La Fleur, S. E., Gomez, F., Houshyar, H., et al. (2003). Chronic stress and obesity: a new view of "comfort food". *Proceedings of the National Academy of Sciences, USA, 100,* 11696–11701.

Davis, J. D., Gallagher, R. J., Ladove, R. F., & Turausky, A. J. (1969). Inhibition of food intake by a humoral factor. *Journal of Comparative and Physiological Psychology, 67,* 407–414.

de Castro, J. M. (1990). Social facilitation of duration and size but not rate of the spontaneous meal intake of humans. *Physiology & Behavior, 47,* 1129–1135.

Denton, D. (1982). *The hunger for salt.* Berlin: Springer-Verlag.

Despres, J. P., Golay, A., & Sjostrom, L. (2005). Effects of rimonabant on metabolic risk factors in overweight patients with dyslipidemia. *New England Journal of Medicine, 353,* 2121–2134.

Deutsch, J. A., Adams, D. W., & Metzner, R. J. (1964). Choice of intracranial stimulation as a function of delay between stimulations and strength of competing drive. *Journal of Comparative and Physiological Psychology, 1964,* 241–243.

Devine, D. P., Leone, P., Pocock, D., & Wise, R. A. (1993). Differential involvement of ventral tegmental mu, delta and kappa opioid receptors in modulation of basal mesolimbic dopamine release: in vivo microdialysis studies. *Journal of Pharmacology and Experimental Therapeutics, 266,* 1236–1246.

Devine, D. P., & Wise, R. A. (1994). Self-administration of morphine, DAMGO, and DPDPE into the ventral tegmental area of rats. *Journal of Neuroscience, 14,* 1978–1984.

de Wit, H., & Stewart, J. (1981). Reinstatement of cocaine-reinforced responding in the rat. *Psychopharmacology, 75,* 134–143.

de Wit, H., & Stewart, J. (1983). Drug reinstatement of heroin-reinforced responding in the rat. *Psychopharmacology, 79,* 29–31.

de Wit, H., & Wise, R. A. (1977). Blockade of cocaine reinforcement in rats with the dopamine receptor blocker pimozide, but not with the noradrenergic blockers phentolamine or phenoxybenzamine. *Canadian Journal of Psychology, 31,* 195–203.

Diamond, J. (1997). *Why is sex fun?: The evolution of human sexuality.* New York: Basic Books.

Dole, V. P., & Nyswander, M. (1965). A medical treatment for diacetylmorphine (heroin) addiction. *Journal of the American Medical Association, 193,* 646–650.

Duncan, E. A., Rider, T. R., Jandacek, R. J., Clegg, D. J., Benoit, S. C., Tso, P., et al. (2006). The regulation of alcohol intake by melanin-concentrating hormone in rats. *Pharmacology, Biochemistry, and Behavior, 85,* 728–735.

Erb, S., Shaham, Y., & Stewart, J. (1996). Stress reinstates cocaine-seeking behavior after prolonged extinction and a drug-free period. *Psychopharmacology, 128,* 408–412.

Ettenberg, A., & Camp, C. H. (1986). Haloperidol induces a partial reinforcement extinction effect in rats: Implications for a dopamine involvement in food reward. *Pharmacology, Biochemistry, and Behavior, 25,* 813–821.

Ettenberg, A., Pettit, H. O., Bloom, F. E., & Koob, G. F. (1982). Heroin and cocaine intravenous self-administration in rats: Mediation by separate neural systems. *Psychopharmacology, 78,* 204–209.

Evans, K. R., & Vaccarino, F. J. (1990). Amphetamine- and morphine-induced feeding: Evidence for involvement of reward mechanisms. *Neuroscience and Biobehavioral Reviews, 14,* 9–22.

Everitt, B. J., & Robbins, T. W. (2005). Neural systems of reinforcement for drug addiction: from actions to habits to compulsion. *Nature Neuroscience, 8,* 1481–1489.

Falk, J. L., Samson, H. M., & Winger, G. (1972). Behavioural maintenance of high concentrations of blood ethanol and physical dependence in the rat. *Science, 177,* 811–813.

Ferrari, P. F., Rozzi, S., & Fogassi, L. (2005). Mirror neurons responding to observation of actions made with tools in monkey ventral premotor cortex. *Journal of Cognitive Neuroscience, 17,* 212–226.

Fiorino, D. F., Coury, A., & Phillips, A. G. (1997). Dynamic changes in nucleus accumbens dopamine efflux during the Coolidge effect in male rats. *Journal of Neuroscience, 17,* 4849–4855.

Fiske, D. W., & Maddi, S. R. (Eds.). (1961). *Functions of varied experience.* Homewood, IL: Dorsey.

Foltin, R. W., Brady, J. V., & Fischman, M. W. (1986). Behavioral analysis of marijuana effects on food intake in humans. *Pharmacology, Biochemistry, and Behavior, 25,* 577–582.

Fouriezos, G., Hansson, P., & Wise, R. A. (1978). Neuroleptic-induced attenuation of brain stimulation reward in rats. *Journal of Comparative and Physiological Psychology, 92,* 661–671.

Fouriezos, G., & Wise, R. A. (1976). Pimozide-induced extinction of intracranial self-stimulation: response patterns rule out motor or performance deficits. *Brain Research, 103,* 377–380.

Fraenkel, G. S. (1959). The raison d'etre of secondary plant substances. *Science, 129,* 1466–1470.

Franklin, K. B. J. (1978). Catecholamines and self-stimulation: Reward and performance effects dissociated. *Pharmacology, Biochemistry, and Behavior, 9,* 813–820.

Franklin, K. B. J., & McCoy, S. N. (1979). Pimozide-induced extinction in rats: Stimulus control of responding rules out motor deficit. *Pharmacology, Biochemistry, and Behavior, 11,* 71–75.

Freed, W. J., & Mendelson, J. (1974). Airlicking: Thirsty rats prefer a warm dry airstream to a warm humid airstream. *Physiology & Behavior, 12,* 557–561.

Freeland, W. J., & Janzen, D. H. (1974). Strategies in herbivory by mammals: The role of plant secondary compounds. *The American Naturalist, 108,* 269–289.

Fulton, S., Woodside, B., & Shizgal, P. (2000). Modulation of brain reward circuitry by leptin. *Science, 287,* 125–128.

Galef, B. G. (2002). Social influences on food choices of Norway rats and mate choices of Japanese quail. *Appetite, 39,* 179–180.

Gallistel, C. R., Boytim, M., Gomita, Y., & Klebanoff, L. (1982). Does pimozide block the reinforcing effect of brain stimulation? *Pharmacology, Biochemistry, and Behavior, 17,* 769–781.

Gallistel, C. R., & Freyd, G. (1987). Quantitative determination of the effects of catecholaminergic agonists and antagonists on the rewarding efficacy of brain stimulation. *Pharmacology, Biochemistry, and Behavior, 26,* 731–741.

Gallistel, C. R., & Karras, D. (1984). Pimozide and amphetamine have opposing effects on the reward summation function. *Pharmacology, Biochemistry, and Behavior, 20,* 73–77.

Gallistel, C. R., Shizgal, P., & Yeomans, J. (1981). A portrait of the substrate for self-stimulation. *Psychological Review, 88,* 228–273.

Garcia, J., Ervin, F. R., & Koelling, R. A. (1966). Learning with prolonged delay of reinforcement. *Psychonomic Science, 5,* 121–122.

Garcia, J., Ervin, F. R., Yorke, C. H., & Koelling, R. A. (1967). Conditioning with delayed vitamin injections. *Science, 155,* 716–718.

Geary, N., & Smith, G. (1985). Pimozide decreases the positive reinforcing effect of sham fed sucrose in the rat. *Pharmacology, Biochemistry, and Behavior, 22,* 787–790.

Ghitza, U. E., Gray, S. M., Epstein, D. H., Rice, K. C., & Shaham, Y. (2006). The anxiogenic drug yohimbine reinstates palatable food seeking in a rat relapse model: a role of CRF1 receptors. *Neuropsychopharmacology, 31,* 2188–2196.

Goeders, N. E., Lane, J. D., & Smith, J. E. (1984). Self-administration of methionine enkephalin into the nucleus accumbens. *Pharmacology, Biochemistry, and Behavior, 20,* 451–455.

Gold, R. M., Kapatos, G., Prowse, J., Quackenbush, P. M., & Oxford, T. W. (1973). Role of water temperature in the regulation of water intake. *Journal of Comparative and Physiological Psychology, 85,* 52–63.

Gratton, A., Hoffer, B. J., & Gerhardt, G. A. (1988). Effects of electrical stimulation of brain reward sites on release of dopamine in rat: An in vivo electrochemical study. *Brain Research Bulletin, 21,* 319–324.

Greenhill, L. L. (2006). The science of stimulant abuse. *Pediatric Annals, 35,* 552–556.

Greenstein, R. A., Fudala, P. J., & O'Brien, C. P. (1997). Alternative pharmacotherapies for opiate addiction. In J. H. Lowinson, P. Ruiz, R. B. Millman, & J. G. Langrod (Eds.), *Substance abuse: A comprehensive textbook* (pp. 415–424). New York: Williams and Wilkins.

Grimm, J. W., Hope, B. T., Wise, R. A., & Shaham, Y. (2001). Incubation of cocaine craving after withdrawal. *Nature, 412,* 141–142.

Grimm, J. W., Shaham, Y., & Hope, B. T. (2002). Effect of cocaine and sucrose withdrawal period on extinction behavior, cue-induced reinstatement, and protein levels of the dopamine transporter and tyrosine hydroxylase in limbic and cortical areas in rats. *Behavioural Pharmacology, 13,* 379–388.

Gross, H., Ebert, M. H., Faden, V. B., Goldbert, S. C., Kaye, W. H., Caine, E. D., et al. (1983). A double-blind trial of delta-9-tetrahydrocannabinol in primary anorexia nervosa. *Journal of Clinical Psychopharmacology, 3,* 165–171.

Hajnal, A., Smith, G. P., & Norgren, R. (2004). Oral sucrose stimulation increases accumbens dopamine in the rat. *American Journal of Physiology – Integrative and Comparative Physiology, 286,* R31–37.

Harlow, H. F. (1953). Mice, monkeys, men and motives. *Psychological Review, 60*, 23–32.

Harper, L. V., & Sanders, K. M. (1975). The effects of adults' eating on young children's acceptance of unfamiliar foods. *Journal of Experimental Child Psychology, 20*, 206–214.

Harris, G. C., Wimmer, M., & Aston-Jones, G. (2005). A role for lateral hypothalamic orexin neurons in reward seeking. *Nature, 437*, 556–559.

Heath, R. G. (1963). Intracranial self-stimulation in man. *Science, 140*, 394–396.

Hebb, D. O. (1980). *Essay on Mind*. New York: Erlbaum.

Herman, C. P., & Polivy, J. (1975). Anxiety, restraint, and eating behavior. *Journal Abnormal Psychology, 84*, 66–72.

Hernandez, G., Hamdani, S., Rajabi, H., Conover, K., Stewart, J., Arvanitogiannis, A., et al. (2006). Prolonged rewarding stimulation of the rat medial forebrain bundle: neurochemical and behavioral consequences. *Behavioral Neuroscience, 120*, 888–904.

Hernandez, L., & Hoebel, B. G. (1988). Food reward and cocaine increase extracellular dopamine in the nucleus accumbens as measured by microdialysis. *Life Sciences, 42*, 1705–1712.

Hollister, L. E. (1971). Hunger and appetite after single doses of marijuana, alcohol and dextroamphetamine. *Pharmacology and Therapeutics, 12*, 44–49.

Holtzman, S. G. (1974). Behavioral effects of separate and combined administrations of naloxone and *d*-amphetamine. *Journal of Pharmacology and Experimental Therapeutics, 189*, 51–60.

Hsia, L. C. & Wood-Gush, D. G. M. (1984). Social facilitation in the feeding behavior of pigs and the effect of rank. *Applied Animal Ethology, 11*, 265–270.

Huestis, M. A., Gorelick, D. A., Heishman, S. J., Preston, K. L., Nelson, R. A., Moolchan, E. T., et al. (2001). Blockade of effects of smoked marijuana by the CB1-selective cannabinoid receptor antagonist SR141716. *Archives of General Psychiatry, 58*, 322–328.

Hull, C. L. (1943). *Principles of Behavior*. New York: Appleton-Century-Crofts.

Jalowiec, J. E., Panksepp, J., Zolovick, A. J., Najam, N., & Herman, B. H. (1981). Opioid modulation of ingestive behavior. *Pharmacology, Biochemistry, and Behavior, 15*, 477–484.

Jenck, F., Gratton, A., & Wise, R. A. (1986). Opposite effects of ventral tegmental and periaqueductal gray morphine injections on lateral hypothalamic stimulation-induced feeding. *Brain Research, 399*, 24–32.

Jenkins, W. O., & Stanley, J. C. (1950). Partial reinforcement: a review and critique. *Psychological Review, 47*, 193–234.

Johanson, C. E. (1978). Drugs as reinforcers. In D. E. Blackman & D. J. Sanger (Eds.), *Contemporary Research in Behavioral Pharmacology* (pp. 325–390). New York: Plenum Press.

Johnson, E. O., Van den Bree, M., Gupman, A. E., & Pickens, R. W. (1998). Extension of a typology of alcohol dependence based on relative genetic and environmental loading. *Alcoholism Clinical and Experimental Research, 22*, 1421–1429.

Josefsson, J.-O., & Johansson, P. (1979). Naloxone-reversible effect of opioids on pinocytosis in Amoeba proteus. *Nature, 282*, 78–80.

Juliano, L. M., & Griffiths, R. R. (2004). A critical review of caffeine withdrawal: empirical validation of symptoms and signs, incidence, severity, and associated features. *Psychopharmacology, 176*, 1–29.

Justinova, Z., Solinas, M., Tanda, G., Redhi, G. H., & Goldberg, S. R. (2005). The endogenous cannabinoid anandamide and its synthetic analog R(+)-methanandamide are intravenously self-administered by squirrel monkeys. *Journal of Neuroscience, 25*, 5645–5650.

Kavaliers, M., & Hirst, M. (1987). Slugs and snails and opiate tales: opioids and feeding behavior in invertebrates. *Federation Proceedings, 46*, 168–172.

Kelleher, R. T., & Morse, W. H. (1968). Schedules using noxious stimuli. III. Responding maintained with response produced electric shocks. *Journal of the Experimental Analysis of Behavior, 11*, 819–838.

Krude, H., Biebermann, H., Luck, W., Horn, R., Brabant, G., & Gruters, A. (1998). Severe early-onset obesity, adrenal insufficiency and red hair pigmentation caused by POMC mutations in humans. *Nature Genetics, 19*, 155–157.

Le, A. D., Harding, S., Juzytsch, W., Funk, D., & Shaham, Y. (2005). Role of alpha-2 adrenoceptors in stress-induced reinstatement of alcohol seeking and alcohol self-administration in rats. *Psychopharmacology, 179*, 366–373.

Le Foll, B., & Goldberg, S. R. (2005). Cannabinoid CB1 receptor antagonists as promising new medications for drug dependence. *Journal of Pharmacology and Experimental Therapeutics, 312*, 875–883.

Lee, B., Tiefenbacher, S., Platt, D. M., & Spealman, R. D. (2004). Pharmacological blockade of alpha2-adrenoceptors induces reinstatement of cocaine-seeking behavior in squirrel monkeys. *Neuropsychopharmacology, 29*, 686–693.

Lester, D., & Freed, E. X. (1973). Criteria for an animal model of alcoholism. *Pharmacology, Biochemistry, and Behavior, 1*, 103–108.

Liang, N. C., Hajnal, A., & Norgren, R. (2006). Sham feeding corn oil increases accumbens dopamine in the rat. *American Journal of Physiology: Integrative and Comparative Physiology, 291*, R1236–1239.

Lopez-Moreno, J. A., Gonzalez-Cuevas, G., & Navarro, M. (2006). The CB1 cannabinoid receptor antagonist rimonabant chronically prevents the nicotine-induced relapse to alcohol. *Neurobiology of Disease, 25*, 274–283

Macenski, M. J., & Meisch, R. A. (1994). Oral drug reinforcement studies with laboratory animals: Applications and implications for understanding drug-reinforced behavior. *Current Directions in Psychological Science, 3*, 22–27.

Martinez, D., Broft, A., Foltin, R. W., Slifstein, M., Hwang, D. R., Huang, Y., et al. (2004). Cocaine dependence and d2 receptor availability in the functional subdivisions of the striatum: relationship with cocaine-seeking behavior. *Neuropsychopharmacology, 29*, 1190–1202.

Martinez, D., Gil, R., Slifstein, M., Hwang, D. R., Huang, Y., Perez, A., et al. (2005). Alcohol dependence is associated with blunted dopamine transmission in the ventral striatum. *Biological Psychiatry, 58*, 779–786.

Mason, R. J., & Reidinger, R. F. (1981). Effects of social facilitation and observational learning on feeding behavior of the red-winged blackbird (Agelaius phoeniceus). *Auk, 98*, 778–784.

Meil, W. M., & See, R. E. (1996). Conditioned cued recovery of responding following prolonged withdrawal from self-administered cocaine in rats: an animal model of relapse. *Behavioural pharmacology, 7*, 754–763.

Mello, N. K. (1973). A review of methods to induce alcohol addiction in animals. *Pharmacology, Biochemistry, and Behavior, 1*, 89–101.

Mendelson, J., & Chillag, D. (1970). Tongue cooling: A new reward for thirsty rodents. *Science, 170*, 1418–1419.

Monroe, R. R., & Heath, R. G. (1954). Psychiatric observations. In R. G. Heath (Ed.), *Studies in schizophrenia* (pp. 345–382). Cambridge, MA: Harvard University Press.

Montague, C. T., Farooqi, I. S., Whitehead, J. P., Soos, M. A., Rau, H., Wareham, N. J., et al. (1997). Congenital leptin deficiency is associated with severe early-onset obesity in humans. *Nature, 387*, 903–908.

Morgan, M. J. (1974). Resistance to satiation. *Animal Behaviour, 22*, 449–466.

Mucha, R. F., & Iversen, S. D. (1986). Increased food intake after opioid microinjections into the nucleus accumbens and ventral tegmental area of rat. *Brain Research, 397*, 214–224.

Noel, M. B., & Wise, R. A. (1993). Ventral tegmental injections of morphine but not U-50,488H enhance feeding in food-deprived rats. *Brain Research, 632*, 68–73.

Noel, M. B., & Wise, R. A. (1995). Ventral tegmental injections of a selective μ or δ opioid enhance feeding in food-deprived rats. *Brain Research, 673*, 304–312.

Nowinski, J., Baker, S., & Carroll, K. M. (1992). *Twelve step facilitation therapy manual: a clinical research guide for therapist treating individuals with alcohol abuse and dependence.* Rockville, MD: National Institute on Alcohol Abuse.

Oldendorf, W. H., Hyman, S., Braun, L., & Oldendorf, S. Z. (1972). Blood-brain barrier: Penetration of morphine, codeine, heroin, and methadone after carotid injection. *Science, 178*, 984–986.

Olds, J. (1958). Self-stimulation of the brain. *Science, 127*, 315–324.

Olds, J. (1962). Hypothalamic substrates of reward. *Physiological Review, 42*, 554–604.

Olds, J., Travis, R. P., & Schwing, R. C. (1960). Topographic organization of hypothalamic self-stimulation functions. *Journal of Comparative and Physiological Psychology, 53*, 23–32.

Olds, M. E. (1982). Reinforcing effects of morphine in the nucleus accumbens. *Brain Research, 237*, 429–440.

Olds, M. E., & Olds, J. (1963). Approach-avoidance analysis of rat diencephalon. *Journal of Comparative Neurology, 120,* 259–295.

Oslin, D. W., Berrettini, W. H., & O'Brien, C. P. (2006). Targeting treatments for alcohol dependence: the pharmacogenetics of naltrexone. *Addiction Biology, 11,* 397–403.

Palmerino, C. C., Rusiniak, K. W., & Garcia, J. (1980). Flavor-illness aversions: the peculiar roles of odor and taste in memory for poison. *Science, 208,* 753–755.

Paly, D., Jatlow, P., Van Dyke, C., Cabieses, F., & Byck, R. (1980). Plasma levels of cocaine in native Peruvian coca chewers. In F. R. Jeri (Ed.), *Cocaine 1980* (pp. 86–89). Lima, Peru: Pacific Press.

Paly, D., Jatlow, P., Van Dyke, C., Jeri, F. R., & Byck, R. (1982). Plasma cocaine concentrations during cocaine paste smoking. *Life Sciences, 30,* 731–738.

Pecina, S., & Berridge, K. C. (2005). Hedonic hot spot in nucleus accumbens shell: where do mu-opioids cause increased hedonic impact of sweetness? *Journal of Neuroscience, 25,* 11777–11786.

Peters, A., Pellerin, L., Dallman, M. F., Oltmanns, K. M., Schweiger, U., Born, J., et al. (2007). Causes of obesity: Looking beyond the hypothalamus. *Progress in Neurobiology, 81,* 61–88

Pfaffmann, C. (1960). The pleasures of sensation. *Psychological Review, 67,* 253–268.

Pickens, R., & Harris, W. C. (1968). Self-administration of *d*-amphetamine by rats. *Psychopharmacologia, 12,* 158–163.

Pollan, M. (2006). *The omnivore's dilemma.* Penguin Press, New York.

Ranaldi, R., Pocock, D., Zereik, R., & Wise, R. A. (1999). Dopamine fluctuations in the nucleus accumbens during maintenance, extinction, and reinstatement of intravenous D-amphetamine self-administration. *Journal of Neuroscience, 19,* 4102–4109.

Reale, D., Festa-Bianchet, M., & Jorgenson, J. T. (1999). Heritability of body mass varies with age and season in wild bighorn sheep. *Heredity, 83,* 526–532.

Rompré, P.-P., & Wise, R. A. (1989). Opioid-neuroleptic interaction in brain stem self-stimulation. *Brain Research, 477,* 144–151.

Rozin, P., & Rodgers, W. (1967). Novel-diet preferences in vitamin-deficient rats and rats recovered from vitamin deficiency. *Journal of Comparative and Physiological Psychology, 63,* 421–428.

Salamone, J. D., Cousins, M. S., & Bucher, S. (1994). Anhedonia or anergia? Effects of haloperidol and nucleus accumbens dopamine depletion on instrumental response selection in a T-maze cost/benefit procedure. *Behavioural Brain Research, 65,* 221–229.

Santos, L. R., Hauser, M. D., & Spelke, E. S. (2001). Recognition and categorization of biologically significant objects by rhesus monkeys (Macaca mulatta): the domain of food. *Cognition, 82,* 127–155.

Schneider, L. H., Davis, J. D., Watson, C. A., & Smith, G. P. (1990). Similar effect of raclopride and reduced sucrose concentration on the microstructure of sucrose sham feeding. *European Journal of Pharmacology, 186,* 61–70.

Schneider, L. H., Gibbs, J., & Smith, G. P. (1986). Selective D-1 or D-2 receptor antagonists inhibit sucrose sham feeding in rats. *Appetite, 7,* 294–295.

Schnoll, R. A., & Lerman, C. (2006). Current and emerging pharmacotherapies for treating tobacco dependence. *Expert Opinion on Emerging Drugs, 11,* 429–444.

Schultz, W., Apicella, P., & Ljungberg, T. (1993). Responses of monkey dopamine neurons to reward and conditioned stimuli during successive steps of learning a delayed response task. *Journal of Neuroscience, 13,* 900–913.

Seligman, M. E. P. (1970). On the generality of the laws of learning. *Psychological Review, 77,* 406–418.

Selley, D. E., Liu, Q., & Childers, S. R. (1998). Signal transduction correlates of mu opioid agonist intrinsic efficacy: receptor-stimulated [35S]GTP gamma S binding in mMOR-CHO cells and rat thalamus. *Journal of Pharmacology and Experimental Therapeutics, 285,* 496–505.

Sem-Jacobsen, C. W. (1959). Depth-electrographic observations in psychotic patients: a system related to emotion and behavior. *Acta Psychiatrica Scandinavica Supplementum, 34*(136), 412–416.

Shaham, Y., Shalev, U., Lu, L., De Wit, H., & Stewart, J. (2003). The reinstatement model of drug relapse: history, methodology and major findings. *Psychopharmacology, 168,* 3–20.

Shaham, Y., & Stewart, J. (1995). Stress reinstates heroin-seeking in drug-free animals: an effect mimicking heroin, not withdrawal. *Psychopharmacology, 119,* 334–341.

Shalev, U., Morales, M., Hope, B., Yap, J., & Shaham, Y. (2001). Time-dependent changes in extinction behavior and stress-induced reinstatement of drug seeking following withdrawal from heroin in rats. *Psychopharmacology, 156*, 98–107.

Shalev, U., Yap, J., & Shaham, Y. (2001). Leptin attenuates acute food deprivation-induced relapse to heroin seeking. *Journal of Neuroscience, 21*, RC129.

Sheffield, F. D., & Roby, T. B. (1950). Reward value of a non-nutritive sweet taste. *Journal of Comparative and Physiological Psychology, 43*, 471–481.

Shepard, J. D., Bossert, J. M., Liu, S. Y., & Shaham, Y. (2004). The anxiogenic drug yohimbine reinstates methamphetamine seeking in a rat model of drug relapse. *Biological Psychiatry, 55*, 1082–1089.

Shettleworth, S. J. (1972). Constraints on learning. In D. S. Lehrman, R. A. Hinde, & E. Shaw (Eds.), *Advances in the study of behavior: IV*. Oxford: Academic Press.

Siegel, R. (1989). *Intoxication: Life in pursuit of artificial paradise*. New York: Dutton.

Sinha, R., Catapano, D., & O'Malley, S. (1999). Stress-induced craving and stress response in cocaine dependent individuals. *Psychopharmacology, 1421*, 343–351.

Steiner, J. E. (1974). Innate, discriminative human facial expressions to taste and smell stimulation. *Annals of the New York Academy of Sciences, 237*, 229–233.

Steiner, J. E. (1979). Human facial expressions in response to taste and smell stimulation. *Advances in Child Devlopment and Behavior, 13*, 257–295.

Strobel, M. G., Freedman, S. L., & Macdonald, G. E. (1970). Social facilitation of feeding in newly hatched chickens as a function of imprinting. *Canadian Journal of Psychology, 24*, 207–215.

Tanda, G., Munzar, P., & Goldberg, S. R. (2000). Self-administration behavior is maintained by the psychoactive ingredient of marijuana in squirrel monkeys. *Nature Neuroscience, 3*, 1073–1074.

Tanda, G., Pontieri, F. E., & Di Chiara, G. (1997). Cannabinoid and heroin activation of mesolimbic dopamine transmission by a common μl opioid receptor mechanism. *Science, 276*, 2048–2050.

Teitelbaum, P., & Epstein, A. N. (1962). The lateral hypothalamic syndrome: recovery of feeding and drinking after lateral hypo-thalamic lesions. *Psychological Review, 69*, 74–90.

Thornton-Jones, Z. D., Vickers, S. P., & Clifton, P. G. (2005). The cannabinoid CB1 receptor antagonist SR141716A reduces appetitive and consummatory responses for food. *Psychopharmacology, 179*, 452–460.

Tinklepaugh, O. L. (1928). An experimental study of representative factors in monkeys. *Journal of Comparative Psychology, 8*, 197–236.

Tucci, S. A., Halford, J. C., Harrold, J. A., & Kirkham, T. C. (2006). Therapeutic potential of targeting the endocannabinoids: implications for the treatment of obesity, metabolic syndrome, drug abuse and smoking cessation. *Current Medicinal Chemistry, 13*, 2669–2680.

Uhl, G. R., Liu, Q. R., & Naiman, D. (2002). Substance abuse vulnerability loci: converging genome scanning data. *Trends in Genetics, 18*, 420–425.

Ungerstedt, U. (1971). Adipsia and aphagia after 6-hydroxydopamine induced degeneration of the nigro-striatal dopamine system. *Acta Psychiatrica Scandinavica Supplementum, 367*, 95–122.

Vaisse, C., Clement, K., Durand, E., Hercberg, S., Guy-Grand, B., & Foroguel, P. (2000). Melanocortin-4 receptor mutations are a frequent and heterogenous cause of morbid obesity. *Journal of Clinical Investigations, 106*, 253–262.

Valenstein, E. S., & Beer, B. B. (1964). Continuous opportunity for reinforcing brain stimulation. *Journal of the Experimental Analysis of Behavior, 7*, 183–184.

Van Dyke, C., Jatlow, P., Ungerer, J., Barash, P. G., & Byck, R. (1978). Oral cocaine: plasma concentrations and central effects. *Science, 200*, 211–213.

Van Gaal, L. F., Rissanen, A. M., Scheen, A. J., Ziegler, O., & Rossner, S. (2005). Effects of the cannabinoid-1 receptor blocker rimonabant on weight reduction and cardiovascular risk factors in overweight patients: 1-year experience from the RIO-Europe study. *Lancet, 365*, 1389–1397.

Visalberghi, E., & Addessi, E. (2000). Seeing group members eating a familiar food enhances the acceptance of novel foods in capuchin monkeys. *Animal Behaviour, 60*, 69–76.

Vocci, F. J., Acri, J., & Elkashef, A. (2005). Medication development for addictive disorders: The state of the science. *American Journal of Psychiatry, 162,* 1432–1440.

Volkow, N. D., Fowler, J. S., Wang, G. J., Hitzemann, R., Logan, J., Schlyer, D. J., et al. (1993). Decreased dopamine D2 receptor availability is associated with reduced frontal metabolism in cocaine abusers. *Synapse, 14,* 169–177.

Walley, A. J., Blakemore, A. I., & Froguel, P. (2006). Genetics of obesity and the prediction of risk for health. *Human Molecular Genetics, 15,* R124–130.

Wang, B., Shaham, Y., Zitzman, D., Azari, S., Wise, R. A., & You, Z. B. (2005). Cocaine experience establishes control of midbrain glutamate and dopamine by corticotropin-releasing factor: a role in stress-induced relapse to drug seeking. *Journal of Neuroscience, 25,* 5389–5396.

Whalen, R. E. (1966). Sexual motivation. *Psychological Review, 73,* 151–163.

White, N. M. (1989). Reward or reinforcement: what's the difference? *Neuroscience and Biobehavioral Reviews, 13,* 181–186.

Will, M. J., Pratt, W. E., & Kelley, A. E. (2006). Pharmacological characterization of high-fat feeding induced by opioid stimulation of the ventral striatum. *Physiology & Behavior, 89,* 226–234.

Wise, R. A. (1973). Voluntary ethanol intake in rats following exposure to ethanol on various schedules. *Psychopharmacologia, 29,* 203–210.

Wise, R. A. (1982). Common neural basis for brain stimulation reward, drug reward, and food reward. In B. G. Hoebel & D. Novin (Eds.), *Neural Basis of Feeding and Reward* (pp. 445–454). Brunswick, ME: Haer Institute.

Wise, R. A. (1987). Intravenous drug self-administration: A special case of positive reinforcement. In M. A. Bozarth (Ed.), *Methods of Assessing the Reinforcing Properties of Abused Drugs* (pp. 117–141). New York: Springer-Verlag.

Wise, R. A. (2002). Brain reward circuitry: Insights from unsensed incentives. *Neuron, 36,* 229–240.

Wise, R. A., & Bozarth, M. A. (1987). A psychomotor stimulant theory of addiction. *Psychological Review, 94,* 469–492.

Wise, R. A., Jenck, F., & Raptis, L. (1986). Morphine potentiates feeding via the opiate reinforcement mechanism. In L. S. Harris (Ed.), *Problems of Drug Dependence 1985* (pp. 228–234). Washington, DC: U.S. Government Printing Office.

Wise, R. A., Leone, P., Rivest, R., & Leeb, K. (1995). Elevations of nucleus accumbens dopamine and DOPAC levels during intra-venous heroin self-administration. *Synapse, 21,* 140–148.

Wise, R. A., Murray, A., & Bozarth, M. A. (1990). Bromocriptine self-administration and bromocriptine-reinstatement of cocaine-trained and heroin-trained lever pressing in rats. *Psychopharmacology, 100,* 355–360.

Wise, R. A., Newton, P., Leeb, K., Burnette, B., Pocock, P., & Justice, J. B. (1995). Fluctuations in nucleus accumbens dopamine concentration during intra-venous cocaine self-administration in rats. *Psychopharmacology, 120,* 10–20.

Wise, R. A., Raptis, L. (1986). Effects of naloxone and pimozide on initiation and maintenance measures of free feeding. *Brain Research, 368,* 62–68.

Wise, R. A., & Rompré, P.-P. (1989). Brain dopamine and reward. *Annual Review of Psychology, 40,* 191–225.

Wise, R. A., & Schwartz, H. V. (1981). Pimozide attenuates acquisition of lever pressing for food in rats. *Pharmacology, Biochemistry, and Behavior, 15,* 655–656.

Wise, R. A., Spindler, J., de Wit, H., & Gerber, G. J. (1978). Neuroleptic-induced "anhedonia" in rats: pimozide blocks reward quality of food. *Science, 201,* 262–264.

Wise, R. A., Yokel, R. A., & de Wit, H. (1976). Both positive reinforcement and conditioned aversion from amphetamine and from apomorphine in rats. *Science, 191,* 1273–1275.

Yeomans, J., Forster, G., & Blaha, C. (2001). M5 muscarinic receptors are needed for slow activation of dopamine neurons and for rewarding brain stimulation. *Life Sciences, 68,* 2449–2456.

Yeomans, J. S., Maidment, N. T., & Bunney, B. S. (1988). Excitability properties of medial forebrain bundle axons of A9 and A10 dopamine cells. *Brain Research, 450,* 86–93.

Yokel, R. A., & Wise, R. A. (1975). Increased lever pressing for amphetamine after pimozide in rats: implications for a dopamine theory of reward. *Science, 187,* 547–549.

You, Z.-B., Chen, Y.-Q., & Wise, R. A. (2001). Dopamine and glutamate release in the nucleus accumbens and ventral tegmental area of rat following lateral hypothalamic self-stimulation. *Neuroscience, 107,* 629–639.

Zaks, A., Jones, T., & Freedman, A. M. (1971). Naloxone treatment of opiate dependence. *Journal of the American Medical Association, 215,* 2108–2110.

Zangen, A., Ikemoto, S., Zadina, J. E., & Wise, R. A. (2002). Rewarding and psychomotor stimulant effects of endomorphin-1: anteroposterior differences within the ventral tegmental area and lack of effect in nucleus accumbens. *Journal of Neuroscience, 22,* 7225–7233.

Zangen, A., Solinas, M., Ikemoto, S., Goldberg, S. R., & Wise, R. A. (2006). Two brain sites for cannabinoid reward. *Journal of Neuroscience,* 26, 4901–4907.

Zhang, M., & Kelley, A. E. (2000). Enhanced intake of high-fat food following striatal mu-opioid stimulation: microinjection mapping and fos expression. *Neuroscience, 99,* 267–277.

Zhang, M., & Kelley, A. E. (2002). Intake of saccharin, salt, and ethanol solutions is increased by infusion of a mu opioid agonist into the nucleus accumbens. *Psychopharmacology, 159,* 415–423.

5 THE LOGIC OF SENSORY AND HEDONIC COMPARISONS: ARE THE OBESE DIFFERENT?

Derek J. Snyder and Linda M. Bartoshuk

Introduction

As a public health concern, the increased global prevalence of obesity is largely the result of sedentary lifestyles and an environment replete with food resources. Obesity occurs when intake significantly exceeds metabolic requirements, which is a highly likely scenario when food is plentiful and activity scant. This failure to maintain homeostasis raises an important question: why are we drawn to consume food that we do not need? Many biological and social factors govern intake, but prominent among them are the sensory and hedonic processes that shape our interactions with the environment. Psychophysical measures of experience have played an essential role in our understanding of these processes, and they have proved exceedingly useful in characterizing fundamental aspects of human behavior.

Measuring experience, however, is a daunting challenge. By definition, individual experience is subjective: we can *describe* our experiences, but we cannot directly *share* the experiences of another person. Is it possible, then, to develop measures that allow us to compare experiences with others? Strictly speaking, we cannot make these comparisons with absolute certainty, yet they have enormous significance and must be measured well. After all, if we are to comprehend the nature of obesity, it behooves us to consider how sensation and affect may differ among the obese.

Toward this goal, this chapter begins with a discussion of sensory and hedonic scales. These powerful tools offer the ability to measure and compare experiences with great accuracy, but only if they are used properly. Inappropriate scaling has become the rule—rather than the exception—in comparisons among individuals and groups. To illustrate, oral sensory research offers several examples of erroneous conclusions arising from poor psychophysical measurement, along with alternative methods that provide more accurate comparisons. Because several long-held beliefs about the experiences of obese individuals stem from flawed sensory and hedonic scaling, this chapter concludes by revisiting some of these themes. As such, refined scaling methods show striking potential to advance scientific views on obesity research, treatment, and prevention.

The Scaling Problem: Sensory and Hedonic Experiences Are Comparable If Measured Properly

Intensity descriptors are relative

In everyday life, we commonly use intensity descriptors to quantify our sensory and hedonic experiences: this tea is *strong*; that salsa is *moderately* spicy; she likes chocolate *a lot*. Investigators measuring the intensity of such experiences often use psychophysical scales that invoke these everyday descriptive terms. For example, a nine-point category scale designed to measure taste sensations includes labels at alternate points: 1 = none, 3 = slight, 5 = moderate, 7 = strong, and 9 = extreme (Kamen et al., 1961). Another, more popular example is the visual analog scale (VAS)—a line labeled in terms of the minimum and maximum of a specific experience. A VAS for sweet taste might be labeled "no sweetness" at one end and "extremely strong sweetness" at the other (Hetherington & Rolls, 1987).

Intensity descriptors are used widely in health and consumer assessments because they appear to be broadly and easily understood, but that familiarity presents a fundamental problem: neither adjective descriptors (e.g., *strong*) nor their adverb modifiers (e.g., *extremely*) denote absolute perceived intensity. Consider an observation made in 1958 by the experimental psychologist S. S. Stevens: "Mice may be called large or small, and so may elephants, and it is quite understandable when someone says it was a large mouse that ran up the trunk of the small elephant" (Stevens, 1958, p. 633). Terms like *large* and *small* are relative; they acquire absolute meaning only when linked to a specific object. In this case, even if we account for individual differences in size, elephants and mice clearly occupy two distinct size ranges. So, when *large* refers to a mouse and *small* to an elephant, we implicitly grasp that the mouse—however large—is the smaller of the two animals.

The flexibility of intensity descriptors is a concept learned early in life. As we develop the ability to describe the world around us, we learn to use these words to describe many different types of experience. What is truly remarkable is that the relationships among descriptors—their positions relative to one another—remain the same across virtually all domains (Borg, 1982; Gracely et al., 1978; Green et al., 1993; Moskowitz, 1977). It is useful to imagine our internal intensity scale as a ruler printed on elastic that stretches or compresses to fit the situation at hand. Some experiences occupy a greater range of absolute intensity than others, but the words describing that range maintain constant relative meaning across various types of experience.

For instance, data indicate that the strongest pain ever experienced is generally more intense than the strongest taste ever experienced (Bartoshuk, Duffy, Fast, Green, Prutkin, & Snyder, 2002). Because we use the same terminology to describe both types of sensation, we are effectively stretching a common intensity ruler to describe pain or compressing it to describe taste. Intensity rulers also stretch and compress to account for individual differences in experience; the discussion that follows will show that an individual born with many taste buds has an expanded "taste ruler" compared to an individual born with few. Consistent with Stevens's observation, the meaning of a word like *strong* varies with both the experience in question and the individual experiencing it.

Despite our implicit understanding that intensity descriptors carry only relative meaning, most of today's scaling practices treat these labels as if they denote equal perceived intensities to all individuals under all conditions. This error does little harm for studies in which individual responses are compared before and after a specific manipulation, or for those in which treatment groups are randomly assigned—but it renders invalid any comparisons between individuals or groups identified by a particular characteristic (e.g., sex, age, medical history, body mass) because that characteristic itself may produce differences in the absolute intensities denoted by scale labels. As the following discussion indicates, this error significantly distorts the appearance and interpretation of experimental data, and it contributes to enduring inaccuracy in the study of human sensation and affect.

Magnitude matching enables valid comparisons

Fortunately, we can make sensory comparisons across groups without assuming that intensity descriptors denote equal perceived intensities to everyone. To illustrate, if two groups of subjects—one with many taste buds, the other with few—sample a sugar solution that is equivalent in concentration to a soft drink and rate its sweetness from 0 (no sweetness) to 100 (strongest sweetness ever tasted),[1] subjects in both groups will select a value near 60. If the experiment ended here, it would imply that both groups experienced similar sweetness, but in fact they do not. If the subjects don headphones and are instructed to set the loudness of a tone to match the sweetness of the sucrose, the group with many taste buds will set the loudness at about 90 decibels (comparable to a train whistle), while the group with few taste buds will set it at about 80 decibels (comparable to a telephone's dial tone). This difference represents a doubling of perceived loudness (because the decibel is a logarithmic unit), indicating that the group with many taste buds experiences twice as much sweetness.

This method, formalized as *magnitude matching* (Marks & Stevens, 1980; Marks et al., 1988; Stevens & Marks, 1980), makes use of our ability to compare (or "match") the intensities of different types of sensations (e.g., sweetness, saltiness,

---

[1]This example is a simplified version of experiments described in Bartoshuk et al., 1992.

loudness, brightness, pain; Stevens, 1959; Stevens & Marks, 1965). In practice, subjects rate the intensity of a sensation of interest (in the sweetness experiment just described, sweetness) relative to an unrelated sensation that serves as a standard (in the sweetness experiment, loudness). Magnitude matching addresses a daunting philosophical hurdle: we cannot compare our sensations directly with those of others, but the use of an independent standard allows us to compare relative differences among stimuli. The sweetness experiment assumed that taste and hearing are unrelated. Logically speaking, this means that any variation in hearing should be roughly the same in the two groups (which, after all, differ systematically only in the number of taste buds that they possess). Thus, expressing sweetness intensity in terms of auditory intensity allows the conclusion that those with the most taste buds experience the greatest sweetness.

Magnitude matching in action: research on oral sensory variation

As the example in the preceding section suggests, observations on intensity scaling owe much to ongoing research on individual differences in oral sensation. Interest in this area began with the phenomenon of *taste blindness*, in which some individuals are congenitally unable to perceive the bitter taste of phenylthiocarbamide (PTC), 6-*n*-propylthiouracil (PROP), and other thiourea compounds (Blakeslee & Fox, 1932; Fox, 1931; Snyder, 1931). Taste blindness has a prevalence of about 25% in the United States, and it is largely the result of point mutations in a single gene, *T2R38* (Kim et al., 2003). Early distinctions between "nontasters" and "tasters" were derived almost exclusively from threshold measures (Harris & Kalmus, 1949), but the rise of magnitude estimation enabled the exploration of suprathreshold differences that more faithfully reflect stimuli found in the real world.

In the suprathreshold scaling methods pioneered by S. S. Stevens (1960), subjects assign numbers to stimuli in a ratio manner, meaning that a stimulus twice as strong as another is assigned a number twice as large. This task shows quite effectively how perceived intensity grows with stimulus concentration, but these ratings by themselves cannot be compared across subjects because we cannot determine the absolute intensities associated with the numbers that subjects use. In an attempt to make such comparisons accurately, nontasters and tasters (defined by threshold) were asked to rate the intensity of suprathreshold PTC and sodium chloride (NaCl). Just as sound was used as a standard in the sweetness experiment described earlier, here NaCl taste was used as a standard because taste blindness was presumed to occur only for thiourea compounds. By this logic, if PTC and NaCl taste are unrelated, any variation in saltiness will be dispersed evenly across nontasters and tasters, so differences in PTC bitterness—actual sensory differences, not procedural artifacts—will emerge as a function of NaCl saltiness. To wit, tasters were predicted to experience the most intense bitterness from suprathreshold PTC, and so they did (Hall et al., 1975).

Surprisingly, expansion of this experiment to other compounds revealed that tasters perceive greater intensity from most oral sensations, not just thiourea bitterness (e.g., Bartoshuk, 1979; Bartoshuk et al., 1988; Gent & Bartoshuk, 1983). Moreover, a subset of tasters, called *supertasters*, perceive the most intense sensations from virtually all taste, oral burn, and oral tactile cues (Bartoshuk, 1991; Prutkin et al., 2000). Individual differences in oral anatomy support these sensory differences, for supertasters have a higher density of fungiform papillae on the tongue (Miller & Reedy, 1990; Bartoshuk et al., 1994); fungiform papillae house taste buds and are innervated by nerve fibers mediating taste and oral somatosensation (Whitehead et al., 1985; Farbman & Hellekant, 1978).[2] These findings refute the assumption that NaCl and PTC/PROP taste are independent. Subsequent use of an auditory standard in place of NaCl revealed that the differences distinguishing nontasters, medium tasters, and supertasters are larger than originally believed (Gent & Bartoshuk, 1983).[3]

Magnitude matching with a labeled scale

Magnitude matching is the only known psychophysical method that permits accurate comparisons among groups, but it does so only if two important conditions are met. First, the standard used must be unrelated to the measure of interest. Suprathreshold scaling uses unrelated stimuli to satisfy this requirement; when labeled scales are used to make such comparisons, the labels themselves act as standards. As demonstrated in the preceding discussion, psychophysical comparisons are irrevocably flawed when they are based on standards that denote different perceived intensities to different groups.

Second, magnitude matching relies on the ratio properties of subject ratings as a reflection of stimulus intensity. If a rating of 10 does not indicate twice as much intensity as a rating of 5, then these ratings are clearly inaccurate, as are any further comparisons based on them. Most category scales lack ratio properties because their intensity labels are spaced evenly, when in fact this spacing fails to reflect actual intensity differences. That said, category scales can acquire ratio properties if the categories are spaced to appropriately reflect the perceived

---

[2]These views on supertasting have been clarified by recent studies showing that specific mutations in the *T2R38* taste receptor gene result in PTC/PROP threshold differences that distinguish tasters from nontasters, thus accounting for taste blindness (Kim et al., 2003). However, these differences alone cannot account for the suprathreshold effect of supertasting (Bartoshuk, Davidson, et al., 2005). Considering that elevated density of fungiform papillae broadly enhances most oral sensations (including PTC/PROP bitterness), PTC/PROP supertasters are probably individuals expressing many fungiform papillae along with the taster form of *T2R38*.

[3]Like NaCl, loudness may be an imperfect standard for oral sensory comparisons. The chorda tympani nerve, which carries taste cues from the anterior tongue, crosses the ear canal just behind the eardrum. Middle-ear disease, therefore, may compromise both hearing and taste perception.

distances among the labels. Several studies accomplished this task using a variety of methods (Borg, 1982; Gracely et al., 1978; Green et al., 1993; Moskowitz, 1977). Importantly, all of these studies obtained similar spacings, suggesting that the relative differences among intensity descriptors remain constant, even when the specific type of experience changes. This constancy of relative spacing forms the basis of the elastic ruler metaphor described earlier.

As these ideas gained traction, investigators sought a labeled scale that would allow valid comparisons among nontasters, medium tasters, and supertasters. The labeled magnitude scale (LMS), a scale created specifically for oral sensations (Green et al., 1993), proved a useful starting point. On this scale, labels were positioned empirically to give the scale ratio properties: 0 = no sensation, 1.4 = barely detectable, 6 = weak, 16 = moderate, 35 = strong, 53 = very strong, and 100 = strongest imaginable sensation. Because intensity descriptors maintain their relative spacing, this sensory ruler can be "stretched" to its maximum by replacing the top label with "strongest imaginable sensation *of any kind.*"[4] This revised scale, known as the *general labeled magnitude scale* (gLMS), allows subjects to rate and compare perceived intensities of any type of sensation on a common scale (e.g., Bartoshuk, Duffy, Green, et al., 2004).

Is the gLMS a labeled-scale form of magnitude matching? To answer this question, subjects rated the most intense sensations they had ever experienced in a variety of sensory domains. The data showed that oral sensory cues are rarely the strongest sensations experienced (Bartoshuk, Fast, Green, Prutkin, et al., 2002), meaning that the top anchor of the gLMS serves as an appropriate independent standard for oral sensory comparisons. Thus, not only does the gLMS satisfy both of the technical requirements of magnitude matching, but it also produces valid comparisons of oral sensation without the need for additional sensory benchmarks (although they may still be used). Further validation of the gLMS came from direct comparisons with magnitude matching using an auditory standard: both methods produce equivalent measures of PROP intensity (Bartoshuk, Duffy, Green, et al., 2004).

THE HEDONIC gLMS   The properties of affective (or hedonic) scaling have been studied much less than those of sensory scaling. Nevertheless, it appears that hedonic experiences can be quantified using the same scaling methods developed for sensory measurement. In other words, hedonic experiences have inten-

---

[4]The term *imaginable* is found in the top anchors of several commonly used scales, yet imagery and experience are markedly different concepts. This term was probably used for the first time in a pain scale described in 1983 (Price et al., 1983), possibly on the assumption that images of extreme pain are similarly intense across individuals, even if their actual pain experiences are different. However, ratings of the strongest imaginable sensation and the most intense sensation ever experienced show significant correlation (Fast, 2004), indicating that imagined sensations are not equally intense to everyone. Apparently, the term *imaginable* fails to confer any added benefit to intensity scales; we plan to remove it in future studies.

sity and may be compared, either with other hedonic experiences (e.g., we can compare our liking for the sweetness of a soft drink with our liking for the odor of a rose) or with sensory ones (e.g., we can compare our liking for the sweetness of a soft drink with the loudness of a tone). These ideas are currently being explored; if they prove correct, valid comparisons of hedonic experience are at hand.

As an intermediate step toward this goal, a hedonic scale closely resembling the gLMS was devised (Bartoshuk, Duffy, Fast, Green, & Snyder, 2002). This *hedonic gLMS* consists of a line labeled "neutral" at its midpoint, "strongest imaginable disliking of any kind" at one end, and "strongest imaginable liking of any kind" at the other. As such, subjects rate their liking or disliking for a given experience—a food, an event, a sensation—in the context of their entire range of affective experience. Later sections of this chapter show how this approach has been useful in measuring food liking among obese versus nonobese individuals.

Inappropriate scaling invalidates comparisons by distorting results

Thus far, this chapter has described the logical flaws of category scaling and recent efforts to correct them, but why is it so important to address these problems? The basic assumption of category scales is that the labels embedded in them mean the same thing to everyone; in more explicit terms, each label must mark a specific intensity experienced equally by all. When this assumption fails, scale ratings cease to provide valid comparisons. Typically, this distortion minimizes or obscures differences that are actually present, but in some cases it leads to an apparent difference in the opposite direction, known as a *reversal artifact*. These distortion effects have been noted by a variety of experts (Aitken, 1969; Biernat & Manis, 1994; Birnbaum, 1999; Narens & Luce, 1983), and it is discouraging that they have been so completely disregarded.

Figure 5.1 illustrates this effect using the example of taste sensation, a modality that shows robust individual variation. Figure 5.1A illustrates observed differences in taste perception among nontasters and supertasters of PROP. (These effects are idealized, but they reflect differences observed in multiple studies.) The three functions represent stimuli that show different degrees of variation across these taste-defined groups: quinine shows a large group difference, but NaCl shows a small difference. Figure 5.1B shows how these real differences are distorted when the label "very strong taste" is erroneously assumed to be equal for everyone. Differences that exceed the variation associated with the label's meaning (quinine) are reduced, those equal to that variation (sucrose) disappear, and those smaller than the label difference (NaCl) become reversal artifacts (Bartoshuk & Snyder, 2004).

Compelling support for this theoretical framework appears in Figure 5.2, which examines several studies comparing perceived taste intensity among nontasters, medium tasters, and supertasters:

(A) Reality

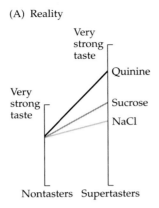

(B) Incorrect assumption that "very strong taste" is the same absolute intensity for nontasters and supertasters of PROP

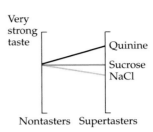

Nontasters Supertasters   Nontasters Supertasters

FIGURE 5.1   Differences in taste perception among nontasters and supertasters of PROP vary depending on the assumptions of the measurement scale used. (A) Individual differences in oral sensation lead to corresponding differences in the absolute intensity conveyed by the label "very strong taste." (B) Sensory differences are compressed—and sometimes reversed—when the scale label is assumed to be equal for everyone. (After Bartoshuk & Snyder, 2004.)

- Figure 5.2A shows data collected using a VAS labeled "none" at one end and "extremely strong" at the other (Tepper & Nurse, 1997). Because the VAS is anchored in terms of the experience judged—in this case, taste—supertasters and medium tasters appear to find high concentrations of PROP equally intense. In fact, magnitude-matching experiments reliably show what the VAS cannot: supertasters find PROP more intense (Bartoshuk et al., 1994), suggesting that the two groups use the VAS term "extremely strong" to indicate very different intensities. For NaCl, the supertaster function represents a reversal artifact, as it actually falls below the functions for nontasters and medium tasters. (Similar examples of reversal artifacts are found in Drewnowski et al., 2007; Drewnowski, Henderson, & Shore, 1997; Drewnowski et al., 1997; Yackinous & Guinard, 2001, 2002.)

- In Figure 5.2B, data were collected using the LMS (Tepper & Ullrich, 2002). Again, PROP functions for supertasters and medium tasters converge at high concentrations, and NaCl shows a reversal artifact—in this case because the top label of the LMS, "strongest imaginable oral sensation," is a poor standard for studies that actually involve oral sensation. As with the VAS, the LMS cannot reveal that supertasters actually experience the strongest taste intensity.

- Figure 5.2C and D reflect data collected using the gLMS (Bartoshuk, Duffy, Green, et al., 2004; Yeomans et al., 2007). Because these studies used scaling methods suitable for measuring individual differences in

(A) VAS

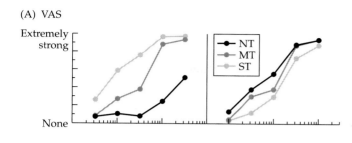

FIGURE 5.2   Taste intensity functions for PROP and NaCl collected with different scaling methods: VAS (A), LMS (B), and gLMS (C and D). Nontasters (NT); medium tasters (MT); supertasters (ST). (A after Tepper & Nurse, 1997; B after Tepper & Ullrich, 2002; C after Yeomans et al., 2007; D after Bartoshuk, Duffy, Green, et al., 2004).

(B) LMS, (100 = strongest imaginable oral sensation)

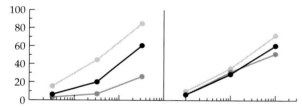

(C) gLMS, (100 = strongest imaginable oral sensation)

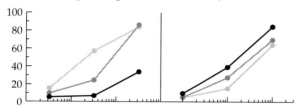

(D) gLMS, (100 = strongest imaginable oral sensation)

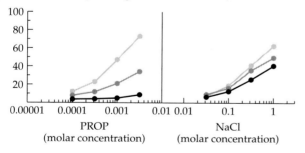

taste perception (i.e., an independent standard), they found that supertasters indeed experience the most intense taste sensations. The gLMS produces a more accurate portrayal of oral sensory variation than do the other scales, so naturally it permits more accurate classification of subjects into taste-related groups.

Sensory and hedonic comparisons—and their broader relevance—are only as valid as the tools used to measure them, so it is hardly surprising that inappropriate scaling has impaired efforts to associate oral sensory variation with intake behavior and other health-related outcomes. Unfortunately, these careless methods persist (e.g., Drewnowski et al., 2007) because they are convenient, even though they fail to capture effects reliably demonstrated by more rigorous techniques.

Intensity Scaling in Obesity Research: How Do Obese Individuals Interact with Food-Related Stimuli?

This section focuses on the impact of inappropriate sensory and affective comparisons on obesity research. As with the oral sensory studies already described, many long-held views on obesity appear to be informed by poor measurement. Careful reconsideration of these views will reveal how refined intensity scales might be used to generate useful comparisons among obese versus nonobese individuals.

Do obese individuals like food more?

It is widely believed that obese individuals consume excess calories because they derive greater pleasure from food. Schachter's (1971) externality theory reflects this view, arguing that obese individuals show an elevated appetitive response for food cues, but this work has been roundly criticized (e.g., Rodin, 1981). Although obesity is characterized by "nonhomeostatic" intake, Mela (2006) concluded that "obesity is not reliably associated with heightened hedonic responses to foods" (p. 10); instead, it may be associated with greater motivation toward eating in general.[5] Is this actually the case? Much of the evidence supporting this conclusion relies on comparisons between obese and nonobese individuals; as demonstrated already, these comparisons are susceptible to comparison errors that encourage us to revisit the issue.

The remainder of this chapter contains data from a questionnaire administered to lecture attendees beginning in 1993 (Bartoshuk, Duffy, Chapo, et al., 2004). These data include demographic information (e.g., sex, age, height, weight), health-related questions related to taste pathology (e.g., head injuries, ear infection), hedonic ratings for 26 foods and beverages (Table 5.1), and intensity ratings for PROP and a butterscotch candy. Consistent with the views on scaling stated thus far, sensory ratings were made with the gLMS and hedonic ratings were made with the hedonic gLMS.

---

[5]This apparent discrepancy derives from evidence supporting a neurobehavioral distinction between "liking" (i.e., hedonic value) and "wanting" (i.e., incentive motivation; Berridge, 1996, 2004).

Table 5.1
Food Groups Resulting from Factor Analysis of Hedonic Ratings

Sweet foods	High-Fat foods	Bitter foods	Salty foods	Remainder
Sugar	Cheddar cheese	Black coffee	Salt	Bananas
Oreo cookies	Mayonnaise	Beer	Salted pretzels	Cooked broccoli
Whipped cream[a]	Whipped cream[a]	Dark chocolate[b]	Popcorn	Margarine
Dark chocolate[b]	Whole milk	Grapefruit juice		Jello
Sweets[c]	Sour cream			Marshmallows
Honey	Sausage			Strawberries
Milk chocolate	Butter			Pecan pie

[a]Whipped cream fell into the sweet and fat food groups.
[b]Dark chocolate fell into the sweet and bitter food groups.
[c]"Sweets" is a food rated by subjects; "sweet foods" is a group identified via factor analysis.

Figure 5.3 shows the highest and lowest food-liking scores for each subject, grouped by body mass index (BMI). Multiple regression showed that BMI contributes to maximum and minimum food-liking ratings independently of age and sex. In other words, contrary to Mela's view, individuals with higher BMIs show a greater hedonic response for food overall; they live in a more palatable

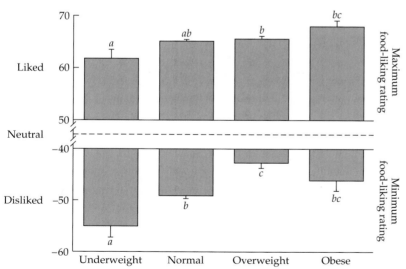

FIGURE 5.3   Maximum and minimum hedonic ratings (hedonic gLMS) for an array of 26 foods and beverages (listed in Table 5.1), plotted by BMI (underweight, <20 kg/m², normal, 20–24.9 kg/m²; overweight, 25–29.9 kg/m²; obese, >30 kg/m²). At each extreme, bars with different letters are significantly different.

food world. This relationship cannot be detected by conventional hedonic scales because these scales assume that the top anchor (i.e., maximal food liking) is equal for everyone; since this experience is actually more intense for the obese, genuine differences are concealed.

Do obese individuals show greater liking for sweet and high-fat foods?

Although the questionnaire data show that obese individuals live in a hedonically more positive food world, does this finding translate to increased liking for the most energy-dense foods? Sweets and fats are, of course, highly palatable and calorie-rich, particularly when combined (Drewnowski & Greenwood, 1983; Smith, 2004); as Pangborn and Simone (1958) observed, "In the mind of the layman, sugar and sweets are 'fattening' and most overweight individuals have a 'sweet tooth'" (p. 24). However, a series of early studies intending to document this idea led to a surprising distinction: fat is liked more by the obese, but sweetness is not (for reviews see Bartoshuk et al., 2006; de Graaf, 2006; Mela & Rogers, 1998). Once again, though, these studies used scales that do not permit comparisons of hedonic ratings across weight groups. What happens when the hedonic gLMS is used?

From the lecture questionnaire database, factor analysis of hedonic gLMS ratings for the 26 foods and beverages surveyed produced four reliable conceptual groups (see Table 5.1). This analysis focused on two of these groups, identified as "sweet foods" (i.e., sugar, Oreo cookies, whipped cream, dark chocolate, sweets, honey, milk chocolate) and "high-fat foods" (i.e., cheddar cheese, mayonnaise, whipped cream, whole milk, sour cream, sausage, butter). Figure 5.4A shows hedonic gLMS ratings for sugar and the two food groups for thin (BMI <18.5) and obese (BMI >30) individuals: contrary to the "distinction" observed in earlier work, obese individuals like all three stimuli significantly more. Of particular interest, Figure 5.4B shows the consequences of assuming that maximum food liking is equally intense for obese and thin individuals. This result—consistent with 50 years of obesity-related dogma—demonstrates the pitfalls of faulty scaling: obese individuals continue to like fats more, but the effects observed in Figure 5.4A disappear for sweets and sugar. In short, when the experiment is performed properly, obese individuals find both sweet and high-fat foods more palatable, but the effect is much greater for fats (Bartoshuk et al., 2006).

Do obese individuals taste sweetness differently?

In much of the existing literature comparing obese versus nonobese individuals, neither threshold nor suprathreshold differences in sweetness were detected (Drewnowski et al., 1991; Enns et al., 1979; Frijters & Rasmussen-Conrad, 1982; Grinker et al., 1972; Malcolm et al., 1980; Rodin, 1975; Rodin et al., 1976; Thomp-

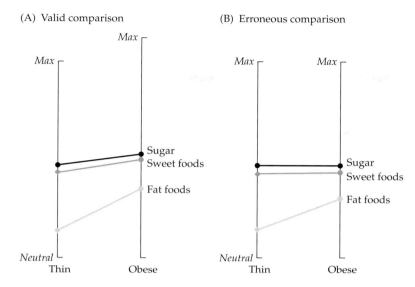

FIGURE 5.4   Differences in hedonic ratings for sweet foods, high-fat foods, and sugar among thin (BMI <18.5; n = 144) and obese individuals (BMI >30; n = 305). (A) Data collected with the hedonic gLMS; differences for all three stimuli are statistically significant ($p < 0.05$). (B) Hedonic differences are compressed (for fats; $p < 0.05$) or eliminated (for sugar and sweets) when the scale label "maximum food liking" is assumed equal for both groups. (After Bartoshuk et al., 2006.)

son et al., 1977; Witherly, 1978; Witherly et al., 1980; Wooley et al., 1972). Threshold studies do not prove that sweetness intensity and BMI are unrelated because sensory thresholds fail to predict suprathreshold sensation (e.g., Bartoshuk, 1988). Meanwhile, the suprathreshold studies cited here employed methods that lead to invalid comparisons between groups. Thus, as with food hedonics, the relationship between sweet taste and obesity must be revisited.

The lecture questionnaire used the gLMS for sensory assessment, thus permitting valid comparisons. Multiple regression showed that sweetness intensity makes a significant contribution to BMI independently of sex and age. Specifically, sweetness intensity shows a negative relationship with BMI; as BMI rises from 20 to 40, perceived sweetness drops by about 10%. If, as these data indicate, obesity is associated with reduced sweet taste, then differences in sweet liking (e.g., Figure 5.4) must be corrected to account for this sensory difference. This task is accomplished by plotting the hedonic value of sweetness as a function of its sensory intensity (Moskowitz, 1971). Figure 5.5 shows that this relationship changes with body mass: at any given sweetness level, sweet liking rises with BMI (Bartoshuk et al., 2006).

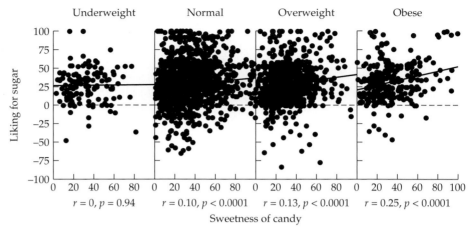

FIGURE 5.5 Hedonic ratings for sugar (hedonic gLMS) plotted against the sweetness of a piece of butterscotch candy (gLMS) for various BMI groups (underweight, <20 kg/m^2; normal, 20–24.9 kg/m^2; overweight, 25–29.9 kg/m^2; obese, >30 kg/m^2). (After Bartoshuk et al., 2006.)

Do obese individuals perceive fat differently?

The neural basis of fat perception remains controversial; it is certainly a tactile stimulus, but it may be a taste stimulus as well (e.g., Chalé-Rush et al., 2007). Consistent with this view, the rewarding properties of fat resemble those of sweet taste (Liang et al., 2006). Yet, although fat intake is widely associated with obesity risk, few data have been collected on fat sensations in obese versus nonobese individuals. One study found no difference in "creaminess" intensity among Pima Indians (who are especially prone to obesity) versus Caucasians (Salbe et al., 2004), but these data were collected using a VAS labeled in terms of fat intensity, rendering the comparison invalid.

To date, data on fat intensity have not been collected using tools that allow direct comparison across BMI groups. This important question remains ripe for further study.

Taste Damage Reveals Complex Interactions that May Promote Obesity

Earlier sections of this chapter focused on invalid comparisons and their impact on current beliefs about obesity. This section, however, reports a new discovery. Although negative correlations between sweet-fat sensations and BMI do not imply a causal direction, mounting evidence suggests that taste damage contributes to obesity risk. This idea is particularly interesting because it represents an environmental rather than a genetic contribution to weight gain. In short, local insults to taste function may alter the sensory properties of foods in ways that boost the hedonic value of energy-dense foods, leading to increased body mass.

Damage to taste perception has consequences that extend far beyond the simple loss of taste sensations. First, taste loss intensifies some oral tactile sensations, including those evoked by fats. This intensification occurs presumably because taste input normally inhibits oral tactile sensations, and taste damage releases this inhibition (Bartoshuk, Snyder, et al., 2005). Second, the links between taste and retronasal olfaction outlined in the next section imply that taste damage compromises food flavor. Together, these changes suggest that taste damage makes sensations evoked by fats more salient.

Taste and retronasal olfaction

Odorants reach the olfactory mucosa by two different routes. When we sniff, odorants enter the nostrils and pass over the turbinate bones; the resulting turbulence causes odorized air to rise to olfactory receptors at the top of the nasal cavity. This process is known as *orthonasal olfaction*. Alternatively, when we put food in our mouths, odorants in the food are forced behind the palate into the nasal cavity by chewing and swallowing. This process is known as *retronasal olfaction*.

The food industry has known for some time that taste and retronasal olfaction are connected (e.g., Noble, 1996); for example, to intensify the pear sensation from pear juice, a manufacturer might add sugar. Recent work has shown that PROP nontasters, with their weaker taste sensations, also experience less intense retronasal olfaction (Bartoshuk, Christensen, et al., 2005; Duffy et al., 2003). In clinical evaluations, some patients who have suffered damage to nerves innervating the oral cavity report a loss of flavor perception, yet orthonasal olfaction remains normal. Similarly, individuals with histories of ear infections experience reduced taste and retronasal olfactory function (Collins et al., 2006). Studies on anesthesia of the oral cavity support these patient reports: unilateral anesthesia of the chorda tympani diminishes retronasal olfaction (Snyder et al., 2001).[6]

Taste damage may increase obesity risk

Infections of the middle ear (i.e., otitis media) may promote taste damage by injuring the chorda tympani nerve as it passes through the middle ear. The association between BMI and the severity of otitis media history[7], first noticed some years ago (Snyder et al., 2004; Snyder et al., 2003a,b; Snyder, Duffy, Chapo,

---

[6]Unilateral anesthesia of the chorda tympani does not diminish whole-mouth taste (because of disinhibition), so the drop in retronasal olfaction cannot be attributed to confusion between taste and retronasal olfactory intensity.

[7]In the lecture questionnaire, those who indicated that they had suffered otitis media requiring antibiotics or tubes were designated as having a moderate to severe history.

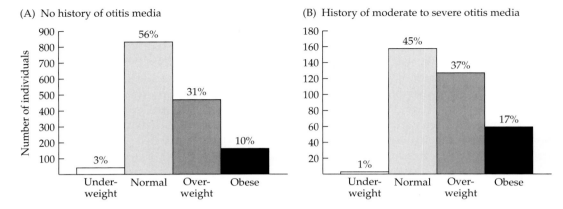

(A) No history of otitis media

(B) History of moderate to severe otitis media

FIGURE 5.6 Number of individuals who are underweight, normal, overweight, or obese among those with a history of moderate to severe otitis media (B) versus those with no history (A). (See Figure 5.5 for BMI group definitions.)

Hoffman, et al., 2003), is both reliable and robust. With multiple regression, age, sex, and otitis media history all contribute independently to BMI. The fact that BMI rises with age is well known; in this data set, BMI was also greater for males. The effect for otitis media history supports previous analyses: individuals with moderate to severe histories of otitis media have higher BMIs, and the magnitude of the effect rises with age. To illustrate, Figure 5.6 shows distributions of BMI for subjects aged 30 and older with a history of moderate to severe otitis media versus those with no history. These distributions are significantly different; indeed, the majority of the individuals with a history of moderate to severe otitis media are overweight or obese.

The relationship between otitis media and increased BMI has now been corroborated by two epidemiological databases (Hoffman et al., 2007; Nelson et al., 2007a,b). In addition, a study examining predictors of obesity in Puerto Rican children showed that obese children were more likely to have experienced ear infections (Tanasescu et al., 2000). Finally, an association between otitis media history and BMI has been described in two separate cohorts of young children (Corcoran et al., 2007; Kim et al., 2007).[8]

TASTE DAMAGE BEYOND OTITIS MEDIA   Also under examination is the possibility that damage to other taste nerves is associated with weight gain. Tonsillectomy

---

[8]Interestingly, one of these studies (Kim et al., 2007) suggested that obesity promotes otitis media. This explanation reverses the model described here; if such an effect exists, it cannot explain the onset of obesity in adults whose otitis media occurred in childhood.

damages the glossopharyngeal nerve, which carries taste and somatosensory input from the rear of the tongue. Two sources of evidence suggest that tonsillectomy is associated with weight gain: the association is evident in the lecture questionnaire database (Bartoshuk et al., 2007) and in an early iteration of the National Health and Nutrition Examination Survey (NHANES; Hoffman et al., 2007).

More generally, those with taste damage arising from many different sources (including otitis media and tonsillectomy) can be identified with *spatial taste testing*, which assesses each of the cranial nerves mediating taste function. In this test, subjects rate the intensities of taste solutions swabbed onto various oral loci; they also rate those solutions when sipped and swallowed (i.e., whole-mouth taste). The ratio of taste intensity on the anterior tongue to whole-mouth taste intensity serves as a measure of anterior taste damage. Hayes and Duffy (2007) have shown that this ratio correlates negatively with adiposity; subjects with higher proportions of body fat show more severe taste damage.

Taste damage alters food choice

If taste damage influences subsequent oral sensations and promotes BMI gain, it probably affects dietary behavior as well. Duffy's laboratory has shown that young children with histories of otitis media consume fewer vegetables and more sweet and salty foods (Arsenault et al., 2004). The consequences of this early pathology—beginning with oral sensory damage—may extend into adulthood: adults with taste damage show reduced liking and intake measures for vegetables (Dinehart et al., 2006), increased intake of alcohol (Duffy et al., 2004), and increased liking and intake measures for sweet-fat foods (Hayes & Duffy, 2007).

Hedonic ratings for the foods in the lecture questionnaire show that individuals aged 30 and older with a history of moderate to severe otitis media show 12% greater overall food liking than do those without that history. Interestingly, among the 26 foods assessed, this increase in liking corresponds to energy density. As Figure 5.7 shows, the hedonic difference between those with and without a history of moderate to severe otitis media rises with caloric load; that is, as energy density increases, those with histories of otitis media show increased food liking. These findings suggest that oral sensory alterations produced by otitis media lead to elevated food liking over time, which in turn may promote greater energy intake and BMI gain.

Thus far, taste damage has been associated with surprisingly broad alterations in the sensory properties of foods. It has also been associated with changes in the hedonic value of foods—changes that favor increased energy intake. However, it is not yet known how these sensory and hedonic changes are linked. What is clear is that continued advances in the psychophysical scaling of hedonic experience will contribute to the solution of this fascinating puzzle.

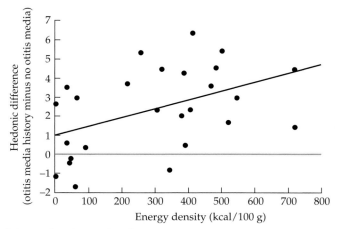

FIGURE 5.7 For each of the 26 foods rated in the lecture questionnaire, the hedonic difference between subjects with and without histories of moderate to severe otitis media is plotted against the energy density of the food ($r = 0.45$, $p < 0.05$).

Conclusion

Obesity is driven by a combination of excessive caloric intake and insufficient energy expenditure, but a fuller understanding of nonhomeostatic intake requires accurate measurements of sensory and hedonic experience. This chapter has provided examples of erroneous conclusions resulting from the use of conventional labeled scales to compare such experiences among obese versus nonobese individuals. Although these scales are suitable under certain circumstances—for example, within-subject comparisons, or comparisons among randomly assigned groups—problems arise when groups differing in a particular characteristic (e.g., sex, age, disease state) are compared because scale labels may not denote the same perceived intensities to members of those groups.

As it turns out, sensory and hedonic labels do not denote the same perceived intensities to obese versus nonobese individuals. Scaling techniques that allow valid comparisons show that the obese live in a more hedonically positive food world than do the nonobese, particularly when it comes to sweet-fat, energy-dense foods. This phenomenon is hardly limited to nontasters (who are most likely to become obese), as taste damage appears to alter the sensory and hedonic properties of foods in ways that promote BMI gain. Together, these findings demonstrate the important role of accurate psychophysical measurement in guiding more refined views of obesity and its enduring impact on health.

References Cited

Aitken, R. C. B. (1969). Measurement of feelings using visual analogue scales. *Proceedings of the Royal Society of Medicine, 62*, 989–993.

Arsenault, M. A., MacLeod, E., Weinstein, J. L., Phillips, V., Ferris, A. M., & Duffy, V. B. (2004, May). *Reported history of otitis media (OM) in children associates with intake of vegetables and sweets.* Paper presented at the International Congress of Dietetics, Chicago, IL.

Bartoshuk, L. M. (1979). Bitter taste of saccharin: Related to the genetic ability to taste the bitter substance 6-*N*-propylthiouracil (PROP). *Science, 205*, 934–935.

Bartoshuk, L. M. (1988). Clinical psychophysics of taste. *Gerodontics, 4*, 249–255.

Bartoshuk, L. M. (1991). Sweetness: History, preference, and genetic variability. *Food Technology, 45*, 108–113.

Bartoshuk, L. M., Christensen, C. M., Duffy, V., Sheridan, K., Small, D. M., & Snyder, D. (2005). PROP and retronasal olfaction. *Chemical Senses, 30*, A236.

Bartoshuk, L., Davidson, A., Kidd, J., Kidd, K., Speed, W., Pakstis, A. et al. (2005). Supertasting is not explained by the PTC/PROP gene. *Chemical Senses, 30*, A87.

Bartoshuk, L. M., Duffy, V. B., Chapo, A. K., Fast, K., Yiee, J. H., Hoffman, H. J. et al. (2004). From psychophysics to the clinic: missteps and Advances. *Food Quality and Preference, 15*, 617–632.

Bartoshuk, L. M., Duffy, V. B., Fast, K., Green, B. G., Prutkin, J. M., & Snyder, D. J. (2002). Labeled scales (e.g., category, Likert, VAS) and invalid across-group comparisons. What we have learned from genetic variation in taste. *Food Quality and Preference, 14*, 125–138.

Bartoshuk, L. M., Duffy, V. B., Fast, K., Green, B. G., & Snyder, D. J. (2002). Hormones, age, genes and pathology: How do we assess variation in sensation and preference? In H. Anderson, J. Blundell, & M. Chiva (Eds.), *Food Selection: From Genes to Culture* (pp. 173–187). Paris: Danone Institute.

Bartoshuk, L. M., Duffy, V. B., Green, B. G., Hoffman, H. J., Ko, C.-W., Lucchina, L. A. et al. (2004). Valid across-group comparisons with labeled scales: the gLMS vs

magnitude matching. *Physiology & Behavior, 82*, 109–114.

Bartoshuk, L. M., Duffy, V. B., Hayes, J. E., Moskowitz, H., & Snyder, D. J. (2006). Psychophysics of sweet and fat perception in obesity: Problems, solutions and new perspectives. *Philosophical Transactions of the Royal Society: Biological Sciences, 361*, 1137–1148.

Bartoshuk, L. M., Duffy, V. B., & Miller, I. J. (1994). PTC/PROP tasting: Anatomy, psychophysics, and sex effects. *Physiology & Behavior, 56*, 1165–1171.

Bartoshuk, L. M., Fast, K., Duffy, V. B., Prutkin, J. M., Snyder, D. J., & Green, B. G. (2000). Magnitude matching and a modified LMS produce valid sensory comparisons for PROP studies. *Appetite, 35*, 277.

Bartoshuk, L. M., Fast, K., Karrer, T. A., Marino, S., Price, R. A., & Reed, D. A. (1992). PROP supertasters and the perception of sweetness and bitterness. *Chemical Senses, 17*, 594.

Bartoshuk, L. M., Green, B. G., Snyder, D. J., Lucchina, L. A., Hoffman, H. J., Weiffenbach, J. M. et al. (2000). Valid across-group comparisons: Supertasters perceive the most intense taste sensations by magnitude matching or the LMS scale. *Chemical Senses, 25*, 639.

Bartoshuk, L. M., Rifkin, B., Marks, L. E., & Hooper, J. E. (1988). Bitterness of KCl and benzoate: related to genetic status for sensitivity to PTC/PROP. *Chemical Senses, 13*, 517–528.

Bartoshuk, L. M., & Snyder, D. J. (2004). Psychophysical measurement of human taste experience. In E. Stricker & S. Woods (Eds.), *Handbook of Behavioral Neurobiology* (Vol. 14, pp. 89–107). New York: Plenum Press.

Bartoshuk, L. M., Snyder, D. J., Catalanotto, F. A., & Hoffman, H. J. (2007, August). *Taste damage (otitis media, head trauma, tonsillectomy) and obesity.* Paper presented at the 7th Pangborn Sensory Science Symposium.

Bartoshuk, L. M., Snyder, D. J., Grushka, M., Berger, A. M., Duffy, V., B, & Kveton, J. F. (2005). Taste damage: previously unsuspected consequences. *Chemical Senses, 30*(Suppl. 1), i218–i219.

Berridge, K. C. (1996). Food reward: Brain substrates of wanting and liking.

Neuroscience and Biobehavioral Reviews, 20, 1–25.

Berridge, K. C. (2004). Motivation concepts in behavioral neuroscience. *Physiology & Behavior, 81,* 179–209.

Biernat, M., & Manis, M. (1994). Shifting standards and stereotype-based judgements. *Journal of Personality and Social Psychology, 66,* 5–20.

Birnbaum, M. H. (1999). How to show that 9 > 221: Collect judgements in a between-subjects design. *Psychological Methods, 4,* 243–249.

Blakeslee, A. F., & Fox, A. L. (1932). Our different taste worlds. *Journal of Heredity, 23,* 97–107.

Borg, G. (1982). A category scale with ratio properties for intermodal and interindividual comparisons. In H. G. Geissler & P. Petzold (Eds.), *Psychophysical Judgment and the Process of Perception* (pp. 25–34). Berlin, Germany: VEB Deutscher Verlag der Wissenschaften.

Chalé-Rush, A., Burgess, J. R., & Mattes, R. D. (2007). Multiple routes of chemosensitivity to free fatty acids in humans. *American Journal of Physiology – Gastrointestinal and Liver Physiology, 292,* G1206–1212.

Collins, S. P., Snyder, D. J., Catalanotto, F., & Bartoshuk, L. M. (2006). Retronasal olfaction and otitis media. *Chemical Senses, 31,* A38.

Corcoran, A., Kneeland, K., Harrington, H., & Duffy, V. (2007, May). *Overweight in preschoolers: Relationships with otitis media exposure and utilization of nutrition assistance programs.* Paper presented at The Connecticut Dietetic Association Spring 2007 Meeting.

de Graaf, C. (2006). Sensory responses, food intake and obesity. In D. J. Mela (Ed.), *Food, Diet and Obesity* (pp. 137–159). Cambridge: Woodhead Publishing.

Dinehart, M. E., Hayes, J. E., Bartoshuk, L. M., Lanier, S. L., & Duffy, V. B. (2006). Bitter taste markers explain variability in vegetable sweetness, bitterness, and intake. *Physiology & Behavior, 87,* 304–313.

Drewnowski, A., & Greenwood, M. R. C. (1983). Cream and sugar: Human preferences for high-fat foods. *Physiology & Behavior, 30,* 629–633.

Drewnowski, A., Henderson, S. A., & Cockroft, J. E. (2007). Genetic sensitivity to 6-*n*-propylthiouracil has no influence on

dietary patterns, body mass index, or plasma lipid profiles of women. *The American Dietetic Association, 107,* 1340–1348.

Drewnowski, A., Henderson, S. A., & Shore, A. B. (1997). Genetic sensitivity to 6-*n*-propylthiouracil (PROP) and hedonic responses to bitter and sweet tastes. *Chemical Senses, 22,* 27–37.

Drewnowski, A., Henderson, S. A., Shore, A. B., & Barratt-Fornell, A. (1997). Nontasters, tasters, and supertasters of 6-n-propylthiouracil (PROP) and hedonic response to sweet. *Physiology & Behavior, 62,* 649–655.

Drewnowski, A., Kurth, C. L., & Rahaim, J. E. (1991). Taste preferences in human obesity: environmental and familiar factors. *American Journal of Clinical Nutrition, 54,* 635–641.

Duffy, V. B., Chapo, A. K., Hutchins, H. L., & Bartoshuk, L. M. (2003). Retronasal olfactory intensity: Associations with taste. *Chemical Senses, 28,* A33.

Duffy, V. B., Peterson, J. M., & Bartoshuk, L. M. (2004). Associations between taste genetics, oral sensation and alcohol intake. *Physiology & Behavior, 82,* 435–445.

Enns, M. P., Van Itallie, T. B., & Grinker, J. (1979). Contributions of age, sex and degree of fatness on preferences and magnitude estimations for sucrose in humans. *Physiology & Behavior, 22,* 999–1003.

Farbman, A. I., & Hellekant, G. (1978). Quantitative analyses of the fiber population in rat chorda tympani nerves and fungiform papillae. *American Journal of Anatomy, 153,* 509-521.

Fast, K. (2004). *Developing a scale to measure just about anything: Comparisons across groups and individuals.* Unpublished medical thesis, Yale University School of Medicine, New Haven, CT.

Fox, A. L. (1931). Six in ten "tasteblind" to bitter chemical. *Science News Letter, 9,* 249.

Frijters, J. E. R., & Rasmussen-Conrad, E. L. (1982). Sensory discrimination, intensity perception, and affective judgment of sucrose-sweetness in the overweight. *Journal of General Psychology, 107,* 233–247.

Gent, J. F., & Bartoshuk, L. M. (1983). Sweetness of sucrose, neohesperidin dihydrochalcone, and saccharin is related to genetic ability to taste the bitter substance 6-*n*-propylthiouracil. *Chemical Senses, 7,* 265–272.

Gracely, R. H., McGrath, P., & Dubner, R. (1978). Ratio scales of sensory and affective verbal pain descriptors. *Pain, 5,* 5–18.

Green, B. G., Shaffer, G. S., & Gilmore, M. M. (1993). A semantically-labeled magnitude scale of oral sensation with apparent ratio properties. *Chemical Senses, 18,* 683–702.

Grinker, J., Hirsch, J., & Smith, D. V. (1972). Taste sensitivity and susceptibility to external influence in obese and normal weight subjects. *Journal of Personality and Social Psychology, 22,* 320–325.

Hall, M. J., Bartoshuk, L. M., Cain, W. S., & Stevens, J. C. (1975). PTC taste blindness and the taste of caffeine. *Nature, 253,* 442–443.

Harris, H., & Kalmus, H. (1949). The measurement of taste sensitivity to phenylthiourea (P.T.C.). *Annals of Eugenics, 15,* 24–31.

Hayes, J. E., & Duffy, V. B. (2007, August). *Explaining variance in central adiposity through taste phenotype and food preference.* Paper presented at the 7th Pangborn Sensory Science Symposium.

Hetherington, M. M., & Rolls, B. J. (1987). Methods of investigating human eating behavior. In F. M. Toates & N. E. Rowland (Eds.), *Feeding and Drinking* (pp. 77–109). New York: Elsevier.

Hoffman, H. J., Losonczy, K., Bartoshuk, L. M., Himes, J. H., Snyder, D. J., & Duffy, V. B. (2007, June). *Taste damage from tonsillectomy or otitis media may lead to overweight children: The U.S. National Health Examination Surveys (NHES), 1963–1970.* Paper presented at the 9th International Symposium on Recent Advances in Otitis Media.

Kamen, J. M., Pilgrim, F. J., Gutman, N. J., & Kroll, B. J. (1961). Interactions of suprathreshold taste stimuli. *Journal of Experimental Psychology, 62,* 348–356.

Kim, J. B., Park, D. C., Cha, C. I., & Yeo, S. G. (2007). Relationship between pediatric obesity and otitis media with effusion. *Archives of Otolaryngology-Head and Neck Surgery, 133,* 379–382.

Kim, U. K., Jorgenson, E., Coon, H., Leppert, M., Risch, N., & Drayna, D. (2003). Positional cloning of the human quantitative trait locus underlying taste sensitivity to phenylthiocarbamide. *Science, 299,* 1221–1225.

Liang, N. C., Hajnal, A., & Norgren, R. (2006). Sham feeding corn oil increases accumbens dopamine in the rat. *American Journal of Physiology – Gastrointestinal and Liver Physiology, 291,* R1236–1239.

Malcolm, R., O'Neil, P. M., Hirsch, A. A., Currey, H. S., & Moskowitz, G. (1980). Taste hedonics and thresholds in obesity. *International Journal of Obesity, 4,* 203–212.

Marks, L. E., & Stevens, J. C. (1980). Measuring sensation in the aged. In L. W. Poon (Ed.), *Aging in the 1980's: Psychological issues* (pp. 592–598). Washington, DC: American Psychological Association.

Marks, L. E., Stevens, J. C., Bartoshuk, L. M., Gent, J. G., Rifkin, B., & Stone, V. K. (1988). Magnitude matching: The measurement of taste and smell. *Chemical Senses, 13,* 63–87.

Mela, D. J. (2006). Eating for pleasure or just wanting to eat? Reconsidering sensory hedonic responses as a driver of obesity. *Appetite, 47,* 10–17.

Mela, D. J., & Rogers, P. J. (Eds.). (1998). *Food, Eating and Obesity: The psychobiological basis of appetite and weight control.* New York: Chapman and Hall.

Miller, I. J., & Reedy, F. E. (1990). Variations in human taste bud density and taste intensity perception. *Physiology & Behavior, 47,* 1213–1219.

Moskowitz, H. R. (1971). The sweetness and pleasantness of sugars. *American Journal of Psychology, 84,* 387–420.

Moskowitz, H. R. (1977). Magnitude estimation: Notes on what, how, when, and why to use it. *Journal of Food Quality, 1,* 195–228.

Narens, L., & Luce, R. D. (1983). How we may have been misled into believing in the interpersonal comparability of utility. *Theory and Decision, 15,* 247–260.

Nelson, H., Daly, K., Davey, C., & Bartoshuk, L. M. (2007a, June). *Otitis media and overweight in toddlers.* Paper presented at the 9th International Symposium on Recent Advances in Otitis Media.

Nelson, H. M., Daly, K. A., Davey, C. S., & Bartoshuk, L. M. (2007b, June). *Otitis media and overweight in toddlers.* Paper presented at the 20th Annual Meeting of the Society for Pediatric and Perinatal Epidemiologic Research.

Noble, A. C. (1996). Taste-aroma interactions. *Trends in Food Science and Technology, 7,* 439–444.

Pangborn, R. M., & Simone, M. (1958). Body size and sweetness preference. *Journal of the American Dietetic Association, 34,* 924–928.

Price, D. D., McGrath, P. A., Rafii, A., & Buckingham, B. (1983). The validation of visual analogue scales as ratio scale measures for chronic and experimental pain. *Pain, 17,* 45–56.

Prutkin, J. M., Duffy, V. B., Etter, L., Fast, K., Gardner, E., Lucchina, L. A. et al. (2000). Genetic variation and inferences about perceived taste intensity in mice and men. *Physiology & Behavior, 69,* 161–173.

Rodin, J. (1975). Effects of obesity and set point on taste responsiveness and ingestion in humans. *Journal of Comparative and Physiological Psychology, 89,* 1003–1009.

Rodin, J. (1981). Current status of the internal-external hypothesis for obesity: What went wrong? *American Psychologist, 36,* 361–372.

Rodin, J., Moskowitz, H. R., & Bray, G. (1976). Relationship between obesity, weight loss, and taste responsiveness. *Physiology & Behavior, 17,* 591–597.

Salbe, A. D., DelParigi, A., Pratley, R. E., Drewnowski, A., & Tataranni, P. A. (2004). Taste preferences and body weight changes in an obesity-prone population. *American Journal of Clinical Nutrition, 79,* 372–378.

Schachter, S. (1971). Some extraordinary facts about obese humans and rats. *American Psychologist, 26,* 129–144.

Smith, J. C. (2004). Gustation as a factor in the ingestion of sweet and fat emulsions by the rat. *Physiology & Behavior, 82,* 181–185.

Snyder, D. J., Bartoshuk, L. M., McKee, S. A., & O'Malley, S. S. (2004). *Tobacco exposure during childhood predicts increased obesity risk in adult men.* Paper presented at the 10th Annual Meeting of the Society for Research on Nicotine and Tobacco, RP-078.

Snyder, D. J., Duffy, V. B., Chapo, A. K., Cobbett, L. E., & Bartoshuk, L. M. (2003a). Food preferences mediate relationships between otitis media and body mass index. *Appetite, 40,* 360.

Snyder, D. J., Duffy, V. B., Chapo, A. K., Cobbett, L. E., & Bartoshuk, L. M. (2003b). Childhood taste damage modulates obesity risk: Effects on fat perception and preference. *Obesity Research, 11*(Suppl.), A147.

Snyder, D. J., Duffy, V. B., Chapo, A. K., Hoffman, H., & Bartoshuk, L. M. (2003). Otitis media influences body mass index by interacting with sex, age and taste perception. *Chemical Senses, 28,* 12.

Snyder, D. J., Dwivedi, N., Mramor, A., Bartoshuk, L. M., & Duffy, V. B. (2001). Taste and touch may contribute to the localization of retronasal olfaction: Unilateral and bilateral anesthesia of cranial nerves V/VII. *Society for Neuroscience Abstracts, 27,* 711–727.

Snyder, L. H. (1931). Inherited taste deficiency. *Science, 74,* 151–152.

Stevens, J. C. (1959). Cross-modality validation of subjective scales for loudness, vibration, and electric shock. *Journal of Experimental Psychology, 57,* 201–209.

Stevens, J. C., & Marks, L. E. (1965). Cross-modality matching of brightness and loudness. *Proceedings of the National Academy of Sciences, 54,* 407–411.

Stevens, J. C., & Marks, L. E. (1980). Cross-modality matching functions generated by magnitude estimation. *Perception and Psychophysics, 27,* 379–389.

Stevens, S. S. (1958). Adaptation-level versus the relativity of judgment. *American Journal of Psychology, 71,* 633–646.

Stevens, S. S. (1960). On the new psychophysics. *Scandinavian Journal of Psychology, 1,* 27–35.

Tanasescu, M., Ferris, A. M., Himmelgreen, D. A., Rodriguez, N., & Perez-Escamilla, R. (2000). Biobehavioral factors are associated with obesity in Puerto Rican children. *Journal of Nutrition, 130,* 1734–1742.

Tepper, B. J., & Nurse, R. J. (1997). Fat perception is related to PROP taster status. *Physiology & Behavior, 61,* 949–954.

Tepper, B. J., & Ullrich, N. V. (2002). Influence of genetic taste sensitivity to 6-n-propylthiouracil (PROP), dietary restraint and disinhibition on body mass index in middle-aged women. *Physiology & Behavior, 75,* 305–312.

Thompson, D. A., Moskowitz, H. R., & Campbell, R. G. (1977). Taste and olfaction in human obesity. *Physiology & Behavior, 19,* 335–337.

Whitehead, M. C., Beeman, C. S., & Kinsella, B. A. (1985). Distribution of taste and general sensory nerve endings in fungiform papillae of the hamster. *American Journal of Anatomy, 173*, 185-201.

Witherly, S. A. (1978). *Eating rates, taste perception and salivary secretion between obese and non-obese subjects.* Unpublished master's thesis, University of California, Davis.

Witherly, S. A., Pangborn, R. M., & Stern, J. (1980). Gustatory responses and eating duration of obese and lean adults. *Appetite, 1*, 53–63.

Wooley, O. W., Wooley, S. C., & Dunham, R. B. (1972). Calories and sweet taste: Effects on sucrose preference in the obese and nonobese. *Physiology and Behavior, 9*, 765–768.

Yackinous, C., & Guinard, J. X. (2001). Relation between PROP taster status and fat perception, touch and olfaction. *Physiology & Behavior, 72*, 427–437.

Yackinous, C. A., & Guinard, J. X. (2002). Relation between PROP (6-*n*-propylthiouracil) taster status, taste anatomy and dietary intake measures for young men and women. *Appetite, 38*, 201–209.

Yeomans, M. R., Tepper, B. J., Rietzschel, J., & Prescott, J. (2007). Human hedonic responses to sweetness: Role of taste genetics and anatomy. *Physiology & Behavior, 91*, 264–273.

6 DEVELOPMENT OF EATING BEHAVIOR: IMMEDIATE AND LONG-TERM CONSEQUENCES

Julie Lumeng

Introduction

Considerable understanding of obesity determinants can be gained through developmental study. Two core developmental issues frame this chapter. First, early culturally determined feeding preferences endure over the life span. Second, childhood body weight strongly predicts lifetime weight. These determinants achieve special urgency now because infants and children are increasingly fed by individuals other than their parents, or fed foods prepared outside the home. Parents exert less control over what children eat today than in previous generations. This trend has broad societal implications because the variety of providers, their differing agendas, and the increasingly restrictive budget constraints that they all face place the child in a feeding situation that lacks a central figure who can *decide and deliver* what children require by way of healthy eating and exercise.

To convey the best understanding of these influences, this chapter focuses particularly on the development of food preferences and controls of hunger and satiety in childhood, and how and by whom they are influenced. The belief that parents are ultimately responsible for what their children eat and how much they weigh will be addressed through discussion of the extent and limits of parental influence on children's eating. The burden is shared by the school system, a major energy provider, and by the advertising campaigns to which children are systematically exposed.

Studying childhood obesity is of particular interest today for three reasons. First, although there have always been obese children, the prevalence has surged significantly in the last two decades: prevalence has tripled in children ages 6 to 19 since 1980, to its current rate of greater than 17% (nearly one in five), and it continues to increase (Ogden et al., 2006). The morbidities associated with childhood obesity raise the harrowing possibility that the life expectancy for children born today, for the first time in history, may be shorter than that of their parents and grandparents. As emphasized throughout this text, the obesity epidemic requires a united approach from a variety of disciplines to address it quickly and effectively.

How has the United States come to a point where nearly one in five children is obese? An excellent place to start looking for answers is sensory processes. Newborns come equipped with basic taste and flavor preferences and aversions that attract them to energy-dense foods and away from potentially toxic foods (Steiner et al., 2001). Cultural and historical influences, as well as certain non-flavor properties of foods (e.g., temperature), can both exaggerate and inhibit these innate preferences. For example, humans have developed preferences for both alcohol and coffee, despite their bitter tastes—possibly for their potent pharmacological effects. Spices and salt, originally used to preserve foods in warm climates, have subsequently become integral parts of many cuisines, even when their preservation properties are no longer needed. Western food industries have exploited the innate preferences for fats and sugars by fabricating countless palatable, low-nutrition, calorie-dense concoctions, aggressively advertising them, and stocking them on supermarket shelves and in fast-food emporiums for purchase by unsuspecting consumers and their children.

Second, humans have recognized for the past century or more that particular foods contain vitamins, minerals, and micronutrients critical to survival, and they have therefore encouraged the consumption of these types of foods (primarily fruits and vegetables), even if they are not calorically dense and are frequently less than optimally palatable. Given that most parents are armed with this knowledge and want to protect their children from becoming obese, one must ask again, What is causing the rapid increase in obesity prevalence?

The tension between our innate food preferences and cultural influences is strongest in childhood. Children naturally reject often bitter and unpalatable vegetables, favoring foods high in sugar and fat that are calorically dense. Parents and grandparents, on the other hand, put a great deal of effort into getting children to eat traditional cuisines that are important to the family culturally, as well as fruits and vegetables, which are important to the children's health.

A third reason why childhood obesity is of particular interest is that the processes underlying cuisine selection, overeating, and overweight parallel those underlying other developmental phenomena, such as language development. Humans begin both their food and their language odysseys as generalists. Newborns can respond like native speakers to all of the languages presented to them, but remarkably soon, even before they start to speak, the window closes and only their native tongue can be readily learned (Polka & Werker, 1994; Werker & Tees, 1984). Developing other languages for many is difficult, even when learning starts relatively early in childhood (Birdsong & Molis, 2001; Johnson & Newport, 1989).

The same holds for feeding development. Children have flexibility early on, accommodating a wide variety of cuisines within the constraint of preferring sweet and disliking bitter. Following the traditions of their native cuisine, children ingest bitter and strong food and drink—for example, coffee in the West, calvados in Normandy, France. Once children have developed a preference for a cuisine, however, shifting to new ones becomes increasingly difficult, particularly for people who are not adventuresome. This pattern parallels the language developmental process of specialization growing out of the initial generalist stance. Almost all people prefer speaking their native language; likewise, they prefer their native cuisine. This pattern of development appears to be true for all domains studied.

Just as eating and flavor preferences become more specific with age, linkage between early weight status and adult weight becomes increasingly strengthened and entrenched through development. The following discussion will describe underlying mechanisms, beginning with specific developmental periods in which children are vulnerable for obesity throughout the life span.

Early-Development Periods Contributing to Lifelong Obesity Risk

Lifelong obesity risk is potentially increased by four primary vulnerable periods in early development: (1) body mass index (BMI) in childhood, (2) maternal weight during pregnancy, (3) rate of weight gain in infancy, and (4) age at adiposity rebound. Each of these is described in detail in the sections that follow.

BMI in childhood predicts BMI in adulthood

Unfortunately, once obesity has taken hold in early childhood, it is likely to persist throughout the life span. The correlation between an individual's weight status as a child and as an adult strengthens over time, as best illustrated by the Bogalusa Heart Study. This study, for which longitudinal data collection began in 1972 in Bogalusa, Louisiana, has examined more than 16,000 individuals of diverse race and socioeconomic status. The data set is an invaluable resource for studying the trajectory of BMI over the life span, as well as cardiovascular risk factors. Using 2600 individuals from this cohort, Freedman and colleagues (2005b) demonstrated the increasing correlation between BMI z-score (one standard deviation unit) measured at different ages in childhood and eventual adult BMI (measured a mean of 17 years later, between ages 18 and 37 years). As illustrated in Figure 6.1, the correlation between childhood BMI z-score and adult BMI is moderate in early childhood, in the range of about 0.40 to 0.50, and gradually increases to a remarkable range of 0.60 to 0.70 by about age 9 years. In general, the tracking of BMI into adulthood was stronger in males than in females.

Older overweight children are more likely to become overweight adults. A classic study by Whitaker and colleagues (1997) reported that the odds ratios for obesity in adults when a child was obese increased as the child grew older, independent of the weight status of the parents: the odds ratio was 4.7 for 3- to 5-year-olds, 8.8 for 6- to 9-year-olds, 22.3 for 10- to 14-year-olds, and 17.5 for 15- to 17-

FIGURE 6.1 Correlation of childhood BMI z-score with adult BMI by age and gender. (After Freedman et al., 2005b.)

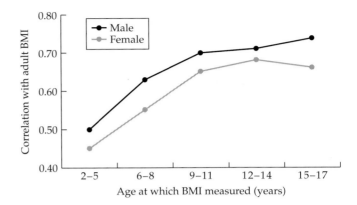

year-olds (Whitaker et al., 1997). BMI tends to continue to track along its present level as children grow older, for reasons that are not entirely clear, but possibly because of increasingly entrenched eating and exercise habits. Alternatively, biological mechanisms triggered by overeating may be the driving element. For example, critical periods for developing a defended weight level (or a concomitant) may be the result of early and continued overeating, as shown in rats.

These findings were refined in a subsequent Bogalusa study, which tracked childhood weight status into adulthood. African Americans tended to be the most vulnerable to the link between childhood and adult obesity (Figure 6.2; Freedman et al., 2005a). Further refinements are called for because this study did not separate race from socioeconomic status. Overweight white children are more likely to escape obesity as an adult if obesity is driven by education and income. White children are more likely to be of higher socioeconomic status, which affords them more opportunities and resources that support changes in

FIGURE 6.2 Proportion of children who became obese adults after being overweight (BMI ≥ ninety-fifth percentile) between ages 5 and 8 years, by gender and race. (After Freedman et al., 2005a.)

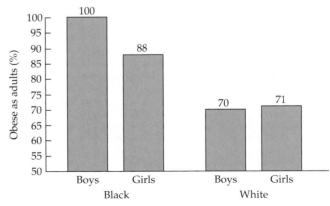

lifestyle and eating habits, compared to African American children, who are more likely to be of lower socioeconomic status. Biological factors that differ by race may also cause stronger long-term overweight tracking. The national increase in BMI reflects changes in the environment that have resulted in increased caloric intake and fewer opportunities for physical exercise. However, these secular changes may interact with biological predispositions and cultural norms to confer differential increases in obesity risk. The consistency of BMI throughout an individual's life may reflect a genetically vulnerable capacity that is realized in an energy-rich society.

Certain factors increase the likelihood that childhood BMI will track into adulthood. These include race, possibly gender, and age at elevated BMI. Future studies need to identify other factors that determine whether childhood BMI will track into adulthood. At least one study has shown a link between the persistence of obesity and psychiatric disorders in children (Mustillo et al., 2003). Additional key potential contributors that merit further study include socioeconomic status, child and parent mental health, maternal education, and availability of community resources that promote dietary and physical activity change. Progress in each area hinges on individual and community resolve to affect change.

Impact of parental weight status: nature or nurture?

Parental obesity increases the likelihood that a child will be obese as an adult (Whitaker et al., 1997). Specifically, at 1 to 2 years of age, if one parent is obese the odds of adult obesity for the child are about 3.2. If *both* parents of a 1- to 2-year-old are obese, the odds of adult obesity for the child shoot up to 13.2, *independent* of the child's own obesity status during childhood. These alarming odds have been replicated in a number of subsequent studies with diverse samples, and the issue remains to determine biological versus environmental determinants and their interactions. Figure 6.3 provides a starting point to determine the relationships among maternal weight status, child's birth weight, and future weight status. The following data support each arrow in the figure.

In a study of nearly 2500 women, maternal prepregnancy weight was associated with birth weight (Jensen et al., 2003): compared to children of normal-weight mothers, the odds of a child having a birth weight of 4 kilograms (about 9 pounds) or greater were 1.4 for mothers who were overweight (BMI ≥ 25)

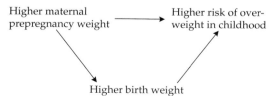

FIGURE 6.3   Relationship between maternal BMI before pregnancy and childhood overweight.

before pregnancy, and 2.2 for mothers who were obese (BMI ≥ 30) before pregnancy. These relationships held after controlling for other factors that could have affected birth weight or influenced maternal weight, including maternal blood sugar levels, age, weight gain during pregnancy, infant gestational age, parity, smoking, screening indicators for diabetes, and ethnic background.

Other work agrees with these findings: Kramer and colleagues (2002), using a sample of about 65,000 Canadian infants born between 1978 and 1996, reported that mean birth weight increased by about 57 grams (about 2 ounces), and the prevalence of infants with birth weights more than two standard deviations above the mean according to national reference data increased from 8% in 1978 to 12% in 1996. The proportion of births to mothers who were obese increased concurrently from 5% to 11%. These increases in infant birth weights were accounted for by decreases in rates of smoking and increases in maternal prepregnancy weights over time (Kramer et al., 2002). From these studies we can conclude the following:

1. Maternal weight predicts birth weight. In a sample of nearly 250,000 children from Denmark, children with birth weights of ≥ 10 pounds were more than twice as likely to be overweight by age 13 years than were children with birth weights of about 7 pounds (Rugholm et al., 2005). The study did not, however, evaluate whether this relationship was independent of maternal weight status. Whitaker and colleagues (2004), using a smaller sample of nearly 8500 mother–child pairs, addressed this issue. He demonstrated that the odds of the child being overweight at age 4 years were significantly linked with the mother's BMI during the first trimester of the pregnancy, as well as the child's own birth weight, independent of one another. These associations held even when the results were controlled for infant gender and birth year, maternal race/ethnicity, parity, smoking during pregnancy, pregnancy weight gain, education, marital status, and age. Figure 6.4 depicts these associations.

The impact of birth weight on weight status at age 4 years, though not depicted in Figure 6.4, was similarly robust. At age 4 years, among children whose birth weight for gestational age was less than the tenth percentile, 9% were obese; among those whose birth weight was between the tenth and eighty-ninth percentiles, 15% were obese; and among those whose birth weight was at the ninetieth percentile or above, 26% were obese. These differences were significant ($p < 0.001$), and independent of the potential confounding variables already described. There were no significant interactions between maternal weight status and birth weight category on future weight status.

The effect of birth weight on future overweight risk in childhood does not seem to interact with the feeding environment. The impact of birth weight on future weight status has remained stable since 1936 (Rugholm et al., 2005). If children of higher birth weight responded to our increasingly obesogenic environment differently from children of

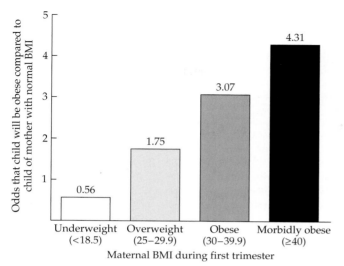

FIGURE 6.4   Odds ratio for overweight (BMI ≥ ninety-fifth percentile for age and gender) at age 4 years by maternal BMI during the first trimester, compared to maternal BMI in normal range (18.5–25 kg/m^2). (After Whitaker, 2004.)

normal birth weight, one would expect the relationship between high birth weight and overweight to have become stronger in the last 50 years. If these children have greater liking for and propensity to ingest the more readily available calorie-dense (sweet and fat) foods, then the link between high birth weight and future overweight would have strengthened in the last 50 years as these types of foods became more commonly available. This has not been the case, however. The link between high birth weight and future overweight has remained stable, suggesting that high birth weight has a direct, as yet unknown, biological impact on future weight status, as opposed to predisposing individuals to a particular behavioral profile that interacts with the obesogenic environment to confer increased overweight risk.

From these data, we can conclude the following:

2. Higher birth weight predicts a higher risk of overweight in children, independent of maternal weight status and demographic factors.

3. Maternal weight status before pregnancy predicts child overweight, independent of birth weight. These effects were additive. Tests of an interactive relationship were not statistically significant.

These findings are summarized in Table 6.1.

In summary, maternal weight status seems to affect birth weight through genetic/metabolic mechanisms (e.g., maternal weight status may lead to different circulating levels of glucose or insulin that traverse the placenta and lay down metabolic predispositions in the infant). Birth weight itself may also affect future adult weight through genetic or biological mechanisms. Maternal weight

Table 6.1
Relationships of Maternal Weight Status, Infant Birth Weight, and Weight Status in Later Childhood

Predictor and outcome	Sample size(n)	Statistical controls	Primary findings[a]
Maternal prepregnancy BMI predicts birth weight.	2459	Maternal blood sugar levels, age, weight gain during pregnancy, gestational age of the infant, parity, smoking, screening indicators for diabetes, and ethnic background	Percentage of infants with a birth weight of ≥4000 grams, depending on mother's prepregnancy BMI: BMI 18.5–24.9: 23% BMI 25–29.9: 31% BMI ≥30: 30%
Higher birth weight predicts higher risk of overweight at age 4 years.	8494	Infant gender and birth year, maternal race/ethnicity, parity, smoking during pregnancy, pregnancy weight gain, prepregnancy weight, education, marital status, and age	Prevalence of obesity at age 4 years, depending on birth weight ($p < 0.001$): BW < 10th percentile: 9% BW ≥ 10th, < 89th percentile: 15% BW ≥ 90th percentile: 26%
Maternal pre-pregnancy weight status predicts child overweight, independent of birth weight.	8494	Infant gender, birth year, birth weight, maternal race/ethnicity, parity, smoking during pregnancy, pregnancy weight gain, education, marital status, and age	Prevalence of obesity at age 4 years, depending on maternal BMI during first trimester ($p < 0.001$): BMI <18.5: 4.7% BMI 18.5–24.9: 9% BMI 25–29.9: 15% BMI 30–39.9: 23% BMI ≥40: 29%

[a]BMI, body mass index; BW, birth weight.

status also affects future risk of overweight independent of birth weight. This effect may be due to (1) genetic influences that have an impact on overweight risk after the infant period; (2) genetic factors that govern eating or physical activity patterns that alter overweight risk; or (3) maternal lifestyle factors that the child adopts by sharing the same environment, which lead to increased obesity risk. In the end, each of these factors likely contributes to the relationship between mother and child obesity.

Patterns of childhood BMI change predict adult BMI

Although weight status itself tracks (e.g., overweight children tend to remain overweight, and thinner children tend to remain thinner) through the life span, as reviewed already, specific *patterns* of growth rate at two sensitive developmental periods also increase long-term obesity risk. These rate effects are also *independent* of parental weight and the child's actual weight at the time of change. The two periods at issue are infancy (birth to 12 months) and 4 to 7 years of age.

Rapid weight gain during the first year of life predicts a higher risk of future overweight in both later childhood and adulthood (Baird et al., 2005). Although rate of weight gain was defined differently among the ten studies in this meta-analysis, infants who gained weight rapidly consistently showed odds ratios or relative risks for obesity ranging from 1.17 to 5.70, depending on the study. The findings in this review have since been replicated twice. *Independent* of birth weight, infants who gained more weight between birth and 6 months were correspondingly heavier at 4 and 7 years of age, (Dennison et al., 2006) and as young adults (Ekelund et al., 2006). In fact, even small newborns are at significantly greater risk of future overweight if they gain at a very rapid rate in the first 6 months of life. The higher risk of future overweight does not simply reflect a high rate of weight gain that persists through early childhood, because even when the initial weight burst stabilizes after 6 months so that the child is at a normal healthy weight at age 1 year, the child's lifetime risk of overweight remains significantly increased (Stettler et al., 2002). Whether this pattern of early weight gain reflects a preexisting risk of overweight based on genetic makeup, or it establishes metabolic dispositions that increase overweight long-term risk (independent of genetic makeup) is unknown.

The period between ages 4 and 7 years, when the so-called adiposity rebound occurs, is also critical for the development of future overweight. Consider the following; BMI naturally *decreases* in all children from infancy into early childhood (a phenomenon commonly referred to as "losing baby fat") and then rebounds. Children lose baby fat from infancy into early childhood, then (in the 4- to 7-year range) accumulate more adipose tissue (though most are not overweight) as they progress toward adolescence. The natural decline in adiposity and subsequent rebound is illustrated for boys between 2 and 12 years of age with the BMI growth chart in Figure 6.5 (girls' patterns are highly similar). This plot represents the "bell curve" of BMI distribution (the fifth to ninety-fifth percentiles) across ages from weights and heights measured in about 10,000 boys participating in the National Health and Nutrition Examination Survey (NHANES) in the five waves between the 1960s and early 1990s. As illustrated by the growth curve, BMI dips to a nadir between about ages 4 and 7 years, and then increases steadily. BMI in earlier childhood (at 2 years) is a robust predictor of BMI in later childhood (age 12 years; Nader et al., 2006). As children grow, they tend to remain relatively near the BMI percentile that they occupied in earlier childhood. Notably, the "range of normal" BMI also expands over the course of childhood. This pattern may, again, reflect biological predispositions, as well as the cumulative effect of experience in the environment over time.

Position is not the only predictor; the exact *timing* of the adiposity rebound is also linked to long-term overweight risk. The younger the child is when the

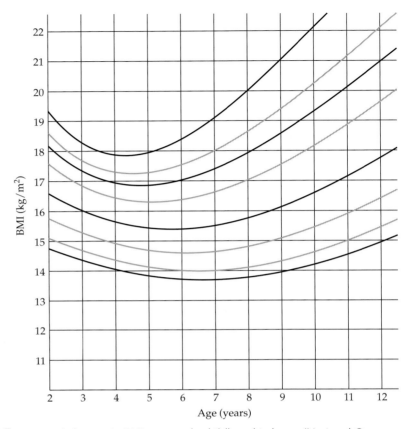

FIGURE 6.5 Normal change in BMI over early childhood in boys. (National Center for Health Statistics, CDC Growth Charts.)

nadir of thinness is reached, the more likely it is that the child will be an overweight adult. Children whose adiposity rebound occurs prior to about age 5 years *are six times more likely to be obese as an adult,* compared to those having adiposity rebound beginning at about 6 years regardless of parental weight or the child's *actual BMI* at the time of rebound (Figure 6.6; Whitaker et al., 1998). Stated differently, even children who remain at a normal BMI throughout this age range or are even on the thinner end of the BMI distribution are considerably more likely to be overweight as an adult if the adiposity rebound occurs early. The child's actual BMI at the time of adiposity rebound predicted future overweight risk, but it did not interact with age at adiposity rebound to alter future overweight risk. Whether early adiposity rebound itself confers increased risk of overweight into adulthood, or it is simply a marker of an existing genetic predisposition to obesity, remains unknown.

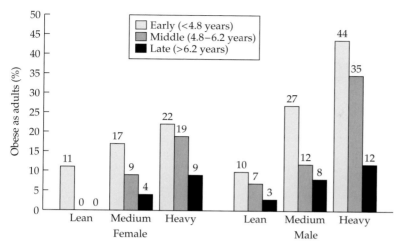

FIGURE 6.6   Percentage of adults who were obese at age 21 to 29 years, by age at adiposity rebound (early, middle, or late) and weight status at time of adiposity rebound (lean (BMI z-score < -0.54), medium (-0.54 ≤ BMI z-score <0.05) , or heavy (BMI z-score > 0.05). (After Whitaker et al., 1998.)

Summary of developmental risk factors

This section has briefly reviewed evidence that maternal BMI predicts children's BMI apparently through both genetic and experiential factors, that BMI tracks throughout life beginning in infancy, that BMI tracks more strongly as the child grows older, and that patterns of growth during particular critical periods, independent of actual weight status, seem to confer obesity risk, though their mechanisms are unclear. The strength of the associations between actual weight status, as well as patterns of growth, and future overweight are summarized in Table 6.2. In short, weight status in early childhood, rate of weight gain in early childhood, weight status in middle childhood, and earlier age at adiposity rebound all confer increased future obesity risk, with odds ratios or relative risks ranging from 1.2 to 17.5. The next section will consider environmental factors that may explain or mediate the persistence of weight status over time.

Infant-Feeding Practices and Overweight

The observation that early-infancy weight gain is associated with lifetime overweight risk has spurred considerable concern about and research on whether infant-feeding practices facilitate later obesity. The putative influence of infant-feeding practices on overweight risk generally falls into one of three categories:

- **Hypothesis 1:** The taste and flavor of infant diet support the development of specific flavor preferences, which continue to track into adult-

Table 6.2

Risk of Adult Obesity by Developmental Period

Developmental period	Specific influence associated with increased later weight status	Degree of risk
Infancy (birth through 24 months)	Weight significantly above the mean (by varying cutoffs) between ages 5 months and 24 months	The odds ratio, or relative risk, of obesity later in childhood or in adulthood is 1.35 to 9.38 (Baird et al., 2005).
	Greater rate of weight gain between varying intervals from birth to age 24 months	The odds ratio, or relative risk, of obesity in later childhood or adulthood based on having a rate of weight gain at the high end of the bell curve is 1.17 to 5.70 (Baird et al., 2005).
		The odds ratio of overweight at age 4 years for every 100 grams per month of infant weight gain, independent of birth weight, is 1.40 (Dennison et al., 2006).
		For each standard deviation increase in infant weight gain between birth and 6 months, BMI at age 17 years increased by about one point, independent of birth weight or maternal BMI (Ekelund et al., 2006).
Childhood (24 months–17 years)	Being overweight during childhood	Being overweight at any point between 24 months and 54 months (BMI ≥ eighty-fifth percentile for age and gender) is associated with an odds ratio for overweight at age 12 years of 6.50 (Nader et al., 2006).
		The odds ratio for being obese as an adult if overweight as a child increases with the age of the child, regardless of parental obesity status, from 4.70 among 3- to 5-year-old obese children to 17.50 among 15- to 17-year-old obese children (Whitaker et al., 1997). The increase occurs in a relatively continuous, or stair-step, fashion between these two age ranges.
	Early adiposity rebound	Children having adiposity rebound at <4.8 years of age, compared to those having adiposity rebound at >6.2 years of age, have an odds ratio of 6.00 for obesity in adulthood, regardless of parental weight or the child's actual BMI at the time of rebound (Whitaker et al., 1998).

hood. These flavor preferences lead to the consumption of foods that either promote or protect against overweight.

- **Hypothesis 2:** A specific, as yet unidentified, compound, when consumed in infancy, confers lifetime overweight protection. When this compound is not eaten, overweight risk is increased.

- **Hypothesis 3:** Early-infancy feeding patterns help establish children's response accuracy to sensations of hunger and satiety. Inappropriate feeding methods and patterns may cause infants to continue eating through otherwise inhibitory sensations arising from stomach, gut, and blood. These patterns, when persisting throughout the life span, increase obesity risk.

Studying the relationship between infant feeding and lifetime overweight risk has so far been limited to evaluating the associations between different types of infant feeding (and the timing of their onset and exclusivity) and overweight risk. The three modes of infant feeding are breast-feeding, feeding of commercial formula, and feeding of solid (pureed) baby food ("beikost")—and any combination of these.

The putative relationship between infant-feeding practices and future overweight risk deserves comment. First, specific types of infant-feeding practices tend to cluster in low-income and minority populations in which obesity is much more prevalent. Second, typical infant-feeding practices have changed dramatically in the past century, overlapping considerably with the emergence of the obesity epidemic. Table 6.3 presents the most current recommendations from the American Academy of Pediatrics regarding infant feeding, along with current feeding practices and changes in feeding practices from the start of the twentieth century onward.

Mothers who have low education levels, are low-income, and are African American are less likely to breast-feed and more likely to introduce solid foods to their infants earlier than recommended. In addition, the prevalence of breast-feeding declined dramatically in the mid twentieth century, and solid food was introduced significantly earlier than in the past in all racial, educational, and economic groups. Although these trends in the timing of certain feeding patterns are currently reversing, it is hypothesized that obesity in the present adult population is related to the feeding practices experienced during infancy 20 or more years earlier. Given the higher prevalence of overweight among lower socioeconomic and minority groups, as well as the increase in obesity prevalence among all groups over time, these differences in feeding practices and their potential relationship to overweight risk have been considered as potential contributors. Because the data regarding the feeding of "solids" are exceedingly sparse and conflicting (Burdette et al., 2006; Ong et al., 2006; Reilly et al., 2005; Wilson et al., 1998; Zive et al., 1992), they will not be a focus of the present discussion. The data supporting these hypotheses in relation to milk from the breast versus formula are reviewed in this section.

Table 6.3
Infant-Feeding Practices: Current Recommendations and Differences in Practices by Race and Socioeconomic Status

American Academy of Pediatrics feeding recommendation	Current feeding practices by race and socioeconomic status	Changes in feeding practices over time
Infants should be exclusively breast-fed for the first 6 months of life. Breast-feeding should be continued at least until age 12 months, and beyond for as long as mutually desired by mother and child (Anonymous, 2005).	African American mothers are much less likely to initiate breast-feeding than white mothers (49% versus 69%; Li, et al., 2005).	In about 1900–1920, most infants breast-fed through out the first year of life; formula feeding was relatively uncommon because of lack of refrigeration and sanitation (Fomon, 2001).
	Mothers in poverty are less likely to initiate breast-feeding than upper-income mothers (56% versus 78%; Li et al., 2005).	In the 1940s, about 70% of infants initially breast-fed (Bain, 1948). By 1970, only 25% of infants initially breast-fed (Hirschman & Hendershot, 1979). In 2001, about 65% of infants initially breast-fed (Li et al., 2003).

Several meta-analyses on the relationship of breast-feeding to child and adult obesity and overweight support an inverse association between breast-feeding and overweight risk (Arenz et al., 2004; Harder et al., 2005; Owen et al., 2005). Each hypothesis identified at the start of this discussion has been invoked to account for the finding. Breast-fed infants are probably exposed to a greater variety of flavors (consumed by the mother in her own diet and transmitted via the breast milk) than are formula-fed infants (Mennella et al., 2001). Breast-fed infants may thus accept a wider variety of flavors (and therefore foods) in their postweaning diets (Mennella & Beauchamp, 1999; Mennella et al., 2001), presumably supporting healthier long-term eating habits, since dietary variety in early childhood predicts later dietary variety (Skinner, Carruth, Bounds, Ziegler, & Reidy, 2002), and greater dietary variety is associated with a more healthful diet (Foote et al., 2004; Murphy et al., 2006).

In addition, breast milk may contain an element that either alters metabolism or alters long-term ingestive behavior to reduce obesity risk over a lifetime. No such compound has been identified to date, and data to support the existence of such a compound are limited at present. Bottle-fed infants have been found to have higher concentrations of plasma insulin following a feeding compared to breast-fed infants (Lucas et al., 1980). Higher insulin levels would theoretically increase fat deposition and adipocyte development. As reviewed by Von Kries and colleagues (1999), breast milk also contains factors that may lead to the inhibition of adipocyte formation, though work remains limited to in vitro studies at this point. The idea that breast milk contains unique compounds that confer specific advantage over formula is not new. Infant formula companies invest a great deal of effort in identifying and replicating these compounds to include in commercial formula. The most recently added compounds in this quest to make formula as similar to breastmilk as possible are docosahexaenoic acid and arachidonic acid, components of membrane lipids in the central nervous system; note, however, that the clinical impact of these compounds remains hotly debated (Lucas et al., 1999; Scott et al., 1998).

Finally, breast-feeding may support a more bounded response to hunger and satiety cues, though this hypothesis is highly speculative with few supporting data. Specifically, the production of breast milk is driven and controlled by infant demand, inducing sensitivity to hunger cues. Moreover, meal volume is rate-limited by milk supply, inducing maternal sensitivity to fullness signals linked to the end of a meal. In contrast, formula is endlessly available, so volume intake may be more determined by remaining bottle contents (and subsequent prompting of the infant to finish) than by the infant's actual hunger.

Several studies have indicated that breast-feeding is associated with less controlling maternal feeding practices (Fisher et al., 2000; Taveras et al., 2004). In other words, mothers who breast-feed seem to allow the infant more control over its own eating behavior, thereby theoretically promoting greater responsiveness in the infant to hunger and satiety by allowing the infant to respond to internal cues, as opposed to external cues from the mother. Accordingly, attentiveness to hunger and satiety cues in the physiological range may normally develop through breast-feeding to cause healthier eating habits. The data in this area, however, remain limited, and much additional work is needed.

Eating Development in Childhood

The ontogeny of childhood eating behavior may be considered a classic developmental problem in several ways. First, there is debate regarding which aspects of the correlation of parent–child weight status (Whitaker et al., 1997) reflect genetic determinism, environmental influences, or, more likely, a complex interaction of the two. Second, a "critical period" may limit the formation of food preferences and the development of responses to internal cues signaling satiety. Third, social functions deeply influence feeding practices, from the perception of body weight to that of food choice. Like all fashions, these change rapidly over the course of development, so appropriate intervention requires understanding which influences are salient at a particular developmental stage. Finally, the most obvious but poorly understood observation reveals that the genesis of childhood eating and food preferences differs fundamentally and dramatically from that of adult eating and food preferences.

This section reviews several of the well-established, possibly innate influences on children's eating behavior and food selection, while describing their developmental trajectories. Given its complexity, the role of parents is discussed in a separate section. This section is guided by Smith's (1998) distinction between primary and secondary influences on ingestion. Primary influences consist of afferents arising from oropharynx, stomach, gut, and blood. Secondary influences reflect neural systems located in the rostral forebrain that are available at birth or come on board differentially during the course of brain maturation. They include the neural systems underlying neophobia and the capacities for classical conditioning at birth (Blass et al., 1984). Importantly, as one would expect, the foods that gain control over these neural systems await particular experiences (i.e. tasting) for their specification.

Food neophobia

Young children, indeed the young of all species studied, only reluctantly sample new foods—a tendency referred to as *food neophobia*. Food neophobia becomes most manifest just as infants become mobile (in about the second year of life). Obviously one cannot deliberately set out to test the earliest time in humans, but it should be noted that in rats, learned avoidance for food and for milk derived from suckling is evident before or by the time of birth. Reluctance to sample new foods by the mobile child likely has evolutionary gain (Cashdan, 1994), because such hesitation would probably protect the child from inadvertently consuming potentially poisonous substances. Indeed, episodes of poisoning reported to poison control centers peak in early childhood (Watson et al., 2003). Interestingly, the infant's propensity to mouth stimuli in an exploratory fashion or to eat nonfood items (a behavior known as *pica*) also wanes after about age 18 months to 24 months, as mobility increases, and this change would also have a protective effect against poisoning.

Several illustrations show why an inherent food neophobia might be protective in young children as they become mobile. Simply put, as means to determine the quality or safety of an unfamiliar food item, taste and smell are unreliable at any age. Adults, however, develop the cognitive ability to differentiate food from nonfood items. Children have not yet learned the ability to differentiate safely edible from unsafe and inedible, and they are often more strongly driven by the appeal of an item's sweetness or bright color than an adult would be. If a substance has immediate negative consequences (e.g., burning the mucosa or inducing nausea and vomiting), the child (if ingestion did not cause death) presumably learns that the substance is not desirable to eat and therefore avoids future ingestion.

A substance that is colorful or colorless, sweet, odorless, and causes no immediate negative consequence of ingestion, but causes dire long-term consequences, is the ultimate potential poison for a child. Two such substances account for a significant proportion of poisonings in childhood. The first is automotive antifreeze (ethylene glycol), which was reported to poison control centers as an ingesta more than 6000 times in 2002 (Watson et al., 2003). The substance is colorless, odorless, and sweet, and ingesting it can actually cause an initial euphoria. Subsequently, however, the ingestion can lead to renal failure and death.

Lead paint is another common ingesta in young children. Lead paint peeling from windowsills in older homes (before lead in paint was banned in 1978) accounts for the majority of exposures, and more than 300,000 US children (2% of children under age 5 years) have excessive blood lead levels (*plumbism*; Woolf et al., 2007). The lead in paint tastes sweet and causes no immediate adverse consequences. Longer-term exposure, however, has clear and well-documented negative impacts on behavior and cognitive development in children. The recognition of these adverse consequences led to extensive legislation to protect children from lead exposure.

The lead paint legislation is a classic example of how policy can be used to shape the environment to make it safer for children and their innate eating behaviors. Such a framework could also be adopted for modifying the food environment to, in some sense, similarly "protect children from themselves" and their own innate predispositions toward consumption. In the examples of antifreeze, lead, and excessive sweet and fat consumption leading to obesity and long-term morbidity, the delay between the ingestion and the negative consequences is long enough that classical conditioning does not create a natural aversion to the offending substances. This delay is crucial because it creates a gap between the ingestion and its consequences that opens the door to a variety of adverse outcomes.

Food neophobia declines with age, as children become somewhat more adventuresome in their food sampling. Food neophobia is typically measured using the Food Neophobia Scale (FNS) developed by Pliner (Pliner & Hobden, 1992). The FNS has a range of 10 to 70, with higher scores indicating greater food neophobia. Work with the FNS has documented that children's food neophobia is rated by parents as declining from the preschool age range (4–7 years; mean FNS score 43), to school age (8–12 years; mean FNS score 38), to adolescence (13–16 years; mean FNS score 33). No further declines in food neophobia occurred in the next age window (17–22 years; Nicklaus et al., 2005). No decline in FNS scores was reported in another study of more than 500 children ages 2 to 6 years (Cooke et al., 2003). Children who are still picky by adolescence are likely to remain so (Marchi & Cohen, 1990). Enduring pickiness has been viewed more as a personality trait (Lien et al., 2001), typically associated with an inhibited or anxious temperament (Galloway et al., 2003; Pliner & Loewen, 1997), as opposed to simply a developmental stage. Thus, the range of foods that a child will accept presumably increases as the child grows older because the innate food neophobia present in nearly all young children is reduced to varying degrees.

However, the expansion of children's repertoire of acceptable foods is limited, naturally, to those foods to which they are exposed. A useful parallel lies in language development. In eating behavior, the child begins with a potentially broad repertoire—a "clean slate" for food preferences (with specific limits, as will be outlined). Infants respond similarly to all languages early on, but by 10 to 12 months they respond only to the language to which they are regularly exposed (Polka & Werker, 1994; Werker & Tees, 1984). Thus, some of the early plasticity in both food preference and language development dissipates within the first 1 to 2 years of life.

Focusing on the development of food preferences, children raised on a very bland diet would be unlikely to easily expand their repertoire to include spicy foods. Similarly, children raised in a culture in which meat is not eaten might be particularly recalcitrant to accepting meat into the diet as they grew older. Culture is one of a host of environmental factors that influence the trajectory and expression of children's food neophobia. Although some have proposed that parents simply wait for the neophobia stage to pass, as opposed to putting a great deal of effort into shaping the child's food preferences during this period of difficult eating behavior, some data indicate that the behavior can be modified. The next section reviews the few available studies.

In a longitudinal study of 70 children followed from 2 to 8 years of age (Skinner, Carruth, Bounds, & Ziegler, 2002), Skinner et al. reported that new foods are more likely to be accepted between ages 2 and 4 than between ages 4 and 8. Figure 6.7 shows that although children had been introduced to an increasingly larger number of foods between ages 2 and 8 years, the number of foods the children actually liked hardly increased at all. The stability of likes and dislikes within individual children over time was also notable. The number of foods that

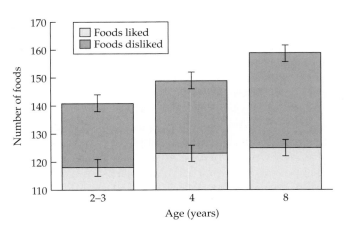

FIGURE 6.7   Number of foods (of a potential 196) that mothers reported children had eaten before and liked, in a sample of 70 children followed longitudinally. (After Skinner, Carruth, Bounds, & Ziegler, 2002.)

children liked at age 2 years was highly correlated with the number of foods that they liked at age 8 years ($r = 0.79$). In contrast, the number of foods that children disliked at age 2 years was not highly correlated with the number disliked at age 8 years ($r = 0.46$). Thus, liking of a food, once established, persists. Dislike of foods, however, is malleable over time, presumably as a result of environmental influences such as parenting practices.

Using this same data set, Skinner sought to determine which of the following variables, alone or in combination, best predicted the number of foods that children liked at age 8 years: (1) number of foods liked at age 2 years; (2) number of foods liked at age 4 years; (3) child temperament; (4) duration of breast-feeding; (5) dietary variety at ages 2, 4, and 8 years; (6) mother's perception of the child's food acceptance at age 8 years; (7) number of times the mother typically exposed a child to a food before deciding that the child didn't like it; and (8) mother's and child's general reluctance to try new things (general neophobia), as well as reluctance to try new foods. Of these covariates, the strongest predictors of the number of foods that a child would like at age 8 years were the number of foods that the child liked at age 4 years and the mother's report of the child's food neophobia. These two factors accounted for 79% of the variance in the number of foods that the child liked at age 8 years. Thus, food preferences present at age 4 years tend to persist in individual children, and that individual variability in food neophobia is a significant and robust predictor of food preferences that appears to be relatively resistant to environmental modification.

If parents are of a mind to promote healthy eating in their children, their efforts toward shaping food preferences and expanding their children's repertoire are best undertaken prior to about age 4 years. Cooke and Wardle (2005) evaluated, in a cohort of nearly 1300 children of ages 4 to 16 years, whether children reported ever having tried each of 115 foods, and whether or not they liked each food. Although older children reported that they had tried a greater number of foods, this broader experience did *not* translate into *liking* a greater number (Cooke & Wardle, 2005); foods tried later in childhood were generally less liked than foods tried earlier in childhood. This translational failure is important because the best predictor of food acceptance is the degree to which a food is liked (Birch, 1979; Resnicow et al., 1997).

Various studies show that the *preschool years are critical for constructing a platform of food diversity upon which food preferences can be built.* Inducing a liking for new foods is more difficult following this period. It is demoralizing that food preferences present at age 4 years are sustained thereafter, despite a willingness to sample new foods. This finding lends urgency to establishing as broad a base as possible in the early childhood years. These data suggest that parents should invest resources to increase the repertoire and quality of foods acceptable to their preschoolers. Most of the healthful foods that parents attempt to include in the child's repertoire are fruits and vegetables. Presumably, if a greater variety of fruits and vegetables are eaten, they should replace unhealthful, obesogenic foods, thereby conferring long-term protection against obesity risk (see Chapter 10).

Unfortunately, the available data addressing the point of actually replacing some of the highly palatable sweet and fat foods in children's diets are not encouraging. It is unknown if these trajectories of food preferences based on gustatory processes in the brainstem are malleable, or if they cannot be moved from dislike into liking. Thus, although preschoolers may expand their repertoire of accepted foods, whether they develop a stable and persistent liking for these foods sufficient to shift them away from a preponderance of calorie-dense foods has proven extremely difficult. Success will require systematically overcoming or bypassing innate flavor preferences for sweet, fat, and oily calorie-dense foods.

Shifting children's preference away from more calorie-dense foods to more healthful options begins with efforts to intensively increase their exposure to more healthful options while systematically decreasing exposure or opportunities to eat "junk food." Although the government regulates the types of foods purchased with government funding, schools can still use their discretion about what other types of foods are made available (not using government funding). Asking schools to serve more healthful meals that preferentially offer relatively costly low-calorie fruits and vegetables over inexpensive, calorie-dense and palatable foods is a challenge in an era of extreme budget restriction (see Chapter 14). Faced with limited budgets, and parents and teachers who often have as a primary goal that children not "go hungry," schools often focus on providing foods that are highly palatable to reduce waste and ensure actual consumption. Food preparation time is also a significant budgetary consideration for schools that is not included in the government allocations. Thus, increasing children's consumption of more healthful foods will likely require as much vigorous advocacy and policy work as it will high-quality research into the controls of eating behavior.

Reports of children overcoming aversion to a variety of blatantly noxious tastes to develop increased liking provide some hope of creating preferences for vegetables that supersede those for sugar and fat. In one of the best examples, the taste preferences of preschool-age children are predicted by the formula that they consumed in infancy (Mennella & Beauchamp, 2002). Infant formulas generally come in one of three varieties: cow's milk–based, soy, and elemental. Compared to cow's milk–based formulas, soy formulas are described as sweeter, more sour, and more bitter. Elemental formulas, which are composed of hydrolyzed proteins, are used for infants with allergies to either milk or soy proteins. Because the proteins in the elemental formulas are hydrolyzed (broken down), they are not allergenic, but the resulting amino acids are quite sour and bitter, leading most adults to perceive elemental formulas as very noxious. Infants readily consume each of the three types of formulas without showing signs of rejection.

At age 4 to 5 years, children were asked to rate their preferences for three types of apple juice: unaltered juice, juice with lemon (sour) added, and juice with grapefruit flavor (bitter) added. According to Menella and Beauchamp

(2002), children's preferences for the different apple juices reflected the formulas that they had been fed as infants. Specifically, only 33% of children fed standard cow's milk formula as infants stated that they liked the sour apple juice, as opposed to 64% of children fed the elemental formula. Contrasts for the bitter apple juice were similar; 30% versus 64% for cow's milk and soy milk, respectively. Moreover, children who had been fed soy or elemental formula in infancy, compared to those fed cow's milk–based formula, had a greater preference for broccoli, implying that there may be long-lasting effects of these early flavor experiences on increasing preferences for vegetables in later childhood (Mennella & Beauchamp, 2002). Note that this example is presented as evidence that early flavor experiences can predict future preferences, but the ideal food for infants is breast milk, and manipulation of formula type in infancy is not considered an appropriate therapeutic intervention for future food preferences.

Preference malleability extends into early childhood; children can also "learn" a preference for the hot-chili burning sensation prevalent in certain cultures. Children in these cultures typically come to like these inherently irritating substances through social modeling by adults and repeated exposure by age 5 years, and not through any material reward or by being "forced" to eat it; the food is simply introduced repeatedly beginning at about age 1 year at increasing intensity, until by age 5 years the children are voluntarily seasoning their food with it themselves (Rozin & Schiller, 1980).

In summary, humans develop liking for a variety of inherently unpalatable substances, including, as reviewed here, bitter and sour tastes as a result of exposure to formulas in infancy; and piquant, spicy flavors from early childhood; as well as coffee and other bitter flavors as adults. These observations support the hopeful view that increasing children's liking for bitter vegetables over sweet, high-fat, or salty foods may be possible to some extent. The difficulty, however, is that sweet and high-fat foods cannot simply be "given up," because their caloric content is an important contributor to children's diets. These foods are also relatively inexpensive and easily available to families, so they continue to contribute a significant portion to the typical child's diet. To bring the point home, a box of macaroni and cheese that can be purchased for a dollar is enough to feed a family of four. One does not have to be an accountant to appreciate the impossibility of providing a healthful meal for a family for the same low cost.

The methods by which children's food preferences can be changed, and how these effects may be modified by the child's age over the course of development, are the subject of the more detailed discussion that follows.

Repeated exposure

Repeated exposure to a new food, at least in middle-class Midwestern preschoolers, increases liking. Unfortunately, about 10 to 15 exposures are needed (Birch & Marlin, 1982). Both 2-year-old (Birch & Marlin, 1982) and 3- to 6-year-old children (Sullivan & Birch, 1999) will start to like a previously neutral food following repeated tastings. Note, however, that the effect of repeated exposure on liking in these studies was relatively modest. Repeated exposure almost never caused a food that was initially aversive to the child to become well liked. Rather, repeated exposure increased the preference for a food ranked relatively neutral to a higher (but still relatively neutral) ranking. Indeed, at least one additional study has shown that repeated exposure will increase liking in children for sweet (i.e., palatable) but not sour flavors (Liem & de Graaf, 2004). This finding is important because, as indicated, the best predictor of food acceptance and intake is how well a food is liked (Birch, 1979). Thus, even relatively modest shifts potentially help balance a child's diet.

The influence of repeated exposures may be limited to young children. Adult data are less consistent, suggesting dissipation or increased specificity with age. Among 24-year-olds, repeated exposure to a bittersweet beverage increased liking (Stein et al., 2003). However, liking of either sweet or sour flavors was *not* increased by repeated exposure (Liem & de Graaf, 2004), and the same was true of unusual foods such as tripe, halva, or chutney (Peryam, 1963). On the other hand, adults develop a liking for bitter substances, such as coffee and alcohol, that are aversive at first taste. This change, however, may reflect the pharmacological properties of these substances, as well as the social milieus in which they are consumed, and not just repeated tasting per se (Cines & Rozin, 1982; Lanier et al., 2005).

How the presence of others influences food selection and quantity consumed

Modeling can affect food consumption in two ways: *food selection* (i.e., increasing liking for a substance) and *quantity consumed*. This section first addresses the effect of others on food selection (see also Chapter 9).

A proven means of increasing a child's (or a chimpanzee's or rat's) willingness to accept a new food is to make sure that the child sees a cohort, especially one of the same age, eat the food. Perhaps observing another individual safely eating the food confers safety on it. A robust animal literature, as well as a small but growing literature in humans, documents the power of a conspecific model for influence on food selection.

Duncker (1938) was the first to consider the specific impact of models on food selection. When a child of about 5 years ate with a child of about 3 years, the younger child was much more likely to follow the eating behavior of the older child than vice versa (Duncker, 1938). The powerful effect of slightly older child peer models on children's eating behavior has been replicated by L. Birch (1980) in an important series of studies that have documented the range and impact of demonstrator-enhanced selection and affect. Importantly, the influence of peer models on children's food selection persists even after the models are no longer present in the food selection situation, and the influence is present as long as 8 weeks later (the longest time period assessed to date; Birch, 1980). The effect is internalized, therefore, and continues to influence food selection even after the initial experience.

Studies identifying the age of onset when the efficacy of a model begins have been inconsistent; starting ages have ranged from 14 months when an adult model was used (Harper & Sanders, 1975), to 32 months in Duncker's early study using child models (Duncker, 1938). Characteristics of the model mediated its effect, with particular characteristics strongly influencing children's food selection (Duncker, 1938). Not surprisingly, mothers are more effective models than strangers, and the model eating the food in front of the child is more effective than the model simply handling the food (Harper & Sanders, 1975). Both of these findings can be understood through familiarity.

Less is known about the impact of models on quantity consumed. Among 3- to 5-year-olds, the mere presence of others eating increases the amount consumed by about 30% (Lumeng & Hillman, 2007). This phenomenon is consistently observed in adults and animals as well (Bayer, 1929; de Castro, 1994; de Castro & Brewer, 1992; de Castro & de Castro, 1989; Harlow, 1932; Herman, et al., 2003). Two hypotheses have been offered concerning underlying mechanisms. According to the arousal/activation hypothesis, activation is greater in larger groups, resulting in a faster eating rate and greater consumption (de Castro, 1990; Zajonc, 1965). The time extension hypothesis asserts that social interaction extends meal duration (i.e., exposure to food), thereby increasing intake. The time extension hypothesis has arisen from human adult research. The distinctions are open to empirical validation. Children, aged 3–5 years, eating in large groups (9 children) initiate meals sooner and eat slightly more quickly than eating in smaller groups (3 children; Lumeng & Hillman, 2007). Group size did not influence meal duration, however. Unlike adults, children eating in large groups actually socialized less than when eating in smaller groups (Lumeng & Hillman, 2007). In summary, although eating in groups increases the amount consumed in both children and adults, the mechanism seems to be an extension of meal duration in adults, but of arousal in children. Additional studies are needed in this area.

Increased consumption in groups of adults is more textured than in children and is moderated by multiple other influences. Adults are much more likely to eat more in the presence of familiar others like family and friends as opposed to strangers. Solitary adults observed by a noneating stranger actually eat less, arguably in conformity to expected social norms (Herman et al., 2003). The youngest children's eating behavior is unlikely to be moderated by social norms, which very likely cast their influence by middle childhood and certainly in adolescence.

Flavor preferences and their ontogeny

Although the potential impact of sensory preferences on obesity risk is evaluated in Chapter 5, this section briefly reviews the ontogeny of gustatory hedonics during the childhood years into adulthood. Efforts to shape eating behavior in children to increase preferences for less obesogenic foods and presumably reduce obesity risk must be informed by taste ontogeny.

This section begins with a brief review of what is known from animal and human studies about taste development in general. As reviewed by Mistretta and Bradley (1985), the ability of the human newborn to differentiate tastes at birth was first described in the 1920s, and the presence of taste buds during fetal development was first documented in the 1960s. Study in the last several decades has focused on the recognition that there is significant development in the human taste system both pre- and postnatally. Rats acquire additional taste buds postnatally, and this morphological maturation is accompanied by significant neurophysiological maturation. The response of the chorda tympani nerve becomes significantly stronger to sodium chloride and sucrose over the course of postnatal development in rats, while the response frequencies to sour and bitter compounds remain constant.

It has been hypothesized that changes in the taste bud cell membrane, in taste bud cell turnover, in synapses between taste cells and afferent fibers, and in the afferent fibers themselves may occur during postnatal development and account for the changing taste patterns. These hypotheses require ongoing study. The solitary nucleus and tract in the brainstem carry and receive visceral sensation and taste from the facial (VII), glossopharyngeal (IX), and vagus (X) cranial nerves, as well as the cranial part of the spinal accessory nerve (XI). The nucleus of the solitary tract (NST) receives projections from the chorda tympani nerve (a branch of the facial nerve), and studies have shown that as development progressed, the NST responded to a wider variety of chemicals and at lower concentrations. In particular, response frequencies to sodium chloride and sucrose increased in the NST over the course of postnatal development (similar to what the studies of the chorda tympani nerve showed), while response frequencies to sour and bitter compounds remained constant (or were fully mature at birth). Note, however, that although rats' response frequencies to sucrose increase postnatally, their preference for very high concentrations of sucrose declines postnatally.

The pontine taste area relays gustatory information from the rostral pole of the solitary nucleus to both the thalamus and the ventral forebrain. For all stimuli, response frequencies mature later in the pontine taste area than in the NST. In short, each level of the central nervous system involved in taste seems to have its own pattern of development. Finally, receptors and ion channels may also mature at the level of the taste cell itself. For example, a receptor in a new taste cell may be responsive only to bitter taste, but as the taste cell matures the receptor may become responsive to sodium chloride. Obviously, basic questions remain unanswered.

Note also that the effects of taste or oral functions on preference are moderated by postingestive or gastric effects. Two central concepts emerge from the literature. First, postingestive effects themselves can directly affect preference. A classic review by Young (1968) describes work in animals on this issue. When chickens have been deprived of food, they develop an increased preference for sucrose solution. Even when provided adequate calories in refeeding, the increased preference for sucrose continues to persist for some time. Similarly, sodium depletion (through dialysis of sodium) results in increased sodium preference. Other studies have shown that when an animal was deficient in a particular vitamin and the vitamin was then provided along with a particular flavor, the animals demonstrated increased and persistent preference for the flavor (Young, 1968). In short, preferences are developed in response to oral sensations that are linked to postingestive changes in health status (Sclafani, 1997; see also Chapter 7).

The second central theme emerging from this literature is that postingestive effects can *moderate* the impact of oral sensations on preference. Mook (1963) conducted experiments in which what was tasted in the mouth differed from what was deposited in the stomach through the use of fistulas, sham feedings, and tube feedings. Typically in rats, the amount of a saline solution consumed differs on the basis of the saline concentration provided, increasing up to a peak of isotonic saline, and then declining once again. Mook found that if pure water is infused into the stomach while differing concentrations of saline are provided via sham feeding for tasting, the effect of saline concentration on amount consumed disappears. Conversely, when isotonic saline is infused into the stomach and the rat is provided differing concentrations of saline by sham feeding, again no change in consumption is observed with the varying saline concentrations that are tasted.

These findings would indicate that the effect of saline concentration on consumption operates at some point that is "post-oral." Furthermore, when hypertonic saline was infused into the stomach and the rat was given even dilute saline solutions to taste, consumption dramatically declined. This finding would indicate that postingestive and oral effects interact in modulating consumption (i.e., the hypertonic saline in the stomach signals supraphysiological sodium concentrations and induces an aversion to a dilute saline taste that is usually preferred). In contrast, taste appears to have more of an independent effect when sucrose or glucose is tasted. In these cases, the rats will continue to increase intake even when plain water is infused into the stomach. In short, postingestive effects clearly both *directly affect* preference and *moderate oral factors* in guiding the formation of food preferences.

A central tenet of the taste system is the concept that its development appears to be relatively plastic and can be modified by environmental influences (Mistretta & Bradley, 1985). The data regarding each of the four primary tastes are reviewed in the sections that follow, and when possible, they are related to the animal data already reviewed.

SWEET   Preference for sweet is present from birth (Desor et al., 1973; Steiner, 1974)—indeed, even in anencephalic infants (infants lacking all or major portions of the brain; Steiner, 1973)—and positive facial expressions in the newborn increase as sweetness intensity increases (Ganchrow et al., 1983). Moreover, newborns can become classically conditioned to touch being followed by sweet taste (Blass et al., 1984). Thus, at birth central mechanisms are in place to savor sweets, and to associate them with the characteristics of the feeder. Sweet preference declines over time: children aged 9 to 15 years have a greater preference for sweetness than do adults (Desor, Greene, et al., 1975), and preferred sweetness intensity declined in individuals tested longitudinally between ages 9 to 10 years and ages 19 to 25 years (Desor, 1987).

Several studies suggest that this preference for higher-intensity sucrose in children compared to adults may be due to children's higher threshold for detecting the sweetness, as well as lesser ability to differentiate subtle differences in sucrose concentration compared to adults (de Graaf, 1999; James et al., 1997; Kimmel et al., 1994; Zandstra & de Graaf, 1998). Children may simply require higher concentrations of sucrose to have the same "sensory experience" of the flavor that adults have. The mechanism underlying this increasing sensitivity to, and decreasing preference for, sucrose among adults remains a mystery. However, some have speculated that the greater preference exhibited by children for higher concentrations of sucrose is biologically plausible in that children also have higher caloric needs, and their preference for sweet, high-calorie foods could confer a survival advantage (de Graaf, 1999), although data on this point are not available.

As reviewed earlier in this discussion, innate and biologically driven influences on sweet liking and its trajectory are also subject to experiential influences, certainly in animals. Human mothers in many cultures, including the United States, feed their young infants water sweetened to their own taste with sugar, honey, or corn syrup. In one diary-based study, 6-month-old infants whose mothers reported feeding them sweet solutions for at least 7 days drank more sweetened water when fed on demand in the laboratory than did control infants who had not received the supplement. In short, human infants' preference for sweet at 6 months reflected their experience of having previously been fed sweetened water by their mothers (Beauchamp & Moran, 1982). The system remains unspecified, however, as to the range of change and the underlying mechanisms. In another study, children's preference for sweet versus salty tofu was contingent on prior repeated exposures to the sweet tofu (Sullivan & Birch, 1999).

Decreased preference for (or aversion to) sweetness can also be learned. Aversions to foods are common and develop through learned associations with adverse consequences of ingesting the food (Logue et al., 1981). For example, eating a food and then developing a gastrointestinal illness, even hours later, will induce an aversion to that food. Both in humans (Logue et al., 1981) and in rats (Kehoe & Blass, 1986a), the aversion develops more commonly when the food is relatively unfamiliar. Food aversions are rapidly formed and have long-lasting effects, whereas the liking for a food develops much more slowly and is much less absolute. Aversions to sweet taste can be formed easily by pairing of the sweet taste with gastrointestinal illness. Rats for which gastrointestinal illness was induced following ethanol ingestion developed a concomitant aversion to a sucrose–quinine (sweet–bitter) solution (presumably because of the similarity in taste; DiLorenzo et al., 1986), and Bernstein and colleagues have repeatedly induced aversion to sweet taste in the form of saccharin by pairing it with gastrointestinal illness (induced by lithium chloride injection; Navarro, et al., 2000; Spray et al., 2000).

Apart from creating an absolute and immediate aversion to sweetness by inducing illness, there appear to be no known methods of slowly decreasing children's liking for sweetness over time, above and beyond the natural decline in preference for sweetness intensity that occurs with age. Efforts to reduce the sugar content of children's diets will likely be a challenge. For reasons discussed earlier, societal and policy changes that lead to an environment less rich in sweet, palatable foods promoted to children will be a challenge. Thus, parents are faced with an added burden, given the availability of sweets on supermarket shelves, the expected and received portion sizes, and the relentless advertising of energy-dense foods on children's TV shows.

SALTY   The importance of sodium cannot be overstated; it plays a critical role in maintaining the volume and composition of every body-fluid compartment and is integral for normal nerve conduction. A number of mechanisms coalesce to regulate sodium intake and output, with taste as the common denominator in mediating salt (sodium) appetite. The system has failed recently because sodium intake in the United States is excessive, contributing to hypertension in those who are genetically predisposed. The individual is not necessarily responsible for elevated intake, which is consequent to a diet of prepared food laden with salt, presumably to enhance food flavor or to serve as a preservative. In other words, much sodium consumption is inadvertent through the intake of prepared foods, as opposed to resulting from individuals using the salt shaker too liberally.

The detection of sodium chloride, unlike some other tastes, is specific to the chorda tympani branch of cranial nerve VII; its transection entirely interrupts sodium detection (Breslin et al., 1993). The normal concentration of sodium in body fluids is 0.9% (isotonic saline). Not surprisingly, then, preference for saline in rats peaks at a concentration of 0.9%. Higher concentrations of saline are aversive to rats (Moe, 1986). Salt appetite is regulated by a variety of complex factors in the body, including baroreceptors that monitor plasma volume and a number of hormones, including aldosterone, that control sodium concentration. As reviewed elsewhere, some work has indicated that the final common pathway is a decreased responsiveness of the chorda tympani nerve to sodium, which leads to less aversion to higher concentrations, and greater intake (Daniels & Fluharty, 2004). Other work has not supported this hypothesis (Nachman & Pfaffmann, 1963), suggesting that other sodium sensors throughout the body play an important role. Additional work to understand the physiological regulation of salt appetite is needed.

As reviewed already, animal data, particularly from the rat, indicate that the ability to detect salty taste develops postnatally, as reflected in response magnitudes in the chorda tympani nerve, the nucleus of the solitary tract (NST), and the pontine area. Neural responses to salt change probably because of intrinsic, developmentally preprogrammed factors rather than because of environmental reorganization (Mistretta & Bradley, 1985). Chorda tympani development may be responsive to experience, very broadly defined. According to Hill (2001), destruction of taste buds in rats at postnatal days 2 through 7 reduces the chorda tympani terminal field in the NST. Impressively, the projection deficit persists even though the taste buds regenerate. Similarly, rats deprived of sodium early in development fail to show caudal migration of the chorda tympani. Restriction of maternal dietary sodium also reduces neurophysiological responses to sodium salts in the chorda tympani, although, remarkably, this impairment is reversible, even in adults, through a single ingestive bout of physiological saline. Clearly, much additional work is needed in this area to improve our understanding of the experiential influences on sodium taste detection.

Indeed, behavioral data from human newborns confirm that the ability to detect salt seems to develop primarily *post*natally. Human newborns appear to be indifferent to salty tastes, as judged by facial expression (Rosenstein & Oster, 1988), and indeed they will consume saline at 0.10 to 0.50 molar (note that isotonic saline is 0.9 molar) in amounts equal to water (Beauchamp & Maller, 1977). A classic report illustrating the indifference of infants to salt, with tragic consequences, described an incident in a newborn nursery in which salt was inadvertently added to formula instead of sugar; the infants continued to readily consume the formula until they became ill from hypernatremia (Finberg et al., 1963).

Notably, in these infants the inability to detect (and appropriately refuse) the high sodium concentration may have been rooted in more than the gustatory system. When infants consume milk via suckling, the flavor may be deposited at the back of the mouth and therefore may largely bypass taste receptors. When stimuli are presented in the posterior pharynx in rats, learning is blocked because the stimulus does not reach the taste receptors on the anterior tongue as readily (Kehoe & Blass, 1986b). Thus the indifference of these infants to a high concentration of sodium in the formula may represent "failure" of not only the gustatory system, but also an unidentified postingestive central function.

The saline concentrations that infants accept with indifference decline by age 4 to 6 months (Beauchamp et al., 1986), and they are rejected by age 18 months (Beauchamp & Maller, 1977). Paradoxically, a preference for higher salt concentrations than that of adults seems to emerge during the preschool age range (Beauchamp & Cowart, 1990), finally taking on the adult pattern during adolescence (Desor, Greene et al., 1975). An interesting study in infant rats by Moe (1986) has shown that the dose–response function for salt preference is extremely shifted to the right before weaning onset. The basis for the emergence of normal preference of isotonicity has not been established in either rats or humans. The interspecies parallels are interesting, since rats and humans are both omnivores. Their generality should also be established in herbivores, such as sheep, about which considerable electrophysiological and histological information during the fetal period is available.

Individual human salt preference seems to be stable over time (Kumanyika & Jones, 1983), although it varies widely between individuals (Beauchamp & Engelman, 1991). Therefore, additional questions have arisen regarding the extent to which salt preference and intake can be modulated. In rats, postnatal exposure to high concentrations of sodium at 7 to 8 days of age (but not 14 days of age) predicted greater acceptance of highly concentrated saline and sucrose (but not sour) in adulthood (Smriga et al., 2002). Testing of norepinephrine concentrations in multiple areas of the brain in the sodium-exposed versus control rats revealed significantly lower norepinephrine concentrations in the amygdala of the sodium-exposed rats compared to controls. The amygdala is fully involved in the integration of emotional responses (in this case, acceptance of high concentrations of saline) with a variety of sensory inputs. This study provided evidence that exposure to a particular sodium concentration in early development causes long-term decreases in amygdala norepinephrine activity, which lead to greater acceptance of high concentrations of saline in adulthood. Indeed, when norepinephrine was infused into the amygdala, the acceptance of high concentrations of saline was diminished.

In humans, inadvertent exposure to a low-chloride formula in infancy was associated with patterns of higher salt preference in adolescence (Stein et al., 1996); and "morning sickness," presumably associated with volume depletion during pregnancy, was associated with higher salt preference in the offspring during both infancy and adolescence (Crystal & Bernstein, 1995, 1998). In short, emerging data suggest that exposure to sodium early in life, in both animals and humans, affects salt preference later, consistent with the work in rats discussed earlier (Hill, 2001).

SOUR   Compared to investigations of sweet, bitter, and salty, studies of sour taste have begun only recently. Preference for sour taste shows considerable variability. The basis for this variability, the manner in which preference for sour taste develops, the potential biological determinants of sour taste, and the implications of sour taste remain unknown. The limited available data are presented here.

Newborns grimace in response to sour tastes (Steiner, 1977) and reduce their intake of sour substances (Desor, Maller, et al., 1975). Oddly, this innate aversion changes to liking in early childhood: children prefer sour flavors in comparison to adults (Liem & Mennella, 2003), although the benefit of the difference remains unclear. Both adults and children who prefer more sour flavors, however, are less food neophobic, and accept a wider variety of foods into the diet (Frank & van der Klaauw, 1994; Liem & Mennella, 2003; Liem et al., 2004). It is not likely that individuals who prefer more sour flavors simply have impaired taste detection (Frank & van der Klaauw, 1994; Liem et al., 2004). Greater willingness to accept sour solutions may simply be a manifestation of lower finickiness.

The few studies on whether experience influences preference for sour may be in conflict. Repeated exposure to sour over a period of 8 days in 8- to 11-year-old children, *did not* lead to increased liking for the sour flavor (though repeated exposure to sweet did lead to increased preference for the sweet flavor; Liem & de Graaf, 2004). In contrast, as just described, prior studies had shown that repeated exposure to sour taste during infancy *does* increase liking for sour by age 4 years (Mennella & Beauchamp, 2002). Early infancy may include a critical period for the development of increased liking for sour taste, or the repeated exposure needed to induce it may need to occur over a prolonged period (e.g., daily exposure for a year, as in infancy, compared to the brief series of eight exposures in the study with school-age children by Liem and deGraaf). This is just the start of the analyses. They gain pragmatic import from the possibility that broadening sour acceptability may, likewise, allow sampling of a wider variety of fruits and vegetables.

BITTER   All studied omnivores (animals that eat a wide variety of substances) have an innate aversion to bitter or "spicy" substances, presumably because these compounds signal potential toxins. Indeed, a negative facial expression with mouth gaping and components of the gag reflex being displayed is observed in newborn infants in response to bitter (Rosenstein & Oster, 1988; Steiner, 1974), confirming that the innate aversion to bitter is present in humans as in other omnivores. Integration of the aversive response is probably subpontine, since Steiner elicited it in an anencephalic infant.

Beyond infancy, however, humans diverge from other omnivores in that we routinely develop likings for bitter or unpalatable substances. Human beings are the *only* omnivores that develop a liking for these substances, as evidenced by the widespread consumption of coffee, alcohol, tobacco, chili, wasabi, pepper, ginger, and horseradish, to name a few. Notably, however, piquant foods make up a small proportion of the diet throughout the life span in most cultures, so the increase in liking is somewhat constrained.

The development of preference for bitter as well as other unpalatable substances in animals and humans has received relatively little research attention. Rarely, animals have been reported as being induced to eat or prefer bitter compounds: rhesus monkeys can be induced to eat bitter quinine voluntarily (Kalmus, 1969), and mere exposure of infant rats to a bitter taste produced a slight and transient increase in preference (Warren & Pfaffmann, 1959). Mennella and Beauchamp (2002) found that children who had consumed a bitter formula during infancy were more likely to accept a bitter apple juice at age 4 years (although, notably, overall the children still preferred the sweeter apple juice over the bitter). Thus, distaste for bitter can be reduced by prior exposure during infancy or childhood under special conditions that only now have started to be explored.

It has been equally challenging to induce acceptance among animals for another inherently unpalatable substance: chili pepper. No method has been effective in increasing acceptance of chili pepper among rats (Rozin et al., 1979), and liking of chili pepper by chimpanzees was induced only if the chimpanzee observed the trainer eating the chili pepper (Rozin & Kennel, 1983). In countries where the consumption of chili pepper is very common, a liking for it among children is induced very gradually, essentially with modeling and without any specific material reward or coercion (Rozin & Schiller, 1980).

The manner in which human beings acquire an acceptance of, and even preference for, bitter substances requires more study at different levels of discourse. These studies are of some urgency, given that vegetables, which are targets for increased consumption from a public health perspective, are frequently inherently bitter. Understanding what helps children overcome their innate aversion would be an important contribution.

UMAMI   Umami, or glutamate, increases the palatability of many different foods, and it has been proposed as a basic, hedonically positive, innate taste preference akin to sweet and salty. On this basis, one would predict that, like salty and sweet, glutamate would be preferred by infants. Although pure glutamate is not preferred by either human infants or adults, both prefer foods with glutamate added, suggesting that glutamate acts as a flavor enhancer (Kemp & Beauchamp, 1994). Exactly how it functions in this manner, however, and how this effect has reached us through natural selection, remains elusive and is an important topic for future study (Beauchamp et al., 1998). In addition, how a preference for umami as a flavor enhancer functions from a neurophysiological standpoint, its ontogeny in both animals and humans, and how environment and experience may mediate its expression remain largely underinvestigated. Making it a widely accepted flavor enhancer for vegetables may be a goal worth exploring by individual families as well as research enterprises.

Perinatal flavor experiences and their impact on future preferences

This chapter has so far reviewed the development of specific discrete tastes, but the topic now turns to the specific impact of exposure to relatively more complex odors or flavors, both prenatally and perinatally, on subsequent behavior. Although the mechanisms of exposure (via the amniotic fluid or breast milk) have been identified, as will be outlined shortly, the neurological mediation of increased preference is not known. In rats, at least, all of the necessary components are present prenatally to respond to olfactory stimuli. Moreover, differential olfactory experiences permanently modify adult neurology and behavior. Specifically, rats exposed to a specific odor during postnatal days 1 through 18 have enhanced neural response to that odor as adults. Early olfactory experiences permit the survival of tufted cells, which stabilize interactions among other neurons in the olfactory bulb. A preference for an odor is also induced more readily when the rat is exposed to the odor in conjunction with stroking (which mimics maternal interaction with the rat pup). Thus, arousal seems to enhance olfactory learning and preference development (Coopersmith & Leon, 1988).

Three essential observations have been made regarding learning about taste and odors in the pre- and perinatal period in animals:

1. **Animals can learn about odors and flavors in utero, which, in turn, can affect in utero behavior.** For example, rats can develop a conditioned aversion to a flavor during gestation that extends into the postnatal period (Smotherman & Robinson, 1985).

2. **What animals learn about odors and flavors prenatally can affect postnatal behavior in other ways.** Pedersen and Blass (1982) exposed rats to a lemon scent in utero via injection into the amniotic fluid and found that pre- and postnatal exposure was necessary for newborn rats to attach to maternal nipples that were lemon-scented and prevented them from attaching to maternal nipples that were not lemon-scented (Pedersen & Blass, 1982). This observation implies that the lemon scent was experienced prenatally in the rat, and validated postnatally (Jacobson, 1991). The impact of prenatal exposure to flavors or odors on postnatal behavior has since been demonstrated in a number of species (Bilko et al., 1994; Schaal et al., 1995).

3. **What animals learn about a flavor or odor during suckling can also strongly affect adult copulatory behavior.** Male rats that had experienced a lemon scent on their mothers' nipple and perivaginal regions during suckling were more vigorous when copulating with lemon-scented female rats, compared to sexually receptive females lacking a lemon scent. Odors that rats experience in association with suckling in infancy help gain control over adult sexual behavior (Fillion & Blass, 1986).

The impact of early odor and flavor experiences on behavior, at least in animals, cannot be overstated. Early observations that original observations that prenatal taste and flavor experiences in human infants affect subsequent behaviors have been recently replicated by Schaal (2000). Schaal and colleagues (2000) demonstrated that infants whose mothers had consumed anise during pregnancy demonstrated greater preference for anise scent than did infants whose mothers had consumed a diet of foods containing no anise. Infants also will develop a preference for odors that they experience in association with breastfeeding (Allam et al., 2006), which has implications for later flavor preferences, as discussed earlier. Specifically, if infants experience a particular odor in human breast milk during suckling, they will be more likely to prefer foods with that odor in the future. It is reasonable to make the provisional suggestion that the range of food preferences is both constrained and expanded through scents transmitted via amniotic fluid and breast milk of foods consumed in the mother's diet. This effect is possible because both fluids are plasma filtrates, such that small elements and compounds can reach the infant through these maternal fluids.

Early infancy may include a critical period. Several recent studies of human infants have demonstrated that flavors experienced by the infant both in utero and postnatally during breast-feeding can affect later feeding behavior. Mennella and colleagues found that infants whose mothers had consumed carrot juice regularly during pregnancy alone or during lactation alone demonstrated fewer negative facial expressions in response to their first taste of carrot-flavored solids, relative to plain solids. In contrast, infants who had not had prior exposure to carrot flavor (during gestation or via breast-feeding) demonstrated no preference for carrot-flavored solid foods compared to plain. Note, however, that the effect was modest, and there was no difference in the amount that the infants actually consumed (Mennella et al., 2001).

This subtle effect of prior exposure to carrot on preference in infancy was presumably due to transmission of the carrot flavor via the amniotic fluid in utero, as well as via the breast milk, since the transmission of flavors in this manner has been demonstrated previously (Mennella & Beauchamp, 1999; Mennella et al., 1995). Thus, the prenatal experience in utero and experience with breast-feeding each had independent effects on postnatal flavor preferences, supporting the common notion that foods eaten during pregnancy and lactation affect the expression of early food preferences.

Development of hunger and satiety controls

Infants appear to respond readily to hunger and satiety cues. Responses to the latter may be more apparent than real, however. Prior work has evaluated the impact of holding the infant during feeding (as opposed to feeding the infant while in an infant seat), as well as social interaction during feeding, on feeding behavior and volume of intake. First, infants readily consumed 43% more formula when feeders interacted socially with them, than when not provided social interaction. Second, when infants were held, the volume ingested was correlated with the time elapsed since they had last eaten ($r = 0.67$), but when infants were not held, volume ingested and time elapsed since the last meal were relatively dissociated ($r = 0.20$; Figure 6.8). In addition, the more the infants looked at the feeder's face during feeding, the less correlated were the volume of intake and the time elapsed since the previous meal. Thus, even among infants as young as 7 to 14 weeks, milk intake can be readily influenced by the milieu in which the milk is delivered (Lumeng et al., 2007).

The conditions that would otherwise bring a meal to its biological end—in bottle-fed infants, at least—are easily overridden by the feeder's behavior. Bottle-fed infants, compared to breast-fed infants, tend to have higher BMIs at age 12 months, and this difference in body fatness tracks to school age (Scholtens et al., 2007). Mothers who bottle-feed also tend to be more controlling of their child's eating behavior at age 12 months than are mothers who breast-feed, suggesting that the maternal tendency to override the child's hunger and satiety cues, through bottle-feeding, may persist (Taveras et al., 2004).

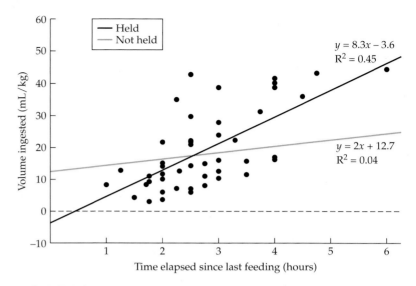

FIGURE 6.8   Volume ingested versus deprivation time in 7- to 14-week-old infants who are held versus not held during feeding. Data points represent the "held" condition only.

We do not know if these overrides cause childhood and adult obesity, or are even linked to them. Needed here are the kinds of detailed data provided by Wolff (1987) in his ethological description of motor ontogeny, in which he meticulously detailed the transitions from one stage to the next. Continuing to encourage intake during bottle-feeding, even when the infant has already exhibited signals for satiety, may weaken the infant's ability to appropriately respond to the sensation of satiety by stopping eating. This chain of events may be extended to the onset of self-feeding. These points have not been addressed empirically, but it is exactly these types of data that are required to gain traction on the contribution of early ingestion to later patterns and choices.

Continuing a palatable meal after declaring satiety is a characteristic of mammalian feeding. As such, it has received considerable attention. Children's responses to portion size provide a clear example of the plasticity of the hunger–satiety physiological system. Environment and cultural norms can easily overwhelm physiological signals. Children 11 months old and younger reduce volume consumed in accord with caloric density, and they will eat less at each eating occasion if more opportunities to eat are provided during the day. These relationships progressively weaken, however, in children 12 to 24 months old (Fox et al., 2006). Indeed, children as young as 2 years old eat more in response to larger portion sizes offered (Fisher, 2007), and the effect of larger portion size on increased consumption is clearly present by age 4 to 5 years (Fisher et al., 2003;

Mrdjenovic & Levitsky, 2005; Rolls et al., 2000). Adults regularly eat more in response to larger portion sizes (Edelman et al., 1986; Rolls et al., 2004). Smith's (1998) view on the segregation of the brainstem from more rostral organizing systems helps explain conceptually how food intake has shifted from control by internal factors operating at pontine/medullary levels (which do not have finely tuned control over intake) to determination by rostral systems that are not engaged by internal monitoring systems, and indeed override them.

Parental Roles

Food preferences and eating behavior start "in the nest." Mammalian infants begin extrauterine life with the perfect nutritious food: mother's milk that has been tailored to nourish the infant by having its fat content adjusted according to the environment (seals, for instance, produce exceedingly high fat milk) and infant age (e.g., kangaroo mothers that simultaneously nurse their newborn and their yearling have two milk sources that provide different consistencies in accord with each joey's needs). Breast milk also provides the infant with information concerning diet. Intake is limited by the mother's milk-synthesizing capacity, and meals are not exaggerated as they can be with bottle-feeding. Even though nutritionally dense, breast milk eventually can no longer meet the child's nutritional needs, and omnivore infants must inevitably face the challenge of food selection. Initial food selections are made by the parents, of course. Even after the child is mobile, the range of food choice is confined by what the parents bring into the home. The child's feeding education from the perspective of choice and amount eaten now goes into full gear.

Feeding the infant (encompassing both the quantity and quality of intake) might be considered a mental preoccupation for most mothers, as evidenced by the frequent report of problems with infants' feeding (Forsyth et al., 1985; Reau et al., 1996). Competent infant feeding, generally reflected in appropriate growth, is viewed (rightly or wrongly) as a fundamental reflection of "good parenting." During scheduled infant checkups, pediatricians always seek to reassure the parents regarding how well the infant is growing. The first information about the doctor's checkup that a proud parent generally shares with friends and family is that the infant's weight is robust—for example, in the ninety-fifth percentile. Feeding infants or children and watching them grow is a defining act of nurturing, so to suggest that parents may be overfeeding their children or that their infants are "too big" or "too heavy" may fly in the face of strong parental convictions about child rearing. Indeed, the documented perception of low-income and minority mothers is that food should never be withheld from preschool-age children when they express hunger (even when they are unlikely to be hungry, given the parent's assessment of their recent intake). Mothers and teachers in focus groups describe providing ample food to children as a rewarding component of caregiving. Limiting portion size is not considered an option (Jain et al., 2001; Lumeng et al., 2007).

Differences in parental feeding practices by race/socioeconomic status and culture

Emerging data relate to patterns of feeding styles in different cultural groups. African American mothers self-report more monitoring, restricting, pressuring, and controlling around children's eating compared to white mothers in most studies (Faith et al., 2003; Spruijt-Metz et al., 2002). Hispanic mothers self-report a feeding style that is both more controlling (demanding, threatening, bribing; Faith et al., 2003; Hughes et al., 2006) and indulgent or child-centered (reasoning, complimenting, encouraging the child to eat; Hughes et al., 2006; Hughes et al., 2005), compared to the style reported by white and African American mothers. Mothers of lower socioeconomic status (SES) seem to prompt their children to eat (Baughcum et al., 2001; Lumeng & Burke, 2006) more than do higher-SES mothers, and it has been hypothesized that this additional prompting may be due to concerns about inconsistent or inadequate food resources in this group. The importance of these cultural differences in belief systems for children's overweight risk remains unclear and is an important area for additional study.

Differences in parental feeding styles in relation to overweight risk

The impact of maternal feeding practices on child overweight risk is an area of active research. Maternal feeding style could be somewhat broadly conceptualized as falling into one of three possible domains: pushing, restricting, and controlling. Each of these types of feeding has been the topic of extensive study in relation to child overweight, and the jury is still out on whether a clear causal relationship between any of these feeding styles and child overweight risk even exists. The data for each domain are briefly reviewed here; a much more extensive review is available elsewhere (Faith et al., 2003a).

Maternal pushing, pressuring, or prompting children to eat has not been consistently linked with children's weight status. Some studies have shown that thinner children are prompted more often to eat (Carnell & Wardle, 2007; Keller et al., 2006; Powers et al., 2006; Spruijt-Metz et al., 2002), others show that heavier children are prompted more to eat (Klesges et al., 1986), and still others demonstrate no relationship (Baughcum et al., 2001; Drucker et al., 1999; Koivisto et al., 1994; Wardle et al., 2002).

Mothers with a restrictive feeding style (restricting access to and consumption of particular foods) tend to have children who are heavier and are more concerned about their children being too heavy (Spruijt-Metz et al., 2002). This link appears to be particularly true for girls, as opposed to boys (Constanzo & Woody, 1985), presumably because mothers may be more concerned about an overweight daughter than an overweight son. Allowing children choice about what they eat has also been inconsistently linked to weight status, with some studies showing that mothers of heavier children allow more choice (Faith et al., 2003), others showing that mothers of thinner children allow more choice (Faith et al., 2003; Hughes et al., 2005), and still others showing no relationship (Baughcum et al., 2001). In short, it simply remains unclear whether there is a particular maternal feeding style that, in and of itself and independent of the child's behavior or response to the mother's feeding style, is associated with a higher risk of obesity.

Feeding style may interact with other factors to lead to an increased risk of overweight in the child. Obese mothers express more concern about their child's eating and becoming overweight (Baughcum et al., 2001) and seem to attune their feeding behavior more carefully to their child's weight status than do nonobese mothers (Lumeng & Burke, 2006; Powers et al., 2006). Obese mothers may be more controlling of their heavier children's eating compared to nonobese mothers because they may be particularly invested in preventing their heavier child from progressing to obesity.

Despite these efforts, genetically mediated behaviors in these mother-child dyads may continue to increase the child's risk for overweight. In one study, for example, although obese mothers didn't prompt their children to eat any more than did nonobese mothers, the children of obese mothers were more compliant with their mothers' prompts (Lumeng & Burke, 2006). In short, children who are genetically predisposed to obesity may respond to the same maternal feeding behaviors differently than do children who are not genetically predisposed to obesity.

Parental versus peer influence on children's food preferences

Even if maternal feeding style has not been consistently linked with a child's overweight risk, mothers still presumably have a strong impact on children's food preferences and the variety of foods that children will accept. Originally through their milk, and then as "gatekeepers of the pantry," mothers have traditionally been thought to exert powerful influence over their children's food preferences and eating behavior. The implication is that children will prefer the same foods as their parents. Interestingly, this has proven not to be the case. The correlation between parents' and children's food preferences is surprisingly low ($r = 0.16$; Rozin, 1991)—a finding consistent with a number of prior studies in the literature reviewed by Rozin.

Correlations among siblings and peers, however, are higher than the generational ones. Pliner and colleagues (1986) reported a correlation of 0.50 for the preferences between siblings (ages 24 months to 83 months)—a value significantly higher than that with their parents, which were in the range of 0.20 to 0.30 (Pliner & Pelchat, 1986). This finding is not surprising, because children are often fed quite similar and standard foods outside the home in school and child care settings, and these foods are presumably less variable than those of the individual home, which reflect different ethnic and religious traditions.

In short, the influence of peers on food preferences seems to be greater than the influence of adults, even when those adults are the parents. Birch and colleagues (1980) had 17 children 2 to 4 years old rank their preferences for nine vegetables. They then seated a child who had ranked, for example, peas as most preferred and corn as least preferred among a group of children in preschool with the opposite preferences for 4 days in a row. When offered the peas or the corn on the first day, only 12% of the pea-preferring target children selected corn. By the fourth day of observing their peers selecting corn over peas, however, the pea-preferring target children were selecting corn 59% of the time. When the children were asked to rank their preferences for the nine vegetables again at the conclusion of the protocol, the nonpreferred vegetable (e.g., corn) moved up on average 2.5 ranks in the list. In short, the vegetable remained relatively nonpreferred, though less strongly so (Birch, 1980).

Subsequent studies have evaluated the strength of the peer effect. In a study of preschoolers whose acceptance of a target food was increased during a meal by the presence of a peer model eating the food, the effect did not last beyond the meal (Hendy, 2002). The fact that peers influence one another's food preferences suggests that peers who spend a lot of time together, or who feel a great affinity for one another, will display closely associated preferences. Rozin, Riklis, and Margolis (2004) addressed this question in third-grade children and found that the correlation of children's preferences with that of their best friends ($r = 0.46$) on a list of 13 foods was no greater than the correlation with any other child in the classroom ($r = 0.50$). Peer influences on food preferences, though greater than that of parents and other adults, seem relatively short-lived and modest. Inducing preferences is difficult, and a relatively long period of time is required to overcome either an innate bias or one acquired through prolonged exposure.

Parents' use of food as a behavior modifier and the social-affective context of eating

Parents are frequently instructed not to use food as a reward. Indeed, a single study demonstrated that a teacher presenting a food to a child in a positive social context ("Hi, Susie. Here, have a cracker.") or using the food as a reward ("Good job cleaning up your toys, John. Here, have a cracker.") increased liking for the food, and the effect endured for at least 6 weeks (Birch et al., 1980). This effect was observed in a classroom setting with teachers, and not with parents.

In a separate study, Birch, Marlin, and Rotter (1984) addressed the effect of *using a reward to induce a child to eat a food* on liking (in contrast to *using food as a reward*). Two types of rewards were evaluated: simple verbal praise (e.g., "You're such a good eater!") and a tangible reward (e.g., "Okay, you ate it; now you get to watch a video."). Although both reward methods increased the child's consumption of the food in the moment, both also modestly *decreased* liking for the food. Thus, rewarding a child for eating his or her vegetables at dinner (e.g., "You can't watch TV until you finish your broccoli."), as well as simply praising a child for eating, (e.g., "Good job eating your spinach, honey!") will *decrease* preference for the vegetable. The decrease in preference in Birch's study occurred after a relatively modest exposure—twice per week for 4 weeks. Whether the decrease in preference persisted after the end of the exposures remains unknown. Nonetheless, the results provide counterintuitive evidence that rewarding a child for eating a food, even in the simplest of manners, may decrease the child's liking of the food over time.

Parents and television viewing

The link between increased television viewing and increased risk of overweight has been well established (see Chapter 12). The role of parents in shaping children's viewing habits, however, deserves mention. A greater amount of television viewing has been linked to an increased prevalence of overweight in children as young as 3 years old (Lumeng et al., 2006). Predictors of increased television viewing in young children are the common indicators of psychosocial risk, including maternal depression, low maternal education, and low income (Burdette et al., 2003; Lumeng et al., 2006). Understanding how to reach mothers in these populations to change this particular parenting behavior is a public health challenge. At minimum, however, providing children in this demographic with opportunities to attend preschool, which presumably would reduce their TV viewing time, would be an important first step.

Life Stressors in Childhood and Lifelong Overweight Risk

A number of studies have demonstrated that childhood mood disturbances predict obesity in adulthood, independent of a number of potential confounders. Pine and colleagues (2001) reported, in a small sample of normal-weight 6- to 17-year-old children, that childhood depression was associated with a higher body mass index in adulthood, regardless of socioeconomic status. Andersen and colleagues (2006) found that anxiety in girls was associated with a consistently higher BMI beginning in childhood that extended into adulthood. The source has not been identified as either increased feeding, decreased activity, or both. The earlier the depression onset appeared in these females, the higher the adult BMI was. Conversely, depression in males was associated with a lower BMI in adulthood that was not influenced by age of onset. These findings are generally consistent with earlier reports that adolescent depression is associated with an increased risk of obesity in women but not men (Richardson et al., 2003).

The mechanism linking stress and mental health disorders with obesity is an area of active research, and a biological mechanism presents itself as a prime hypothesis. Chronic stress is believed to increase abdominal obesity through alterations in the hypothalamic–pituitary–adrenal (HPA) axis and chronic excessive cortisol secretion (Dallman et al., 2003). A number of animal studies support this view. The perspective that overeating energy-dense foods can be viewed as addiction (see Chapters 4 and 14) predicts that stress will cause and maintain overeating. This is certainly true for the classic addictions to substances such as nicotine, alcohol, and illicit drugs. Likewise, stress would also be predicted to trigger relapse of overeating.

Eating foods high in fat and carbohydrates ("comfort foods") seems to reduce the body's response to stress. Physically restrained (and therefore stressed) rats that were given access to lard and sucrose consumed a greater proportion of the "comfort food" compared to control rats, and consumption of comfort food reduced activity of the HPA axis (Pecoraro et al., 2004). In another study in rats, chronic stress and high corticosterone levels were correlated with greater caloric intake of palatable food, which, in turn, led to preferential deposition of abdominal fat (Dallman et al., 2003). Sweet tastes and fat flavors cause endogenous opioid release, which might be a source of comfort.

In all likelihood, these observations in rats apply directly to humans and the obesity epidemic. It is especially notable that the effect on stress reduction seems to occur specifically with sucrose and fat. These calorie-dense foods are likely to predispose individuals in particular to excessive weight gain and the development of obesity. Regrettably, consumption of fruits, vegetables, and whole grains is not known to affect the cortisol response or reduce stress.

A few human studies are consistent with the animal findings. Individuals who identified themselves as "stress eaters" tended to gain more weight during stressful periods (final exams, in this case), and they demonstrated increases in insulin, cortisol, and total/HDL cholesterol ratio, although the direction of causality cannot be established (Epel et al., 2004). All of these changes characterize abdominal obesity and "the metabolic syndrome." Chronic stress (chronic excessive cortisol secretion) in childhood may induce "coping" feeding patterns that have the unfortunate consequence of adult obesity.

Endogenous neuropeptides are involved in the reward processes in eating behavior. Indeed, in animals and human infants, the ingestion of sweet and fatty foods alleviates crying and distress (Gibson, 2006). Even into adulthood, sweet taste increases pain tolerance, and a number of naturalistic studies have demonstrated that, during periods of stress, individuals consume more sweet and fatty foods (but not more vegetables). As a result, through classical conditioning, a craving for comfort foods can develop and be strengthened in situations and places in which stress had been previously been eased by ingestion of such foods. Furthermore, in situations of stress and a need to relax, consumption of sweet or fatty food will have been proven to be relaxants. Understanding the bases of these conditioned cravings will be of considerable help in normalizing intake.

Summary

This chapter has identified specific influences on obesity risk and eating behavior in childhood. Multiple studies indicate that factors influencing overeating and obesity risk in childhood exert their influence throughout the life span. Because the early years well predict future BMI, as well as the breadth of food selection and liking, infancy and childhood provide the natural intervention milieu for shaping food choice and eating patterns and, hopefully, obesity prevention.

A recurrent theme has been the need to experimentally and formally disentangle the roles of genetics and environment in shaping behavior and conferring obesity risk. This area must continue to receive attention in the coming decades. Stemming obesity prevalence is possible, but it will require a multi-pronged approach with a focus on early childhood to *prevent* obesity. Any intervention program will also require an appreciation for the ways in which eating behavior is deeply rooted in different cultures and for the need to understand and respect these cultural differences before any intervention is undertaken.

This as an attainable goal that will require action on many levels—by parents, by school systems, in neighborhoods to improve facilities and provide a safe ambience, and politically to help remedy the support provided to certain industries that have disproportionately contributed to the current obesity epidemic in the United States.

References Cited

Allam, M., Marlier, L., & Schaal, B. (2006). Learning at the breast: Preference formation for an artificial scent and its attraction against the odor of maternal milk. *Infant Behavior & Development, 29*, 308–321.

Anderson, S., Cohen, P., Naumova, E., & Must, A. (2006). Association of depression and anxiety disorders with weight change in a prospective community-based study of children follow up into adulthood. *Archives of Pediatrics & Adolescent Medicine, 160*, 285–291.

Anonymous. (2005). Policy Statement: Breastfeeding and the use of human milk. *Pediatrics, 115*, 496–506.

Arenz, S., Ruckerl, R., Koletzko, B., & von Kries, R. (2004). Breast-feeding and childhood obesity — a systematic review. *International Journal of Obesity, 28*, 1247–1256.

Bain, K. (1948). The incidence of breast feeding in hospitals in the United States. *Pediatrics, 2*, 313–320.

Baird, J., Fisher, D., Lucas, P., Kleijnen, J., Roberts, H., & Law, C. (2005). Being big or growing fast: Systematic review of size and growth in infancy and later obesity. *BMJ, 331*, 929.

Baughcum, A., Powers, S., Johnson, S., Chamberlin, L., Deeks, C., Jain, A., et al. (2001). Maternal feeding practices and beliefs and their relationships to over- weight in early childhood. *Journal of Developmental and Behavioral Pediatrics, 22*, 391–408.

Beauchamp, G., Bachmanov, A., & Stein, L. (1998). Development of taste genetics of glutamate taste preference. *Annals of the New York Academy of Sciences, 855*, 412–416.

Beauchamp, G., & Cowart, B. (1990). Preference for high salt concentrations among children. *Developmental Psychology, 26*, 539–545.

Beauchamp, G., Cowart, B., & Moran, M. (1986). Developmental changes in salt acceptability in human infants. *Developmental Psychobiology, 19*, 75–83.

Beauchamp, G., & Engelman, K. (1991). High salt intake: Sensory and behavioral factors. *Hypertension, 17*(Suppl. 1), 181.

Beauchamp, G., & Maller, O. (1977). The development of taste preferences in humans: A review. In M. Kare & O. Maller (Eds.), *The chemical senses and nutrition.* New York: Academic Press.

Beauchamp, G., & Moran, M. (1982). Dietary experience and sweet taste preference in human infants. *Appetite, 3*, 139–152.

Bilko, A., Altbacker, V., & Hudson, R. (1994). Transmission of food preference in the rabbit: The means of information transfer. *Physiology & Behavior, 56*, 907–912.

Birch, L. (1979). Preschool children's food preferences and consumption patterns. *Journal of Nutrition Education, 11,* 189–192.

Birch, L. (1980). Effects of peer models' food choices and eating behaviors on preschoolers' food preferences. *Child Development, 51,* 489–496.

Birch, L., & Marlin, D. (1982). I don't like it; I never tried it: effects of exposure on two-year-old children's food preferences. *Appetite, 3,* 353–360.

Birch, L., Marlin, D., & Rotter, J. (1984). Eating as the "means" activity in a contingency: effects on young children's food preference. *Child Development, 55,* 432–439.

Birch, L., Zimmerman, S., & Hind, H. (1980). The influence of social-affective context on the formation of children's food preferences. *Child Development, 51,* 856–861.

Birdsong, D., & Molis, M. (2001). On the evidence for maturational constraints in second-language acquisition. *Journal of Memory and Language, 44,* 235–249.

Blass, E., Ganchrow, J., & Steiner, J. (1984). Classical conditioning in newborn humans 2–48 hours of age. *Infant Behavior & Development, 7,* 223–235.

Breslin, P., Spector, A., & Grill, H. (1993). Chorda tympani section decreases the cation specificity of depletion-induced sodium appetite in rats. *American Journal of Physiology, 264,* R319–R323.

Burdette, H., Whitaker, R., Hall, W., & Daniels, S. (2006). Breastfeeding, introduction of complementary foods, and adiposity at 5 years of age. *American Journal of Clinical Nutrition, 83,* 550–558.

Burdette, H., Whitaker, R., Kahn, R., & Harvey-Benino, J. (2003). Association of maternal obesity and depressive symptoms with television-viewing time in low-income preschool children. *Archives of Pediatrics & Adolescent Medicine, 157,* 894–899.

Carnell, S., & Wardle, J. (2007). Associations between multiple measures of parental feeding and children's adiposity in United Kingdom preschoolers. *Obesity, 15,* 137–144.

Cashdan, E. (1994). A sensitive period for learning about food. *Human Nature, 5,* 279–291.

Cines, B., & Rozin, P. (1982). Some aspects of the liking for hot coffee and coffee flavor. *Appetite, 3,* 23–34.

Constanzo, P., & Woody, E. (1985). Domain-specific parenting styles and their impact on the child's development of particular deviance: The example of obesity proneness. *Journal of Social and Clinical Psychology, 3,* 425–445.

Cooke, L., & Wardle, J. (2005). Age and gender differences in children's food preferences. *British Journal of Nutrition, 93,* 741–746.

Cooke, L., Wardle, J., & Gibson, E. (2003). Relationship between parental report of food neophobia and everyday food consumption in 2–6-year-old children. *Appetite, 41,* 205–206.

Coopersmith, R., & Leon, M. (1988). The neurobiology of early olfactory learning. In E. Blass (Ed.), *Handbook of Behavioral Neurobiology* (Vol. 9, pp. 283–308). New York: Plenum Press.

Crystal, S., & Bernstein, I. (1995). Morning sickness: Impact of offspring salt preference. *Appetite, 25,* 231–240.

Crystal, S., & Bernstein, I. (1998). Infant salt preference and mother's morning sickness. *Appetite, 30,* 297–307.

Dallman, M., Pecoraro, N., Akana, S., LaFleur, S., Gomez, F., Houshyar, H., et al. (2003). Chronic stress and obesity: A new view of "comfort food". *Proceedings of the National Academy of Sciences, USA, 100,* 11696–11701.

Daniels, D., & Fluharty, S. (2004). Salt appetite: A neurohormonal viewpoint. *Physiology & Behavior, 81,* 319–337.

de Castro, J. (1990). Social facilitation of duration and size but not rate of the spontaneous meal intake of humans. *Physiology & Behavior, 47,* 1129–1135.

de Castro, J. M. (1994). Family and friends produce greater social facilitation of food intake than other companions. *Physiology & Behavior, 56,* 445–455.

de Castro, J. M., & Brewer, E. M. (1992). The amount eaten in meals by humans is a power function of the number of people present. *Physiology & Behavior, 51,* 121–125.

de Castro, J. M., & de Castro, E. S. (1989). Spontaneous meal patterns in humans: influence of the presence of other people. *American Journal of Clinical Nutrition, 50,* 237–247.

de Graaf, C. (1999). Sweetness intensity and pleasantness in children, adolescents, and adults. *Physiology & Behavior, 67,* 513–520.

Dennison, B., Edmunds, L., Stratton, H., & Pruzek, R. (2006). Rapid infant weight gain predicts childhood overweight. *Obesity, 14*, 491–499.

Desor, J. (1987). Longitudinal changes in sweet preferences in humans. *Physiology & Behavior, 39*, 639–641.

Desor, J., Greene, L., & Maller, O. (1975). Preferences for sweet and salty in 9- to 15-year-old and adult humans. *Science, 190*, 686–687.

Desor, J., Maller, O., & Andrews, K. (1975). Ingestive responses of human newborns to salty, sour, and bitter stimului. *Journal of Comparative and Physiological Psychology, 89*, 966–970.

Desor, J., Maller, O., & Turner, R. (1973). Taste in acceptance of sugars by human infants. *Journal of Comparative and Physiological Psychology, 84*, 496–501.

DiLorenzo, P., Kiefer, S., Rice, A., & Garcia, J. (1986). Neural and behavioral responsivity to ethyl alcohol as a tastant. *Alcohol, 3*, 55–61.

Drucker, R., Hammer, L., Agras, W., & Bryson, S. (1999). Can mothers influence their child's eating behavior? *Journal of Developmental and Behavioral Pediatrics, 20*, 88–92.

Duncker, K. (1938). Experimental modifcation of children's food preferences through social suggestion. *Journal of Abnormal Child Psychology, 33*, 490–507.

Edelman, B., Engell, D., Bronstein, P., & Hirsch, E. (1986). Environmental influences on the intake of overweight and normal-weight men. *Appetite, 7*, 71–83.

Ekelund, U., Ong, K., Linne, Y., Neovius, M., Brage, S., Dunger, D., et al. (2006). Upward weight percentile crossing in infancy and early childhood independently predicts fat mass in young adults: The Stockholm Weight Development Study (SWEDES). *American Journal of Clinical Nutrition, 83*, 324–330.

Epel, E., Jiminez, S., Brownell, K., Stroud, L., Stoney, C., & Niaura, R. (2004). Are stress eaters at risk for the metabolic syndrome? *Annals of the New York Academy of Sciences, 1032*, 208–210.

Faith, M., Heshka, S., Keller, K., Sherry, B., Matz, P., Pietrobelli, A., et al. (2003). Maternal-child feeding patterns and child body weight— Findings from a population-based sample. *Archives of Pediatrics & Adolescent Medicine, 157*, 926–932.

Fillion, T., & Blass, E. (1986). Infantile experience with suckling odors determines adult sexual behavior in male rats. *Science, 231*, 729–731.

Finberg, L., Kiley, J., & Luttrell, C. (1963). Mass accidental salt poisoning in infancy. *Journal of the American Medical Association, 184*, 121–124.

Fisher, J. (2007). Effects of age on children's intake of large and self-selected food portions. *Obesity, 15*, 403–412.

Fisher, J., Birch, L., Smiciklas-Wright, H., & Picciano, M. (2000). Breast-feeding through the first year predicts maternal control in feeding and subsequent toddler energy intakes. *Journal of the American Dietetic Association, 100*, 641–646.

Fisher, J., Rolls, B., & Birch, L. (2003). Children's bite size and intake of an entree are greater with larger portions than with age-appropriate or self-selected portions. *American Journal of Clinical Nutrition, 77*, 1164–1170.

Fomon, S. (2001). Infant feeding in the 20th century: Formula and beikost. *Journal of Nutrition, 131*, 409S–420S.

Foote, J., Murphy, S., Wilkens, L., Basiotis, P., & Carlson, A. (2004). Dietary variety increases the probability of nutrient adequacy among adults. *Journal of Nutrition, 134*, 1779–1785.

Forsyth, B., Leventhal, J., & McCarthy, P. (1985). Mother's perceptions of problems of feeding and crying behaviors. A prospective study. *American Journal of Diseases of Childhood, 139*, 269–272.

Fox, M., Devaney, B., Reidy, K., Razafindrakoto, C., & Ziegler, P. (2006). Relationship between portion size and energy intake among infants and toddlers: Evidence of self-regulation. *Journal of the American Dietetic Association, 106*, S77–S83.

Frank, R., & van der Klaauw, N. (1994). The contribution of chemosensory factors to individual differences in reported food preferences. *Appetite, 22*, 101–123.

Freedman, D., Khan, L. K., Serdula, M., Dietz, W., Srinivasan, S., & Berenson, G. (2005a). Racial differences in the tracking of childhood BMI to adulthood. *Obesity Research, 13*, 928–935.

Freedman, D., Khan, L. K., Serdula, M., Dietz, W., Srinivasan, S., & Berenson, G. (2005b). The relation of childhood BMI to adult adiposity: The Bogalusa Heart Study. *Pediatrics, 115*, 22–27.

Galloway, A., Lee, Y., & Birch, L. (2003). Predictors and consequences of food neophobia and pickiness in young girls. *Journal of the American Dietetic Association, 103,* 692–698.

Ganchrow, J., Steiner, J., & Daher, M. (1983). Neonatal facial expressions in reponse to different qualities and intensities of gustatory stimuli. *Infant Behavior & Development, 6,* 473–484.

Gibson, E. (2006). Emotional influences on food choice: Sensory, physiological and psychological pathways. *Physiology & Behavior, 89,* 53–61.

Harder, T., Bergmann, R., Kallischnigg, G., & Plagemann, A. (2005). Duration of breast-feeding and risk of overweight: A meta-analysis. *American Journal of Epidemiology, 162,* 397–403.

Harlow, H. (1932). Social facilitation of feeding in the albino rat. *Journal of Genetic Psychology, 43,* 211–221.

Harper, L., & Sanders, K. (1975). The effect of adults' eating on young children's acceptance of unfamiliar foods. *Journal of Experimental Child Psychology, 20,* 206–214.

Hendy, H. (2002). Effectiveness of trained peer models to encourage food acceptance in preschool children. *Appetite, 39,* 217–225.

Herman, P., Roth, D., & Polivy, J. (2003). Effects of the presence of others on food intake: A normative interpretation. *Psychological Bulletin, 129,* 873–886.

Hill, D. (2001). Taste Development. In E. Blass (Ed.), *Developmental Psychobiology* (Vol. 13). New York: Plenum.

Hirschman, C., & Hendershot, G. (1979). *Trends in breast feeding among American mothers.* Hyattsville, MD: Department of Health, Education, and Welfare.

Hughes, S., Anderson, C., Power, T., Micheli, N., Jaramillo, S., & Nicklas, T. (2006). Measuring feeding in low-income African-American and Hispanic parents. *Appetite, 46,* 215–223.

Hughes, S., Power, T., Fisher, J., Mueller, S., & Nicklas, T. (2005). Revisiting a neglected construct: Parenting styles in a child-feeding context. *Appetite, 44,* 83–92.

Jacobson, M. (1991). *Developmental Neurobiology* (3rd ed.). New York: Plenum Press.

Jain, A., Sherman, S., Chamberlin, L., Carter, Y., Powers, S., & Whitaker, R. (2001). Why don't low-income mothers worry about their preschoolers being overweight? *Pediatrics, 107,* 1138–1146.

James, C., Laing, D., & Oram, N. (1997). A comparison of the ability of 8–9-year-old children and adults to detect taste stimuli. *Physiology & Behavior, 62,* 193–197.

Jensen, D., Damm, P., Sorensen, B., Molsted-Pedersen, L., Westergaard, J., Ovesen, P., et al. (2003). Pregnancy outcome and prepregnancy body mass index in 2459 glucose-tolerant Danish women. *American Journal of Obstetrics and Gynecology, 189,* 239–244.

Johnson, J., & Newport, E. (1989). Critical period effects in second language learning: The influence of maturational state on the acquisition of English as a second language. *Cognitive Psychology, 21,* 60–99.

Kalmus, H. (1969). The sense of taste of chimpanzees and other primates. *Chimpanzee, 2,* 130–141.

Kehoe, P., & Blass, E. (1986a). Behaviorally functional opioid systems in infant rats: I. Evidence for olfactory and gustatory classical conditioning. *Behavioral Neuroscience, 100,* 359–367.

Kehoe, P., & Blass, E. (1986b). Conditioned aversions and their memories in 5-day-old rats during suckling. *Journal of Experimental Psychology: Animal Behavior Processes, 12,* 40–47.

Keller, K., Pietrobelli, A., Johnson, S., & Faith, M. (2006). Maternal restriction of children's eating and encouragements to eat as the 'non-shared' environment: A pilot study using the child feeding questionnaire. *International Journal of Obesity, 30,* 1670–1675.

Kemp, S., & Beauchamp, G. (1994). Flavor modification by sodium chloride and monosodium glutamate. *Journal of Food Science, 59,* 687–696.

Kimmel, S., Sigman-Grant, M., & Guinard, J. (1994). Sensory testing with young children. *Food Technology, 94,* 92–99.

Klesges, R., Malott, J., Boschee, P., & Weber, J. (1986). The effects of parental influences on children's food intake, physical activity, and relative weight. *International Journal of Eating Disorders, 5,* 335–346.

Koivisto, U., Fellenius, J., & Sjoden, P. (1994). Relations between parental mealtime practices and children's food intake. *Appetite, 22,* 245–257.

Kramer, M., Morin, I., Yang, H., Platt, R., Usher, R., McNamara, H., et al. (2002). Why are babies getting bigger? Temporal trends in fetal growth and its determinants. *Journal of Pediatrics, 141*, 538–542.

Kumanyika, S., & Jones, D. (1983). Patterns of week-to-week table salt use by men and women consuming constant diets. *Human Nutrition, 37A*, 348–356.

Lanier, S., Hayes, J., & Duffy, V. (2005). Sweet and bitter tastes of alcoholic beverages mediate alcohol intake in of-age undergraduates. *Physiology & Behavior, 83*, 821–831.

Li, R., Darling, N., Maurice, E., Barker, L., & Grummer-Strawn, L. (2005). Breastfeeding rates in the United States by characteristics of the child, mother, or family: The 2002 National Immunization Survey. *Pediatrics, 115*, e31–e37.

Li, R., Zhao, Z., Mokdad, A., Barker, L., & Grummer-Strawn, L. (2003). Prevalence of breastfeeding in the United States: The 2001 National Immunization Survey. *Pediatrics, 111*, 1198–1201.

Liem, D., & de Graaf, C. (2004). Sweet and sour preferences in young children and adults: Role of repeated exposure. *Physiology & Behavior, 83*, 421–429.

Liem, D., & Mennella, J. (2003). Heightened sour preferences during childhood. *Chemical Senses, 28*, 173–180.

Liem, D., Westerbeek, A., & Wolternik, S. (2004). Sour taste preferences of children relate to preference for novel and intense stimuli. *Chemical Senses, 29*, 713–720.

Lien, N., Lytle, L., & Kleep, K. (2001). Stability in consumption of fruit, vegetables, and sugary foods in a cohort from age 14 to 21. *Preventive Medicine, 33*, 217–226.

Logue, A., Ophir, I., & Strauss, K. (1981). The acquisition of taste aversions in humans. *Behaviour Research and Therapy, 19*, 319–333.

Lucas, A., Sarson, D., Blackburn, A., Adrian, T., Aynsley-Green, A., & Bloom, S. (1980). Breast vs. bottle: Endocrine responses are different with formula feeding. *Lancet, 1*, 1267–1269.

Lucas, A., Stafford, M., Morley, R., Abbott, R., Stephenson, T., MacFayden, U., et al. (1999). Efficacy and safety of long-chain polyunsaturated fatty acid supplementation of infant-formula milk: A randomized trial. *Lancet, 354*, 1948–1954.

Lumeng, J., & Burke, L. (2006). Maternal prompts to eat, child compliance, and mother and child weight status. *Journal of Pediatrics, 149*, 330–335.

Lumeng, J., & Hillman, K. (2007). Larger group size increases consumption in children. *Archives of Disease in Childhood*, in press.

Lumeng, J., Kaplan-Sanoff, M., Shuman, S., & Kannan, S. (2007). Head Start teachers' perceptions of children's eating behavior, food insecurity, and overweight. *Journal of Nutrition Education and Behavior*, in press.

Lumeng, J., Patil, N., & Blass, E. (2007). Social influences on formula intake via suckling in 7- to 14-week-old infants. *Developmental Psychobiology, 49*, 351–361.

Lumeng, J., Rahnama, S., Appugliese, D., & Bradley, R. (2006). Television exposure and overweight risk in preschoolers. *Archives of Pediatrics & Adolescent Medicine, 160*, 417–422.

Marchi, M., & Cohen, P. (1990). Early childhood eating behaviors and adolescent eating disorders. *Journal of the American Academy of Child and Adolescent Psychiatry, 29*, 112–117.

Mennella, J., & Beauchamp, G. (1999). Experience with a flavor in mother's milk modifies the infant's acceptance of flavored cereal. *Developmental Psychobiology, 35*, 197–203.

Mennella, J., & Beauchamp, G. (2002). Flavor experiences during formula feeding are related to preferences during childhood. *Early Human Development, 68*, 71–82.

Mennella, J., Jagnow, C., & Beauchamp, G. (2001). Prenatal and postnatal flavor learning by human infants. *Pediatrics, 107*, e88.

Mennella, J., Johnson, A., & Beauchamp, G. (1995). Garlic ingestion by pregnant women alters the odor of amniotic fluid. *Chemical Senses, 20*, 207–209.

Mistretta, C., & Bradley, R. (1985). Development of taste. In E. Blass (Ed.), *Handbook of Behavioral Neurobiology, Vol. 8, Developmental Processes in Psychobiology and Neurobiology* (pp. 205–236). New York: Plenum Press.

Moe, K. (1986). The ontogeny of salt preference in rats. *Developmental Psychobiology, 19*, 185–196.

Mook, D. (1963). Oral and postingestional determinants of the intake of various solutions in rats with esophageal fistulas. *Journal of Comparative and Physiological Psychology, 56*, 645–659.

Mrdjenovic, G., & Levitsky, D. (2005). Children eat what they are served: The imprecise regulation of energy intake. *Appetite, 44*, 273–282.

Murphy, S., Foote, J., Wilkens, L., Basiotis, P., Carlson, A., White, K., et al. (2006). Simple measures of dietary variety are associated with improved dietary quality. *Journal of the American Dietetic Association, 106*, 425–429.

Mustillo, S., Worthman, C., Erkanli, A., Keeler, G., Angold, A., & Costello, E. (2003). Obesity and psychiatric disorder: Developmental trajectories. *Pediatrics, 111*, 851–859.

Nachman, M., & Pfaffmann, C. (1963). Gustatory nerve discharge in normal and sodium deficient rats. *Journal of Comparative and Physiological Psychology, 56*, 1007–1011.

Nader, P., O'Brien, M., Houts, R., Bradley, R., Belksy, J., Crosnoe, R., et al. (2006). Identifying risk for obesity in early childhood. *Pediatrics, 118*, e594–e601.

Navarro, M., Spray, K., Cubero, I., Thiele, T., & Bernstein, I. (2000). cFos induction during conditioned taste aversion expression varies with aversion strength. *Brain Research, 887*, 450–453.

Nicklaus, S., Boggio, V., Chabanet, C., & Issanchou, S. (2005). A prospective study of food variety seeking in childhood, adolescence and early adult life. *Appetite, 44*, 289–297.

Ogden, C., Carroll, M., Curtin, L., McDowell, M., Tabak, C., & Flegal, K. (2006). Prevalence of overweight and obesity in the United States, 1999–2004. *Journal of the American Medical Association, 295*, 1549–1555.

Ong, K., Emmett, P., Noble, S., Ness, A., Dunger, D., & Team, A. S. (2006). Dietary energy intake at the age of 4 months predicts postnatal weight gain and childhood body mass index. *Pediatrics, 117*, e503–e508.

Owen, C., Martin, R., Whincup, P., Smith, G., & Cook, D. (2005). Effect of infant feeding on the risk of obesity across the life course: A quantitative review of published evidence. *Pediatrics, 115*, 1367–1377.

Pecoraro, N., Reyes, F., Gomez, F., Bhargava, A., & Dallman, M. (2004). Chronic stress promotes palatable feeding, which reduces signs of stress: Feedforward and feedback effects of chronic stress. *Endocrinology, 145*, 3754–3762.

Pedersen, P., & Blass, E. (1982). Prenatal and posnatal determinants of the first suckling episode in albino rats. *Developmental Psychobiology, 15*, 349–355.

Peryam, D. (1963). The acceptance of novel foods. *Food Technology, 17*, 33–39.

Pine, D., Goldstein, B., Wolk, S., & Weissman, M. (2001). The association between childhood depression and adulthood body mass index. *Pediatrics, 107*, 1049–1056.

Pliner, P., & Hobden, K. (1992). Development of a scale to measure the trait of food neophobia in humans. *Appetite, 19*, 105–120.

Pliner, P., & Loewen, E. (1997). Temperament and food neophobia in children and their mothers. *Appetite, 28*, 239–254.

Pliner, P., & Pelchat, M. (1986). Similarities in food preferences between children and their siblings and parents. *Appetite, 7*, 333–342.

Polka, L., & Werker, J. (1994). Developmental changes in perception of nonnative vowel contrasts. *Journal of Experimental Psychology: Human Perception and Performance, 20*, 421–435.

Powers, S., Chamberlin, L., vanSchaick, K., Sherman, S., & Whitaker, R. (2006). Maternal feeding strategies, child eating behaviors, and child BMI in low-income African American preschoolers. *Obesity, 14*, 2026–2033.

Reau, N., Senturia, Y., & Lebally, S. (1996). Infant and toddler feeding patterns and problems: normative data and a new direction. *Journal of Developmental and Behavioral Pediatrics, 17*, 149–153.

Reilly, J., Armstrong, J., Dorosty, A., Emmett, P., Ness, A., Rogers, I., et al. (2005). Early life risk factors for obesity in childhood: Cohort study. *BMJ, 330*, 1157.

Resnicow, K., Hearn, M., & Smith, M. (1997). Social cognitive predictors of children's fruit and vegetable intake. *Health Psychology, 16*, 272–276.

Richardson, L., Davis, R., Poulton, R., McCauley, E., Moffitt, T., Caspi, A., et al. (2003). A longitudinal evaluation of adolescent depression and adult obesity. *Archives of Pediatrics & Adolescent Medicine, 157*, 739–745.

Rolls, B., Engell, D., & Birch, L. (2000). Serving portion size influences 5-year-old but not 3-year-old children's food intakes. *Journal of the American Dietetic Association, 100*, 232–234.

Rolls, B., Roe, L., Meengs, J., & Wall, D. (2004). Increasing portion size of a sandwich increases energy intake. *Journal of the American Dietetic Association, 104,* 367–372.

Rosenstein, D., & Oster, H. (1988). Differential facial responses to four basic tastes in newborns. *Child Development, 59,* 1555–1568.

Rozin, P. (1991). Family resemblance in food and other domains: The family paradox and the role of parental congruence. *Appetite, 16,* 93–102.

Rozin, P., Gruss, L., & Berk, G. (1979). Reversal of innate aversions: Attempts to induce a preference for chili peppers in rats. *Journal of Comparative and Physiological Psychology, 93,* 1001–1014.

Rozin, P., & Kennel, K. (1983). Acquired preferences for piquant foods by chimpanzees. *Appetite, 4,* 69–77.

Rozin, P., Riklis, J., & Margolis, L. (2004). Mutual exposure or close peer relationships do not seem to foster increased similarity in food, music or television program preferences. *Appetite, 42,* 41–48.

Rozin, P., & Schiller, D. (1980). The nature and preference for chili pepper by humans. *Motivation and Emotion, 4,* 77–101.

Rugholm, S., Baker, J., Olsen, L., Schack-Nielsen, L., Bua, J., & Sorensen, T. (2005). Stability of the association between birth weight and childhood overweight during the development of the obesity epidemic. *Obesity Research, 13,* 2187–2194.

Schaal, B., Marlier, L., & Soussignan, R. (2000). Human foetuses learn odours from their pregnant mother's diet. *Chemical Senses, 25,* 729–737.

Schaal, B., Orgeur, P., & Arnould, C. (1995). Olfactory preferences in newborn lambs: possible influence of prenatal experience. *Behaviour, 132,* 351–365.

Scholtens, S., Gehring, U., Brunekreef, B., Smit, H. A., de Jongste, J. C., Kerkhof, M., et al. (2007) Breastfeeding, Weight Gain in Infancy, and Overweight at Seven Years of Age: The Prevention and Incidence of Asthma and Mite Allergy Birth Cohort Study. *American Journal of Epidemiology, 165,* 919–926.

Sclafani, A. (1997). Learned controls of ingestive behavior. *Appetite, 29,* 153–158.

Scott, D., Janowsky, J., Carroll, R., Taylor, J., Auestad, N., & Montalto, M. (1998). Formula supplementation with long-chain polyunsaturated fatty acids: Are there developmental benefits? *Pediatrics, 102,* e59.

Skinner, J., Carruth, B., Bounds, W., & Ziegler, P. (2002). Children's food preferences: A longitudinal analysis. *Journal of the American Dietetic Association, 102,* 1638–1647.

Skinner, J., Carruth, B., Bounds, W., Ziegler, P., & Reidy, K. (2002). Do food-related experiences in the first 2 years of life predict dietary variety in school-aged children? *Journal of Nutrition Education and Behavior, 34,* 310–315.

Smith, G. (1998). *Satiation: From gut to brain.* New York: Oxford University Press.

Smotherman, W., & Robinson, S. (1985). The rat fetus in its environment: Behavioral adjustments to novel, familiar, aversive, and conditioned stimuli presented in utero. *Behavioral Neuroscience, 99,* 521–530.

Smriga, M., Kameishi, M., & Torii, K. (2002). Brief exposure to NaCl during early postnatal development enhances adult intake of sweet and salty compounds. *Neuroreport, 13,* 2562–2569.

Spray, K., Halsell, C., & Bernstein, I. (2000). cFos induction in response to saccharin after taste aversion learning depends on conditioning method. *Brain Research, 852,* 225–227.

Spruijt-Metz, D., Lindquist, C., Birch, L., Fisher, J., & Goran, M. (2002). Relation between mothers' child-feeding practices and children's adiposity. *American Journal of Clinical Nutrition, 75,* 581–586.

Stein, L., Cowart, B., Epstein, A., Pilot, L., Laskin, C., & Beauchamp, G. (1996). Increased liking for salty foods in adolescents exposed during infancy to chloride-deficient feeding formula. *Appetite, 27,* 65–77.

Stein, L., Nagai, H., Nakagawa, M., & Beauchamp, G. (2003). Effects of repeated exposure and health-related information on hedonic evaluation and acceptance of a bitter beverage. *Appetite, 40,* 119–129.

Steiner, J. (1973). The gustofacial response: Observation on normal and anencephalic newborn infants. In J. Bosma (Ed.), *Oral sensation and perception: Development in the fetus and infant: Fourth Symposium.* Bethesda, MD: U.S. Department of Health, Education and Welfare, National Institute of Health.

Steiner, J. (1974). Innate discriminative human facial expressions to taste and smell stimuli. *Annals of the New York Academy of Sciences, 237,* 229–233.

Steiner, J. (1977). Facial expressions of the neonate infant indicate the hedonics of food-related stimuli. In J. Weiffenbach (Ed.), *Taste and development: The genesis of sweet preference.* Washington, DC: U.S. Government Printing Office.

Steiner, J., Glaser, D., Hawilo, M., & Berridge, K. (2001). Comparative expression of hedonic impact: Affective reactions to taste by human infants and other primates. *Neuroscience and Biobehavioral Reviews, 1,* 53–74.

Stettler, N., Zemel, B., Kumanyika, S., & Stallings, V. (2002). Infant weight gain and childhood overweight status in a multi-center, cohort study. *Pediatrics, 109,* 194–199.

Sullivan, S., & Birch, L. (1999). Pass the sugar, pass the salt: Experience dictates preference. *Developmental Psychology, 26,* 546–551.

Taveras, E., Scanlon, K., Birch, L., Rifas-Shiman, S., Rich-Edwards, J., & Gillman, M. (2004). Association of breastfeeding with maternal control of infant feeding at age 1 year. *Pediatrics, 114,* e577–e583.

von Kries, R., Koletzko, B., Sauerwald, T., vonMutius, E., Barnert, D., Grunert, V., et al. (1999). Breastfeeding and obesity: Cross sectional study. *BMJ, 319,* 147–150.

Wardle, J., Sanderson, S., Guthrie, C., Rapoport, L., & Plomin, R. (2002). Parental feeding style and the inter-generational transmission of obesity risk. *Obesity Research, 10,* 453–462.

Warren, R., & Pfaffmann, C. (1959). Early experience and taste aversion. *Journal of Comparative and Physiological Psychology, 52,* 263–266.

Watson, W., Litovitz, T., Rodgers, G., Klein-Schwartz, W., Youniss, J., Rose, S., et al. (2003). Annual report of the American Association of Poison Control Centers Toxic Exposure Surveillance System.

American Journal of Emergency Medicine, 21, 353–421.

Werker, J., & Tees, R. (1984). Cross-language speech perception: Evidence for perceptual reorganization during the first year of life. *Infant Behavior & Development, 7,* 49–63.

Whitaker, R. (2004). Predicting preschooler obesity at birth: The role of maternal obesity in early pregnancy. *Pediatrics, 114,* e29–e36.

Whitaker, R., Pepe, M., Wrigt, J., Seidel, K., & Dietz, W. (1998). Early adiposity rebound and the risk of adult obesity. *Pediatrics, 101,* e5.

Whitaker, R., Wright, J., Pepe, M., Seidel, K., & Dietz, W. (1997). Predicting obesity in young adulthood from childhood and parental obesity. *New England Journal of Medicine, 337,* 869–873.

Wilson, A., Forsyth, J., Greene, S., Irvine, L., Hau, C., & Howie, P. (1998). Relation of infant diet to childhood health: Seven year follow up of cohort of children in Dundee infant feeding study. *BMJ, 316,* 21–25.

Wolff, P. (1987). *The development of behavioral states and the expression of emotions in early infancy: New proposals for investigation.* Chicago, IL: University of Chicago Press.

Woolf, A., Goldman, R., & Bellinger, D. (2007). Update on the clinical management of childhood lead poisoning. *Pediatric Clinics of North America, 54,* 271–294.

Young, P. (1968). Evaluation and preference in behavioral development. *Psychological Review, 75,* 222–241.

Zajonc, R. (1965). Social facilitation. *Science, 149,* 269–274.

Zandstra, E., & de Graff, C. (1998). Sensory perception and pleasantness of orange beverages from childhood to old age. *Food Quality and Preference, 9,* 5–12.

Zive, M., McKay, H., Frank-Spohrer, G., Broyles, S., Nelson, J., & Nader, P. (1992). Infant-feeding practices and adiposity in 4-y-old Anglo- and Mexican-Americans. *American Journal of Clinical Nutrition, 55,* 1104–1108.

7 LEARNING AND HEDONIC CONTRIBUTIONS TO HUMAN OBESITY

Martin R. Yeomans

Introduction

Obesity results from a positive energy balance, with energy from food ingested exceeding energy expended. To understand the causes of obesity, on both individual and population scales we need to understand the factors that lead to overeating. This chapter focuses on the idea that pleasure derived from the sensory qualities of food (sensory hedonics) contributes importantly to short-term overeating and thereby to positive energy balance. Although it is easy to demonstrate that animals, including humans, eat more food that is perceived as pleasurable, the bases of differential pleasure are less clear. Accordingly, the majority of this chapter explores the learning processes that underlie acquired food likes and dislikes. Although most research in this area has been conducted in normal-weight animals and humans, the implications of these findings and ideas may provide insights into obesity, including how to prevent and treat it.

Introduction to Hedonic Stimulation of Appetite

Hedonics, or liking, is a critical determinant of how much we eat. First, hedonics guide food *choice*: whether a potential food item is accepted or rejected is largely derived by sensory hedonics. A potential food with an unpleasant flavor (one that "tastes" bad) is likely to be rejected unless the organism is heavily food-deprived and has no alternative food source. Second, *volume consumed* is determined in part by the hedonic qualities of the food. This section briefly reviews these two influences, and in particular considers the potential role of hedonically driven overeating in the genesis of obesity. But first it is important to clarify the terminology used in descriptions of hedonic aspects of eating and the qualities of food that elicit sensory pleasure.

Palatability and food preference: key concepts in hedonic aspects of eating

Palatability is one of the most widely used terms in descriptions of the pleasurable aspects of eating. Yet, despite many reviews (Naim & Kare, 1991; Drewnowski, 1998; Le Magnen, 1987; Young, 1967; Kissileff, 1976; Yeomans, 1998) and theories (Berridge, 1996; Davis & Levine, 1977; Cabanac, 1989; Berridge & Robinson, 1998), there remains a lack of consensus on the nature of palatability. Although describing a food as palatable clearly denotes that it is liked, the basis of this positive evaluation remains unclear. Palatability *is not simply a consequence of the chemical constitution of a food*. Palatability reflects an evaluation of a particular food by its consumer: as in all things, what may be palatable to one person may be aversive to another. This observation itself is critical to understanding why some people may show strong affective responses to a food and consequently be prone to overeat that food, while others may show little interest, or even a strong aversive response, to the same food. In essence, the perception that a food tastes "good" (i.e., is palatable) reflects an interaction between the chemical structure of the food, a person's prior experience with that food, current nutritional needs, and the point at which the food is tasted during a meal.

An early observation on the nature of obesity and its relation to feeding indicated that obese people tend to react more to the taste of food (i.e., they were finicky). They ate more palatable foods but less bland food (Nisbett, 1968). This difference may explain why some people have difficulty resisting food cues, overeat, and consequently become obese. Yet many resist these cues and do not overeat, even in environments where palatable foods are abundant.

Food preferences are manifested in the selection of one food over another when both are presented simultaneously. Preference is a common measure in animal studies in which objective measures of "liking" are difficult to come by. Although palatability and preference overlap, because in general the chosen food can be interpreted as the more palatable, preference makes less direct reference to the hedonic quality of the food, and at any one time a less "palatable" item may be preferred—for example, because it is perceived as more healthful, more cost-effective, or more appropriate to specific dietary needs. If all else were equal, however, the more palatable choice would be predicted to be the preferred choice. Because of the difficulty in measuring hedonic responses in animals, *preference* and *palatability* are often taken to mean the same thing, but this mistaken impression could both lead to circularity in defining palatability (suggesting that the reason animals prefer one food is that it is more palatable) and generate spurious results if the actual choice were based on factors other than flavor hedonics.

The relationship between sensory and hedonic evaluations of foods

Another important influence on sensory hedonics is the nature of the sensory components being evaluated—that is, the "taste" of the food. In reality, "taste

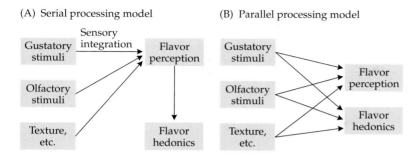

(A) Serial processing model   (B) Parallel processing model

FIGURE 7.1   Two conceptual models of how sensory input, flavor perception, and flavor hedonics are related. (A) Serial processing. (B) Parallel processing.

hedonics" (as in "this ice cream tastes really good") consists of complex interactions between many sensory components (Prescott, 1999; Verhagen & Engelen, 2006). The general term *flavor* is thus preferred to denote the multisensory nature of this experience. A detailed description of the primary sensory qualities of taste and smell that are the main contributors to food flavor is provided in Chapter 5, but a brief summary here will help clarify the relationship between flavor components and sensory hedonics. Food flavor arises from a complex integration of primary gustatory (taste) and olfactory (smell) information along with other sensory inputs, temperature, and pain perception (generated by oral irritants such as carbon dioxide and food constituents such as pepper or chili), including the anticipation of flavor generated by visual appearance and sound (think crackling cereal or popcorn; Zampini & Spence, 2004).

An alternative brain-imaging techniques have advanced our understanding of these processes (Kringelbach, 2004; Small & Prescott, 2005), how sensory qualities are integrated into flavor perception remains distant. Two alternatives for central integration are presented in Figure 7.1. One idea holds that hedonic evaluation reflects a serial process that operates after a food has been identified according to the incoming sensory information (Figure 7.1A). Support for a serial processing model includes findings that food liking, but not its sensory characteristics, can be altered by the association of a flavor with illness or pharmacological challenge. The dissociation between sensory and hedonic qualities of food can be obtained through opiate receptor antagonists. People who had received these drugs reported no change in their ability to identify the food, or in their ratings of the sensory quality of the food, but they reliably rated foods as having a less pleasant flavor (Yeomans & Gray, 2002).

An alternative formulation of the relationship between sensory quality and hedonic evaluation is one of parallel processing (Figure 7.1B): sensory inputs lead to flavor perception by one pathway and to hedonic experience by a separate pathway. Our understanding of the neural pathways stimulated by sensory inputs in rodents can be interpreted in this way (Sewards, 2004), but in humans a serial process seems more plausible because the brain areas most implicated in hedonic evaluations (e.g., the pre-orbitofrontal cortex; see Small & Prescott, 2005) are downstream of the primary sensory flavor inputs.

A good example came from a recent study of the interaction between perception of a food-related odor and the "umami" taste (the taste qualities generated by monosodium glutamate, or MSG; McCabe & Rolls, 2007). On its own, ingestion of MSG was not a pleasant experience, and the experience of a vegetable odor alone was rated as unpleasant. However, presentation of MSG and the same vegetable odor together was experienced as very pleasant and was associated with significantly greater activation of the orbitofrontal cortex than the activation generated by either stimulus alone. So, in humans, the hedonic experience of flavors appears to involve the downstream integration of sensory information relating to the food to be ingested. At the end, as anticipated, the critical determinant of choice and intake appears to be hedonic evaluation: more is eaten of liked food, and disliked food will probably be rejected. At issue are the bases upon which foods are liked or disliked.

Hedonic evaluation and food acceptance

The first reaction to the sensory qualities of a food is to either accept or reject that food. Indeed, the natural wariness toward new potential foods (neophobia) means that a new food may be rejected even before being placed in the mouth (the "I don't like it, I never tried it" effect reported in children; Birch & Marlin, 1982). Given the variety of potential foods available to omnivores like us, this gatekeeping process is vital because failing to identify poisonous items rapidly and correctly, and to accept only safe, nutritious foods, is a potentially fatal liability.

Hedonic stimulation of appetite

Eating is a source of pleasure, and anticipation of pleasure alone may be sufficient to stimulate it. In the short term, the hedonic quality of a food determines the amount consumed. Feeding on an energy-dense diet rich in fat, sugar, or both induces overeating and consequent obesity in previously lean animals (Sclafani, 1993; Warwick & Schiffman, 1992; Woods et al., 2003). This dietary-induced obesity leads to subsequent insulin resistance and diabetes in rats (Kraegen et al., 1991), just as the current obesity epidemic is leading to huge increases in the incidence of dietary-induced diabetes in humans. As discussed in Chapter 10, dietary variety is also a cause of overeating. Indeed, a reliable model of diet-induced obesity remains the "cafeteria diet," in which lean rats become obese on a diet of energy-rich fatty and sweet foods (Rogers & Blundell, 1984). Remarkably, even a change in diet texture can lead to short-term overeating, and thus overcome satiety. The impact is so profound that after drinking a glucose solution to satiety, rats readily consumed more glucose presented in powdered form. Thus, taste hedonics can stimulate intake even in sated rodents.

Although applying a strict definition of sensory hedonics to insects is tricky, some parallels in the way sugar solutions can stimulate ingestion in flies fit with the idea of sensory stimulation of appetite (Dethier, 1976). Feeding by the fruit fly is stimulated by the detection of sugar (most effectively sucrose) by specific sugar receptors on the legs. The degree to which feeding is stimulated, and the duration of the feeding bout, is proportional to the concentration of sucrose: flies initiate the feeding sequence faster, and continue feeding for longer, with more concentrated sugar sources. However, flies do not feed to the point of obesity; presumably extra weight impairs the ability to fly. To prevent overfeeding, postingestive neural signals from the gut in flies counteract the stimulation of feeding by sweetness. When this signal was removed (by the nerve from the gut being severed), flies overfed to the point of bursting (Dethier & Boderstein, 1958; Dethier & Gelperin, 1967). Thus, for a fly the hedonic stimulus to overfeed is normally countered by signals indicating how full the gut is. The extent to which analogous controls are found in humans will be discussed later. But even the constrained appetite system of the fly shows evidence that sensory stimulation allows opportunistic utilization of sugar that would lead to obesity if not countered by an efficient gut-based satiety system.

Manipulated palatability also affects short-term eating in humans. In experimental investigations, the test food flavor is made more or less palatable while the nutritional components remain unaltered. Volunteers consume more food that is rated as palatable (Bobroff & Kissileff, 1986; Bellisle et al., 1984; Zandstra et al., 2000). The relationship between differences in palatability of test conditions and associated differences in food intake can be readily determined. Figure 7.2 shows a clear linear relationship between differences in hedonic evaluation of two foods and consequent difference in intake. The consistency of this

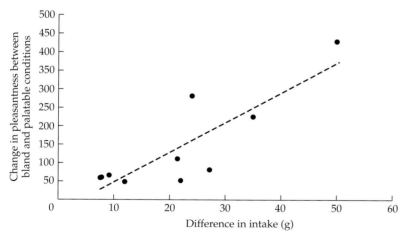

FIGURE 7.2   The relationship between differences in food pleasantness and consequent increases in food intake in humans. (After Yeomans, 2007.)

FIGURE 7.3 Effects of manipulated palatability on the experience of appetite during a meal. (After Yeomans, 1996.)

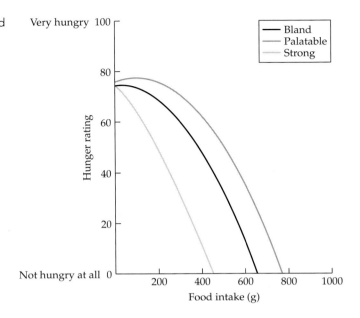

relationship is impressive across a wide range of foods, differences in nutrient content, testing situations, and so on.

The relationship between palatability and appetite gives some clue about the mechanisms underlying this effect. For example, the acceptability of food "taste" influences perceptions of our own hunger and desire to eat. Figure 7.3 shows average responses to the question "how hungry do you feel?" recorded across a meal. The pattern of hunger change depends on liking for the flavor of food (Yeomans, 1996; Yeomans et al., 1997) hunger ratings increase during the early stages of meals when the food being consumed is rated as palatable, but not when the food is rated as bland or unpleasantly strong-tasting. These findings suggest that food palatability, whether gustatory or acquired, exerts positive feedback on our perception of need (hunger) and our urgency to satisfy it.

Because our diet has become more energy-dense and palatable, the hedonic attributes of foods can and do cause overeating, since appetite stimulation by palatability has a greater impact on the consumption of energy-dense foods than of other foods. This effect is illustrated in Figure 7.4. Here, volunteers ate a simple food (porridge) in either a bland or palatable (sweetened) form, and with either low or high energy density. As Figure 7.4A shows, increased palatability resulted in more being eaten, but increased energy density did not decrease intake. This combination of active overeating (driven by palatability) and passive overeating (due to differences in energy density) meant that nearly three times as much energy was consumed of the palatable high-energy version than the bland low-energy one (Figure 7.4B).

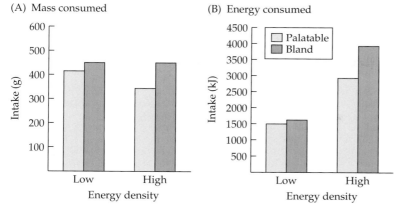

FIGURE 7.4   Mass (A) and energy (B) consumed by volunteers eating high- or low-energy breakfasts served in both bland and palatable form. (After Yeomans et al., 2005.)

The Bases of Food Preference

Palatability is the end result of complex interactions among sensory qualities of food, the individual's feeding history, and the particular characteristics of the individual. This is a tripartite approach to individual differences and their particular interactions with different foods. Sorting out these factors provides a salient means for understanding how affect, overeating, and obesity are related.

Given that survival depends on eating, and that food is generally hard to come by, it follows that the most energy-dense foods should be sought out, and consumed heartily when available. Because almost all food sources in the wild contain needed nutrients, nutritional requirements can be met equally from the food and intestinal specializations. As a backup for hard times of specific nutrient shortage, followed by replenishment, improved health is associated with the foods that helped restore the deficit. Foods that are reliable, safe, and energy-rich may generate innate preferences, and foods that are potentially harmful or poor sources of nutrition either are innately disliked or result in rapid acquired dislikes. For omnivores such as us, however, the range of potential foods is very large and foods do not always telegraph their toxic status. Thus, our diet is anything but predetermined, so we must find a way to utilize potential new food items.

Evolutionary pressures have favored the development of an appetite system that incorporates a small number of innate hedonic responses to some of the five primary tastes (liking for sweet, potential to like salty when salt-deprived, dislike for sour and bitter), coupled with a learning system that allows rapid learning of which foods are safe and beneficial. The evolution of this complex learning system is now hypothesized as a major driving force for cognitive evolution:

the complexity of the advanced ability of humans to learn is likely to have been shaped by the need to compete for food, and to make optimal use of scarce food resources in the environment. Moreover, as we will see later, even our innate tendency to like sweet and dislike bitter and sour tastes can be modified by experience, so that people come to like bitter flavor components such as those produced by alcohol, caffeine, and so on. We are able to learn through experience that, in these contexts, bitterness predicts not only a safe (nonpoisonous) item, but also one that has some form of desirable postingestive effect.

The overall conclusion is that, for humans and other omnivores, the majority of our food likes and dislikes are acquired by learning, and hedonic responses to food are primarily a reflection of this past learning. However, an appetite system that was adaptive when valuable food sources were scarce and insecure becomes a liability when food is freely available. Our appetite control system did not develop to cope with a diet of energy-dense palatable foods, since these are rare in nature. As we have manufactured foods designed to have maximal appeal to our sensory systems, so have we unwittingly generated stimuli that promote overconsumption. Thus, the current obesity crisis may be an inevitable consequence of the mismatch between an appetite system that evolved to deal with the problem of securing safe, nutrient-rich food in an environment where such food was scarce and a modern-day environment where safe, palatable, energy-dense food is readily available (Ulijaszek, 2007).

Innate preferences and aversions

How can we determine whether a preference is innate or acquired? The nature/nurture debate has been hotly contested in every area of human activity, and it remains a source of contention in our understanding of food preferences. One approach examines preferences before exposure to flavors to preclude modulation by experience. Consider the preference of some populations of garter snakes for their most common prey, the banana slug (Arnold, 1977). Coastal garter snakes eat banana slugs, but mountain garter snakes avoid them. Naive, newly hatched snakes from coastal parents showed appetitive tongue protrusions when presented with banana-slug odors, but offspring of mountain snakes did not. Crossbreeding further modified banana slug preference. This rare example of an innate food preference is possible because of the unique sensory qualities of banana slugs and a specific predator–prey relationship.

The human diet is highly varied and offers less opportunity to evaluate innate flavor preferences. Moreover, unequivocal tests of innate response to flavors are confounded by flavor exposure. One widely cited approach has been to examine responses of human neonates to flavor components. Classic studies tested such responses by applying sweet tastants to the tongues of newborn babies (Desor et al., 1973; Steiner, 1979; Berridge, 2000). The outcome was consistent with clear acceptance of sweet tastes, as indicated most notably in the facial expressions of the human neonates and other species given similar tests. As Fig-

(A) Positive responses to sweet

(B) Negative responses to bitter

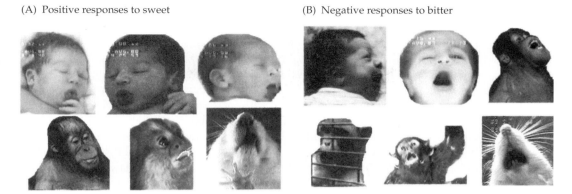

FIGURE 7.5   Orofacial responses to sweet (A) and bitter (B) tastes by human neonates, apes, monkeys, and rats. (After Berridge, 2000, with permission from Elsevier.)

ure 7.5 shows, human, rat, and monkey facial responses to sweet taste (Figure 7.5A) are all consistent with flavor acceptance, and they include appetitive tongue protrusions; whereas the responses to bitter (Figure 7.5B) show expressions typical of dislike, including gaping, and rejection of the substance.

The near universal preference for sweet tastes has been explained in terms of the reliable relationship in nature between a sweet taste and safe, nutritious foods rich in sugars (Hladik et al., 2002). Mammals have specific sweet-taste receptors (Matsunami et al., 2000); indeed, as noted earlier, even fruit flies have specific receptors to detect sweet molecules (Dahunukar et al., 2001). Although the genetic bases of the sweet receptors in fruit flies and in mammals are distinct, the ability to detect and accept sweetness appears strongly conserved, and it is likely to be a primitive component of our food preferences. In this regard, the molecular structure of the vertebrate sweet-taste receptor has been conserved across species from fishes to humans, with only rare examples of sweet-insensitive species such as chickens (Shi & Zhang, 2006).

Of course, the presence of a gene showing detection of sweet substances is not direct evidence of liking for the sweet taste, and a counterargument to the interpretation of neonatal responses to sweet taste is that they could reflect the consequences of the stimulation of sweet receptors in utero, and so may be a consequence of exposure rather than of genetics, although this conclusion is contradicted by sweet preferences in premature babies (Maone et al., 1990). The strongest evidence that sweet-taste preferences are genetically predetermined comes from breeding studies in which separate lines of sweet-preferring and sweet-disliking rats have been selected (Bachmanov et al., 2002).

Sweet taste also exerts powerful effects on behavior in newborn animals. Most striking is analgesia generated by simple application of sweet tastes to the tongue of newborn rats (Blass & Fitzgerald, 1988) and humans (Blass & Watt, 1999). But even innate sweet preference can be modified by experience, as discussed in more detail later. For example, a study by Beauchamp and Moran (1984) assessed sweet preference in 2-year-old children who had never consumed sweetened water, had had less than 6 months experience of sweetened water, or had had more than 6 months experience. The unexposed group showed the least preference for sweetened over plain water, with increasing preference as level of exposure increased. In this case it could be argued that the innate sweet preference either was lost when unreinforced or required exposure to become sufficient to be expressed in the choice test used. Another factor here may be neophobia, discussed more later, in which even a liked taste such as sweet may be treated with caution when first experienced in a novel context.

Complicating the evaluation of innate flavor preferences is the fact that some preferences may be latent: they are not expressed until specific nutritional circumstances make the preference valuable. The classic example is salt preference. Most species do not show a preference for the taste of salt if tested while salt-replete. However, in many animals—including rats (Bertino & Tordoff, 1988; Leshem, 1999), nonhuman primates (Denton et al., 1993), and humans (Leshem, 2000)—liking for salt increases when they are salt-deprived. This is a highly adaptive response: increased liking for salt promotes intake and so acts to counter salt depletion (Berridge et al., 1984; Denton, 1982; Epstein, 1991; Schulkin, 1991). For example, in a remarkable study by Kriekhaus and Wolf (1968), rats explored a complex environment that included a concentrated salt source. Their reaction was to avoid the salt. Following salt depletion induced by adrenalectomy, the rats now actively sought out and consumed the salt. This increased intake is matched by increased preference in choice tests, and the orofacial reaction of salt-deprived rats becomes similar to those seen in response to sweet taste (Berridge et al., 1984; Curtis et al., 2001). Although acute salt deprivation does not generate robust increases in salt intake in humans (Mattes, 1997), dietary uses of salt in a need-free state are higher in individuals with a history of salt depletion (Leshem, 1998).

Countering the idea of a latent salt preference is a learning model arguing that the experience of reversal of salt depletion by consumption of salty foods leads to a learned salt preference, possibly through latent learning of the effects of salt when replete being expressed during subsequent salt deprivation. Modified salt preference following exercise in humans fits better with a learned than an innate account (Wald & Leshem, 2003), and overall, any innate component of salt preference is clearly modified by subsequent experience of salty foods.

The dislike for bitter tastes shown in Figure 7.5B has been interpreted as reflecting the avoidance of items that are poisonous (Behrens & Meyerhof, 2006; Fischer et al., 2005), since most poisons have strong, bitter tastes. Again significant progress has been made in identifying the relevant receptors and associated genes (Shi et al., 2003). Bitter-taste perception is complex: in humans, 25 different bitter-taste receptor genes have been identified so far (Behrens & Meyerhof,

2006). These findings fit with the variability of poisonous molecules in the environment. The strong link between a bitter taste and an aversive hedonic reaction, as shown by the facial expressions of human neonates and others in Figure 7.5B, ensures immediate rejection of potentially poisonous items. But even this response can be overcome: as discussed more fully later, the bitter tastes of alcohol and caffeine do not prevent humans from developing a predilection for alcoholic beverages and coffee, either through personal experience or through mere observation of a confederate showing enjoyment while consuming a bitter-tasting food or drink (Rozin & Schiller, 1982). This evidence suggests that innate preferences are a useful first reaction to new foods, but that experience ultimately shapes our food preferences.

Acquired food preferences

A number of theories explain how learning principles may be applied to the problem of food preference development. Three of these theories—mere exposure, flavor–consequence learning, and flavor-based evaluative conditioning—are widely accepted and are seen as major components of the learning system that underlies the acquisition of flavor preferences and aversions. Social factors also influence flavor preference development. For example, social modeling in humans characterized by observation that another individual shows a positive hedonic response to a food may counter the normal neophobic response to a new food, particularly in children (Birch, 1999).

Mexican children show a strong aversion to the burning sensation generated by capsaicin, the irritant in chili, but exposure to chili in the context of family members enjoying chili peppers promotes experimentation with chili, facilitating preference acquisition over the course of a number of meals (Rozin & Schiller, 1980). Likewise, the odor of a new food on the breath of one rat increases the likelihood that the new food will be tried by other rats (Galef & Laland, 2005). However, these social effects appear to be more involved in overcoming neophobic responses to new foods, rather than directly enhancing food palatability. Because this chapter focuses on how hedonic responses relate to overeating rather than to food acceptance, social effects are not considered further here; several excellent reviews of social influences in food preference development are available (e.g., Birch, 1999; Conner & Arimitage, 2002).

MERE EXPOSURE   *Mere exposure* (Zajonc, 1968) refers to repeated nonreinforced exposure to any stimulus that results in an increase in preference for that stimulus (the converse of the classic adage that familiarity breeds contempt). Mere exposure has been widely demonstrated outside the food preference literature (Bornstein, 1989), but specific studies examining this phenomenon in humans with food stimuli are more limited (Pliner, 1982; Stevenson & Yeomans, 1995; Crandall, 1984). Mere exposure remains a useful description of familiarity effects, but in itself it does not explain the nature of the underlying change. Thus, explanations for mere-exposure effects usually make reference to reduced neophobia or other explanations, such as opponent-process affective responses (Solomon & Corbit, 1974).

FLAVOR–CONSEQUENCE LEARNING Affective responses to food may be acquired through conditioned taste aversion learning (CTA; Garcia & Koelling, 1966). While working on bait shyness in rats, researchers noted that typically the rats consumed a very small quantity of a new food; if the food was poisonous and the animal became ill, it avoided the *flavor* of the food that had poisoned it. In a seminal series of studies, Garcia demonstrated that even a single pairing between exposure to a flavor and illness caused rats to subsequently avoid that flavor. In a study that challenged our understanding of the fundamental nature of associative learning, Garcia and Koelling (1966) demonstrated that rats are predisposed to associate flavors with illness.

The design of this complex study is illustrated in Figure 7.6, which shows that all rats drank a flavored solution (either salty or sweet). Drinking also triggered cues unrelated to flavor (a combination of noise and light, which resulted in the phrase "noisy-bright tasty water" to describe the cues the rats experienced). These cues can be viewed as a complex conditioned stimulus, or CS, in conditioning terms. The researchers then induced illness in half the rats (either by switching the salty-taste solution from harmless sodium chloride to nausea-inducing lithium chloride, or by exposing the rats to mild radiation). The remaining rats experienced a different aversive outcome when they drank: each lick triggered a mild electric foot shock. These biological consequences can be interpreted as unconditioned stimuli, or USs, in conditioning terms.

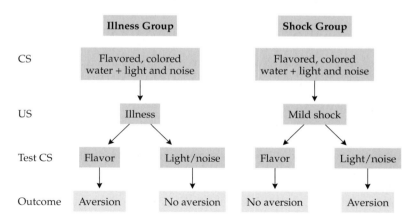

FIGURE 7.6 The design and outcome of Garcia and Koelling's classic study on conditioned taste aversion development in rats.

Figure 7.6 also shows that after training, the cues from drinking were divided so that half the rats in each US group were offered either the flavored water without the light/noise, or normal water with the light/noise, to drink. This generalization testing allowed Garcia and Koelling to determine the extent to which the cues were now associated with either illness or shock. The crucial finding was that rats trained with illness readily drank water in the presence of the light/noise cues, but drank little of the flavored water. In contrast, rats that had been trained with the electric shock US readily drank the flavored water but avoided the normal water with light/noise cues. The conclusion is important: rats are *predisposed to learn to associate flavors with illness, and external visual/auditory cues with external harm.* Stated differently, the linkage of somatic information is constrained. Its accessibility for behavioral actions is limited through the context in which the information was obtained. Moreover, delays of up to 24 hours (Garcia et al., 1966; Smith & Roll, 1967) between the experience of the new-flavor CS and the experience of illness did not compromise CTA formation.

At the time, these findings led to the belief that CTA was a unique form of learning. Although the linkage of associations between flavor and illness could be seen as analogous to Pavlovian conditioning, typical learning studies required close temporal contiguity between the neutral CS and the biologically significant US for learning to proceed. However, further research confirmed that differences between CTA and other forms of associative learning were more quantitative than qualitative (Logue, 1979), though the long delay between CS and US is unique to flavor-based learning.

Does CTA apply to humans? Although anecdotal accounts for acquired flavor aversions in humans are common, conducting actual experimental studies in which people experience novel flavors and are then made to feel ill raises clear ethical concerns. In a classic study, Bernstein (1978) sidestepped these ethical issues by studying children with cancer who were undergoing chemotherapy as part of their treatment. Such children stop eating and lose weight—a condition described as *cancer anorexia*. The treatment drugs are toxic, of course, so weight loss was thought to reflect the combined effects of the disease and toxic effects of the chemotherapy. Bernstein reasoned that cancer anorexia might reflect the development of CTA to food consumed prior to each treatment session. To test this hypothesis, she contrasted acceptance of a novel, homemade ice cream by children undergoing chemotherapy for cancer relative to controls. The outcome was clear: children who underwent chemotherapy associated with nausea showed an acquired aversion to the ice cream, evidenced by their reduced preference for the test ice cream in a choice test (Figure 7.7) relative to children who received alternative treatments not associated with nausea and, importantly, to those whose treatment was not associated with the ice cream. This finding not only demonstrated the importance of CTA in humans, but also led to novel ways of countering cancer anorexia.

One may pose the reciprocal question: if the experience of illness after consuming a food leads to a conditioned dislike for that food flavor, then would a

FIGURE 7.7 The proportion of children selecting an ice cream that they had consumed previously either during treatment sessions for cancer chemotherapy [ice cream plus GI (gastrointestinal) toxicity], had consumed ice cream in the absence of GI toxicity (ice cream alone), or had not previously consumed ice cream (GI toxicity alone). (After Bernstein, 1978.)

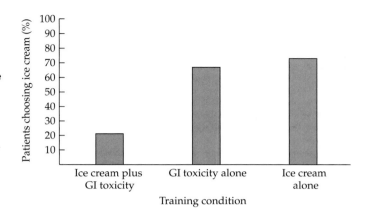

positive experience cause that flavor to be liked? The idea of flavor–consequence learning (FCL) places CTA into a broadened model for understanding changes in liking and preference based on a capacity to associate flavors with postingestive consequences. This concept rests on the constraint of linking the perceived sensory characteristics (flavor) of the ingested food or drink (acting as CS) to the postingestive effects of that food or drink (US).

The associative substructure of FCL is shown in Figure 7.8, which suggests that several critical features are needed for the manifestation of clear likes and dislikes. The first of these is whether the consequence of eating or drinking (the unconditioned response, or UR) is liked or disliked. It follows that the strongest learning will be for foods and drinks with the largest negative (e.g., gastric malaise) or positive (e.g., alcohol intoxication) effects.

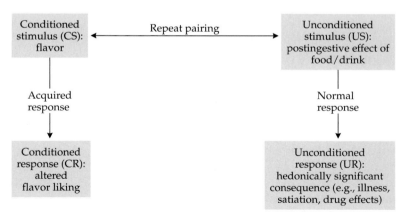

FIGURE 7.8 The associative substructure underlying flavor–consequence learning.

Second, learning will be progressive, so repeated experiences of flavor and consequence will strengthen the underlying association. Even though a single experience of a flavor and illness can lead to CTA, repeated pairings of flavor with illness increase aversion. For example, chocolate contains multiple sources of energy, along with caffeine, all of which could reverse short-term feelings of lethargy. FCL predicts that repeated experience of these effects of chocolate would lead to strong liking for chocolate flavor.

Third, the strength of the association of flavor and consequence will determine the degree to which the flavor comes to control behavior. For example, if a person has a strong association between chocolate and mood elevation generated by past experience of the effects of chocolate, feelings of sluggishness may lead to chocolate being sought out and consumed. Thus, the FCL model provides clear hypotheses about how flavors may modify behavior, reflecting past experiences. The FCL paradigm lends itself well to identifying the nature of postingestive effects (the US) which promote increased liking.

From a nutritional perspective, the primary requirement of a food is that it be a safe source of nutrition and energy. The FCL model, therefore, predicts that major sources of energy would strongly reinforce or induce a flavor preference. The clear relationship between energy density and liking for foods supports this prediction (Drewnowski, 1998). This relationship also holds in children's preferences for fruits that have higher energy density (Gibson & Wardle, 2003), consistent with the importance of energy as the primary reinforcer of FCL. Likewise, in times of nutritional deficit, foods that contain the missing commodity would be preferentially selected and ingested. They are, but a number of pairings are needed. Thus, FCL could induce or sustain food preferences to reflect the extent to which these foods had provided nutritional benefits.

The clearest evidence that energy can reinforce changes in flavor preferences comes from animal studies in which neutral flavors are selectively paired with postingestive nutrient delivery (Sclafani, 1999; Capaldi, 1972). The consequence of eating nutritional foods is increased satiety or a more specific nutritional outcome, perhaps correcting a nutritional deficit. Early studies confirmed that pairing a novel flavor (the CS+) with intake of energy led to a preference for the CS+ relative to a second flavor, which was tasted as often but not paired with energy (Booth, 1972; Fedorchak & Bolles, 1987; Mehiel & Bolles, 1984). These studies were all based on coexperience of the flavor CS+ and the paired nutrient, consumed orally.

A problem with this design is that these studies confound experience of the CS+ and US in the mouth, so they open the possibility for associations between the CS+ and US flavor apart from consequences. Experiments providing the most convincing evidence for FCL in animals avoid this problem by delivering nutrients into the stomach, thereby precluding any oral effects of the US (Figure 7.9). To assess flavor preference, rats are given free access to two flavored, non-nutritive solutions. Consumption of one solution (the positive flavor cue, or CS+ in Pavlovian conditioning terms) triggers intragastric infusion of an energy-bearing

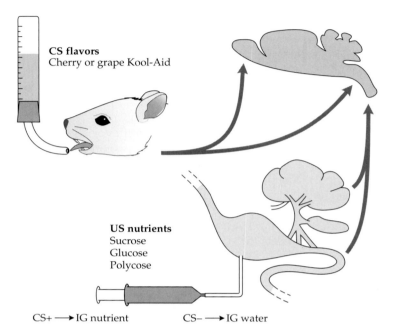

FIGURE 7.9   The two-bottle choice training method used extensively by Sclafani and colleagues in studies of flavor-nutrient learning in rats. IG, intragastric. (Courtesy of Anthony Sclafani.)

liquid. Consuming the alternative flavor (the negative flavor cue, or CS–) leads to intragastric infusion of water. Note that this design also gives the animal control of nutrient infusion: the intragastric infusion is contingent on the rat's drinking the relevant flavored liquid. Any emerging preference for CS+ over CS– must then be due to post-oral effects of the nutrient, acting as US. This design then precludes explanations for emerging preference for the CS+ in terms of oral response to the nutrient, so it provides a clear test of FCL.

The outcome of these studies is a profound and durable preference for the CS+ over the CS– with all the major dietary sources of energy: sucrose (Sclafani, 2002;), glucose (Myers & Sclafani, 2001a,b), starch (Sclafani & Nissenbaum, 1988; Elizalde & Sclafani, 1988), fats (Lucas & Sclafani, 1989), and alcohol (Ackroff & Sclafani, 2002b; Ackroff & Sclafani, 2001). The magnitude of the preference for CS+ over CS– depends on various factors, including length of training and nutrient infused, but these effects are all consistent with a conditioning model of FCL in which the strength of the CS and US, as well as the number of CS–US pairings, affects the rate of CS–US association.

For example, Figure 7.10 shows relative preference for the CS+ over CS– flavor following intragastric infusion of various nutrients, including sugars, oil

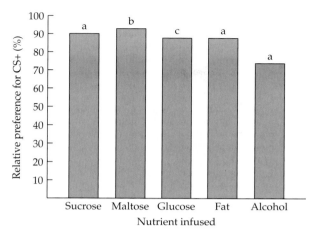

FIGURE 7.10   Flavor preferences acquired by associations between oral exposure to flavors and intragastric delivery of different nutrients in rats. Data are intake of CS+ flavor as a percentage of total intake from two-bottle choice tests following extended training. A ratio of 50% would reflect indifference. [Data sources: (a) Ackroff et al., 2004; (b) Azzara and Sclafani, 1998; (c) Myers and Sclafani, 2001.]

emulsions, and alcohol. In all cases the relative preference is strong, although alcohol in general seems less effective than other nutrients at supporting FCL in this paradigm (Ackroff & Sclafani, 2002b; Ackroff et al., 2004). These preferences persist even when CS+ consumption no longer leads to nutrient delivery (Drucker et al., 1994), and they can be learned even when the rats are not food-deprived at the time they are exposed to pairings of CS+ with US (Yiin et al., 2005).

Another important feature of this learning is that the preference for CS+ over CS– is seen in the context of rats drinking these solutions while they have unrestricted access to solid food. Thus, even when other sources of energy are being ingested that are not contingent on the CS+ flavor, rats are able to discriminate the CS+/US association and alter preference accordingly. Earlier we noted that preference need not be the same as liking. In the case of FCL supported by intragastric glucose infusion, analysis of orofacial responses following training found greater positive hedonic facial reactions to the CS+ (Myers & Sclafani, 2001b), consistent with increased palatability of the CS+ as a consequence of association with the post-oral effects of glucose.

Human studies also provide evidence for equivalent changes in flavor preference. For example, children showed a much larger increase in preference for the flavor of a yogurt that they had consumed repeatedly in a high-fat version than they did for a second flavor consumed in a low-fat, low-energy version (Figure 7.11; Birch et al., 1990). That said, however, the status of FCL as a vehicle for change in flavor preference based on delivery of energy-containing nutrients in adults remains unclear, since many studies have failed to find these effects (Brunstrom, 2005). We should remain open to the possibility, however, that the flavor of "new" foods is not sufficiently distinct to be recognized as new by adults with broad eating habits, and that most significant food preferences are established early in life (Birch, 1999).

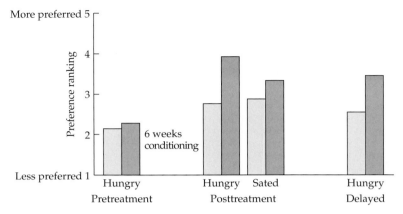

FIGURE 7.11 Changes in children's preference for the flavors of yogurts consumed in low- or high-fat form. (After Kern et al., 1993, with permission from Elsevier.)

The range of potential foods available to humans leads to huge variety in liking for different flavors. However, our liking for the flavors of drinks containing alcohol and caffeine is more consistent, and it seems contrary to our inherent inclination to dislike bitter tastes. FCL provides an obvious framework for explaining this acquired liking: the specific flavor of the drink becomes a reliable and contingent predictor of the positive postingestive effect of the drink. It is likely that FCL with alcohol as US in rats is based on both the pharmacological effects of alcohol and the number of calories ingested (Ackroff & Sclafani, 2001, 2002a, 2002b, 2003), but despite its parsimony as an explanation of how humans acquire a like for the flavor of alcoholic drinks, no studies have explicitly reported FCL with alcohol as US in humans. In contrast, the use of caffeine for its postingestive consequence is now well established in laboratory models of FCL in humans (Rogers et al., 1995; Richardson et al., 1996; Yeomans et al., 1998; Yeomans et al., 2005), and caffeine has also been reported to condition flavor preferences in rats (Fedorchak et al., 2002).

FLAVOR–FLAVOR MODELS OF EVALUATIVE CONDITIONING A second form of conditioned association that may contribute to changes in liking is *evaluative conditioning (EC)*. In EC, evaluation of one stimulus changes through association with a second stimulus, which is already liked or disliked (De Houwer et al., 2001; Field & Davey, 1999). In flavor-based EC paradigms, a neutral flavor CS is paired with a liked or disliked flavor US. The key features of this form of learning (usually known as *flavor–flavor learning*, or *FFL*) are highlighted in Figure 7.12. The essential idea is that association of a previously hedonically neutral flavor or flavor component (interpreted as the CS) with a second flavor or fla-

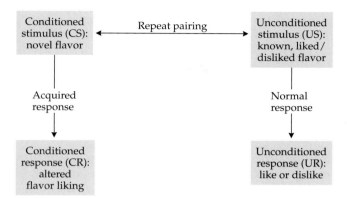

FIGURE 7.12 The associative substructure underlying flavor–flavor learning.

vor element that is already liked or disliked (interpreted as the US) results in an equivalent change in liking for the previously neutral flavor CS.

For example, Baeyens and colleagues (1996) examined changes in liking for the flavor and color of solutions that had either been paired with an aversive flavor (the soapy taste of the detergent Tween) or nothing. As Figure 7.13 shows, liking for flavors paired with an unpleasant flavor element decreased regardless of whether the solution was colored, whereas liking for the appearance (color) was unaffected by learning. Thus, coexperience of a disliked flavor element (Tween) and a novel flavor (the CS+) results in dislike for the flavor of the CS+. The specificity of these effects to the flavor but not color of the trained stimuli is reminiscent of the specificity of CTA to gustatory cues.

Evaluative conditioning is not restricted to learning about foods or drinks but is generally seen as the explanation for changes in liking in any situation where a novel, neutral stimulus (CS) is contingently paired with a second, hedonically

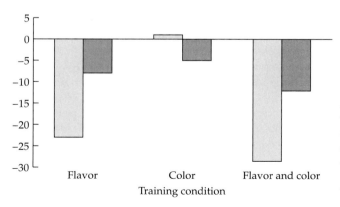

FIGURE 7.13 Acquired-dislike novel solutions paired either with a disliked flavor (detergent: CS+) or with water (CS–). Both CS+ and CS– were two solutions differing in flavor only, color only, or both flavor and color. (After Baeyens et al., 1996, with permission from Elsevier.)

significant stimulus (US). Thus, EC may represent a general form of affective learning yet may be an important element of flavor preference development. EC can also explain examples of increased liking for foods generated by seeing others consume and like those foods—for example, with children acquiring a like for novel vegetables after seeing peers consume and like them (Addessi et al., 2005; Addessi et al., 2007).

Earlier we discussed the idea of an innate sweet preference. It follows that adding sweetness to a novel-flavored food or drink will increase its immediate palatability. In FFL, the contingent pairing of the novel flavor components (seen as CS) and sweetness (acting as US) will promote increased liking for the flavor CS on its own. Studies in animals strongly support this idea: repeated experience of a novel flavor along with sweetness in the mouth yields a conditioned preference for the sweet-paired flavor relative to flavors paired with water (Capaldi et al., 1994; Fanselow & Birk, 1982; Warwick & Weingarten, 1996). Unlike FCL, FFL does not require postingestive effects: the liking change is based purely on the hedonic qualities of the CS and US before ingestion.

It has proven more difficult, however, to find empirical evidence to support FFL based on sweetness resulting in acquired liking for sweet-paired flavors (Zellner et al., 1983; Yeomans et al., 2006; compare Baeyens et al., 1990; Rozin et al., 1998). One explanation for this inconsistency is individual variability in liking for the sweet-taste US. Indeed, FFL would predict opposing changes in liking for flavors paired with sweetness between sweet likers and sweet dislikers, and this prediction has been confirmed experimentally (Looy & Weingarten, 1991). Associations between flavor and sweetness are likely to facilitate liking for flavors of any food or drink that has been experienced with added sweetness. Because most sweetness arises from sugars, the flavors of foods with added sugar may generate two types of flavor-based associations: FFL at the gustatory level, and FCL arising from postingestive effects of sugars. The acquired liking may in turn promote greater intake, leading to overeating.

In contrast to studies of FFL in which the US is sweetness, studies examining liking for a novel flavor that has been paired with an aversive US—such as the aversive, soapy flavor produced by the surfactant Tween (see Figure 7.13)—find consistent evidence of acquired dislike (Baeyens et al., 1996; Baeyens et al., 1990; Baeyens et al., 1995). As with the contrast between CTA and liking acquired by FCL, the pressure to avoid potential poisons may selectively promote aversive learning, whereas acquired liking proceeds at a slower rate.

In summary, FFL may provide a vehicle through which both positive and negative hedonic responses to flavors may be acquired. As with FCL, liking change with FFL in humans and animals requires relatively few pairings of CS and US flavors. Whether EC has properties distinct from more classic examples of conditioning is currently a topic of debate fueled by reports that EC is less dependent on contingency effects and may not show extinction (De Houwer et al., 2001). In the context of this chapter, however, the key finding is that liking for novel flavor components can be increased by the presence of already liked flavors.

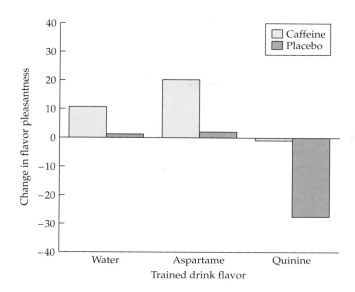

FIGURE 7.14 Change in rated pleasantness of drink flavors before and after repeated pairing with caffeine or placebo and with added sweetness (aspartame), added bitterness (quinine), or no added flavoring (water). (After Yeomans et al., 2007.)

How Do FCL and FFL Interact?

In the laboratory it is possible to design studies that explicitly pair flavors with nutrients (such as the paradigm shown in Figure 7.9) or pair a novel flavor with a second liked or disliked flavor with no consequence. But our real-life experience of food allows both types of associations to occur simultaneously. For example, rats prefer the taste of a pure glucose solution over an equally caloric solution of glucose with citric acid. But if a rat drank these solutions with an added novel flavor, the rat could potentially associate the new flavor with the hedonic quality of the solutions (FFL) or the nutrient effects of glucose (FCL). Tests reveal greater preference for the flavor paired with glucose alone, clearly showing that FFL occurs alongside FCL (Warwick & Weingarten, 1996). In humans, too, FCL and FFL co-occur. Figure 7.14 shows changes in liking for a flavor following association with either a liked (the sweet taste of aspartame) or a disliked (bitter taste of quinine) flavor (FFL) and the effects of caffeine (FCL). The effects of caffeine increased flavor liking, whereas the taste of quinine induced disliking, so quinine and caffeine together resulted in less change in liking than did caffeine without quinine (Yeomans et al., 2007).

The Relationship between Liking and Satiety: How Acquired Likes May Lead to Overeating

Theories about the relationship between palatability and homeostatic controls of eating fall into two broad groupings. One group views palatability as the affective expression generated by the sensory and informational attributes of a food in relation to satisfying nutritional and energetic needs. In this view, food intake is primarily under homeostatic control, explaining why palatability is a determinant of short-term feeding. In principle, this idea could apply equally to food flavors for which liking is innate (e.g., sweetness) or acquired, as indicated. Liking, therefore, should be enhanced by hunger and diminished by satiety. Although some evidence is consistent with this view (Cabanac, 1989; Cabanac, 1971), the ability of flavor manipulation to enhance appetite through palatability described in detail earlier contradicts this view because it suggests that hunger state and palatability have separate effects. The distinction between the effects of hunger state and palatability was shown clearly in studies of diary records of eating: both rated hunger and palatability of the meal predicted the size of the meal, but these effects were independent, so food was not more palatable when hungry than sated (De Castro et al., 2000).

The second group of theories relates palatability to reward processes that may operate independently of need state. The idea here is that meal size results from two sets of integrative processes. One is based on negative feedback, as described already, and acts to terminate the meal. The second, a positive feed-forward system that is driven hedonically, stimulates appetite, thereby increasing meal size (Smith, 2000). This idea fits with the data on palatability effects discussed earlier.

Feed-forward (palatability) and negative feedback (satiety effects) may operate independently, in which case simultaneous manipulations should have additive effects. Alternatively, low levels of satiety may actually magnify the effects of orosensory reward, thereby promoting overeating of palatable foods. One test of this idea is to combine manipulations of satiety in a prelunch preload with manipulations of palatability at the test meal (Yeomans et al., 2001; Robinson et al., 2005). In the study by Yeomans and colleagues (2001), increasing palatability of a test meal decreased the ability of a moderate energy preload to reduce test-meal intake. Note in Figure 7.15A that voluntary lunch intake was lower after a high-energy than low-energy soup preload, but no such effect is seen when the lunch was palatable. When preload energy is included, overall energy intake was greatly increased in both (bland and palatable) high-energy soup conditions (Figure 7.15B), consistent with a large literature suggesting that consumption of hidden energy obtained as a preload does not accurately compensate for the added energy at a subsequent test meal. Couple this effect with the stimulation of appetite by palatability, and total energy intake from the combination of an energy-dense soup followed by a palatable lunch was three times greater than for a low-energy soup and a bland lunch.

These effects of palatability may be irrelevant to energy balance if short-term overeating induced by palatability results in less being eaten at subsequent meals. But laboratory data suggest that any subsequent short-term compensation in intake is weak; for example, increasing intake of a preload by manipulating palatability did not result in reduced intake at a subsequent test meal

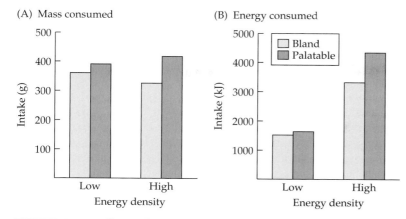

FIGURE 7.15 Effects of low-energy (60-kilojoule) and high-energy (360-kilojoule) soup preloads on mass (A) and energy (B) consumed in a lunch presented in bland or palatable forms. (After Yeomans et al., 2001.)

(de Graaf et al., 1999). So energy-dense, palatable snacks eaten between meals are predicted to add to overall energy intake and thus promote weight gain.

Whereas stimulation of appetite by palatability overrides satiety, expression of liking for flavors that is acquired through FCL is stronger when we are hungry than when sated. Look again at Figure 7.11. Notice that the acquired preference for the high-fat paired yogurt flavor was much stronger when the children tasted the food while hungry than while sated. Likewise, rats that had developed a preference for a flavor paired with energy when they were hungry showed less preference for the energy-paired flavor when they were sated (Fedorchak & Bolles, 1987). However, this state-dependent expression of acquired flavor preferences may depend on how hungry the individual was when the association was acquired.

As noted earlier, flavor preferences acquired through FCL can develop in rats that have unrestricted access to their normal diet, chow, suggesting that hunger is not necessary for the acquisition of flavor liking through FCL (Sclafani, 2004). Moreover, if rats acquire liking for a novel flavor when they are sated, they continue to express this liking when sated. So, with FCL it appears that acquired likes do depend on how hungry we are both when we acquire the association (acquisition) and subsequently when we experience the flavor again (expression).

The sensitivity of FCL-acquired likes to hunger state has implications for understanding overeating. Because, as we have seen, intake is driven by absolute liking, we should consequently eat less of flavors that we have learned to like through FCL if we acquired our liking when we were hungry and experience the food when we are sated. However, this pattern should hold true only if the flavor is a reliable predictor of consequence. If a flavor is an unreliable predictor of consequence, no reliable association can develop, so liking will remain unchanged. For example, increased consumption of sweetened caloric beverages is recognized as a contributory factor to obesity (van Dam & Seidall, 2007). Most of these beverages are available in both high- and low-energy forms, and if consumers use a mixture of flavor-matched high- and low-energy versions, flavor is not a reliable predictor of energy (Stubbs & Whybrow, 2004). Sweetness would, however, tend to increase flavor liking through FFL. Since FFL appears insensitive to hunger state, flavor liking would become insensitive to need state; and as liking increased, so would overconsumption. Thus, paradoxically, the development of energy-free products such as diet sodas may unwittingly promote intake.

With FFL, except when liking for the US is hunger-dependent, there is no reason for acquired liking to depend on current hunger. So flavor liking developed through FFL should be expressed regardless of hunger state, and consequently the liked food should be overconsumed even in the sated condition. If the preferred food is energy-rich, overeating will occur and, if done regularly, will result in weight gain. This hypothesis has been supported by laboratory findings. In hungry rats, preferences for flavors acquired by associations with sucrose, in which both FFL and FCL likely operate, were sensitive to hunger, but a flavor preference acquired by association with a non-nutritive sweetener (saccharin) was not (Fedorchak & Bolles, 1987). Likewise, in hungry people, liking for the flavor of a drink that had been acquired by association with sucrose was hunger-sensitive, whereas liking for the same flavor acquired by association with the non-nutritive sweetener aspartame was not (Figure 7.16; Mobini et al., 2007). So, whereas expression of liking for flavors acquired by FCL depends on hunger state during training, liking acquired by FFL is independent of hunger.

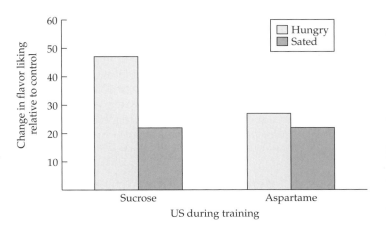

FIGURE 7.16 The effects of hunger at test time on changes in relative preference for a flavored drink acquired by association with either a caloric sweetener (sucrose) or a noncaloric sweetener (aspartame). (After Mobini et al., 2007.)

Palatability, Learning, and Obesity

How might food pleasures translate into overeating, with its morbid consequences? The current obesity epidemic reflects, in part, the increased availability, low price, and aggressive marketing of palatable, energy-dense foods (Drewnowski, 1998; Stubbs & Whybrow, 2004; Blundell & Cooling, 2000). The link between palatability and energy density can explain these associations. Ingestion of foods with high energy density induces flavor liking through FCL. Furthermore, the widespread use of sweetening agents promotes increased flavor liking through FFL. Both conditioned aspects of ingestion, of course, top off the already robust intakes through innate sweet preference. Once a flavor is liked, it will be overconsumed. Thus, overconsumption could be explained as the inevitable clash between an appetite control system that has evolved to maximize energy-rich sources of food, especially when scarce, and a modern environment in which energy-dense foods are common (unlike the diets that shaped the development of our appetite control system).

As mentioned at the start of this chapter, a classic finding was that obese individuals overrespond to hedonic cues from food (Nisbett, 1968). It might then follow that obesity is a consequence of oversensitivity to the hedonic stimulus to eat. Obese subjects show normal sensory responses to taste stimuli (de Graaf, 2005; Nasser, 2001). Because the only innate components of palatability are taste-related, any differences in hedonic response between obese and normal-weight individuals must reflect differences arising from learned food preferences. Most relevant is liking for fat, because obese subjects have greater liking for the sensory qualities of fat (Mela & Sacchetti, 1991; Gibney et al., 1995), show abnormally strong liking for mixtures of fat and sugar (Drewnowski, 1992), and overconsume fatty foods (Blundell & Cooling, 2000; Blundell & Macdiarmid, 1997; Golay & Bobbioni, 1998). Liking for the sensory qualities of fats is likely to be acquired, probably through FCL, since fat is a reliable source of energy and fat has been shown to support flavor preference development in experimental studies with rats (Lucas & Sclafani, 1989; Ackroff et al., 2004; Lucas et al., 1998; Acroff et al., 2005) and humans (Johnson et al., 1991).

Earlier we noted the association between palatability and energy density, and the association between fat intake and obesity can be explained accordingly. Energy-dense foods promote flavor liking through FCL, but they may generate weak satiety cues, thus leading to passive overconsumption (Westerterp, 2006). Stimulation of appetite by acquired liking for the flavor of energy-dense foods would be predicted to compound this effect. For example, Salbe and colleagues (2004) examined liking for the sensory quality of energy-dense mixtures of fat and sugar in an obese-prone population: Pima Indians. Hedonic responses to these solutions were a predictor of subsequent weight gain: those with higher liking scores gained more weight in the subsequent 5 years.

One of the few dietary correlates of weight gain, particularly in adolescents, is increased consumption of both sugar-based and artificially sweetened low-energy drinks (Berkey et al., 2004; Wollitzer et al., 2004). These beverages could act to promote overconsumption in three ways. First, evidence suggests that energy consumed as a beverage has weak satiety effects (Almiron-Roig et al., 2003). Second, our preference for sweet tastes could lead to stimulation of appetite and thus directly promote short-term overconsumption. Third, incorporation of sweet tastes into products will promote increased liking for the product flavor by both FFL and FCL, and thus will increase the tendency to overconsume the sweet-associated flavor.

Summary

This chapter has confirmed that pleasure is an important driver of food intake, with clear evidence that intake increases as a linear function of flavor pleasantness. Overeating in response to palatability overrides satiety cues based on what we have consumed beforehand, and palatability-driven overeating does not lead to reductions in subsequent short-term intake. Because palatability and energy density go together, increased availability of palatable, energy-dense foods is likely to be one of the environmental causes of the current obesity crisis (Drewnowski & Specter, 2004; Wansink, 2004).

The link between palatability and energy density is driven partly by an innate sweet preference, but mainly by learned associations between flavor and energy. Flavor preference is also partly driven by associations between new flavors and existing liked flavor components. Although expression of these acquired preferences does depend to some extent on how hungry we are when we eat, this control appears inadequate to allow us to adjust intake to maintain body weight.

The overall conclusion is that we have developed an appetite system that responds well to deprivation by stimulating appetite, but that is less able to prevent overconsumption in the face of a diet of energy-dense, palatable foods. Successful treatment of obesity must therefore include mechanisms to help individuals resist food cues to counter hedonically-driven overeating.

References Cited

Ackroff, K., Lucas, F., & Sclafani, A. (2005). Flavor preference conditioning as a function of fat source. *Physiology & Behavior, 85,* 448–460.

Ackroff, K., Rozental, D., & Sclafani, A. (2004). Ethanol-conditioned flavor preferences compared with sugar- and fat-conditioned preferences in rats. *Physiology & Behavior, 81,* 699–713.

Ackroff, K., & Sclafani, A. (2001). Flavor preferences conditioned by intragastric infusion of ethanol in rats. *Pharmacology Biochemistry, and Behavior, 68,* 327–338.

Ackroff, K., & Sclafani, A. (2002a). Ethanol flavor preference conditioned by intragastric carbohydrate in rats. *Pharmacology, Biochemistry, and Behavior, 74,* 41–51.

Ackroff, K., & Sclafani, A. (2002b). Flavor quality and ethanol concentration affect ethanol-conditioned flavor preferences. *Pharmacology, Biochemistry, and Behavior, 74,* 229–240.

Ackroff, K., & Sclafani, A. (2003). Flavor preferences conditioned by intragastric ethanol with limited access training. *Pharmacology, Biochemistry, and Behavior, 75,* 223–233.

Addessi, E., Chiarotti, F., Visalberghi, E., & Anzenberger, G. (2007). Response to novel food and the role of social influences in common marmosets (Callithrix jacchus) and Goeldi's monkeys (Callimico goeldii). *American Journal of Primatology 69*, 1210–1222

Addessi, E., Galloway, A. T., Visalberghi, E., & Birch, L. L. (2005). Specific social influences on the acceptance of novel foods in 2–5-year-old children. *Appetite, 45*, 264–271.

Almiron-Roig, E., Chen, Y., & Drewnowski, A. (2003). Liquid calories and the failure of satiety: how good is the evidence? *Obesity Reviews, 4*, 201–212.

Arnold, S. J. (1977). Polymorphism and geographic variation in the feeding behavior of the garter snake Thamnophis elegans. *Science, 197*, 676–678.

Azzara, A. V., & Sclafani, A. (1998). Flavor preferences conditioned by intragastric sugar infusions in rats: maltose is more reinforcing than sucrose. *Physiology & Behavior, 64*, 535–541.

Bachmanov, A. A., Reed, D. R., Li, X., & Beauchamp, G. K. (2002). Genetics of sweet taste preference. *Pure & Applied Chemistry, 7*, 1135–1140.

Baeyens, F., Crombez, G., De Houwer, J., & Eelen, P. (1996). No evidence for modulation of evaluative flavor-flavor associations in humans. *Learning and Motivation, 27*, 200–241.

Baeyens, F., Crombez, G., Hendrickx, H., & Eelen, P. (1995). Parameters of human evaluative flavor-flavor conditioning. *Learning and Motivation, 26*, 141–160.

Baeyens, F., Eelen, P., Van Den Burgh, O., & Crombez, G. (1990). Flavor-flavor and color-flavor conditioning in humans. *Learning and Motivation, 21*, 434–455.

Beauchamp, G. K., & Moran, M. (1984). Acceptance of sweet and salty tastes in 2-year old children. *Appetite, 5*, 291–305.

Behrens, M., & Meyerhof, W. (2006). Bitter taste receptors and human bitter taste perception. *Cellular and Molecular Life Sciences, 63*, 1501–1509.

Bellisle, F., Lucas, F., Amrani, R., & Le Magnen, J. (1984). Deprivation, palatability and the micro-structure of meals in human subjects. *Appetite, 5*, 85–94.

Berkey, C. S., Rockett, H. R., Field, A. E., Gillman, M. W., & Colditz, G. A. (2004). Sugar-added beverages and adolescent weight change. *Obesity Research, 12*, 778–788.

Bernstein, I. L. (1978). Learned taste aversions in children receiving chemotherapy. *Science, 200*, 1302–1303.

Berridge, K. C. (1996). Food reward: brain substrates of wanting and liking. *Neuroscience and Biobehavioral Reviews, 20*, 1–25.

Berridge, K. C. (2000). Measuring hedonic impact in animals and infants: microstructure of affective taste reactivity patterns. *Neuroscience and Biobehavioral Reviews, 24*, 173–198.

Berridge, K. C., Flynn, F. W., Schulkin, J., & Grill, H. J. (1984). Sodium depletion enhances salt palatability in rats. *Behavioral Neuroscience, 98*, 652–660.

Berridge, K. C., & Robinson, T. E. (1998). What is the role of dopamine in reward: hedonic impact, reward learning, or incentive salience? *Brain Research Bulletin, 28*, 309–369.

Berridge, K. C., & Schulkin, J. (1989). Palatability shift of a salt-associated incentive during sodium depletion. *Quarterly Journal of Experimental Psychology, 41B*, 121–138.

Bertino, M., & Tordoff, M. G. (1988). Sodium depletion increases rats preferences for salted food. *Behavioral Neuroscience, 102*, 565–573.

Birch, L. L. (1999). Development of food preferences. *Annual Review of Nutrition, 19*, 41–62.

Birch, L. L., & Marlin, D. W. (1982). "I don't like it; I never tried it." effects of exposure on two-year-old children's food preferences. *Appetite, 3*, 353–360.

Birch, L. L., McPhee, L., Steinberg, L., & Sullivan, S. (1990). Conditioned flavor preferences in young children. *Physiology & Behavior, 47*, 501–505.

Blass, E. M., & Fitzgerald, E. (1988). Milk-induced analgesia and comforting in 10-day old rats: opioid mediation. *Pharmacology, Biochemistry, and Behavior, 29*, 9–13.

Blass, E. M., & Watt, L. B. (1999). Suckling- and sucrose-induced analgesia in human newborns. *Pain, 83*, 611–623.

Blundell, J. E., & Cooling, J. (2000). Routes to obesity: phenotypes, food choices and activity. *British Journal of Nutrition, 83* (Suppl. 1), S33–38.

Blundell, J. E., & Macdiarmid, J. I. (1997). Fat as a risk factor for overconsumption: Satiation, satiety, and patterns of eating. *Journal of the American Dietetic Association, 97*(Suppl. 7), S63–S69.

Bobroff, E. M., & Kissileff, H. (1986). Effects of changes in palatability on food intake and the cumulative food intake curve of man. *Appetite, 7*, 85–96.

Booth, D. A. (1972). Conditioned satiety in the rat. *Journal of Comparative and Physiological Psychology, 81*, 457–471.

Bornstein, R. F. (1989). Exposure and affect: overview and meta-analysis of research, 1968–1987. *Psychological Bulletin, 106*, 265–289.

Brunstrom, J. M. (2005). Dietary learning in humans: directions for future research. *Physiology & Behavior, 85*, 57–65.

Cabanac, M. (1971). Physiological role of pleasure. *Science, 173*, 1103–1107.

Cabanac, M. (1989). Palatability of food and the ponderostat. *Annals of the New York Academy of Sciences, 575*, 340–352.

Capaldi, E. D. (1992). Conditioned food preferences. *Psychology of Learning and Motivation, 28*, 1–33.

Capaldi, E. D., Owens, J., & Palmer, K. A. (1994). Effects of food deprivation on learning and expression of flavor preferences conditioned by saccharin or sucrose. *Animal Learning and Behavior, 22*, 173–180.

Conner, M., & Arimitage, C. J. (2002). *The social psychology of food*. Buckingham: Open University Press.

Crandall, C. S. (1984). The liking of foods as a result of exposure: eating doughnuts in Alaska. *Journal of Social Psychology, 125*, 187–194.

Curtis, K. S., Krause, E. G., & Contreras, R. J. (2001). Altered NaCl taste responses precede increased NaCl ingestion during Na(+) deprivation. *Physiology & Behavior, 72*, 743–749.

Dahunukar, A., Foster, K., Van der Goes Van Naters, W. M., & Carlson, J. R. (2001). A Gr receptor is required for response to the sugar trehalose in taste neurons of *Drosophila*. *Nature Neuroscience, 4*, 1182–1186.

Davis, J. D., & Levine, M. W. (1977). A model for the control of ingestion. *Psychological Review, 84*, 379–412.

de Castro, J. M., Bellisle, F., Dalix, A.-M., & Pearcey, S. M. (2000). Palatability and intake relationships in free-living humans:
characterization and independence of influence in North Americans. *Physiology & Behavior, 70*, 343–350.

de Graaf, C. (2005). Sensory responses, food intake and obesity. In D. J. Mela (Ed.), *Food, diet and obesity* (pp. 137–159). Cambridge: Woodhead Publishing.

de Graaf, C., de Jong, L. S., & Lambers, A. C. (1999). Palatability affects satiation but not satiety. *Physiology & Behavior, 66*, 681–688.

De Houwer, J., Thomas, S., & Baeyens, F. (2001). Associative learning of likes and dislikes: a review of 25 years of research on human evaluative conditioning. *Psychological Bulletin, 127*, 853–869.

Denton, D. A. (1982). *The hunger for salt*. Berlin, Germany: Springer-Verlag.

Denton, D. A., Eichberg, J. W., Shade, R., & Weisinger, R. S. (1993). Sodium appetite in response to sodium deficiency in baboons. *American Journal of Physiology, 264*, R539–543.

Desor, J. A., Maller, O., & Turner, R. E. (1973). Taste in acceptance of sugars by human infants. *Journal of Comparative and Physiological Psychology, 84*, 496–501.

Dethier, V. G. (1976). *The hungry fly*. Cambridge, MA: Harvard University Press.

Dethier, V. G., & Boderstein, D. (1958). Hunger in the blowfly. *Zeitschrift fur Tierpsychologie, 15*, 129–140.

Dethier, V. G., & Gelperin, A. (1967). Hyperphagia in the blowfly. *Journal of Experimental Biology, 47*, 191–200.

Drewnowski, A. (1992). Sensory preferences and fat consumption in obesity and eating disorders. In D. J. Mela (Ed.), *Dietary fats: determinants of preference, selection and consumption* (pp. 59–77). London: Elsevier.

Drewnowski, A. (1998). Energy density, palatability and satiety: implications for weight control. *Nutrition Reviews, 56*, 347–353.

Drewnowski, A., & Specter, S. E. (2004). Poverty and obesity: the role of energy density and energy costs. *American Journal of Clinical Nutrition, 79*, 6–16.

Drucker, D. B., Ackroff, K., & Sclafani, A. (1994). Nutrient-conditioned flavor preferences and acceptance in rats: effects of deprivation state and nonreinforcement. *Physiology & Behavior, 56*, 701–707.

Elizalde, G., & Sclafani, A. (1988). Starch-based conditioned flavor preferences in rats: influence of taste, calories and CS–US delay. *Appetite, 11,* 179–200.

Epstein, A. N. (1991). Thirst and salt intake: a personal view and some suggestions. In D. J. Ramsay & D. A. Booth (Eds.), *Thirst – physiological and psychological aspects* (pp. 481–501). Berlin, Germany: Springer-Verlag.

Fanselow, M. S., & Birk, J. (1982). Flavor-flavor associations induce hedonic shifts in taste preference. *Animal Learning and Behavior, 10,* 223–228.

Fedorchak, P. M., & Bolles, R. C. (1987). Hunger enhances the expression of calorie- but not taste-mediated conditioned flavour preferences. *Journal of Experimental Psychology: Animal Behavior Processes, 13,* 73–79.

Fedorchak, P. M., Mesita, J., Plater, S., & Brougham, K. (2002). Caffeine-reinforced flavor preferences in rats. *Behavioral Neuroscience, 116,* 334–346.

Field, A. P., & Davey, G. C. L. (1999). Re-evaluating evaluative conditioning: an exemplar comparison model of evaluative conditioning effects. *Journal of Experimental Psychology: Animal Behavior Processes, 25,* 211–224.

Fischer, A., Gilad, Y., Man, O., & Paabo, S. (2005). Evolution of bitter taste receptors in humans and apes. *Molecular Biology and Evolution, 22,* 432–436.

Galef, B. G., & Laland, K. N. (2005). Social learning in animals: empirical studies and theoretical models. *Bioscience, 55,* 489–499.

Garcia, J., Ervin, F. R., & Koelling, R. A. (1966). Learning with prolonged delay of reinforcement. *Psychonomic Science, 5,* 121–122.

Garcia, J., & Koelling, R. A. (1966). Relation of cue to consequence in avoidance learning. *Psychonomic Science, 4,* 123–124.

Gibney, M., Sigman-Grant, M., Stanton, J. L., Jr., & Keast, D. R. (1995). Consumption of sugars. *American Journal of Clinical Nutrition, 62*(Suppl. 1), 178S–193S; discussion, 194S.

Gibson, E. L., & Wardle, J. (2003). Energy density predicts preferences for fruit and vegetables in 4-year-old children. *Appetite, 41,* 97–98.

Golay, A., & Bobbioni, E. (1997). The role of dietary fat in obesity. *International Journal of Obesity, 21*(Suppl. 3), S2–S11.

Harris, J. A., Gorissen, M. C., Bailey, G. K., & Westbrook, R. F. (2000). Motivational state regulates the content of learned flavor

preferences. *Journal of Experimental Psychology: Animal Behavior Processes, 26,* 15–30.

Hladik, C. M., Pasquet, P., & Simmen, B. (2002). New perspectives on taste and primate evolution: the dichotomy in gustatory coding for perception of beneficent versus noxious substances as supported by correlations among human thresholds. *American Journal of Physiological Anthropology, 117,* 342–348.

Johnson, A. K., & Thunhorst, R. L. (1997). The neuroendocrinology of thirst and salt appetite: visceral sensory signals and mechanisms of central integration. *Frontiers in Neuroendocrinology, 18,* 292–353.

Johnson, S. L., McPhee, L., & Birch, L. L. (1991). Conditioned preferences: young children prefer flavors associated with high dietary fat. *Physiology & Behavior, 50,* 1245–1251.

Kauffman, N. A., Herman, C. P., & Polivy, J. (1995). Hunger-induced finickiness in humans. *Appetite, 24,* 203–218.

Kern, D. L., McPhee, L., Fisher, J., Johnson, S., & Birch, L. L. (1993). The postingestive consequences of fat condition preferences for flavors associated with high dietary fat. *Physiology & Behavior, 54,* 71–76.

Kissileff, H. R. (1976). Palatability. In B. Wolman (Ed.), *International encyclopedia of psychiatry, psychology, psychoanalysis and neurology* (Vol. 10, p. 172). New York: Academic Press.

Kraegen, E. W., Clark, P. W., Jenkins, A. B., Daley, E. A., Chisholm, D. J., & Storlien, L. H. (1991). Development of muscle insulin resistance after liver insulin resistance in high-fat-fed rats. *Diabetes, 40,* 1397–1403.

Krieckhaus, E. E., & Wolf, G. (1968). Acquisition of sodium by rats: interaction of innate effects and latent learning. *Journal of Comparative and Physiological Psychology, 65,* 197–201.

Kringelbach, M. L. (2004). Food for thought: hedonic experience beyond homeostasis in the human brain. *Neuroscience, 126,* 807–819.

Le Magnen, J. (1987). Palatability: concept, terminology and mechanisms. In R. A. Boakes, D. A. Popplewell, & M. J. Burton (Eds.), *Eating Habits: Food, Physiology and Learned Behaviour* (pp. 131–154). Chichester, UK: Wiley.

Leshem, M. (1998). Salt preference in adolescence is predicted by common prenatal and infantile mineralofluid loss. *Physiology & Behavior, 63,* 699–704.

Leshem, M. (1999). The ontogeny of salt hunger in the rat. *Neuroscience and Biobehavioral Reviews, 23,* 649–659.

Leshem, M. (2000). Human salt appetite. *Appetite, 35,* 298.

Logue, A. W. (1979). Taste aversion and the generality of the laws of learning. *Psychological Bulletin, 86,* 276–296.

Looy, H., & Weingarten, H. P. (1991). Effects of metabolic state on sweet taste reactivity in humans depend on underlying hedonic response profile. *Chemical Senses, 16,* 123–130.

Lucas, F., Ackroff, K., & Sclafani, A. (1998). High-fat diet preference and overeating mediated by postingestive factors in rats. *American Journal of Physiology, 275,* R1511–R1522.

Lucas, F., & Sclafani, A. (1989). Flavor preferences conditioned by intragastric fat infusions in rats. *Physiology & Behavior, 46,* 403–412.

Maone, T. R., Mattes, R. D., Bernbaum, J. C., & Beauchamp, G. K. (1990). A new method for delivering a taste without fluids to preterm and term infants. *Developmental Psychobiology, 23,* 179–191.

Matsunami, H., Montmayeur, J.-P., & Buck, L. B. (2000). A family of candidate taste receptors in human and mouse. *Nature, 404,* 601–604.

Mattes, R. D. (1997). The taste for salt in humans. *American Journal of Clinical Nutrition, 65,* 692S–697S.

McCabe, C., & Rolls, E. T. (2007). Umami: a delicious flavor formed by convergence of taste and olfactory pathways in the human brain. *European Journal of Neuroscience, 25,* 1855–1864.

Mehiel, R., & Bolles, R. C. (1984). Learned flavor preferences based on caloric outcome. *Journal of Experimental Psychology–Animal Behavior Processes, 12,* 421–427.

Mela, D. J., & Sacchetti, D. A. (1991). Sensory Preferences for Fats – Relationships with Diet and Body-Composition. *American Journal of Clinical Nutrition, 53,* 908–915.

Mobini, S., Chambers, L. C., & Yeomans, M. R. (2007). Interactive effects of flavour-flavour and flavour-consequence learning in development of liking for sweet-paired flavours in humans. *Appetite, 48,* 20–28.

Myers, K. P., & Sclafani, A. (2001a). Conditioned enhancement of flavor evaluation reinforced by intragastric glucose. I.

Intake acceptance and preference analysis. *Physiology & Behavior, 74,* 481–493.

Myers, K. P., & Sclafani, A. (2001b). Conditioned enhancement of flavor evaluation reinforced by intragastric glucose. II. Taste reactivity analysis. *Physiology & Behavior, 74,* 495–505.

Naim, M., & Kare, M. R. (1991). Sensory and postingestional components of palatability in dietary obesity: an overview. In M. I. Friedman, M. G. Tordoff, & M. R. Kare, *Appetite and Nutrition* (Vol. 4, pp. 109–126). New York: Dekker.

Nasser, J. (2001). Taste, food intake and obesity. *Obesity Reviews, 2,* 213–218.

Nisbett, R. E. (1968). Taste, deprivation and weight determinants of eating behavior. *Journal of Personality and Social Psychology, 10,* 107–116.

Pliner, P. (1982). The effect of mere exposure on liking for edible substances. *Appetite, 3,* 283–290.

Prescott, J. (1999). Flavour as a psychological construct: implications for perceiving and measuring the sensory qualities of foods. *Food Quality and Preference, 10,* 349–356.

Ramirez, I. (1994). Flavor preferences conditioned with starch in rats. *Animal Learning and Behavior, 22,* 181–187.

Richardson, N. J., Rogers, P. J., & Elliman, N. A. (1996). Conditioned flavour preferences reinforced by caffeine consumed after lunch. *Physiology & Behavior, 60,* 257–263.

Robinson, T. M., Gray, R. W., Yeomans, M. R., & French, S. J. (2005). Test-meal palatability alters the effects of intragastric fat but not carbohydrate preloads on intake and rated appetite in healthy volunteers. *Physiology & Behavior, 84,* 193–203.

Rogers, P. J., & Blundell, J. E. (1984). Meal patterns and food selection during the development of obesity in rats fed a cafeteria diet. *Neuroscience and Biobehavioral Reviews, 8,* 441–453.

Rogers, P. J., Richardson, N. J., & Elliman, N. A. (1995). Overnight caffeine abstinence and negative reinforcement of preference for caffeine-containing drinks. *Psychopharmacology, 120,* 457–462.

Rozin, P. (1982). Human food selection: the interaction of biology, culture and individual experience. In L. M. Barker (Ed.), *The psychobiology of human food selection* (pp. 225–254). Westport, CT: AVI Publishing.

Rozin, P., & Schiller, D. (1980). The nature and acquisition of a preference for chili pepper in humans. *Motivation and Emotion, 4,* 77–101.

Rozin, P., Wrzesniewski, A., & Byrnes, D. (1998). The elusiveness of evaluative conditioning. *Learning and Motivation, 29,* 397–415.

Salbe, A. D., DelParigi, A., Pratley, R. E., Drewnowski, A., & Tataranni, P. A. (2004). Taste preferences and body weight changes in an obesity-prone population. *American Journal of Clinical Nutrition, 79,* 372–378.

Schulkin, J. (1991). *Sodium hunger, the search for a salty taste.* Cambridge: Cambridge University Press.

Sclafani, A. (1993). Dietary obesity. In A. J. Stunkard & T. A. Wadden (Eds.), *Obesity: theory and therapy* (pp. 125–136). New York: Raven.

Sclafani, A. (1999). Macronutrient-conditioned flavor preferences. In H.-R. Berthoud & R. J. Seeley (Eds.), *Neural control of macronutrient selection* (pp. 93–106). Boca Raton: CRC Press.

Sclafani, A. (2002). Flavor preferences conditioned by sucrose depend upon training and testing methods: two-bottle tests revisited. *Physiology & Behavior, 76,* 633–644.

Sclafani, A. (2004). Oral and postoral determinants of food reward. *Physiology & Behavior, 81,* 773–779.

Sclafani, A., & Nissenbaum, J. W. (1988). Robust conditioned flavor preference produced by intragastric starch infusions in rats. *American Journal of Physiology, 255,* R672–R675.

Sewards, T. V. (2004). Dual separate pathways for sensory and hedonic aspects of taste. *Brain Research Bulletin, 62,* 271–283.

Shi, P., & Zhang, J. (2006). Contrasting modes of evolution between vertebrate sweet/umami receptor genes and bitter receptor genes. *Molecular and Biological Evolution, 23,* 292–300.

Shi, P., Zhang, J., Yang, H., & Zhang, Y. P. (2003). Adaptive diversification of bitter taste receptor genes in Mammalian evolution. *Molecular and Biological Evolution, 20,* 805–814.

Small, D. M., & Prescott, J. (2005). Odor/taste integration and the perception of flavor. *Experimental Brain Research. 166,* 345–357

Smith, G. P. (2000). The controls of eating: a shift from nutritional homeostasis to behavioral neuroscience. *Nutrition, 16,* 814–820.

Smith, J. C., & Roll, D. L. (1967). Trace conditioning with X-rays as the aversive stimulus. *Psychonomic Science, 9,* 11–12.

Solomon, R. S., & Corbit, J. D. (1974). An opponent-process theory of motivation: 1. Temporal dynamics of affect. *Psychological Review, 81,* 119–145.

Steiner, J. E. (1979). Human facial expressions in response to taste and smell stimulation. In H. W. Reese & L. P. Lipsitt (Eds.), *Advances in Child Development and Behavior* (Vol. 13, pp. 257–295). New York: Academic Press.

Stevenson, R. J., & Yeomans, M. R. (1995). Does exposure enhance liking for the chilli burn? *Appetite, 24,* 107–120.

Stubbs, R. J., & Whybrow, S. (2004). Energy density, diet composition and palatability: influences on overall food energy intake in humans. *Physiology & Behavior, 81,* 755–764.

Ulijaszek, S. J. (2007). Obesity: a disorder of convenience. *Obesity Reviews, 8*(Suppl. 1), 183–187.

van Dam, R. M. & Seidell, J. C. (2007). Carbohydrate intake and obesity. *European Journal of Clinical Nutrition, 61*(Suppl.1), S75–S99.

Verhagen, J. V., & Engelen, L. (2006). The neurocognitive bases of human multimodal food perception: sensory integration. *Neuroscience and Biobehavioral Reviews, 30,* 613–650.

Wald, N., & Leshem, M. (2003). Salt conditions a flavor preference or aversion after exercise depending on NaCl dose and sweat loss. *Appetite, 40,* 277–284.

Wansink, B. (2004). Environmental factors that increase the food intake and consumption volume of unknowing consumers. *Annual Review of Nutrition, 24,* 455–479.

Warwick, Z. S., & Schiffman, S. S. (1992). Role of dietary fat in calorie intake and weight gain. *Neuroscience and Biobehavioral Reviews, 16,* 585–596.

Warwick, Z. S., & Weingarten, H. P. (1996). Dissociation of palatability and calorie effects in learned flavor preferences. *Physiology & Behavior, 55,* 501–504.

Westerterp, K. R. (2006). Perception, passive overfeeding and energy metabolism. *Physiology & Behavior, 89,* 62–65.

Wollitzer, A. O., Jovanovic, L., & Petitt, D. J. (2004). Adolescent obesity is associated with excess consumption of diet soda. *Diabetes, 53,* A599–A600.

Woods, S. C., Seeley, R. J., Rushing, P. A., D'Alessio, D., & Tso, P. (2003). A controlled high-fat diet induces an obese syndrome in rats. *Journal of Nutrition, 133,* 1081–1087.

Yeomans, M. R. (1996). Palatability and the microstructure of eating in humans: the appetiser effect. *Appetite, 27,* 119–133.

Yeomans, M. R. (1998). Taste, palatability and the control of appetite. *Proceedings of the Nutrition Society, 57,* 609–615.

Yeomans, M. R. (2007). The role of palatability in control of food intake: implications for understanding and treating obesity. In S. J. Cooper & T. C. Kirkham (Eds.), *Appetite and Body Weight: Integrative systems and the Development of Anti-Obesity Drugs* (pp. 247–269). Amsterdam, Holland: Elsevier.

Yeomans, M. R., Durlach, P. J., & Tinley, E. M. (2005). Flavour liking and preference conditioned by caffeine in humans. *Quarterly Journal of Experimental Psychology, 58B,* 47–58.

Yeomans, M. R., & Gray, R. W. (2002). Opioids and human ingestive behaviour. *Neuroscience and Biobehavioral Reviews, 26,* 713–728.

Yeomans, M. R., Gray, R. W., Mitchell, C. J., & True, S. (1997). Independent effects of palatability and within-meal pauses on intake and subjective appetite in human volunteers. *Appetite, 29,* 61–76.

Yeomans, M. R., Lee, M. D., Gray, R. W., & French, S. J. (2001). Effects of test-meal palatability on compensatory eating following disguised fat and carbohydrate preloads. *International Journal of Obesity, 25,* 1215–1224.

Yeomans, M. R., Mobini, S., & Chambers, L. C. (2007). Additive effects of flavour-caffeine and flavour-flavour pairings on lik-ing for the smell and flavour of a novel drink. *Physiology & Behavior,* in press.

Yeomans, M. R., Mobini, S., Elliman, T. D., Walker, H. C., & Stevenson, R. J. (2006). Hedonic and sensory characteristics of odors conditioned by pairing with tastants in humans. *Journal of Experimental Psychology–Animal Behavior Processes, 32,* 215–228.

Yeomans, M. R., Spetch, H., & Rogers, P. J. (1998). Conditioned flavour preference negatively reinforced by caffeine in human volunteers. *Psychopharmacology, 137,* 401–409.

Yiin, Y. M., Ackroff, K., & Sclafani, A. (2005). Flavor preferences conditioned by intra-gastric nutrient infusions in food restricted and free-feeding rats. *Physiology & Behavior, 84,* 217–231.

Young, P. T. (1967). Palatability: the hedonic response to foodstuffs. In C. F. Code (Ed.), *Handbook of Physiology, section 6: Alimentary canal, Vol. 1, Control of food and water intake* (pp. 353–366). Washington, DC: American Physiology Society.

Zajonc, R. B. (1968). Attitudinal effects of mere exposure. *Journal of Personality and Social Psychology, 9,* 1–27.

Zampini, M., & Spence, C. (2004). The role of auditory cues in modulating the perceived crispness and staleness of potato chips. *Journal of Sensory Studies, 19,* 347–363.

Zandstra, E. H., de Graaf, C., Mela, D. J., & Van Staveren, W. (2000). Short- and long-term effects of changes in pleasantness on food intake. *Appetite, 34,* 253–260.

Zellner, D. A., Rozin, P., Aron, M., & Kulish, C. (1983). Conditioned enhancement of human's liking for flavor by pairing with sweetness. *Learning and Motivation, 14,* 338–350.

8 EXERCISE FOR OBESITY TREATMENT AND PREVENTION: CURRENT PERSPECTIVES AND CONTROVERSIES

Shaun M. Filiault

Introduction

Daily energy balance reflects the relationships among several variables, including the energy derived from food, the energy used to fuel necessary body functions and metabolism, and the energy used to power body movement. Accordingly, changes in any of these variables affect energy balance.

Energy balance influences body mass.[1] When energy consumed equals energy expended, body mass remains roughly stable. When caloric intake exceeds caloric expenditure, however, a positive energy balance emerges and body mass increases, thereby potentially launching a trajectory toward obesity. Conversely, when energy expended exceeds energy consumed, body mass decreases, potentially moving an overweight or obese person toward a more healthy body mass. Thus, in principle, treatment for obesity involves creating a daily negative energy balance.

Negative energy balance can be achieved by the manipulation of either energy intake or energy expenditure. Cutting down on energy intake means caloric restriction ("dieting"), which can be accomplished through a variety of methods, such as reducing or eliminating specific macronutrients (e.g., low-carbohydrate diets), decreasing portion sizes, or cutting down on between-meal snacks. By itself, dieting can substantially reduce body mass; however,

---

[1]A common indicator of body mass is a ratio between an individual's weight and height, a statistic called the *body mass index (BMI)*, which is the weight in kilograms, divided by height in square meters. On a population level, some research has linked elevated BMI (i.e., a BMI greater than 30) to health problems such as cardiovascular disease and insulin-resistant diabetes, among other negatives, but elevated body mass, in and of itself, is *not* a disease. BMI is a particularly poor indicator of health because it fails to account separately for fat and muscle. Furthermore, as discussed in this chapter, BMI does not account for health behaviors that can enhance or mitigate the risk of disease. In that sense, elevated body mass (i.e., overweight and obesity) should be thought of as one of many factors that can *predispose* an individual to disease, but *not* as a disease in its own right.

such reductions are only very rarely sustained, reflecting the difficulty in beginning and adhering to a diet (Volek et al., 2005; Foster et al., 2003). A more efficacious approach, then, may be to increase energy expenditure to promote a negative energy balance and fight obesity. Physical activity—and particularly exercise—is one method of increasing caloric expenditure.

Even though physical activity increases energy expenditure, the efficacy of increased physical activity to promote weight loss is *at best equivocal*, as will be discussed. Although physical activity on its own may not be an entirely effective vehicle for weight loss, it can enhance dietary adherence and efficiency, can promote a host of medical and psychological benefits apart from weight loss, and is a potent preventive measure against obesity. Therefore, an understanding of how to initiate an exercise program and ensure adherence, and the ability to create effective programs that increase physical activity, are indispensable skills in the battle against obesity.

After a brief introduction to some key concepts in the physical activity literature, this chapter examines exercise recommendations by the US government and expert organizations, physical activity levels in the population, the efficacy of exercise as a weight reduction tool, additional health benefits of exercise, and issues related to exercise initiation, adherence, and programming.

Physical Activity and Measurements of Energy Expenditure

Definitions

Organisms require energy to support life and interact with their environments. Animals require energy to carry out metabolic and essential body functions such as respiration and neurological activity. The daily total energy use of all these life-sustaining functions is called the *basal metabolic rate* (*BMR*). An individual's BMR is approximately 1 kilocalorie per kilogram of body weight per hour; thus, heavier individuals have higher BMRs than their lighter peers.[2] BMR, however, is only one contributor to the overall energy budget. Additional energy expenditure derives from the myriad daily tasks that require postural adjustment or movement, such as walking, dusting, or biking, all of which are accommodated under the umbrella term *physical activity*. The breadth of physical activity is captured by the definition given in the 2005 edition of the American *Dietary Reference Intakes* (hereafter referred to as the *DRI*): physical activity is "bodily movement that is produced by the contraction of muscle that substantially increases energy expenditure" (FNB/IOM, 2005, p. 891).

---

[2]For example, an individual who weighs 80 kilograms will have a BMR of approximately 80 kcal/h. By contrast, an individual who weights 50 kilograms will have a BMR of about 50 kcal/h. This difference reflects the increased energy needs of maintaining life-sustaining functions in a larger individual.

Types of physical activity

There are two general categories of physical activity: unplanned and planned. Unplanned activities are the tasks of daily independent living that are generally utilitarian in nature. Walking to the car, taking out the garbage, and mopping the floor are all examples of unplanned physical activity. Each expends energy and generally serves as a means to another end, not as an end in itself. By contrast, planned physical activity consists of "planned structured and repetitive bodily movements done to promote or maintain one or more components of physical fitness" (FNB/IOM, 2005, p. 891). Planned physical activity, commonly referred to as *exercise* or *leisure-time physical activity*, can be further categorized into endurance and resistance, as Table 8.1 shows.

Endurance exercises involve repeated, rhythmic motions of integrated skeletal groups that are sustained by, and therefore enhance, the cardiovascular system (e.g., heart, lungs, circulatory networks). Endurance training, more commonly called *cardiovascular exercise*, or simply *cardio* (because of its targeted beneficiary), involves long-term movement (10 minutes or more) and is therefore highly aerobic in nature (i.e., uses large amounts of oxygen). *Resistance* training, in contrast, is characterized by short bursts of energy use, primarily by skeletal muscles, and is generally anaerobic in nature (i.e., relies primarily on the creatine system—the body system that powers short-term movements). This intense use of skeletal muscle generates considerable force and ultimately results in muscular growth and increased strength. Circuit and weight training are examples of resistance training.

Measures that express energy consumption: absolute versus relative

By definition, both unplanned and (both forms of) planned physical activities consume energy, and sustained increases in either area increase daily energy expenditure. However, some forms of physical activity place a greater energy demand on the body to sustain the desired movements. Simply stated, the more intense

Table 8.1
Types of Physical Activity

Types of physical activity	Target body systems	Examples
Unplanned	Cardiovascular, skeletal, muscular	Mopping, bed making, walking to the car
Planned		
Endurance	Cardiovascular, skeletal	Running, swimming, rowing, biking
Resistance	Skeletal, muscular	Sit-ups, bench press, pin-weight circuit

an exercise is, the greater is its energy demand. Similarly, the longer an activity lasts, the greater is its energy demand. Thus the relationship between exercise intensity and duration provides a basis for estimating the amount of energy needed for a particular exercise. One measure of the cost of exercise is absolute: energy expended as expressed in kilocalories (kcal) or kilojoules (kJ).[3] The other measure, metabolic equivalents (METs) is more relative. Let's examine both measures.

ABSOLUTE   Probably the most obvious way to express energy use is in energy units used per unit of time (e.g., kilocalories per hour). Because increased intensity and increased duration require more energy, it is possible to determine the energy requirements for exercise based on the intensity and duration of any activity. This method is useful on a personal level, but not on a population level, for determining the energy costs of exercise. The reason the method does not work on the population level is that proportionally more energy is required to move a heavier object than a lighter one over a given distance. Thus, a 70-kilogram individual will expend more energy than a 50-kilogram individual for any given task. Likewise, the 70-kilogram individual will expend more energy more quickly than a 50-kilogram individual will, thus requiring less physical activity to achieve that energy output goal. Therefore, a generic recommendation to, for example, burn 100 kilocalories per day, will require less physical activity by a heavier person than by a lighter person.

The relationship between body mass index (BMI) and total daily energy expenditure is linear (Schulz & Schoeller, 1994). Heavier individuals have a higher BMR and also burn more energy when engaged in physical activities. In general, heavier individuals expend more energy per unit of time. Yet an increased level of energy expenditure does not shift the energy balance, because the number of calories burned is proportional to the body weight for a given task. Consequently, expressing energy expenditure in absolute terms, though useful to an individual at a constant weight, proves methodologically impractical on a population level, or to someone whose weight is in flux. Therefore, a measurement was devised to hold stable the relationship between energy expenditure and body mass.

RELATIVE: MET   The relational aspect of energy expenditure and body mass is captured by the concept of metabolic equivalents (METs), which standardizes exercise intensity. METs take into account body mass by describing energy expenditure in reference to the BMR (a measure that inherently accounts for body mass). A MET of 1 means that no energy is being expended beyond that supplied by the BMR (i.e., 1 MET = BMR), and a MET of 3 means that energy expenditure is three times greater than the BMR. In caloric terms,

$$1 \text{ MET} = 1 \text{ kcal/kg of body weight/hour of exercise} \tag{8.1}$$

---

[3]There are approximately 4.2 kilojoules per kilocalorie.

The Compendium of Physical Activities (Ainsworth et al., 2000) provides MET values associated with thousands of different physical activities—ranging from sprinting to shuffling cards. The compendium makes it possible to determine the exercise intensity of a given activity and use that MET to calculate actual caloric output using equation (8.1). Standardizing exercise intensity through METs readily allows planning by individuals of different BMIs to target caloric loss relative to their body mass. Moreover, the MET allows for population guidelines for particular physical activities that do not stumble over the proportionality issue already described.

Physical activity level and daily energy expenditure

Exercise intensity expands readily to physical activity level (PAL), which is a ratio reflecting overall daily energy expenditure. Calculating PAL first requires determining one's resting energy expenditure (REE), an estimate of the body's overall daily energy expenditure while at rest. The following examples REE equations vary by biological sex and age:

Males:

Ages 18–29: (15.3 × body weight in kg) + 679 $\qquad$ (8.2)

Ages 30–60: (11.6 × body weight in kg) + 879 $\qquad$ (8.3)

Females:

Ages 18–29: (14.7 × body weight in kg) + 496 $\qquad$ (8.4)

Ages 30–60: (8.7 × body weight in kg) + 829 $\qquad$ (8.5)

This information enables the calculation of PAL, which is a comparison of one's overall daily energy expenditure (DEE)—including calories expended through exercise—to one's REE:

$$PAL = (REE + DEE)/BMR + 0.1 \qquad (8.6)^{4}$$

Equation (8.6) presents the relationship between exercise (planned and unplanned) and daily caloric expenditure. This relationship provides a rule of thumb for targeting one's daily estimated energy requirement (EER) to maintain the desired level of energy balance for either weight maintenance or weight loss. There are four categories of PAL:

---

[4] A PAL of 1 would imply that the individual burns no calories beyond those associated with basic life functions. Although a PAL of 1 is theoretically possible, in normal practice a minimal PAL would be 1.1, because a "bonus" of 0.1 is added to the calculated ratio to account for calories expended digesting food and the slight metabolic boost experienced after a meal (called the *thermic effect of a meal*).

1. **Sedentary:** PAL 1.10–1.39

2. **Low active:** PAL 1.40–1.59

3. **Active:** PAL 1.60–1.89

4. **High active:** PAL 1.9–2.5

This categorization can help approximate individual EER, which can then be compared to actual energy intake. EER is determined by separate equations on the basis of one's PAL grouping and biological sex, and it takes into account body mass and height (see Table 8.2).

In obese people, by definition, energy intake exceeds EER. If an obese person wishes to lose weight, then either intake must be reduced (by caloric restriction) or EER must be increased through physical activity, or both. Regular exercise is encouraged as a path toward matching EER to actual intake. Indeed, both gov-

---

Table 8.2
Estimated Energy Requirement Equations

Males: EER = 662 − 9.53 × age + [PAC × (15.91 × weight in kg × height in m)]
Females: EER = 354 − 6.91 × age + [PAC × (9.361 × weight in kg + 726 × height in m)]
where PAC (physical activity coefficient) is based on PAL:

	PAC	
PAL	Males	Females
Sedentary	1.00	1.00
Low active	1.11	1.12
Active	1.25	1.27
High active	1.48	1.45

Example: A 20-year-old man weighs 70 kg and is 1.70 m tall. His PAL is 1.45. Find his PAC. A male with a PAL of 1.45 is "low active." Therefore, his PAC is 1.11.
Using the equation for males:

EER =   662 − 9.53 × 20 + [1.11 × (15.91 × 70 × 1.7)]
          662 − 190.6 + [1.11 × 1893.29]
          471.4 + 2101.55
          2572.95

Therefore, on the basis of this man's current age, height, weight, and activity level, he requires 2573 kilocalories a day to maintain his current weight and level of activity. Energy consumption above this amount may cause him to gain weight; energy consumption below this amount may cause him to lose weight. Note that as his age, body mass, or activity level changes, so will his EER.

ernment panels and expert professional organizations have developed recommendations regarding the optimal level of physical activity for healthy living (which, as will be shown, is not the same as losing weight).

Exercise Recommendations and Population Activity Levels

Recommendations

The 2005 *DRI* (FNB/IOM, 2005) recommends that individuals engage in 60 minutes daily of accumulated moderate-intensity activity (3–4 METs) to help maximize exercise benefits for health and disease prevention. Daily accumulated activity allows one to engage in exercise bursts throughout the day, rather than requiring a more restrictive 60-minute block that may be difficult for some individuals to achieve because of work or fitness restrictions (FNB/IOM, 2005). Indeed, Murphy and colleagues (2002) demonstrated that, in middle-aged women, three daily 10-minute bursts of moderate-intensity walking yielded similar cardiovascular and psychological benefits, including reduced anxiety and depressive symptoms as did one half-hour exercise session. Such results reify the *DRI*'s message that accumulated activity can be just as effective as a single, prolonged exercise session.

As one might expect of attempts at population-level recommendations, there are some differences among guidelines published by different groups. The American College of Sports Medicine (ACSM), for example, recommends moderate-intensity (based on heart rate) exercise for a daily accumulation of 20 to 60 minutes, with minimum bouts of 10 minutes, 3 to 5 days a week, to achieve cardiovascular fitness. Although the ACSM acknowledges that more frequent exercise would burn more calories—a defining component of weight loss— additional exercise provides disproportionately increasing risk for injury and burnout (ACSM, 1998). In its 2001 statement, the ACSM acknowledges that obese individuals may need to exercise approximately 200 to 300 minutes per week to achieve energy balance, meaning that they must exercise at the higher end of the 1998 population recommendations, though not nearly as much as recommended by the 2005 *DRI*. A 1996 report by the US surgeon general provides a midpoint between these two recommendations, suggesting 30 minutes of moderate-intensity physical activity most days of the week (Pate et al., 1995). Thus, although there is some disagreement concerning ideal daily exercise levels to maximize health, there is unanimity on the benefit of exercise and on the need for Americans to become more active.

Population activity levels

Most Americans do not begin to meet even the most relaxed physical activity guideline. Sixty percent are not regularly physically active, and an astonishing 25% report no planned physical activity in the preceding month (FNB/IOM,

2005). Indeed, only 22% of Americans exercise for at least 30 minutes daily (Rippe & Hess, 1998). Generally, people who live in developed countries have PALs in the "low active" range (Schulz & Schoeller, 1994).

Activity levels in obese people are of particular concern because, in association with poor eating habits, low activity levels may accelerate weight gain. Activity reports among the obese are conflicting. The *DRI* suggests that most obese people are at least "low active" (FNB/IOM, 2005). In a well-designed study using doubly labeled water,[5] Westerterp (1999b) did not establish a relationship between PAL and BMI, suggesting that obese individuals are no more likely to be sedentary than are their nonobese peers. These views are described in Westerterp's (1999a) comprehensive review of PAL in relation to obesity, which concludes that "the majority of obese subjects is [sic] moderately active and an increase in the activity level of obese subjects is limited by the ability to perform exercise of higher intensity" (p. 24). In contrast, Schulz and Schoeller (1994) reported a negative relationship between BMI and PAL, especially in men. Of note, however, very few individuals in that study reported a PAL of 1.1, and most were clustered below 1.50, suggesting that although very few individuals were entirely sedentary, most were not highly active either. Finally, Wessel and colleagues (2004) found a negative relationship between measures of adiposity and self-reported exercise.

Although the data regarding activity levels in the obese are conflicting, there is agreement that obese people are not fully sedentary as a group and do engage in modest levels of activity. Therefore, exercise programming for the obese requires a focus on increasing PAL from "low active" to "active," rather than the more difficult task of transitioning from "sedentary" to "low active." However, the practicality and sustainability of such an increase is questionable, especially given the modest efficacy of exercise in producing weight loss in the obese (discussed next). As will be detailed later in the chapter, establishing obesity prevention programs holds greater promise on a population level.

Exercise Efficacy in Weight Loss

Endurance exercise

Given the potential benefit of exercise in generating a negative energy balance, it is not surprising that exercise as an obesity intervention has drawn considerable attention. Studies in this area have often focused on endurance exercise, which, because of its prolonged and aerobic nature, can generate greater caloric benefits than resistance training can. Although using greater energy per unit of time, resistance training is characterized by short bursts of explosive energy,

---

[5]The use of doubly labeled water (DLW) is considered to be one of the highest quality research methods for assessing metabolism and physical activity. Although theoretically complex, the DLW method is based on assessing the turnover of body gases and fluids during energy use. DLW provides a marker of such turnover. Although the DLW method is the "gold standard" in this area of research, its high cost limits its use.

rather than prolonged, consistent energy expenditure; that character of resistance training diminishes its overall caloric use.

The potential of exercise for helping obese people lose weight has been best characterized by a commonly cited analysis of 784 individuals in the US National Weight Control Registry.[6] These participants reported exercising for at least 60 minutes daily (i.e., were "active" to "high active") and reported burning 2800 kilocalories a week through mostly endurance exercise (Klem et al., 1997). They were also dieting intensively. The retrospective nature of the study precludes disentangling the weight loss generated by exercise from that brought about by caloric restriction. Still, it does point to exercise as being an integral part of weight loss. Some other, less commonly cited studies also point to exercise as being beneficial in producing weight loss (Table 8.3).

The weight loss described by Klem and colleagues (1997) is unusual for its success. Indeed, a considerable literature exists that poses a substantial challenge to the notion that exercise alone can treat obesity. A comprehensive review of such exercise research programs (Wing, 1999) reported that in studies comparing an exercise intervention group versus a control obese group, exercisers expe-

---

[6]Individuals listed in the registry are highly successful at weight loss, having maintained at least 30 pounds of weight loss over a 1-year period. Those included in the study by Klem and colleagues (1997) were remarkably successful, averaging an approximate 65-pound weight loss over 5 years.

Table 8.3
Five Selected Studies Demonstrating Weight Loss Induced by Exercise Only

Study	Population	Study design	Results[a]
Klem et al., 1997	Men and women in National Weight Control Registry	Retrospective surveys	Mean 30-lb weight loss was maintained for at least 5 years
Anderssen et al., 1995	219 men and women	Control vs. exercise vs. diet/exercise vs. diet groups	C gained 1.1 kg; E lost 0.9 kg ($p < 0.05$)
Donnelly et al. 2003	131 men and women	Control vs. exercise groups	Men: C lost 0.5 kg; E lost 5.2 kg Women: C gained 2.9 kg; E gained 0.6 kg ($p < 0.05$ for both)
Irwin et al., 2003	173 women	Control vs. exercise groups	C gained 0.1 kg; E lost 1.3 kg ($p < 0.05$).
Stewart et al., 2005	115 men and women	Control vs. exercise groups	C lost 0.5 kg; E lost 2.3 kg ($p < 0.05$).

Note: All studies utilized a randomized design and had an intervention period of at least 4 months. Exercise groups consumed diets with similar daily caloric values. See Catenacci & Wyatt, 2007 for a complete review.

[a]C, control group; E, exercise group.

rienced an average weight loss of 2.4 kilograms over the 4- to 12-month course of the studies. In light of the their duration, Wing concludes that these programs yield "modest" effects (1999, p. 548). Similarly, Miller and colleagues (1997), in a meta-analysis of 493 studies evaluating the relationship between exercise efficacy and weight loss, reported a mean weight loss of just 0.2 pound per week.

Given such lackluster results, Hill and Wyatt (2005) conclude that "although it is possible to lose weight with physical activity alone, the amount of physical activity required for substantial weight loss is well beyond what is feasible for most Americans in today's environment" (p. 766). Catenacci and Wyatt (2007) concur, stating that although exercise *can* generate some degree of weight loss, that weight loss is typically modest, and the level of exercise required to maintain those losses may well be beyond the capabilities of most people. These conclusions provide an intriguing, albeit sad, insight into today's obesity epidemic.

Though potentially helpful if one stays the course, a slow rate of weight loss can be discouraging; indeed, the majority of individuals exercising for weight loss terminate their programs within 6 months (Dishman, 1982; Miller et al., 1997). This attrition rate is unfortunate because (1) exercise programs are most effective at producing weight loss when maintained for longer than 12 months (Jakicic & Otto, 2005) and (2) exercise has other health-related benefits for the obese besides weight loss, as will be discussed later.

Exercise may also help prevent the return of lost weight. In a 12-month follow-up study of 34 women who had lost at least 12 kilograms (26.5 pounds) through a variety of exercise programs, 30 of the 34 women regained at least some weight (a mean of 7.1 kilograms, approximately 15 pounds), with one individual regaining 40 kilograms (about 88 pounds). Highly active participants regained the lowest amount of weight but had engaged in a minimum of 1.3 hours daily of moderate-intensity (4 METs) physical activity (Schoeller et al., 1997). This level exceeds the upper bounds of even the *DRI* recommendations. Long-term sustainability of such high levels of physical activity is questionable, given that almost all the women exercising gained back some weight.

These exercise activities may simply have been of insufficient intensity to induce energy balance (e.g., match PAL to EER). Eighty minutes a day is well beyond the reach of almost all (Miller, 2004). High-intensity activity, however, does not require as long a period of daily commitment. Unfortunately, many obese individuals are unable to sustain high-intensity physical activity (Ekkekakis & Lind, 2006; Miller, 2004; Westerterp, 1999a). Accordingly, the ability of low-intensity exercise for more reasonable periods of time to generate weight loss is questionable.

Resistance exercise

Although endurance exercise has commonly been used in weight reduction programs, resistance exercise may also provide benefit. The sections that follow describe the mechanisms conferring that benefit, and review some studies that have used resistance exercise to generate weight loss.

MECHANISMS   The influence of endurance exercise on weight loss is limited by the natural processes of the weight loss itself, particularly as induced either by dieting or by endurance exercise. Both fat mass and lean mass contribute to total weight loss, with its concomitant reduction in body mass. What matters, though, is the *type* of weight loss, not simply weight loss per se. Because lean mass has a higher basal metabolic rate (BMR) than does fat mass, it requires more energy to sustain (Forbes & Welle, 1983; Hill & Wyatt, 2005). It follows, therefore, that a loss of lean mass causes a sharper BMR decline than would an equal loss of fat mass. From the perspective of energy balance, loss of lean mass results in a sharper decline in daily energy requirement than would an equal loss of fat mass. Accordingly, if a person maintains a stable diet, having lost lean mass, then in comparison with a person who has lost fat mass, the former will have to work harder to maintain the same rate of weight loss because consumed food will not be as fully metabolized and will be preferentially stored as fat. Thus, a loss of lean mass requires the individual to either (1) reduce caloric intake or (2) increase PAL so as not to regain weight.

Unlike endurance exercise, resistance exercise, through its capacity to hypertrophy skeletal muscle, can protect or even enhance muscle mass. Thus, the inclusion of resistance exercise in a weight loss program helps protect lean mass and, in principle, safeguards against sharp declines in BMR and EER. However, as with endurance exercise, research results on the efficacy of resistance exercise in assisting weight loss are mixed.

EFFICACY OF RESISTANCE EXERCISE IN WEIGHT LOSS   In a comparison of the impact of resistance exercise (RE), diet (D), and a combination of the two (RED) on body composition, Ballor and colleagues (1988) divided 40 female subjects into one of four groups: RE, D, RED, or a nonexercising, nondieting control. Groups that included exercise as part of the intervention experienced statistically significant gains in muscle mass (1.08 kilograms and 0.42 kilogram, respectively) compared to the D group and controls. Dieting groups (D, RED) lost significant amounts of fat mass and experienced a reduction in body fat percentage and body mass, compared to nondieting groups. These results suggest the importance of resistance exercise in maintaining lean mass, especially when engaging in other activities (e.g., dieting) that may otherwise reduce lean mass. Indeed, the RED group was not only able to prevent loss of lean mass, but actually gained lean mass while reducing fat mass, resulting in what would be, theoretically, an improved metabolic profile. However, metabolic variables were not included in this study.

Van Etten and colleagues (1997) evaluated RE effects on sedentary men of a high body fat percentage (BF%; mean preintervention BF% = 24)[7] and included metabolic profiles as outcome variables. Participants engaged in an 18-week

---

[7]Normal body fat percentage in men is less than 20.

weight-training program while consuming an isocaloric diet. Although body mass remained roughly stable over the course of the study (+0.1 kilogram), exercising men lost 2.0 kilograms of fat mass and gained 2.1 kilograms of lean mass, resulting in a 2.6% reduction in BF%. Note, however, that an inactive control group, during the same period, lost 1.4 kilograms of fat mass, yielding a 1.6% difference in BF%. These body composition changes resulted in an average daily metabolic rate (ADMR)[8] increase of approximately 1 megajoule (about 240 kilocalories).

Together, these and other studies argue for a complementary role between resistance exercise and traditional methods of weight loss such as dieting. Compliance issues aside, exercise, particularly resistance exercise, may enhance the effects of dieting by protecting lean mass and thus partially ameliorating changes to EER. Indeed, diet and exercise can be a powerful combination in combating obesity, not only because of their complementary physiological effects, but also because exercise may enhance diet compliance and increase efficiency in metabolizing ingested food.

Diet and exercise

Traditional thought on the relation between exercise and diet held that increased exercise resulted in increased energy intake so as to compensate for energy loss, thereby resulting in no net gain (Mayer et al., 1956). If such a relationship were true, it would augur poorly for exercise as an obesity treatment. Fortunately, such is not the case. Koulouri and colleagues (2006) reported that, for adult women enrolled in a walking program, increased exercise did not result in increased food intake. This decoupling between exercise and energy intake is not surprising. As noted by Blundell and King (1999) and argued elsewhere in this volume, food intake is loosely coupled with physiological triggers, and psychosocial influences often drive food intake. Thus, although a prolonged bout of exercise may induce hunger, it does not provoke a 1:1 ratio of intake to expenditure, as Mayer and colleagues (1956) had suggested. Decoupling of exercise losses and eating gains strengthens a two-pronged approach of exercise and diet in obesity treatment.

Combined exercise and diet programs yield better weight loss results than does either method alone. For example, a meta-analysis of diet programs, exercise programs, and diet-plus-exercise programs on weight loss demonstrated that diet and exercise yielded the greatest loss in body mass (11.0 kilograms, compared to 10.7 and 2.9 kilograms for diet and exercise alone, respectively) and the greatest loss in BF% (9.0%, compared to 7.8% and 3.3%; Miller et al., 1997). In recent reviews of literature on exercise as obesity treatment, both Jakicic and Otto (2005) and Catenacci and Wyatt (2007) came to a similar conclusion, asserting that diet and exercise combined have the greatest effect on weight loss.

---

[8]ADMR = BMR + caloric cost of exercise + thermic effect of food.

Note from the meta-analysis by Miller and colleagues (1997), as well as the study on resistance training by Baylor and colleagues (1988), that diet produced the bulk of weight loss. For Miller, exercise yielded only an additional 0.3 kilogram lost over diet alone (not a statistically significant difference); and for Ballor, the diet-only group actually lost 0.58 kilogram more than the combined group (also not statistically significant). Thus, the role of exercise may be to protect resting metabolic rate from the deleterious effects of weight loss by protecting lean mass. However, exercise may also promote better diet adherence. As noted already, diets have particularly poor adherence rates, especially in the long term (Volek et al., 2005; Foster et al., 2003); thus, any benefit that caloric restriction may provide is lost when the diet ends. For instance, Jakicic, Wing, and Winters-Hart (2002) demonstrated that increases in physical activity were related to decreases in energy intake in overweight women. Similarly, Villanova and associates (2006) note that physical activity can be used to promote weight loss after a behavioral intervention focusing on the intake of healthful foods. Individuals who engaged in the greatest amount of exercise after the end of the intervention lost the most weight in the long term. Given the equivocal effect of exercise on weight loss, these results suggest that exercise acted as a proxy for other healthy behaviors included in the program, such as dieting.

Exercise and weight loss maintenance

Finally, exercise plays an important role in maintaining weight loss (Hill & Wyatt, 2005). However, as outlined in the preceding discussion (Klem et al., 1997; Schoeller et al., 1997), the amount of exercise necessary to maintain weight loss is quite high, and may not be sustainable. Thus, although diet and exercise combined may facilitate weight loss, the long-term fate of that weight loss is questionable. Ultimately, then, exercise, paired with diet or on its own, may not provide a viable long-term solution to obesity treatment. Yet although exercise may not facilitate weight loss—and levels of exercise that do facilitate weight loss may be unrealistic—even at low levels exercise provides important metabolic, physiological, and psychological benefits that should not be ignored. Indeed, although exercise may not treat obesity per se, it can assist in treating the medical complications often associated with the condition.

Health Benefits of Exercise

Cardiovascular health

Although exercise programs may not routinely produce substantial weight loss, *they do provide health-related benefits*.

CARDIAC EVENTS AND HEART ATTACK   A groundbreaking epidemiological study of 908 individuals conducted by Wessel and associates (2004) assessed the relationships among physical fitness, BMI, and both the incidence of adverse cardiac events (e.g., congestive heart failure, unstable angina) and major adverse cardiac events (death, heart attack, stroke) in women. Fitness was defined by self-reported ability to engage in physical activities that approximate at least 7 METs,[9] as well as by answers to a questionnaire regarding average activity levels. Interestingly, both fit nonobese and fit obese women experienced statistically similar incidences in both categories of adverse events. In the all-events category, the incidence was 23.9% for nonobese versus 28.4% for obese; for the major-events category, 5.6% for nonobese and 9.5% for obese, respectively. In contrast, the nonfit nonobese and the nonfit obese women reported all-events incidences of 42.9% for nonobese versus 41.6% for obese; and for major events, 16.8% for nonobese versus 14.3% for obese, respectively.

The incidence differences between obesity statuses for the nonfit women were not statistically significant, but those incidences were significantly greater than the ones reported in either category of fit women. In summarizing, the authors claimed that "level of physical activity and functional capacity are more important than weight status or body habitus for CV [cardiovascular] risk stratification in women" (Wessel et al., 2004, p. 1185). Accordingly, risk of cardiovascular obesity-related problems may be better explained by low levels of fitness than by obesity per se.

Laukkanen and colleagues (2004) concur. They found that even a 1-MET increase in the level of peak oxygen consumption—a marker of physical fitness—was linked with reduced risk of death due to coronary artery disease and other adverse cardiac events, such as stroke or heart failure. Given these research findings, the American Heart Association issued a position statement (AHA, 2003), endorsed by the ACSM, asserting that physical activity can help lower the risk of cardiac problems. Although the association's statement does not address weight loss, it provides a role for exercise in mitigating the risk of bad cardiovascular health, including that caused by obesity.

HYPERTENSION   High blood pressure (hypertension) is associated with many of the lifestyle patterns of obese people, including high salt intake, a fatty diet, and low levels of exercise. Considerable research suggests that regular (mean of three sessions per week for 15 to 70 minutes each), moderate-intensity exercise not only prevents future blood pressure problems, but helps correct hypertension in those already afflicted (Fagard, 1999).

---

[9]This is not to say these women regularly engage in endurance exercise at an intensity of 7 METs (which would be considered vigorous activity). Instead, this measure signifies that these women have the cardiovascular capacity to circulate adequate oxygen to engage, for at least several minutes, in a 7-MET endurance activity. A rough linear relationship exists between exercise intensity (METs) and liters of oxygen required by the body, per minute, to sustain that intensity of activity (about 3.5 L/min per MET). According to Ainsworth and colleagues' (2000) *Compendium*, 7 METs is equivalent to walking at a pace of 5 miles per hour.

Abdominal fat and metabolic profile

Exercise preferentially reduces abdominal obesity, thereby improving an individual's metabolic profile. This is important because abdominal obesity, in particular visceral abdominal fat, enhances risk for type 2 diabetes, the metabolic syndrome, and adverse cardiac events (Matsuzawa et al., 1995; Okura et al., 2004; Tanaka et al., 2004).

Exercise may also reduce abdominal fat. Ross and Katzmarzyk (2003) assessed BMI, fitness level, and body and abdominal fat in over 7500 adults. Within any BMI group, those who exhibited greater aerobic capacity had lower levels of both body fat and abdominal fat. These results suggest that exercise may reduce the harm associated with obesity by generating a more favorable body composition. Note, however, that regardless of fitness level, higher BMIs were positively related to higher waist circumference (a measure of abdominal fat). Thus, although exercise can produce favorable changes in body composition, even in the obese, it may be favorable to be both fit *and* trim.

These results are supported by recent work on obese and overweight European children (Nassis et al., 2005). Cardiovascular fitness level, measures of body and abdominal fat, and BMI were assessed in 742 boys and 620 girls. Individuals with higher levels of cardiovascular fitness level (after accounting for sex and age) had lower levels of abdominal and total fat when compared to others of a similar BMI. The review by Mayo, Grantham, and Balasekaran (1999) also suggests that exercise can reduce abdominal fat. They note, however, that research in this area is limited and conclusions should be made accordingly. Overall, exercise seems to decrease abdominal adiposity, but these are early findings.

Type 2 diabetes, glucose metabolism, and insulin resistance

Another problem associated with elevated BMI is insulin resistance (type 2 diabetes) and elevated blood glucose levels. Regular physical activity may diminish type 2 diabetes. According to Kelley and Goodpaster's (1999) review, exercise affects insulin action and glucose metabolism and reduces both obesity-related insulin resistance and glucose intolerance. Significantly, both endurance and resistance exercise help. Exercise influences were independent of weight loss: even when exercise did not induce weight loss, it improved insulin action and reduced blood glucose to more normal levels.

Subsequent studies have been supportive. For instance, Slentz and colleagues (2002) enrolled five dyslipidemic adults in a 9-month endurance exercise program that involved four weekly 60-minute endurance exercise sessions at moderate to high intensity (70% to 80% of VO_2 max, or maximal oxygen consumption). Body mass, fasting glucose, insulin sensitivity, and cholesterol levels were measured during pre- and post-training, at 0, 5, and 30 days. Although body mass was reduced by approximately 3 kilograms immediately following training, by 30 days the loss had been reclaimed. Fasting glucose levels, however, dropped significantly (from 5.39 to 4.46 millimoles) during training, and remained stable for 30 days. This study was typical: exercise did not induce a lasting change in body mass, but it persistently improved other metabolic factors on a longer-term basis. The benefits of exercise on insulin and glucose have been codified. As such, frequent (three to five times a week, for 30 to 60 minutes each time), moderate-intensity exercise, among other population guidelines, such as a healthful diet, is encouraged to help prevent type 2 diabetes (Kirska, 2003).

Dyslipidemias and fat metabolism

Associated with insulin resistance and high blood glucose are high levels of free fatty acids that contribute to the development of triglyceride production (such as cholesterol), excess glucose production by the liver, and poor fat metabolism (Perez-Martin, Raynaud & Mercier, 2001). Exercise-induced improvements in insulin action help mitigate these changes. Goodpaster, Katsiaras, and Kelley (2003) studied these changes in 25 obese participants in a 16-week endurance exercise program of four to six weekly sessions of 30 to 40 minutes per session. Both visceral and subcutaneous body fat depots were diminished by an average of 5.1 kilograms (11.25 pounds). Insulin action improved by 49% because of a 159% improvement in nonoxidative glucose disposal. Moreover, the loss of body fat and improvement in insulin sensitivity were strongly positively correlated ($r = 0.62$). Moreover, participants lost about 8 kilograms (17.6 pounds) of body mass (as anticipated, given the diet-and-exercise regimen). Importantly, an exercise-only group did not lose weight. Nonetheless, their insulin action also improved, although significantly less than was observed in the combined intervention group (16% improvement versus 61% improvement). See also Perez-Martin, Raynaud, and Mercier, 2001 for corroborative data on exercise effects on lipid metabolism and free fatty acid levels.

While exerting an influence on insulin-based mobilization of fat stores, exercise may produce a more modest impact on cholesterol levels. Stefanick (1999) provided a muted conclusion in this regard, asserting that exercise alone, at best, produces minimal changes in an individual's cholesterol profile, with most studies demonstrating only a quite modest change of between 0.11 and 0.25 millimole. However, Stefanick notes that exercise, when paired with a low-fat diet, can promote positive changes in these triglycerides, though the amount of that impact depends on the saturated fat content of the diet. These results, while providing a mixed image of the efficacy of exercise on cholesterol levels, do hint at the importance of an intervention based on both diet and exercise, and do not unequivocally negate the importance of exercise in this regard.

Other benefits, total morbidity, and mortality

Exercise provides benefits beyond the cardiovascular and metabolic benefits identified in the previous sections. It increases bone mineral density, thereby reducing the risk of osteoporosis (Kraemer et al., 2002; Warburton et al., 2006).

Furthermore, regular exercise reduces the risk of a wide host of hormonally linked cancers (including breast, prostate, colon, and endometrial cancers (Hewitt et al., 2005; Wu et al., 2006; Hanna & Adams, 2006; Irwin, 2006; Rissanen & Fogelholm, 1999), and it helps improve the outcomes of factors that are more difficult to evaluate, such as quality of life and satisfaction with life (Blissmer et al., 2006; Bowen et al., 2006). Exercise has proven useful in preventing and treating clinical depression (Ernst et al., 2006; Tsang et al., 2006; Harris et al., 2006), and it may help arrest cigarette smoking (Schneider et al., 2007).

Although the underlying mechanisms differ for each benefit, the inescapable conclusion is that physical fitness helps prolong life, in ways that can be more fully enjoyed by individuals. According to Blair and colleagues (1989), physical fitness level was a better predictor than BMI for all-cause mortality in both men and women. Exercise especially reduced risks related to cardiovascular disease, cancer, and type 2 diabetes. Thus, as discussed earlier, a substantial literature has established the health benefits of exercise and suggests that they can be reaped independently of weight loss.

Backlash

The notion that exercise does not have to bring about weight loss to significantly improve an individual's health challenges the traditional emphasis on the centrality of weight loss for recapturing good health, and it has generated a flurry of research that places many of these findings in a larger perspective. For example, Mora and colleagues (2006) examined BMI, physical activity, and cardiovascular biomarkers in a sample of 27,158 middle-aged women. As Table 8.4 shows, physically active individuals were at lower risk for health negatives, as were individuals with lower BMIs. However, risk was reduced in lower-BMI categories regardless of exercise status. In particular, inactive normal-weight women were at lower risk than were active obese women, with no overlap in variance between the two categories for many risk factors. Mora's group concedes, however, that "physical activity and BMI were only weakly and inversely correlated" (p. 1414), suggesting, as argued earlier in the chapter, that the obese are no more likely to be sedentary than are their thinner peers. These results are similar to the findings of Christou and colleagues (2005), who assessed 135 men for various cardiovascular health markers, BMI, and other measures of adiposity, in addition to aerobic capacity. Although aerobic capacity mitigated some risk factors, obesity status was a stronger predictor of cardiovascular health.

Finally, an epidemiological study (Hu et al., 2004) of over 116,000 individuals found that both adiposity and physical activity were strong, independent predictors of premature death. However, physical inactivity (less than 3.5 hours of exercise per week) and elevated BMI (>25), when combined, accounted for 31% of premature deaths in their sample. Thus, different experimental and epidemiological studies agree on improved health benefits through exercise, which mitigate but do not eliminate the negative consequences of elevated BMI.

Table 8.4
Impact of Physical Activity and BMI on Selected Measures of Cardiovascular Health

	Physical Activity					
	Group					
Biomarker	5 (most active)	4	3	2	1 (least active)	p
C-reactive protein (mg/L)[a]	1.78	1.78	1.9	2.11	2.54	<0.001
LDL cholesterol (mg/dL)[b]	119.2	120.1	121.1	122.1	124.6	<0.001
Fibrinogen (mg/dL)[c]	345	346	349	354	362	<0.001

	BMI					
	Group					
Biomarker	<21.9	21.9–23.8	23.8–25.8	25.8–29.3	>29.3	p
C-reactive protein (mg/L)	0.87	1.31	1.85	2.64	4.49	<0.001
LDL cholesterol (mg/dL)	112.7	18.4	123.7	126	125.9	<0.001
Fibrinogen (mg/dL)	322	335	350	362	393	<0.001

Source: After Mora et al., 2006.
[a]Raised levels of C-reactive protein, a marker of inflammation, are related to cardiovascular disease.
[b]LDL cholesterol (low-density lipoprotein, or "bad cholesterol") is a lipoprotein associated with vascular congestion and cardiovascular disease.
[c]Excess levels of fibrinogen, a blood-clotting agent, are related to cardiovascular disease.

On these grounds, it is reasonable to recommend that all individuals be physically active (adhering to the guidelines reviewed earlier) with the goal of fitness and *not necessarily of attaining a normal BMI*. Recall that exercise provides only modest benefit in regard to weight loss because weight loss is not rapid enough to sustain the behavior, and, like diet regimes, exercise programs are marred by adherence problems, especially in the "obesogenic culture" of contemporary American society. These two trends signal difficulty in achieving, and maintaining, a normal body mass. Unfortunately, these predictions have been repeatedly borne out in the consistent failure of exercise to sustain weight loss.

Physical Activity as Obesity Prevention

As demonstrated, exercise potently combats the ill health outcomes often associated with obesity, but it is not a useful tool for weight reduction; indeed, exercise-only weight reduction programs generally produce negligible outcomes.

Although a few investigators have raised the possibility of being healthy and heavy (e.g., Blair & LaMonte, 2005), debate on that issue is ongoing. All would agree that good health is best achieved through exercise and a normal BMI, and no literature suggests that being fit and thin is unhealthy. The overall lack of benefit of exercise to weight reduction, and the reversal of gain when exercise programs are suspended or contracted, suggest the low efficiency of exercise in generating long-term changes in body mass. However, exercise may still be effective in preventing obesity, a subject to which we now turn.

Exercise as a preventive

Exercise may help prevent weight gain (Grundy, Blackburn, Higgins, et al, 1999). For example, a 10-year investigation on the relationship between leisure-time physical activity and BMI (Haapanen et al., 1997) that tracked 2564 men and 2695 women in Finland from 1980 to 1990 evaluated the consequences of different physical activity patterns. On the basis of self-report, participants were classified into one of four groups: (1) active throughout the 10-year span; (2) no reported leisure-time activity in 1980, but active at least once a week in 1990; (3) active at least once a week in 1980 but inactive in 1990; or (4) inactive throughout. Over the 10-year duration, those who became inactive, or were always inactive, gained 1.5 and 1.2 kilograms, respectively, when compared to the always-active group. There was no statistical difference between the always-active and became-active groups. Furthermore, the odds ratio (relative risk) of gaining more than 5 kilograms over the duration was 1.96 for those who became inactive and 1.62 for those who were always inactive, using the always-active group as a comparison. The odds ratio for the group that became active was 1.15, which was not statistically different from the 1.00 reference for the always-active group.

In a 5-year longitudinal study assessing PAL and body mass in American adult men and women (DiPietro et al., 2003), participants' self-reported leisure-time activities were each assigned a MET value. PAL value was estimated on the basis of the energy expenditure associated with METs. Three groups based on PALs were formed: low (<1.45), moderate (1.46 × 1.59) and high (×1.60). Individuals who increased their PAL from low to moderate, or from low to high, lost, respectively, 0.16 and 0.26 kilogram per year when compared to those who maintained a low PAL. Those who maintained a moderate PAL gained 0.12 kilogram per year; finally, individuals whose activity level dipped from high to moderate gained 0.31 kilogram per year more than those who maintained their high PALs for the duration. The authors thus conclude that a PAL of 1.45 may be the minimum value necessary to maintain healthy body weight. Although the clinical significance of this level of weight gain, even for the nonexercisers, is questionable, these results do signify that exercise can help attenuate weight gain, and substantiate the notion that all individuals should at least engage in a moderate level of physical activity.

A prospective trial on the efficacy of physical activity to prevent weight gain was conducted on American undergraduates who are prone to considerable weight gain during their first undergraduate year ("the freshman 15"; Donnelly, et al., 2003). Overweight American college students were randomized into either a nonexercising control group or an exercise intervention group that engaged in 45 minutes, of moderate- to high-intensity exercise 5 days a week. At the end of 16 months, men in the intervention had lost about 5 kilograms and had lowered their BMIs by 1.6 kg/m^2, while the nonexercisers had maintained weight. The women's exercise group had maintained their weights, while the controls had gained weight (2.9 kilograms) and increased their BMI by 1.1 kg/m^2. These results do demonstrate that a high level of physical activity, maintained for the long term, can assist not only in the prevention of weight gain, but perhaps also in weight loss. However, the long-term sustainability of this high level of activity is questionable (e.g., Miller, 2004).

Children and adolescents

Activity levels in children and adolescents may contribute to obesity prevention. Poor levels of physical activity increase obesity risk. A cross-sectional study of 780 European children assessed BMI, skin-fold thickness (a measure of body fat), pubertal development, cardiovascular fitness, and frequency of different intensities of physical activity (Ruiz et al., 2006). Engagement in vigorous physical activity (greater than 6 METs) was significantly and negatively correlated with total body fat; children who engaged in only 10 to 18 minutes a day of vigorous activity exhibited approximately 40 millimeters of skin-fold thickness, versus about 35 millimeters for those who engaged in more than 40 minutes of vigorous activity a day. However, total duration of physical activity, and engagement in intermediate exercise intensities, did not share a relationship with body fat.

Despite these results, all intensities of physical activity did share a significant, positive relationship with the level of cardiovascular fitness, though engagement in vigorous activity had the strongest relationship. Intensity of physical activity, rather than duration, may be the more significant parameter in preventing body fat accumulation. Although the duration of exercise practiced by the least-fat group (40 minutes per day) is at the higher end of the population guidelines discussed earlier, the intensity (6 METs) is much greater than that in the guidelines (3–4 METs). Indeed, if exercise is to work as an obesity preventive, engagement in high-intensity exercise for long periods may be required.

Limitations

High levels of intense exercise may help prevent weight gain. Indeed, exercise as a path for obesity prevention (Saris et al., 2003) requires a PAL of 1.70—about 45 to 60 minutes daily of moderate exercise. Given the fairly low average PAL levels in most industrialized nations (see the earlier discussion of population activity levels), a goal of 1.70 PAL may be setting the bar too high. Thus, although exercise can help prevent weight gain, the amount of exercise needed to achieve that goal may be beyond the capabilities of many people, given job and family demands on time and resources. Ruiz and associates (2006) favor introducing high levels of activity when children are young, and teaching lifelong habits of physical activity and healthy eating. This recommendation has not yet been put to formal test.

Nonexercise activity thermogenesis (NEAT)

An intriguing line of research is that concerning *nonexercise activity thermogenesis (NEAT)*. NEAT capitalizes on the fact that energy transfer between food and the body's energy stores is not entirely efficient; some energy is *not* harnessed as adipose tissue, glycogen, or muscle protein. This excess energy *must* be transferred to another form of energy sink. NEAT suggests that this energy is dissipated to the surround through unplanned body movements such as fidgeting and minor postural adjustments (Levine et al., 1999).

Higher daily levels of NEAT may help prevent weight gain and, thereby, obesity. Levine and colleagues (1999) overfed 16 normal-weight individuals by 1000 kilocalories a day for 8 weeks; participants were instructed not to exercise. As a result of the overfeeding, the participants gained an average of 4.7 kilograms.[10] In addition to body mass, participants' baseline and postintervention BMR, the thermic effect of food (TEF), and overall daily energy expenditure (DEE) were assessed.[11] DEE increased by 531 kilocalories, meaning that on average, 432 kilocalories of energy was stored in the body. Of the 531-kilocalorie increase, 79 kilocalories were explained by an increase in resting metabolic rate (as is to be expected with weight gain; see the earlier discussion), and 139 were explained by increases in TEF. Therefore, the remaining 313 kilocalories must have been consumed by the other component of DEE: physical activity. Given that volitional physical activity was held at a minimum, the authors infer that levels of NEAT rose. These results suggest that NEAT increases as a response to overfeeding, which is not surprising, given the first law of thermodynamics.

As anticipated, there was a strong negative correlation ($r = -0.77$) between increased activity energy expenditure and weight gain: participants whose activity levels increased the most gained the least weight. The authors conclude, "As humans overeat, those with effective activation of NEAT can dissipate the excess

---

[10]Given that an average of 7700 excess kilocalories of energy is required for a gain of 1 kilogram, participants would have gained 7.25 kilograms if the system had been "closed" (i.e., all calories consumed were stored or burned through physical activity).

[11]TEF is the energy required to power digestive processes related to eating. DEE is the total daily energy expended by an individual, which includes the basal metabolic rate, TEF, and energy used by physical activity.

energy so that it is not available for storage as fat, whereas those with lesser degrees of NEAT activation will likely have greater fat gain and be predisposed to develop obesity" (Levine et al., 1999, pp. 213). Increased NEAT activities—such as postural adjustments and fidgeting—might help combat obesity. Indeed, some investigators have begun to consider methods of increasing NEAT in individuals by, for instance, using stability balls as chairs in offices and classrooms. Results are forthcoming.

Although exciting, NEAT may not be the silver bullet for obesity prevention that some hope. Later work by Levine and colleagues (2005) demonstrates that there may be a strong genetic predisposition to individuals' levels of NEAT. Twenty physically inactive volunteers participated—10 normal-weight and 10 obese (based on BMI). Participants' movements were tracked every half second for 10 days, through radiotelemetry, and metabolic rates were assessed using doubly labeled water. Obese participants sat for 164 minutes per day longer than their thin peers; by contrast, lean participants maintained an upright posture 152 minutes per day more than the obese individuals. Total body movement was negatively correlated with both body fat percentage ($r = -0.52$) and kilograms of body fat ($r = -0.57$). If the obese and lean participants had similar postural patterns, the obese persons would have burned an additional 352 kilocalories per day.[12] These results again suggest the value of NEAT in preventing obesity.

However, seven of the obese individuals then underwent a supervised weight reduction (via dieting) of 8 kilograms; nine of the lean volunteers underwent a supervised weight gain of 4 kilograms. Despite these changes in body mass, individual levels of NEAT remained roughly the same ($r = 0.80$ for weight gainers; $r = 0.83$ for weight losers). The authors concluded that although NEAT may help prevent obesity, individual levels of NEAT are at least partially intrinsic to the individual and perhaps biologically determined.

Thus, physical activity—even NEAT-related activity—can help prevent obesity. However, individual predisposition to NEAT may be genetically determined. If that is true, then intervention programs using NEAT as a mechanism for weight loss may be fighting an uphill battle. A more promising manner of preventing obesity—or mitigating the health negatives encountered by those who are already obese—may be to increase voluntary levels of both planned and unplanned physical activity. As will be shown, however, the manner in which individuals are prompted to exercise, and the health-related messages distributed to a population, can dramatically affect exercise efficacy and adherence.

---

[12]Assuming a body mass of 80 kilograms, 352 kilocalories of energy is roughly the equivalent of taking a leisurely bike ride (4 METs, based on the *Compendium*; Ainsworth et al., 2000) for an hour.

Health at Any Size (H@AS)

As indicated earlier, the possibility of being both fit and fat has caused a stir within the exercise science community. This controversy has immediacy beyond academic research, because it affects exercise choice and duration, and the goals related to physical activity. The more traditional position holds that the overweight and obese should be encouraged to lose weight for the sake of good health (e.g., Christou et al., 2005; Mora et al., 2006).

Basic tenets

The traditional viewpoint has come under recent challenge. First, a number of sources in the literature have suggested that physical fitness is a greater determinant of health than is BMI (Blair & LaMonte, 2005), so weight loss should be less of a treatment focus than exercise behavior is. Second, focus on body mass and body shape is more reflective of Western society's obsession with the svelte—and irrational hate for fat—than of substantive, evidence-based practice. This shape-based focus can be psychologically catastrophic (Lindeman, 1999; Lyons & Miller, 1999 Miller & Jacob, 2001; Campos, 2004). Finally, programs whose sole focus is weight loss are riddled with problems such as poor adherence and lackluster efficacy (Miller, 1999, 2005; Miller et al., 1997).

An alternative to weight loss–based programs is the *health at any size (H@AS)*[13] paradigm. The idea of H@AS asserts that it is possible to be healthy at any level of BMI, given a prudent lifestyle that includes wise food choices and regular physical activity (Miller & Jacob, 2001; Kratina, 2004). As such, body mass does not matter as much as individual behavior in determining health. The trick, then, is to encourage individuals to take up, and maintain, healthy behaviors—itself not an easy task.

The H@AS approach is based in cognitive and clinical psychology. According to Kratina (2004, p. 8), H@AS has five tenets: (1) health enhancement, (2) size and self acceptance, (3) the pleasure of eating well, (4) the joy of movement, and (5) an end to weight bias. H@AS uses cognitive-behavioral techniques to encourage engagement in healthy, sustainable eating behaviors rather than reactive, nonsustainable dieting sequences. Exercise is promoted for fun and health, rather than for weight loss or out of fear. Reinforcement for these behaviors is the enjoyment of the activity. These facets promote not only physical health, but psychological well-being through self-acceptance (Kratina, 2004). Miller (2004) says of H@AS, "The goal should be to integrate physical activity into one's lifestyle with behavioral techniques that result in long-term adherence and attainment of that individual's goals" (p. 53). Accordingly, H@AS treatments are individual in nature and take into account personal differences in exercise history, bar-

---

[13]Also commonly referred to as *health at every size (HAES)*.

riers to exercise, and exercise goals. A one-model-fits-all formula, like those advocated in the exercise recommendations earlier in this chapter, is simply unrealistic, say proponents of H@AS (Miller, 2004).

H@AS program efficacy

H@AS-oriented treatments seem to work. According to Miller and Jacob (2001), clients treated using H@AS protocols actually lose body mass. However, unlike individuals in programs aimed specifically at shedding pounds—who tend to gain back mass over time—H@AS-treated individuals sustain body weight loss and continue to lower their BMI at a modest rate. Furthermore, those adhering to an H@AS protocol sustain their exercise behaviors over time.

For instance, Sbrocco and colleagues (1999) assessed 24 obese women, each of whom was assigned to either a traditional weight-conscious obesity program or a program founded on H@AS principles. Treatment lasted 13 weeks and involved weekly group psychotherapy. The traditional group focused on weight loss, diet, and exercise adherence. The H@AS group centered on sustainable choices that promote health and happiness and focused on behavioral change rather than weight loss. Participants' BMI, exercise adherence, self-reported eating patterns, eating disorder symptoms, and self-esteem were assessed before intervention and 3, 6, and 12 months after intervention. Although immediately after treatment the traditional group exercised a mean of 49.6 minutes per week, compared to 44.1 minutes per week for the H@AS group, by the 12-month follow-up the H@AS group was exercising a mean of 42.0 minutes per week compared to 35.9 for the traditional group. Similarly, although the traditional group lost 5.6 kilograms after treatment, versus 2.5 kilograms for the H@AS group, at the 1-year follow-up the traditional group had regained 1.3 kilograms and the H@AS group had lost an additional 7.5 kilograms. Most importantly, from an H@AS perspective, both immediately following treatment and 6 months later the H@AS group had significantly lower scores on measures of eating pathology and depression, and higher scores on a measure of self-esteem.

Another example of an H@AS program is Feel Wonder*full* (FWF) [sic], an exercise initiative geared toward obese women (Watkins et al., 2005). A 12-week, qualitative study examined 13 middle-aged, obese women who attended a private health club (FWF) that emphasized fitness over thinness (i.e., operated on an H@AS model). Accordingly, the facility did not provide beauty magazines—which tend to emphasize thinness—and it employed female fitness instructors who had a build similar to that of the participants. Thus the participants were provided with positive role models who were healthy and heavy, and they were not exposed to thinness-exalting media. Finally, exercise programs were individually designed to best meet each participant's ability and needs. Results suggest that the program improved the affect and self-esteem of these women. Further, the participants felt empowered to exercise, perceiving fewer psychological barriers to participation when the emphasis was on individual fitness rather than general thinness. Finally, the women reported greater mobility and less pain. Results such as these—especially with regard to increased exercise adherence—should be of obvious appeal to those interested in improving public health through increased physical activity.

The H@AS paradigm holds promise for assisting people to lead active, healthy lives. Although debate continues about the validity of the H@AS approach, there is unanimous agreement that people need to become physically active, and remain active over time. The field of exercise and health psychology has put forth a number of theories regarding why and how people initiate exercise programs, as well as the psychosocial factors that help foster adherence.

Theories of Exercise Initiation and Adherence

A number of programs to initiate and sustain exercise are available. As reviewed by Heath (2003), the approaches are (1) the health belief model, (2) the transtheoretical model, (3) relapse prevention, and (4) planned behavior. Although distinct in their emphases, each model attempts to provide the motivational antecedents needed to initiate exercise and/or the attitudinal factors that promote exercise adherence.

Health belief

According to Rosenstock's (1974; Strecher & Rosenstock, 1997) health belief model, only internal cues can prompt an individual to take up exercising. These cues must be related to one's perception of disease risk. In particular, an individual will initiate an exercise program if he or she (1) perceives himself to be at risk for an illness, (2) perceives the illness to be serious, (3) perceives action to be beneficial in avoiding/treating that illness; and (4) sees no substantial barriers to action. In these regards, the health belief model is reactive and fear-based because it focuses entirely on avoiding disease rather than attaining good health or having fun. Accordingly, Rosenstock is closer to traditional weight loss programming than to the H@AS model.

Transtheoretical model

The transtheoretical model of behavior change (Prochaska & DiClemente, 1994) takes a broader perspective on exercise initiation and maintenance. Individuals are thought to "move" through stages of readiness and ability to engage in an exercise program. Movement is not necessarily linear; there is a "natural" tendency to move back and forth between levels. The first stage, *precontemplation*, depicts people before thought has been given to initiate an exercise program. The second stage, *contemplation*, refers to an individual who has started to consider exercising. The transtheoretical model does not distinguish between attitudinal and other factors that push an individual from precontemplation to contemplation. The motivation may be intrinsic and fear-based, as in the health belief model; may consist of more positive attitudinal beliefs toward exercise (e.g., H@AS); or may be external, such as social support or pressure from friends, family, or the community. Although this ambiguity regarding the bases of contemplation makes the transtheoretical model applicable to many individuals, it also weakens its predictive or utilitarian value in determining why and when a person will opt to initiate an exercise program.

In the third phase, *preparation*, the individual undertakes the life changes and initiates the contacts necessary to begin a program. Joining a gym or scheduling an appointment with an exercise physiologist are examples of preparation activities. People in the fourth phase, *action*, have completed the preparation work and regularly engage in an exercise program. The fifth phase, *maintenance*, is the long-term adherence (longer than 6 months) to the program. As indicated, the transtheoretical model is a circular rather than linear process. The maintenance phase is not an end point, but rather a phase in an individual's lifetime of physical activity. The system is naturally bidirectional, so two-way movement across boundaries is expected, does not pose a matter for concern, and is not viewed as a setback. An individual can move from contemplation to precontemplation, or from maintenance to contemplation, without discouragement.

Relapse prevention

Another theory is the relapse prevention model (Collins 2005; Marcus & Stanton, 1993). This model focuses exclusively on the cyclical nature of exercise behaviors after initiation. It is strictly a maintenance model that encourages individuals to develop psychological tools to mitigate challenges to exercise continuation, and strategies to avoid or cope with situations that have a high risk for relapse. The model fosters awareness of differences between a lapse in exercise behaviors (a missed workout) and a relapse of exercise behaviors (multiple missed workouts). As such, the relapse prevention model attempts to provide the psychological resources necessary to sustain or reinitiate exercise through the lifetime, despite the various stressors and challenges that arise. For example, a high-stress situation, such as being sick, may prompt an individual to cease exercising. The relapse prevention model encourages individuals to develop strategies for coping with that stress—such as shortened workouts—that best allow for either continued exercise during the stressful period or ideas that could lead to speedy resumption of exercise behavior soon thereafter, such as setting a target date for resumption.

Theories of reasoned action and planned behavior

Two well-established models of exercise behavior are Ajzen's theory of reasoned action (TRA; e.g., Ajzen & Fishbein, 1980, Fishbein & Ajzen, 1975) and the TRA's offspring, the theory of planned behavior (TPB; Ajzen, 1985, 1988, 1991; see

Hausenblas et al., 1997, for an update of both). These theories address a number of factors related to exercise initiation, but they do not account specifically for long-term adherence.

Specifically, the TRA identifies two contributing factors to exercise intention: attitudes and subjective norms. *Attitudes* are the individual's beliefs about the exercise process (e.g., whether it hurts or is fun), its benefits (e.g., weight loss, heart health), and its disadvantages (e.g., time-consuming, boring). Related to attitude is attitude *strength*, which refers to the intensity of the individual's beliefs regarding exercise. *Subjective norms* are the ways in which the beliefs of others—family, friends, and the community—about exercise (e.g., importance, acceptability, safety) affect intention. The TPB further suggests that *perceived control* over exercise (e.g., whether a gym is affordable or whether it's safe to jog locally) influences intention to exercise.

The calculus of attitude, strength, subjective norm, and perceived control determines the likelihood of actually initiating an exercise program. Consider an individual who perceives a number of benefits to exercise, believes strongly in those benefits, is surrounded by friends who are fit, and has the money to join a gym. The TPB would predict that the individual would begin exercising, given positive attitudes, strong strength of attitudes, encouraging subjective norms, and no perceived barriers. Contrast that situation with an individual who weakly acknowledges that exercise might help his blood pressure but strongly believes that exercise will hurt and will be boring, whose family members are also sedentary, and who lives in a neighborhood where it may be unsafe to take an evening jog. The likelihood that that individual will begin an exercise program is diminished, says the TPB.

Predictive value of models

In a meta-analysis of 31 studies comparing the utility of the TRA and the TPB in predicting expressed intent to exercise with actual exercise behavior, Hausenblas and colleagues (1997) showed that attitudes toward exercise were strongly and significantly associated to both intention to exercise and actual exercise behavior, and that these attitudes were a better predictor than were perceived norms. However, perceived behavioral control exhibited a significant relationship to both intent and behavior. These results demonstrate not only the utility of the TPB in determining exercise behavior, but the importance of individual beliefs and perceived control at the start of an exercise program.

Another study compared several major theories of behavior change, including the transtheoretical model and the TPB (Palmeira et al., 2007). In one program, 142 overweight and obese women participated in 16 weeks of counseling that featured information on exercise and nutrition, as well as promoted self-esteem and positive body image. At the beginning and end of the program, participants completed a questionnaire that included questions regarding attitudes toward exercise, motivations for weight loss, and general self-concept. Facets of both the transtheoretical and the TPB models accounted for exercise behaviors and weight loss; important to both models was an understanding of and sense of control over the change process, and positive attitudinal facets.

Comparing the models

Despite some obvious differences, the theories described in the preceding sections do have similarities. First, an understanding of exercise goals and attitudes is critical to the initiation of exercise behavior. Some models, like the health belief model, focus more on avoidance of health negatives as motivating; other models, such as the TRA/TPB, allow for positive facets of exercise—like fun—to factor into the equation as well. Although the former might be of more appeal to traditional thought on obesity, the latter is more in line with the H@AS camp. In both cases, however, it is acknowledged that some benefit of exercise—whether disease avoidance or improved self-esteem—must be perceived in order for an individual to actually start a program.

Second, exercise initiation and maintenance are best achieved when construed as a lifelong process. Participants should anticipate lapses and relapses from which recovery and resumption of activity can and should be the norm. Indeed, exercise should be conceptualized as integral to a program that promotes health, and part of a lifetime of healthy behavior rather than a reactive behavior motivated by fear. The transtheoretical and relapse prevention models acknowledge that setbacks happen, are natural, and do not have to be seen as failures. The H@AS paradigm would agree because exercise is better conceived of as part of a healthy life than as a focused medical treatment to which stringent adherence is mandatory.

Finally, health-related behaviors depend on social norms and support. This facet is encouraged by the relapse prevention model and the TPB, and it is given cursory nod by the transtheoretical model. Indeed, explicit in the TPB is the idea that perceived social norm and perceived behavioral control determine exercise initiation. That fact is powerfully demonstrated in groundbreaking research by Christakis and Fowler (2007) that examined the impact of social relationships on obesity. The study analyzed changes in obesity status over a 32-year period in a group of 5124 subjects and their spouses, relatives, friends, and neighbors (total sample size: 12,067). Results indicated that having a mutual same-sex friend who was obese increased one's own chance of becoming obese by 171%. Having an obese spouse or sibling likewise increases one's odds of becoming obese, but to a lesser degree (37% and 40%, respectively; see Table 8.5). Importantly, geographical proximity to obese friends, or the presence of an obese neighbor, did not increase one's chances of becoming obese. Therefore, it is the social relationship between individuals that can be obesogenic, *not* a similar geographical location. The authors thus conclude that relationships with obese individuals may alter a person's "general perception of the social norms regarding the acceptability of obesity" (Christakis and Fowler, 2007, p. 377).

Table 8.5
Relative Risk of Developing Obesity Based on Type of Social Relationship with Obese Individuals

Type of relationship	Risk increase (%)[a]
Mutual friends (either sex)	171
Male, same-sex friends	100
Same-sex siblings	58
Husbands	44
Female, same-sex friends	38
Wives	37
Immediate neighbors	NS
Opposite-sex friends	NS

Source: After Christakis & Fowler, 2007.
[a]NS, not significant.

Findings such as those by Christakis and Fowler hold great promise for health promotion. They signal—as is suggested by the theories described earlier—that social norms affect health behavior. Therefore, if a community's norms can be altered to recognize the importance of regular exercise, individuals may be prompted to become more physically active, *especially if their friends become active.* Exercise promotion must target communities. *Support from others, and a safe place to exercise, are critical to exercise behavior.*

These facets can be achieved through community-based initiative. Even when a community does not have the means to open a gym or subsidize membership, community support for group walks or exercise sessions at little or no community cost can promote activity in a social and safe manner.

Community Programming

The preceding considerations have furthered development and implementation of community-based approaches as a means of promoting physical activity. Such endeavors seek structural changes on the community level through social, political, economic, and educational programs that promote and reward physical activity and provide facilities for their expression. King (1994) describes individual exercise programming as a "waiting" stance (the personal trainer or exercise physiologist "waits" for a client), but public health exercise programming adopts a "seeking" stance that provides opportunities for exercise supported by the community. The seeking approach exploits both planned and unplanned physical activity as sources of caloric expenditure. Calories can be lost anywhere at any time, if communities are designed to support unplanned activities. The idea is for exercise to shift away from the health club to the variegated facets of daily living.

Simple community-based changes can significantly influence exercise efforts. For example, Brownell and colleagues (1980) placed a small sign stating "Your heart needs exercise … Here's your chance" (p. 1541) at a point of choice between escalator or staircase in several pedestrian-heavy areas of a major city. Using an ABAB reversal design[14] they discovered that the sign encouraged a threefold increase in stair use, and this gain was reversed when the sign was removed. Although stair use remained modest even during intervention (roughly 15%), these findings are hopeful because the increase in stair use occurred within the framework of physical inactivity. Community-wide implementation of such inexpensive and benign interventions could create an ambience that would increase unplanned activity, thereby magnifying the impact of individual efforts such as Brownell's. Such a change in attitude could result in improved public health.

Larger-scale interventions such as these have been undertaken in two US naval bases. After obtaining baseline indices of physical fitness and exercise frequency, a number of significant organizational changes to promote leisure-time activity were implemented on one base. These included commendations for improved fitness, increased opportunity for exercise, and renovation of trails and exercise facilities. The other base served as a control. After 1 year, the exercise-promoting base witnessed significant improvements in various measures of physical fitness, such as 1-mile run time, and pectoral and abdominal strength. Although levels of adiposity did not change for the intervention group, the average body fat percentage of control participants increased slightly (Linenger et al., 1991). Even in populations that are extremely fit, opportunities to further the incidence of both planned and unplanned exercise yielded positive physical benefits and underscore the importance of political/organizational support of community changes to encourage physical fitness.

Indianapolis, Indiana, has launched a massive public health campaign titled *HealthierINDY* that seeks to streamline physical activity promotion programs in the city through collaboration among various departments and agencies responsible for physical activity programming. This collaboration involves regular meetings of relevant parties, joint advertising of community exercise programs, attempts at cost reduction, and recruiting of media support to publicize these

---

[14]An ABAB design involves a baseline measurement of the target variable (A) followed by the introduction of an intervention (in this instance, the poster design) and subsequent remeasurement of the target variable ("B"). The intervention is then removed, followed by further measurement of the target variable. Finally, the intervention is reintroduced, and a final assessment of the variable is conducted. If changes in the variable consistently follow the introduction of the treatment, and removal of the treatment returns the variable to baseline levels, the intervention is assumed to be effective.

efforts. In addition to regular weekly programming, the initiative hosts a yearly weeklong festival to distribute information about the various programs available during the year and sponsor outdoor exercise programs to increase not only awareness, but on-the-spot physical activity. The program, still in its infancy, has not yet been formally evaluated. Interest is high, however—at least judging from the substantial increases in annual festival attendance (Hendrick, 2003).

Other new and innovative programs are using technology to help obese individuals. Van Wormer (2004) describes an e-counseling program designed to encourage physical activity. Participants were given pedometers and asked to record their daily number of steps as a baseline. Later, participants were e-mailed weekly by a counselor to discuss issues related to adherence, goal setting, and praise. Even though the sample studied was small ($n = 3$), all participants showed promising results: all had increased their daily number of steps, and two of the participants had more than doubled their daily pedometer readings. Weight loss was positively correlated with increase in the number of steps. Such a program model is attractive because it is inexpensive and can be accessed privately, at an individual's convenience.

However, results of another study question the efficacy of the Internet in assisting individuals with maintaining weight loss (Wing et al.,2006). In that study, individuals who had lost an average of 19.3 kilograms (42.5 pounds) were assigned to one of three weight loss maintenance counseling programs for 18 months: face-to-face, Internet-based, or a no-contract control. After the intervention period, the Internet and control groups both regained nearly 5 kilograms (11 pounds), but the face-to-face group regained only 2.5 kilograms (5.5 pounds). Clearly, more research is needed regarding Internet-based interventions, though results such as those by Van Wormer suggest promise in using the Internet to promote physical activity, even if such activity may not be accompanied by weight loss.

The preceding examples, among others, have demonstrated that community-based programming can positively influence public health by making available safe facilities, by structuring programs that promote healthy behaviors, and by providing accurate and accessible information about exercise and its relationship to health. Community-based programs, therefore, can help individuals initiate and maintain physical activity by developing positive social norms, removing barriers to exercise, and disseminating accurate health-related information about exercise. Indeed, the sign posted by Brownell and colleagues (1980) focused on heart health, not weight loss, and the HealthierINDY program has encouraged exercise to improve overall health. Although these programs may not lead to weight loss per se, they can improve health, as demonstrated by the naval program (Linenger, et. al., 1991). A paradigmatic shift is required to crystallize this difference. That said, this approach is in its infancy and as yet has neither gained a widespread following nor been critically evaluated. The initial reports are hopeful, especially regarding program adherence.

Exercise Risks

Although exercise can promote positive health outcomes, it is not risk-free. Cardiovascular incidents can result from exercise, especially endurance activities. Yet the risk of heart attack is low, and heart attack almost always occurs in people already predisposed to cardiovascular disease. In general, exercise is not contraindicated; people at cardiovascular risk, however, should undergo exercise testing with a physician before commencing an exercise program (Brukner & Brown, 2005).

Exercise-induced musculoskeletal injury, especially during resistance training, is a possible risk factor. The risk of injury is quite low, however, especially if the guidelines for exercise frequency presented by the ACSM are followed (Kraemer et al., 2002) Elderly individuals' risk of musculoskeletal injuries is higher, especially for people with preexisting bone problems, such as osteoporosis (Brunker & Brown, 2005). Such individuals should first consult with a physician or exercise physiologist and should develop a reasonable exercise plan with a professional trainer before commencing any exercise routine (Kraemer et al., 2002).

Finally, any discussion of exercise would be incomplete if it did not address issues of body image, eating disorders, and exercise addiction. Dissatisfaction with one's physique, and a desire to change one's body to meet social standards—a phenomenon commonly called *body image dissatisfaction*—provides an important attitudinal basis for exercise in both women (Lindeman, 1999; McDonald & Thompson, 1992) and men (Drummond, 2001, 2002). However, individuals exercising for those reasons commonly drop out of their exercise programs because of a lack of short-term gratification—a problem that we encountered earlier in people who exercise to lose weight. The change is too slow to sustain the operant. People who drop out may further perceive themselves as failures or endure dampened self-esteem or affect (Lindeman, 1999; Miller & Jacob, 2001; Drummond, 2001).

At the other end of the spectrum, people who studiously follow or exceed the guidelines may become exercise-dependent, possibly putting themselves at risk of eating disorders and other health problems (Cockerill, 1996). This relationship of exercise to both body image problems and disturbed eating again suggest the importance of having accurate knowledge regarding exercise efficacy and of evaluating and challenging inaccurate exercise attitudes through programs such as H@AS.

Conclusion

In summary, physical activities, both unplanned and planned, require energy expenditure beyond basal metabolic demands. Intense caloric expenditure alone could induce weight loss in determined individuals for whom systematic food reduction has proven problematic. Although most obese individuals are not inactive, their levels of caloric output are less than their caloric intake. A number of programs that differ in strategy and tactics for weight loss advocate frequent physical activity, the benefits of which are cumulative. However, although theoretically important to weight loss, exercise programming has shown mixed results in producing actual weight loss; and those who successfully lose weight on exercise programs typically exercise at frequencies and intensities beyond those recommended for optimal health. Such a program is likely not sustainable in the long run.

A sea change in attitudes toward health and exercise is required—from a motivational stance of altering body weight and body shape, to a stance that seeks optimal health as ideal. This approach holds greater promise for developing a healthy and sustainable lifestyle that can withstand occasional reversals and setbacks. Community-based initiatives can help sustain exercise behaviors, all of which can improve public health.

Acknowledgments

The author wishes to acknowledge Drs. Murray Drummond and Grant Tomkinson, as well as Claire Drummond—all of the University of South Australia human movement program—for their comments, suggestions, and encouragement.

References Cited

Ainsworth, B. E., Haskell, W. L., Whitt, M. C., Irwin, M. L., Swartz, A. M., Strath, S. J., et al. (2000). Compendium of physical activities: An update of activity codes and MET intensity. *Medicine & Exercise in Sports & Exercise, 32*, S498–S516.

Ajzen, I. (1985). From intention to actions: A theory of planned behavior. In J. Kuhl & J. Beckman (Eds.), *Action control: From cognition to behavior* (pp. 11–39). Heidelberg, Germany: Springer-Verlag.

Ajzen, I. (1988). *Attitudes, personality, and behavior.* Chicago, IL: Nasey.

Ajzen, I. (1991). The theory of planned behavior. *Organization Behavior and Human Decision Processes, 50*, 179–211.

Ajzen, I., & Fishbein, M. (1980). *Understanding attitudes and predicting social behavior.* Englewood Cliffs, NJ: Prentice Hall.

American College of Sports Medicine. (1998). The recommended quantity and quality of exercise for developing and maintaining cardiorespiratory and muscular fitness, and flexibility in healthy adults. *Medicine & Science in Sports & Exercise, 30*, 975–991.

American College of Sports Medicine. (2001). Appropriate intervention strategies for weight loss and prevention of weight regain for adults. *Medicine & Science in Sports & Exercise, 33*, 2145–2156.

American College of Sports Medicine. (2002). Progression models in resistance training for healthy adults. *Medicine & Science in Sports & Exercise, 34*, 364–380.

American Heart Association. (2003). Exercise in physical activity in the treatment and prevention of atherosclerotic cardiovascular disease. *Circulation, 107*, 3109–3316.

Anderssen, S., Holme, I., Urdal, P., & Hjermann, I. (1995). Diet and exercise intervention have favorable effects on blood pressure in mild hypertensives: the Oslo Diet and Exercise Study (ODES). *Blood Pressure, 4*, 343–349.

Astrup, A. (1999). Physical activity and weight gain and fat distribution with menopause: Current evidence and research issues. *Medicine & Science in Sports & Exercise, 31*, S564–S567.

Ballor, D. J., Katch, V. K., Becque, M. D., & Marks, C. R. (1998). Resistance weight training during caloric restriction enhances lean body weight maintenance.

American Journal of Clinical Nutrition, 47, 19–25.

Blair, S. N., & Brodney, S. (1999). Effects of physical activity and obesity on morbidity and mortality: Current evidence and research issues. *Medicine & Science in Sports & Exercise, 31,* S646–S662.

Blair, S. N., Kohl, H. W., III, Paffenberger, R. S., Jr., Clark, D. G., Cooper, K. H., & Gibbons, L. W. (1989). Physical fitness and all-cause mortality: A prospective study of healthy men and women. *Journal of the American Medical Association, 262,* 2395–2401.

Blair, S. N., & LaMonte, M. J. (2005). Commenatary: Current perspectives on obesity and health: Black and white, or shades of grey? *International Journal of Epidemiology, 35,* 69–72.

Blissmer, B., Riebe, D., Dye, G., Ruggiero, L., Greene, G., & Caldwell, M. (2006). Health-related quality of life following a clinical weight loss intervention among overweight and obese adults: intervention and 24 month follow-up effects. *Health and Quality of Life Outcomes, 4,* 43. Retrieved July 20, 2006 from http://www.pubmed-central.nih.gov/articlerender.fcgi?artid=1553435

Blundell, J. E., & King, N. A. (1999). Physical activity and regulation of food intake: Current evidence. *Medicine & Science in Sports & Exercise, 31,* S573–S583.

Bowen, D. J., Fesinmeyer, M. D., Yasui, Y., Tworoger, S., Ulrich, C. M., Irwin, M. L., et al. (2006). Randomized trial on physical activity in sedentary middle aged women: Effects on quality of life. *International Journal of Behavioral Nutrition, 3,* 34.

Brownell, K. D., Stunkard, A. J., & Albaum, J. M. (1980). Evaluation and modification of exercise patterns in the natural environment. *American Journal of Psychiatry, 137,* 1540–1545.

Brukner, P. D., & Brown, W. J. (2005). Is exercise good for you? *Medical Journal of Australia, 183,* 538–541.

Campos, P. F (2004). *The obesity myth: Why America's obsession with weight is hazardous to your health.* New York: Gotham.

Cantenacci, V. A., & Wyatt, H. R. (2007). The role of physical activity in producing and maintaining weight loss. *Endocrinology & Metabolism, 3,* 518–529.

Christakis, N. A., & Fowler, J. H. (2007). The spread of obesity in a large social network over 32 years. *New England Journal of Medicine, 357,* 370–379.

Christou, D. D., Gentile, C. L., DeSouza, C. A., Seals, D. R., & Gates, P. E. (2005). Fatness is a better predictor of cardiovascular disease risk factor profile than aerobic fitness in healthy men. *Circulation, 111,* 1904–1914.

Cockerill, I. M. (1996). Exercise dependence and associated disorders: A review. *Counseling Psychology Quarterly, 9,* 119–129.

Collins, R. L. (2005). Relapse prevention for eating disorders and obesity. In G. A. Marlatt & D. M. Donovan (Eds.), *Relapse Prevention: Maintenance Strategies in the Treatment of Addictive Behaviors* (2nd ed., pp. 248–275). New York: Guilford Press.

DiPietro, L., Dziura, J., & Blair, S. N. (2003). The relation of estimated physical activity level (PAL) to 5-year weight change in middle-aged adults. *Medicine & Science in Sports & Exercise, 35,* S72.

Dishman, R. K. (1982). Compliance/adherence in health-related exercise. *Health Psychology, 1,* 237–267.

Donnelly, J. E., Hill, J. O., Jacobsen, D. J., Potteiger, J., Sullivan, D. K., Johnson, S. L., et al. (2003). Effects of a 16-month randomized controlled exercise trial on body weight and composition in young, overweight men and women. *Archives of Internal Medicine, 163,* 1343–1350.

Drummond, M. J. N. (2001). Boys' bodies in the context of sport and physical activity: Implications for health. *Journal of Physical Education New Zealand, 34,* 53–64.

Drummond, M. J. N. (2002). Men, body image, and eating disorders. *International Journal of Men's Health, 1,* 89–98.

Ekkekakis, P., & Lind, E. (2006). Exercise does not feel the same when you are overweight: The impact of self-selected and imposed intensity on affect and exertion. *International Journal of Obesity, 30,* 652–660.

Ernst, C., Olson, A. K., Pinel, J. P., Lam, R. W., Christie, B. R. (2006). Antidepressant effects of exercise: Evidence for an adult-neurogenesis hypothesis? *Journal of Psychiatry and Neuroscience, 31,* 84–92.

Fagard, R. H. (1999). Physical activity in the prevention and treatment of hypertension in the obese. *Medicine & Science in Sports & Exercise, 31,* S624–630.

Fishbein, M., & Ajzen, I. (1975). *Belief, attitude, intention, and behavior.* Don Mills, NY: Addison Wesley.

Food and Nutrition Board/ Institute of Medicine (2005). Physical Activity. In *Dietary Reference Intakes for Energy, Carbohydrate, Fiber, Fat, Fatty Acids, Cholesterol, Protein, and Amino Acids* (pp. 880–935). Washington, DC: National Academy of Sciences.

Forbes, G. B., & Welle, S. L. (1983). Lean body mass in obesity. *International Journal of Obesity, 7*, 99–107.

Foster, G. D., Wyatt, H. R., Hill, J. O., McGuckin, B. G., Brill, C., Mohammed, B. S., et al. (2003). A randomized trial of a low-carbohydrate diet for obesity. *New England Journal of Medicine, 348*, 2082–2090.

Goodpaster, B. H., Katsiaras, A., & Kelley, D. E. (2003). Enhanced fat oxidation through physical activity is associated with improvements in insulin sensitivity in obesity. *Diabetes, 52*, 2191–2197.

Hanna, L., & Adams, M. (2006). Prevention of ovarian cancer. *Clinical Obstetrics & Gynecology, 20*, 339–362.

Haapanen, N., Miilunpalo, S., Pasanen, M., Oja, P., & Vuori, I. (1997). Association between leisure time physical activity and 10-year body mass change among working-aged men and women. *International Journal of Obesity, 21*, 288–296.

Harris, A. H., Cronkite, R., & Moss, R. (2006). Physical activity, exercise coping, and depression in a 10-year cohort study of depressed patients. *Journal of Affective Disorders, 73*, 79–85.

Hausenblas, H. A., Carron, A. V., Mack D. E. (1997). Application to the theories of reasoned action and planned behavior to exercise behavior: A meta-analysis. *Journal of Sport and Exercise Psychology, 19*, 36–51.

Heath, G. W. (2003). Behavioral approaches to physical activity promotion. In J. K. Ehrman, P. M. Gordon, P. S. Visich, & S. J. Keteyian (Eds.), *Clinical Exercise Physiology* (pp. 11–24). Champaign, IL: Human Kinetics.

Hendrick, H. (2003). HealthierINDY awareness week: A first step in implementing the HealthierUS initiative in Indianapolis. *ACSM's Health and Fitness Journal, 7*, 6–9.

Hewitt, J. A., Mokbel, K., van Someren, K. A., Jewell, A. P., & Garrod, R. (2005). Exercise for breast cancer survival: The effect on cancer risk and cancer-related fatigue (CRF). *International Journal of Fertility and Women's Medicine, 50*, 231–239.

Hill, J. O., & Wyatt, H. R. (2005). Role of physical activity in preventing and treating obesity. *Journal of Applied Physiology, 99*, 765–770.

Hu, F. B., Willet, W. C., Li, T., Stampfer, M. J., Colditz, G. A., & Mason, J. E. (2004). Adiposity as compared with physical activity in predicting mortality among women. *New England Journal of Medicine, 351*, 2694–2703.

Irwin, M. L. (2006). Randomized controlled trials of physical activity and breast cancer prevention. *Exercise and Sport Science Reviews, 43*, 182–193.

Irwin, M. L. Yasui, Y., Ulrich, C. M., Bowen, D., Rudolph, R. E., Schwartz, R. S., et al. (2003). Effect of exercise on total and intra-abdominal body fat in postmenopausal women: A randomized controlled trial. *Journal of the American Medical Association, 266*, 323–330.

Jakicic, J. M., & Otto, A. D. (2005). Physical activity considerations for the treatment and prevention of obesity. *American Journal of Clinical Nutrition, 82*, 226S-229S.

Jakicic, J. M., Wing, R. R., Winters-Hart, C. (2002). Relationship of physical activity to eating behaviors and weight loss in women. *Medicine & Science in Sports & Exercise, 34*, 1653–1659.

Kelley, D. E., & Goodpaster, B. H. (1999). Effects of physical activity on insulin action and glucose tolerance in obesity. *Medicine & Science in Sports & Exercise, 31*, S619–S623.

King, A. C. (1994). Community and public health approaches to the promotion of physical activity. *Medicine & Science in Sports & Exercise, 26*, 1405–1412.

Kirska, A. (2003). Can a physically active lifestyle prevent type 2 diabetes? *Exercise and Sports Sciences Review, 31*, 132–137.

Klem, M. L., Wing, R. R., McGuire, M. T., Seagle, H. M., & Hill, J. O. (1997)A descriptive study of individuals successful at long-term maintenance of substantial weight loss. *American Journal of Clinical Nutrition, 66*, 239–246.

Kraemer, W. J., Adams, K., Cafarelli, E., Dudley, G. A., Dooly, C., Feigenbaum, M. S. et al. (2002). American college of sports medicine position stand: Progression models in Resistance training for healthy adults. *Medicine & Science in Sports & Exercise, 34*, 364–380.

Kratina, K. (2004). Holding constant: Health at every size. *Health at Every Size, 18*, 8–10.

Laukkanen, J. A., Kurl, S., Salonen, R., Rauramaa, R., & Salonen, J. T. (2004). The predictive value of cardiorespiratory fitness for cardiovascular events in men with various risk profiles: A prospective population-based cohort study. *European Heart Journal, 25*, 1428–1437.

Levine, J. A., Eberhardt, N. L & Jensen, M. D. (1999). Role of nonexercise activity thermogenesis in resistance to fat gain in humans. *Science, 283*, 212–214.

Levine, J. A., Lanningham-Foster, L. M., McCrady, S. K., Krizan, A. C., Olson, L. R., Kane, P. H., et al. (2005). Interindividual variation in posture allocation: Possible role in human obesity. *Science, 307*, 584–586.

Lindeman, A. K. (1999). Quest for ideal weight: Costs and consequences. *Medicine & Science in Sports & Exercise, 31*, 1135–1140.

Linenger, J. M., Chesson, C. V., & Nice, D. S. (1991). Physical fitness gains following simple environmental change. *American Journal of Preventative Medicine, 7*, 298–310.

Lyons, P., & Miller, W. C. (1999). Effective health promotion and clinical care for large people. *Medicine & Science in Sports & Exercise, 31*, 1141–1146.

Marcus, B. H., & Stanton, A. L. (1993). Evaluation of relapse prevention and reinforcement interventions to promote exercise adherence in sedentary females. *Research Quarterly for Exercise and Sport, 64*, 447–452.

Matsuzawa, Y, Nakamura, T., Shimomura, I., & Kotani, K. (1995). Visceral fat accumulation and cardiovascular disease. *Obesity Research, 3*, 645S-647S.

Mayer, J., Roy, P., & Mitra, K. P. (1956). Relation between caloric intake, body weight, and physical work: Studies in an industrial male population in West Bengal. *American Journal of Clinical Nutrition, 4*, 169–175.

Mayo, M. J., Grantham, J. R., & Balasekara, G. (2003). Exercise-induced weight loss preferentially reduces abdominal fat. *Medicine & Science in Sports & Exercise, 35*, 207–213.

McDonald, K., & Thompson, J. K. (1992). Eating disturbance, body image dissatisfaction, and reasons for exercising: Gender differences and correlation findings.

International Journal of Eating Disorders, 11, 289–292.

Miller, W. C. (1999). How effective are traditional dietary and exercise interventions in weight loss? *Medicine & Science in Sports & Exercise, 31*, 1129–1134.

Miller, W. C. (2004). Exercise as a treatment for obesity. *Health at Every Size, 18*, 51–53.

Miller, W. C. (2005). Exercise and weight: Fit or fat or fit and fat? *Health at Every Size, 19*, 71–81.

Miller, W. C., & Jacob, A. V. (2001). The health at any size paradigm for obesity treatment: The scientific evidence. *Obesity Review, 2*, 37–45.

Miller, W. C., Koceja, D. M., & Hamilton, E. J. (1997). A meta-analysis of the past 25 years of weight loss research using diet, exercise, or diet plus exercise intervention. *International Journal of Obesity, 21*, 941–947.

Mora, S., Lee, I., Bring, J. E., & Ridker, P. (2006). Association of physical activity and body mass index with novel and traditional cardiovascular biomarkers in women. *Journal of the American Medical Association, 295*, 1412–1419.

Murphy, M., Nevill, A., Neville, C., Biddle, S., & Hardman, A. (2002). Accumulating brisk walking for fitness, cardiovascular risk, and psychological health. *Medicine & Science in Sports & Exercise, 34*, 1468–1474.

Nassis, G. P., Pssara, G., Sidossis, L. S. (2005). Central and total adiposity are lower in overweight and obese children with high cardiorespiratory fitness. *European Journal of Clinical Nutrition, 59*, 137–141.

Okura, T., Nakata, Y., Yamabuki, K., Tanaka, K. (2004). Regional body composition changes exhibit opposing effects on coronary heart disease risk factors. *Arteriosclerosis, Thrombosis, and Vascular Biology, 24*, 923–929.

Palmeira, A. L. Teixeira, P. J., Branco, T. L., Martins, S. S., Minderico, C. S., Barata, J. T., et al. (2007). Predicting short-term weight loss using four leading health behavior change theories. *International Journal of Behavioral Nutrition and Physical Activity, 4*, 4–14.

Pate, R. R., Pratt, M., Blair, S. N., Haskell, W. L., Macera, C. A., Bouchard, D., et al. (1995). Physical activity and public health: A recommendations from the Centers of Disease Control and Prevention from the American College of Sports Medicine.

Journal of the American Medical Association, *273,* 402–407.

Perez-Martin, A., Raynaud, E., & Mercier, J. (2001). Insulin resistance and associated metabolic abnormalities in muscle: Effects of exercise. *Obesity Review, 2,* 47–59.

Pollock, M. L., Gaesser, G. A., Butcher, J. D., Despres, J. P., Dishman, R. K., Franklin, B. A., Garber, C. E. (1998). ACSM position stand: The recommended quality and quantity of exercise for developing and maintaining cardiorespiratory and muscular fitness, and flexibility in healthy adults. *Medicine & Science in Sports & Excise, 30,* 975–991.

Prochaska, J. O., & DiClemente, C. C. (1994). *The Transtheoretical Approach: Crossing Traditional Boundaries of Therapy,* [originally published in 1984]. Malabar, FL: Krieger.

Rippe, J. M., & Hess, S. (1998). The role of physical activity in the prevention and management of obesity. *Journal of the American Dietetic Association, 98,* S31–S38.

Rissanen, A., & Fogelhom, M. (1999). Physical activity in the prevention and treatment of other morbid conditions and impairments associated with obesity: Current evidence and research issues. *Medicine & Science in Sports & Exercise, 31,* S635–S645.

Rosenstock, I. M. (1974). The health belief model and preventative health behavior. *Health Education Monographs, 2,* 354–386.

Ross, R., & Katzmarzyk, P. T. (2003). Cardiorespiratory fitness is associated with diminished total and abdominal obesity independent of body mass index. *International Journal of Obesity, 27,* 204–210.

Ruiz, J. R., Rizzo, N. S., Hurtig-Wennlof, A., Ortega, F. B., Wurnberg, J., & Sjostrom, M. (2006). Relations of total physical activity and intensity to fitness and fatness in children: The European Youth Heart Study. *American Journal of Clinical Nutrition, 84,* 299–303.

Saris, W. H. M., Blair, S. N., van Baak, M. A., Eaton, S. B., Davies, P. S. W., Di Pietro, L., et al. (2003). How much physical activity is enough to prevent unhealthy weight gain? Outcome of the IASO 1st Stock Conference and consensus statement. *Obesity Review, 4,* 101–114.

Sbrocco, T., Nedegaard, R. C., Stone, J. M., Lewis, E. (1999). Behavioral choice treatment promotes continuing weight loss: Preliminary results of cognitive-behavioral decision-based treatment for obesity.

Journal of Consulting Clinical Psychology, 67, 260–266.

Schneider, K. L., Spring, B., & Pagoto, S. L. (2007). Affective benefits of exercise while quitting smoking: Influence of smoking-specific weight concern. *Psychology of Addictive Behaviors, 21,* 255–260.

Schoeller, D. A, Shay, K., & Kushner, R. F. (1997). How much physical activity is needed to minimize weight gain in previously obese women? *American Journal of Clinical Nutrition, 66,* 551–556.

Schulz, L. O., & Schoeller, D. A. (1994). A compilation of total daily energy expenditures and body weight in healthy adults. *American Journal of Clinical Nutrition, 60,* 676–681.

Slentz, C. A., Torgan, C. E., Houmard, J. A., Tanner, C., & Kraus, W. E. (2002). Long-term effects of exercise training and detraining on carbohydrates metabolism in overweight subjects. *Clinical Exercise Physiology, 4,* 22–28.

Stefanick, M. L. (1999). Physical activity for preventing and treating obesity-related dyslipoproteinemias. *Medicine & Sciences in Sports & Exercise, 31,* S609–S618.

Stewart, K., Bacher, A., Turner, K., Lim, J., Hees, P., Shapiro, E., et al. (2005). Exercise and risk factors associated with metabolic syndrome in older adults. *American Journal of Preventative Medicine, 28,* 9–18.

Strecher, V. J., and Rosenstock, I. M. (1997). The Health Belief Model. In K. Glanz, F. M. Lewis, & B. K. Rimer (Eds.), *Health Behavior and Health Education: Theory, Research, and Practice* (pp. 41–59). San Francisco: Jossey-Bass.

Tanaka, K., Okura, T., Shigematsu, R, Nakata, Y, Jun Lee, D., Wan Wee, S. et al. (2004). Target value of intraabdominal fat area for improving coronary heart disease risk factors. *Obesity Research, 12,* 695–703.

Tsang, H. W., Fung, K. M., Chan, A. S., Lee, G., & Chan, F. (2006). Effect of a qigong exercise programme on elderly with depression. *International Journal of Geriatric Psychiatry, 21,* 890–897.

van Etten, L. M. L. A., Westerterp, K. R., Verstappen, F. T. J., Boon, B. J. B., & Saris, W. H. M. (1997). Effect of an 18-wk weight-training program on energy expenditure and physical activity. *Journal of Applied Physiology, 82,* 298–304.

van Warmer, J. J. (2004). Pedometers and brief e-counseling: Increasing physical activity for overweight adults. *Journal of Applied Behavior Analysis, 37*, 421–425.

Villanova, N., Pasqui, F., Burzacchini, S., Forlani, G., Manini, R., Suppini, A., et al. (2006). A physical activity program to reinforce weight maintenance following a behavior program in overweight/obese subjects. *International Journal of Obesity, 30*, 697–703.

Volek, J. S., vanHeest, J. L., & Forsythe, C. E. (2005). Diet and exercise for weight loss: A review of current issues. *Sports Medicine, 35*, 1–9.

Warburton, D. E. R., Nicol, C. W., & Bredin, S. S. D. (2006). Prescribing exercise as preventative therapy. *Canadian Medical Journal Association Journal, 174*, 961–974.

Watkins, P. L., Ebbeck, V., & Levy, S. S. (2005). Feel wonder*full* fitness: A tailored exercise program for larger women. *Health at Every Size, 19*, 101–120.

Wessel, T. R., Arant, C. B., Olson, M. B., Johnson, B. D., Reis, S. E., Sharaf, B. L., et al. (2004). Relationship of physical fitness vs. body mass index with coronary artery disease and cardiovascular events in women. *Journal of the American Medical Association, 292*, 1179–1187.

Westerterp, K. R. (1998). Alterations in energy balance with exercise. *American Journal of Clinical Nutrition, 68*, 970S-974S.

Westerterp, K. R. (1999a). Assessment of physical activity level in relation to obesity: Current evidence and research issues. *Medicine & Science in Sports & Exercise, 31*, S522–S525.

Westerterp, K. R. (1999b). Obesity and physical activity. *International Journal of Obesity, 23*, 59–64.

Wing, R. R. (1999). Physical activity in the treatment of the adult overweight and obesity: Current evidence and research issues. *Medicine & Science in Sports & Exercise, 31*, S547–S552.

Wing, R. R., Tate, D. F., Gorin, A. A., Raynor, H. A., & Fava, J. L. (2006). A self-regulation program for maintenance of weight loss. *New England Journal of Medicine, 355*, 1563–1571.

Wu, K., Hu, F. B., Willet, G. C., Giovannucci, E. (2006). Dietary patterns and risk of prostate cancer in US men. *Cancer Epidemiology Biomarkers and Prevention, 15*, 167–171.

Zelasko, C. J. (1995). Exercise for weight loss: What are the facts? *Journal of the American Dietetic Association, 95*, 1414–1417.

9 BUILT ENVIRONMENTS AND OBESITY

Jeffery Sobal and Brian Wansink

Introduction

Obesity is a complex condition influenced by many diverse types of factors that intersect and interact. Understanding obesity requires multiple approaches that range from narrow examination of the smallest mechanisms to broad consideration of global processes.

Considerable research on obesity takes a biological perspective, examining physiological, genetic, and other characteristics and processes involved in feeding and body weight maintenance. Supplementing those perspectives are behavioral, cognitive, and other psychological analyses that provide information about motivations, attitudes, and other reasons for why people are fatter or thinner. In addition, social science investigations have revealed how social structure, culture, and economics, among other factors, markedly affect food intake and body weight stability or lability. This chapter will move past physiology, beyond behavior, and separate from the social to consider how physical environments influence obesity.

An environmental perspective (Chang & Christakis, 2002) has recently emerged as a way to both frame and interact with other approaches. Environmental approaches consider how the physical environment determines and, in turn, is itself influenced by body weight. For example, clothing provides a "portable environment" (Watkins, 1995) that substitutes for body fat as insulation against the cold, and it is chosen according to the fatness or thinness of a person's body. Environmental thinking is represented in the emergence of terms like *obesogenic environment* (Boehmer et al., 2006; Swinburn et al., 1999) and *toxic food environment* (Brownell & Horgen, 2004).

The present chapter defines the built environment, presents a framework for classifying it into three levels of scale that influence energy intake and energy expenditure, and discusses patterns and mechanisms of environmental influence. Finally, the discussion will cover the implications and applications of built-environment influences on energy balance and body weight and their possible modifications.

Defining the Built Environment

The *built environment* is "everything humanly made, arranged, or maintained" (Bartsuka & Young, 1994, p. 5). Built environments represent the physical world that is modified by humans, in contrast to natural environments that have few human alterations. This inclusive definition includes all that humans have changed from natural materials and natural environments into built environments, which range widely in size from tiny tools to highway systems that span continents. The scope and diversity of built environments in the lives of people are extensive, intensive, and diverse. Using tools and building structures are cultural universals for humans (Brown, 1991). People in contemporary postindustrial societies spend 90% of their time inside buildings (Evans & McCoy, 1998).

The influences of built environments on body weight may be direct or indirect. For example, it may be obvious that a lack of a home refrigerator directly limits the consumption of fresh, low-calorie foods. However, it may be less obvious that a lack of exercise facilities in a neighborhood indirectly inhibits physical activity of the residents in that community. Both storage and exercise constraints can contribute to obesity.

Classifying Built Environments

Built environments can be classified according to their scale (relative size), which forms a spectrum of units of analysis from very small (such as utensils or containers) to extremely large (like regional farm irrigation channels or international shipping networks; Marston, 2000; Sheppard & McMaster, 2004). Most analyses of the built environment and body weight focus on a narrow range of the full spectrum of environmental scale, typically neighborhoods and communities, and do not consider other scales, such as eating utensils or global communication networks (e.g., Booth et al., 2005). However, some investigators also have begun to make scalar distinctions (Swinburn et al., 1999; Wells et al., 2007), such as considering the influence of rooms, tables, and plates on food intake (Sobal & Wansink, 2007).

Built environments can also be classified by conceptual and analytical differentiation of their influences on energy intake and on energy expenditure. For example, a neighborhood with good sidewalks both promotes walking rather than driving to local stores and might also encourage recreational walking that improves fitness and expends calories. By definition, the balance between energy intake and expenditure influences body weight levels and shapes weight gain and weight loss (Hill & Peters, 1998). Influences on energy intake focus on at least two ways by which the built environment shapes the food and nutrition system (Sobal et al., 1998). One approach determines what foods actually come to market, as well as their quantity and price. This approach assesses food availability—some-

Table 9.1
Influences of Built-Environment Scale on Energy Intake and Expenditure

| | | Energy intake and expenditure | |
		Intake	Expenditure
Built-environment scale	Macro scale	Food systems	Transportation
		Commodity chains	Communications
		Food complexes	Mass media
	Meso scale	Food landscapes	Exercise landscapes
		Foodsheds	Neighborhoods
		Food deserts	Facilities
	Micro scale	Kitchenscapes	Rooms
		Tablescapes	Furniture
		Platescapes	Clothing

times in response to past demand and sometimes in anticipation of a change in demand (as with new products). Another approach evaluates accessibility through individuals' food choices and their amount of food consumption.

Table 9.1 presents a classification of built environments on three scales (macro, meso, and micro) and by two components of energy balance (intake and expenditure). This classification provides a useful framework for considering major perspectives on how the built environment influences body weight. The following sections are organized according to this framework and review current ideas about built environments and energy balance, first examining how different scales of the built environment influence energy intake through foods, and next considering how energy expenditure through physical activity is influenced by the built environment.

Energy Intake and Built Environments

To take in energy, people ingest foods and beverages, and all intake takes place within particular environments. As a physical act, eating is connected to the built infrastructure provided by many types and levels of built environments, ranging from farms to plates. Built-environment influences on energy intake will be reviewed here for three scales: macro, meso, and micro.

Energy intake: macro scale

Macro-scale built-environment influences on energy intake represent structures on a very large scale that cannot be observed by a specific individual but can be represented by diagrams, graphs, or other images (Sobal & Wansink, 2007).

Examples of macro-scale built environments are the infrastructures for food systems, pathways of food commodity chains, and facilities of food complexes for particular crops and comestibles (see Table 9.1). All of these influence how and how much energy is consumed by populations and individuals.

FOOD SYSTEMS   *Food systems* are the "sets of operations and processes involved in transforming raw materials into foods and transforming nutrients into health outcomes, all of which functions as a system within biophysical and sociocultural contexts" (Sobal et al., 1998, p. 853). As such, food systems include all of the technologies used to provide resources to raise and harvest animals and plants, process these into foodstuffs, distribute food products for purchase by consumers, acquire and prepare foods, and eat foods in meals and snacks (Sobal, 2004; Tansey & Worsley, 1995). The agricultural revolutions involving the domestication of plants and animals and industrialization of food production have created built environments that are increasingly efficient at capturing energy in food commodities that will eventually be eaten as foods by consumers (Sobal, 1999; Sobal & Lee, 2003).

Food systems are increasingly being transformed by development of the built infrastructure for growing, harvesting, storing, selling, buying, cooking, and eating. New transportation and preservation technologies permit present food systems to offer foods from around the world that are available at all hours of the day or night and can be preserved to cook or consume days or weeks in the future. The processing of perishable meats and preparation of instant microwave dinners are embedded within a complex and evolving set of built environments that facilitates eating a greater variety and larger amount of food than has ever before been possible. Hot foods are now available from vending machines, and most convenience stores are able to leverage the extended perishability of foods to offer both fruits and meat-related foods that were not widely available even 5 years ago.

COMMODITY CHAINS   *Commodity chains* are the pathways that food products follow as they flow from production to consumption (Friedland, 1984, 2001). They include the built infrastructure that developed to move and process foods from the point at which energy is captured during farming to the point at which food energy is ingested by consumers. Analysis of commodity chains is particularly useful because it focuses on tracing foods and the energy they contain upstream to prior origins, as well as downstream to the impacts on body weight and health outcomes (Dixon, 2002; Wilkins, 2005). Longer commodity chains provide more steps at which foods may be modified, with the pragmatic consequence for consumers that increased chain length modifies simple, fresh, whole foods that are generally less calorie-dense into processed, preserved, refined foods that are dense with calories. For example, whereas a short commodity chain might involve a purchase of whole potatoes from a farm stand, a long commodity chain might include buying French fries from a fast-food outlet. To give an idea of the extent of involvement in a commodity chain, consider tomato soup. At one point, 53 different companies were involved in the production required to bring one can of tomato soup to market (Wansink, 2007). These included not only the companies that grew the tomatoes, but those that produced the spices, preservatives, cans, and labels. Each source and step required built-environment infrastructure to play a particular role in the commodity chain.

The delocalization of food production (Pelto & Pelto, 1983) into global food and nutrition systems (Sobal, 1999) has increased commodity chains not only in length (distance from producer to consumer) but also in duration (time from production to consumption). To process and store foods along these paths, the food durability must be increased, often by the addition of sugars and oils at one or many steps in the commodity chain to preserve the foods (Thompson & Cowan, 1995). Fruits and vegetables, such as bananas, are often picked very early and shipped green. Others, such as cucumbers, are waxed to help deter a loss of moisture.

Processing often adds energy to fresh foods so that they can withstand the time spent in different sites through the full length of contemporary commodity chains without spoiling, which also increases the number of calories in the food supply. For example, adding sugar, oil, and salt to oats may make a durable and transportable snack bar that has "value added" because it does not require cooking and can withstand passage from farm to consumers, but it also leads to "value subtracted" from the fresh oats that have fewer calories and preservatives. Individuals interested in preventing weight gain or in losing weight can benefit from consuming foods earlier and in shorter commodity chains. Shopping in built environments like farmers' markets or simply buying supermarket food that is less processed can help people move toward healthier eating with fewer added calories.

FOOD COMPLEXES   *Food complexes* are webs of relationships representing sectors of the agrifood industry that link raw materials to final goods in a web of production, processing, and distribution of particular food types (Friedmann, 1982, 1991; Friedmann & McMichael, 1989). Food complexes include the global wheat complex, livestock complex, durable-food complex, and others. These complexes have developed facilities that determine how much of a particular type of food eventually reaches consumers. In particular, the mass production of standardized, processed durable foods uses manufacturing and transportation infrastructure to obtain sugar and oil substitutes that can be used to provide many of the foods that are most implicated in body weight gain, such as candies, sweet baked goods, fast foods, and similar items (Friedmann, 1991). Although they make many foods inexpensive, food complexes can also sometimes make it more expensive—in terms of dollars and effort—to take in less energy during eating.

Food complexes are crucial portions of the global food environment that reduce the variety and quality of foods because of the centralization of large-scale food production into standardized and highly processed facilities. Food complexes increase the number of calories stored in many foods by creating economies of scale and scope that homogenize highly processed food products. For food consumers, food complexes have made high-calorie processed foods containing substantial amounts of fats and sugars extremely cheap and convenient, while fresh fruits and vegetables remain much more expensive and less readily available (Drewnowski, 2005).

Energy intake: meso scale

Meso-scale built-environment influences on energy intake represent human-scale infrastructures that can typically be seen at one time by a particular individual (Sobal & Wansink, 2007). These include the food landscapes, foodsheds, and food deserts in which people are embedded when they make food choices (see Table 9.1).

FOOD LANDSCAPES   *Food landscapes* include the wide range of distribution points at which food is available for acquisition by consumers as eating outlets available for choosing foods (Guptill & Wilkins, 2002; Sobal & Wansink, 2007). Food landscapes represent the view of food outlets in neighborhoods and communities, and they influence food intake and obesity through the number and types of food outlets that serve a community, such as supermarkets, fast-food restaurants, and beverage outlets (Edmonds et al., 2001; Morland, Wing, & Roux, 2002; Morland, Wing, Roux, & Poole, 2002; LaVeist & Wallace, 2000). In addition to the presence or absence of food outlets in food landscapes, the mix of types of built environments where food is provided through supermarkets and restaurants influences food consumption (Block & Kouba, 2006).

For example, Cheadle and colleagues (1991) reported that the amount of supermarket shelf space devoted to healthful foods was associated with actual consumption of nutritious foods. However, it is not clear how much the supply of food influences consumption, or how much the demand for healthful food influences the supply provided by grocers or restaurateurs in the food landscape (Sallis & Glanz, 2006). Individuals may personally become sensitive to the food landscapes in the built environment in which they reside and obtain foods, and seek to change the landscape of offerings to more healthful foods or seek out healthier landscapes when they acquire foods. They may try to buy locally grown foods or travel a little farther to find a restaurant or food store that best fits their needs.

FOODSHEDS   *Foodsheds* are areas in which food flows from global or regional sources to specific sites of consumption such as a city or town (Kloppenberg et al., 1996). Foodsheds include built-environment infrastructures that serve as smaller subunits in larger food and nutrition systems (Sobal, 1999, 2004). Foodsheds are seen as analogous to watersheds in the larger hydrological system, where channels exist for particular types and amounts of food to flow to where it is acquired by consumers. For example, fresh milk may be trucked from the periphery of a foodshed into central markets where consumers purchase dairy products; the infrastructure of that milkshed is a system of built environments (Durand, 1964). For perishable foods like meat, milk, eggs, and fruit, cities traditionally had distinct foodsheds that included built roads and other forms of transportation used by city residents (Hedden, 1929; Scola, 1992).

With the increasing globalization of the agrifood system, durable manufactured foods (with high energy content from added fats and sugars) do not necessarily need to originate from sources near cities, because foodsheds have expanded in size and scope to include worldwide food sources traveling through a variety of built environments. Food miles are the distance that food travels from production to consumption. Industrially produced, processed, and distributed food products travel about 1500 miles from source to supermarket; local foods travel about 50 miles to farmers' markets (Pirog et al., 2001), with different numbers and types of built environments involved in the foodshed for each category of food. Individuals may adapt their food choices to the built environment of their local foodsheds to acquire fewer processed foods from distant areas and more foods produced locally and seasonally that may be less calorically dense (but typically more expensive).

FOOD DESERTS   *Food deserts* are defined as areas where healthful food is not available, because markets and restaurants do not locate in (or have withdrawn from) low-income or high-crime areas (Cummins & Macintyre, 2002; Wrigley, 2002). Built environments that are food deserts tend to offer highly processed, high-fat, high-calorie foods with few vitamins and minerals, or little fiber, which contribute to high energy intake and constitute a risk for obesity. Types of outlets in food deserts include global fast-food chain restaurants and convenience stores, as well as individually owned food shops and corner stores that offer food high in energy but low in nutrient density (Pearce et al., 2007). For example, food deserts include small urban grocery stores (bodegas) that rarely stock lower-calorie foods like fresh fruits and vegetables or skim milk (Wechsler et al., 1995). Health-conscious individuals residing in food deserts may cope by traveling to other built environments where more healthful and often cheaper foods are more available, or by encouraging the existing local food purveyors to offer more healthful foods.

Energy intake: micro scale

Micro-scale built-environment influences on energy intake represent the immediate contexts in which actual eating is embedded. These small-scale environments include kitchenscapes, tablescapes, platescapes, and other proximate-scale built environments (see Table 9.1; Sobal & Wansink, 2007).

KITCHENSCAPES   *Kitchenscapes* are rooms within architectural structures that offer bounded foodspaces (Bove & Sobal, 2006) for preparing, serving, and consuming foods. Kitchenscapes as built environments include many dimensions that shape what people choose to eat and how much they consume (Sobal & Wansink, 2007). Closer proximity of food sources within a room leads to greater volume of consumption (Wansink, Painter, et al., 2006). Similarly, greater visibility of foods within a room leads to more consumption of conspicuous foods (Painter et al., 2002). The overall ambience of the built environment, characterized by smell, color, lighting, sound, and other characteristics, combines to enhance food intake or suppress food consumption (Stroebele & de Castro, 2004).

Kitchens and other rooms where food is consumed offer behavior settings (Barker, 1968; Schoggin, 1989) that facilitate patterns of eating, including what to eat and how much to eat. Individuals can make healthier food choices and reduce the amount of food intake in kitchenscapes by not provisioning kitchens with energy-dense foods, avoiding stockpiling of unhealthful foods, storing foods out of the view of most people in the room, placing food sources distant from sites of consumption like tables, and removing distractions such as televisions (Sobal & Wansink, 2007).

TABLESCAPES *Tablescapes* include the appearance of furniture or surfaces from which food is consumed (Sobal & Wansink, 2007). Tablescapes offer small-scale built environments that make food immediately available for direct consumption and serve as sites for eating. Many characteristics of tablescapes as built environments both facilitate and inhibit food intake. The visibility of foods as part of the tablescape shows which comestibles are available and provides cues to eat (Wansink, Painter, et al., 2006). The arrangement of foods influences how much food is consumed, with people taking less food for themselves when foods are presented in disorganized rather than organized patterns (Kahn & Wansink, 2004).

The sizes of serving containers dramatically influence food consumption, and people are typically not aware of this influence (Wansink, 2004, 2006; Wansink & Sobal, 2007). For example, people take more snacks, ice cream, and popcorn from larger vessels and consume more of what they take (Wansink & Cheney, 2005; Wansink & Kim, 2005; Wansink, Van Ittersum, et al., 2006). Individuals can reduce caloric intake from tablescapes by avoiding putting serving containers within easy access to eaters, limiting visibility of food sources by using opaque containers and covers for food containers, using smaller food source containers, and having fewer different food sources available (Sobal & Wansink, 2007).

PLATESCAPES *Platescapes* include small-scale built environments in the form of containers and implements for eating foods (Sobal & Wansink, 2007). Up to 71% of the total calories eaten by people in contemporary postindustrial societies are consumed after being transferred from another source to a vessel such as a plate, bowl, glass, or other utensil (Wansink, 1996), and people tend to eat about 92% of the food that they personally serve for themselves (Wansink & Cheney, 2005). The shapes of containers exert a consistent effect on how much food is taken and later consumed; for example, people tend to pour more liquids into wider glasses than into taller glasses that hold the same volume

Table 9.2
Selected Micro-Level Scapes Influencing Food Intake

Roomscapes	Furniturescapes	Containerscapes
Kitchenscapes	Tablescapes	Platescapes
Officescapes	Deskscapes	Bowlscapes
Carscapes	Surfacescapes (counterscapes, etc.)	Cupscapes
Yardscapes	Chairscapes	Packagescapes (boxscapes, bagscapes, canscapes, bottlescapes, etc.)
Storagescapes (shelfscapes, cabinetscapes, pantryscapes)	Trayscapes	Utensilscapes
Others	Blanketscapes at picnics	Others
	Others	

(Wansink & Van Ittersum, 2003, 2005). People eat and drink more from larger containers, such as big popcorn boxes (Wansink & Kim, 2005), higher-volume canteens (Wansink et al., 2005), and larger food packages (Wansink, 1996). In addition, people consume more food when using larger eating implements, such as bigger spoons (Wansink, Van Ittersum, et al., 2006). Individuals can control caloric intake by modifying platescapes, using smaller dishes, serving smaller portions into these containers, not eating directly from large commercial packages, and using smaller utensils in eating (Sobal & Wansink, 2007).

The range of micro-scale built environments that can influence food intake stretches far beyond what can be sufficiently discussed here. Table 9.2 notes some micro-level built environments for further consideration.

Summary of built-environment influences on energy intake

Overall, macro-scale, meso-scale, and micro-scale built environments exert many influences on what foods are available, how accessible they are to consumers, how people choose particular foods, and how much of a food is consumed. These built-environment influences on energy intake are balanced by built-environment influences on expenditure, which are reviewed in the next section.

Energy Expenditure and Built Environments

Energy is used both by internal metabolic processes that operate within the body and by external physical activities in which the body moves to perform various tasks. Built environments influence some internal forms of energy expenditure involuntarily, such as thermoregulation to maintain body temperature in cold buildings (Keith et al., 2006; Sobal, 2001). However, the greatest concern about the influence of built environments on energy expenditure has to do with body movements, where built environments enhance or lessen the activity of individuals. Built-environment influences on energy expenditure will be reviewed here for three scales: macro, meso, and micro.

Energy expenditure: macro scale

Macro-scale built-environment influences on energy expenditure represent infrastructures on a very large scale that cannot be easily observed at one time by individuals (Sobal & Wansink, 2007). Examples of macro-scale built environments are the infrastructures for transportation systems, communications networks, and mass media environments (see Table 9.1), all of which influence how populations and individuals behave and therefore how and how much energy they expend.

TRANSPORTATION *Transportation* infrastructures include walking paths, roads, rail systems, water and air networks, and other large-scale built environments that move people and objects from one place to another. The development of transportation technologies since the industrial revolution has systematically substituted mechanically produced energy for human muscle-powered energy (Sobal, 2001) in a shift from active to passive personal transportation, which on a large scale is correlated with a rise in body fat (Lee & Sobal, 2003). For example, the more people travel in vehicles, the more likely they are to be obese in the United States (Lopez-Zetina et al., 2006). Bell and Popkin (2002) found that in Chinese households, men who acquired a car doubled their likelihood of becoming obese compared to those who did not acquire an automobile. Frank and colleagues (2004) reported a 6% increase in likelihood of obesity for every hour per day spent in a car, and a 5% reduction in likelihood of obesity for every kilometer walked per day.

The design of transportation networks is also important, with urban sprawl providing poor accessibility that inhibits or prevents walking and is associated with greater population-level obesity (Ewing et al., 2003, 2006; Lopez, 2004). Individuals can deal with transportation infrastructures in many ways, including voluntarily traveling by foot or bicycle rather than in motorized vehicles whenever it is feasible, both for utilitarian activities like shopping and for leisure-time recreation. For example, throughout Europe built transportation environments include widely available and accessible public bicycle parking and designated bicycle paths separate from automobile traffic.

COMMUNICATION *Communication* infrastructures involve built technologies that permit the exchange of messages between individuals in different places, saving the energy needed to travel to engage in face-to-face communication. The development of mail, telegraph, telephone, computer, and other electronic technologies lets people exchange information and ideas without having to expend calories by traveling across vast distances or even to an adjacent room. Some studies suggest that using computers to communicate is associated with over-weight in young girls (Kautiainen et al., 2005). In addition, time spent in seden-tary forms of communication activities is an opportunity cost that displaces active behavior, so that people writing, telephoning, or text-messaging are less likely to be engaged in other, more vigorous forms of physical activity. Indi-viduals can deal with the low energy expenditure that is typical of sedentary communication technologies by developing awareness of their low activity; mul-titasking energetic activity while communicating; lessening the time they spend in passive, motionless communication; and seeking active communication envi-ronments rather than passive communication settings.

MASS MEDIA   *Mass media* facilities include built-environment networks that send information and entertainment across space in large volumes to exten-sive audiences, and have a considerable infrastructure that delivers and trans-mits media and permits individuals to consume and interact with the media. Mass media include print forms (newspapers, magazines, books, and other types) and electronic forms (radio, television, computer, and other types). Con-sumption of mass media is typically a sedentary activity in which people sit down and inactively read or view what has become a vast array of media options. The macro-scale development of global mass media infrastructures has created populations of readers, listeners, and viewers who have displaced more active forms of work and entertainment with largely motionless use of their time that does not expend energy beyond basal metabolic needs.

A great deal of evidence suggests that television viewing is a sedentary activi-ty that is associated with higher levels of body fat (e.g., Booth et al., 2005; Car-oli et al., 2004). Individuals can exercise control over mass media influences on their physical activity by eliminating, minimizing, and being selective in mass media consumption; multitasking active pursuits with normally passive mass media use; controlling the presence of media objects and devices available and accessible to them; and seeking built environments that offer active rather than passive media consumption.

Energy expenditure: meso scale

Meso-scale built-environment influences on energy expenditure represent middle-level structures that can be observed in an individual's viewshed (Etzenhouser et al., 1998). Meso-scale built environments include exercise landscapes, neighborhoods, and facilities (see Table 9.1), all of which influence how individuals embedded within these structures behave and consequently how much energy they expend.

EXERCISE LANDSCAPES   An *exercise landscape* is the visual appearance of a par-ticular area or place in the built or natural environment that can be examined for possibilities to engage in physical activity. For example, the aesthetic attrac-tiveness of safe and scenic sites for walking, such as parks and trails, provides a positive association with more physically active behaviors (Giles-Corti et al.,

2005). The presence of trees and other landscaping, scenic views, adequate lighting, and low levels of automobile traffic facilitate pedestrian and human-powered travel (Humpel et al., 2002). Individuals can enhance physical activity by becoming aware of sites for exercise, developing appropriate perceptions of how close those sites are, improving visual attractiveness of existing sites to be appealing and user-friendly, and encouraging the development of additional desirable sites for physical activity. Some community efforts have reclaimed inner-city neighborhoods for walking paths.

NEIGHBORHOODS *Neighborhoods* have infrastructures consisting of local built environments that influence human physical activity (Humpel et al., 2002). These include the availability of sidewalks, parking spaces, and destinations within a walkshed (Cervero et al. 1995). Neighborhood design is an important component of connectivity (the ability to walk between points), with grid street patterns facilitating more pedestrian access and use than do isolated neighborhoods with few street or path connectors. Studies of neighborhood activity report positive influence of neighborhood design on pedestrian walking activity (Saelens et al., 2003). Individuals can enhance physical activity in neighborhoods by becoming aware of and attempting to change neighborhood environments that may discourage walking or bicycling; increasing their pedestrian and cycling travel for commuting, errands, and leisure; and becoming involved in planning new neighborhood infrastructure and modification of existing built environments to make them more pedestrian-oriented than automobile-focused. Current efforts to work with communities, local governments, and companies have yielded collaborations to support local agriculture, to develop promising alliances with companies, and to make physical activity more possible through the help of government investments in safe walking paths and other efforts.

FACILITIES *Facilities* are built environments used for voluntary exercise; they include gymnasiums, health clubs, running/jogging/walking tracks, swimming pools, tennis and basketball courts, playgrounds, playing fields, and other sites designed for recreational activity. Existing studies suggest that the availability of exercise facilities as part of the built environment of an area is associated with greater facility utilization and more individual exercise (Sallis et al., 1986). Access to facilities is crucial for use, and perceived proximity to exercise sites may be at least as important as objective distance (Jilcott et al., 2007). Individuals can enhance facility activities by increasing their awareness of facilities and learning how to use them; increasing the availability and accessibility of facilities; and overcoming space, time, and cost barriers to facility use.

Energy expenditure: micro scale

Micro-scale built-environment influences on energy expenditure represent small physical structures and objects that form the most immediate environments of an individual's world. Examples of micro-scale built environments include rooms, furniture, clothing, and other small-scale built environments that influence how people behave and consequently how much energy they expend (see Table 9.1).

ROOMS   *Rooms* afford many opportunities for activity (Gibson, 1979) that people perceive and use in engaging with built environments in everyday life. Rooms constitute behavior settings (Barker, 1968; Schoggen, 1989) that carry expectations about engaging or not engaging in particular activities. In private homes, for example, formal living rooms facilitate quiet, sedentary behavior, whereas informal recreation rooms provide appropriate settings for activity. Larger rooms require more movement to accomplish everyday tasks; smaller rooms confine and restrict physical activity, encouraging more sedentary behavior.

The floor plan of a building is often designed for energy and building-material efficiency, but it can also be built to encourage physical activity by the inclusion of well-designed, uncluttered, and safe hallways and stairways that facilitate movement between rooms. Regular stair use increases physical activity, and 2 minutes of stair climbing per day can prevent 1 pound of weight gain per year (Zimring et al., 2005). Individuals can enhance physical activity in rooms by treating them as built environments that can be easily entered and exited, and increasing the ability to move freely in rooms without impediments or restrictions.

FURNITURE   *Furniture* is a form of built environment that provides objects for supporting bodies and other things, offering an immediate infrastructure for people and their possessions. Furniture in postindustrial societies has become widely available and relatively inexpensive, so people can easily save energy in everyday life by sitting rather than standing (Sobal, 2001). Furniture is increasingly ergonomically designed, padded, and adjustable, making sitting, reclining, and lying more comfortable and decreasing fidgeting and shifting, thus requiring less caloric output from body micromovements (Sobal, 2001; Wells et al., 2007). Individuals can deal with physical activity and furniture by consciously standing rather than sitting for some tasks; taking breaks from sitting to stand, stretch, and move around; and having ergonomically sound furniture that does not contribute to back problems or other impairments that may inhibit physical activity at other times. Seeking out built environments where furniture makes energy expenditure possible and even encourages it, such as choosing rocking chairs versus fixed chairs, can reduce sedentarism.

CLOTHING   *Clothing* has been labeled the "portable environment" (Watkins, 1995) and provides the most immediate built environment for human bodies. Comfortable clothing requires less adjustment and movement in response to the clothing itself, thus conserving energy (Sobal, 2001). Contemporary clothing weighs considerably less, has fewer layers, and has less friction against the body than did the clothing of past historical eras, and therefore simply sitting, standing, or moving around requires less energy expenditure (Duggan, 1988; Teitlebaum & Goldman,

1972). For example, Wells and colleagues (2007) report that a typical US women's clothing ensemble in the 1880s weighed approximately 9.8 pounds, whereas a contemporary women's outfit weighs only about 2.4 pounds. Thus, contemporary clothing may provide a built environment that requires only one-fourth of the energy of clothing of past eras to carry around through daily activities. Individuals may manage clothing to encourage physical activity by purchasing garments, undergarments, and footwear that fit appropriately and facilitate physical activity by being durable, comfortable, easy to care for, and compatible with walking, moving around, and engaging in other forms of active life.

Conclusion

The multiscalar built environment has a variety of potential influences on energy intake and energy expenditure. The built environment provides an infrastructure that offers opportunities to take in energy or conserve energy in everyday life, as well as to voluntarily limit food consumption or expend energy. Consideration of the pervasive influence of built environments on energy intake and expenditure is crucial for understanding patterns and trends in body weight, as well as for planning and executing activity and weight management interventions. Examples of how different scales of built environments are embedded within each other are presented in Figure 9.1.

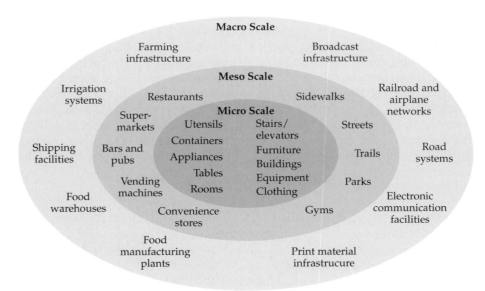

FIGURE 9.1   Selected built environments that influence food intake (left) and energy expenditure (right) at the macro, meso, and micro scales.

Note that research about relationships of built environments, food intake, and physical activity is a very new topic, so an extensive, replicated knowledge base has not yet accumulated, as indicated by critical reviews of the literature in this area (Ferreira et al., 2007; Gebel et al., 2007; White, 2007). Therefore, application of these ideas should proceed with caution until strong, replicated research becomes available (Brug et al., 2006).

Uses of current ideas and information about the built environment and energy balance offer potential in many domains. *Policies* have been proposed to limit the addition of food energy in macro-scale food systems (e.g., Brownell & Horgen, 2004). *Planning* is considering meso-scale built environments involved in food systems (Pothukuchi, 2004; Pothukuchi & Kaufman, 1999, 2000). *Reengineering* of micro-scale food environments like platescapes has been proposed as a way for individuals to successfully manage food intake (Wansink, 2006).

In summary, built environments are multiscalar and multifaceted, and they will need multidisciplinary insights to be fully understood as influences on energy balance and body weight. Assessments and interventions that consider built environments should be incorporated both independently and in conjunction with other strategies and tactics for managing body weight. Policy makers, planners, administrators, clinicians, and citizens all can contribute to planning, designing, maintaining, and using built environments to encourage healthy eating and physical activity, manage body weight, and promote health.

References Cited

Barker, R. G. (1968). *Ecological Psychology: Concepts and methods for studying the environment of human behavior*. Stanford, CA: Stanford University Press.

Bartuska, T. J., & Young, G. L. (Eds). (1994). *The built environment: A creative inquiry into design & planning*. Menlo Park, CA: Crisp Publications.

Bell, A. C., & Popkin, B. M. (2002). The road to obesity or the path to prevention: Motorized transportation and obesity in China. *Obesity Research, 10*, 277–283.

Block, D., & Kouba, J. (2006). A comparison of the availability and affordability of a market basket in two communities in the Chicago area. *Public Health Nutrition, 9*, 837–845.

Boehmer, T. K., Lovegreen, S. L., Haire-Joshu, D., & Brownson, R. C. (2006). What constitutes an obesogenic environment in rural communities? *American Journal of Health Promotion, 20*, 411–421.

Booth, K. M., Pinkston, M. M., & Poston, W. S. (2005). Obesity and the built environment. *Journal of the American Dietetic Association, 105*(5, Suppl. 1), S110–117.

Bove, C. A., & Sobal, J. (2006). Foodwork in newly married couples: Making family meals. *Food, Culture, and Society, 9*, 69–89.

Brown D. E. (1991). *Human Universals*. New York: McGraw-Hill.

Brownell, K. D., & Horgen, K. B. (2004). *Food Fight*. New York: Contemporary Books.

Brug, J., van Lenthe, F. J., & Kremers, S. P. J. (2006). Revisiting Kurt Lewin: How to gain insight into behavioral correlates of obesogenic environments. *American Journal of Preventive Medicine, 31*, 525–529.

Caroli, M., Argentieri, L, Cardone, M., & Masi, A. (2004). Role of television in childhood obesity prevention. *International Journal of Obesity, 28*(Suppl. 3), S104–108.

Cervero, R., Round, A., Goldman, T., & Wu, K. (1995). *Rail access modes and catchment areas for the BART system*. Working Paper No. 307. Berkeley CA: University of California Transportation Center, Department of City and Regional Planning, University of California at Berkeley.

Chang, V. W., & Christakis, N. A. (2002). Medical modeling of obesity: A transition from action to experience in a 20th Century American medical textbook. *Sociology of Health and Illness, 24*, 151–177.

Cheadle, A., Psaty, B. M., Curry, S., Wagner, E., Diehr, P., Koepsell, T., et al. (1991). Community-level comparisons between the grocery store environment and individual dietary practices. *Preventive Medicine, 20*, 250–261.

Cummins, S., & Macintyre, S. (2002). A systematic study of an urban foodscape: The price and availability of food in greater Glasgow. *Urban Studies, 39*, 2115–2130.

Dixon, J. (2002). *The changing chicken: Chooks, cooks and culinary culture.* Sydney, Australia: UNSW Press.

Drewnowski, A. (2005). The economics of obesity: dietary energy density and energy cost. *American Journal of Clinical Nutrition, 82*, 265S–273S.

Duggan, A. (1988). Energy cost of stepping in protective clothing ensembles. *Ergonomics, 31*, 3–11.

Durand, L. (1964). The major milksheds of the Northeastern quarter of the United States. *Economic Geography, 40*, 9–33.

Edmonds, J., Baranowski, T., Baranowski, J., Cullen, K. W., & Myers, D. (2001). Ecological and socioeconomic correlates of fruit, juice, and vegetable consumption among African-American boys. *Preventive Medicine, 32*, 476–481.

Etzenhouser, M. T., Owens, M. K., Spalinger, D. E., & Murden, S. B. (1998). Foraging behavior of browsing ruminants in a heterogeneous landscape. *Landscape Ecology, 13*, 55–64.

Evans, G. W., & McCoy, J. M. (1998). When buildings don't work: The role of architecture in human health. *Journal of Environmental Psychology, 18*, 85–94.

Ewing, R., Brownson, R. C., & Berrigan, D., (2006). Relationships between urban sprawl and weight of United States youth. *American Journal of Preventive Medicine, 31*, 464–474.

Ewing, R., Schmid, T., Killingsworth, R., Zlot, A., & Radenbush, R. (2003). Relationship between urban sprawl and physical activity, obesity, and morbidity. *American Journal of Health Promotion, 18*, 47–57.

Ferreira, I., van der Horst, K., Wendel-Vos, W., Kremers, S., van Lenthe, F. J., & Brug, J. (2007). Environmental correlates of physical activity in youth-a review and update. *Obesity Reviews, 8*, 129–154.

Frank, L. D., Andersen, M. A., & Schmid, T. L. (2004). Obesity relationships with community design, physical activity, and time spent in cars. *American Journal of Preventive Medicine, 27*, 87–96.

Friedland, W. (2001). Reprise on commodity systems methodology. *International Journal of Sociology of Agriculture and Food, 9*, 82–103.

Friedland, W. H. (1984). Commodity systems analysis: An approach to the sociology of Agriculture. In H. K. Schwarzweller (Ed.), *Research on Rural Sociology and Development* (pp. 221–235). Greenwich, CT: JAI Press.

Friedmann, H. (1982). The political economy of food: The rise and fall of the postwar international food order. *American Journal of Sociology, 88* (Suppl.), S248–S286.

Friedmann, H. (1991). Changes in the international division of labor: Agri-food complexes and export agriculture. In W. H. Friedland, L. Busch, F. H. Buttel, & A. P. Rudy (Eds.), *Towards a new political economy of agriculture* (pp. 65–93). Boulder, CO: Westview Press.

Friedmann, H., & McMichael, P. (1989). Agriculture and the state system: The rise and decline of national agricultures, 1870 to the present. *Sociologia Ruralis, 29*, 93–117.

Gebel, K., Bauman, A. E., & Petticrew, M. (2007). The physical environment and physical activity: A critical appraisal of review articles. *American Journal of Preventive Medicine, 32*, 361–365.

Gibson, J. J. (1979). *The ecological approach to visual perception.* Boston: Houghton Mifflin.

Giles-Corti, B., Broomhall, M. H., Knuiman, M., Collins, C., Douglas, K., Ng, K., et al. (2005). Increasing walking: How important is distance to, attractiveness, and size of public open space? *American Journal of Preventive Medicine, 28*, 169–176.

Guptill, A., & Wilkins, J. L. (2002). Buying into the food system: Trends in food retailing and implications for local foods. *Agriculture and Human Values, 19*, 39–51.

Hedden, W. P. (1929). *How great cities are fed.* Boston: D. C. Heath.

Hill, J. O., & Peters J. C. (1998). Environmental contributions to the obesity epidemic. *Science, 280*, 1371–1374.

Humpel, N., Owen, N., & Leslie, E. (2002). Environmental factors associated with adults' participation in physical activity: A review. *American Journal of Preventive Medicine, 22*, 188–199.

Jilcott, S. B., Evenson, K. R., Laraia, B. A., & Ammerman, A. S. (2007). Association between physical activity and proximity to physical activity resources among low-income, midlife women. *Preventing Chronic Disease, 4*, 1–16.

Kahn, B. E., & Wansink, B. (2004). The influence of assortment structure on perceived variety and consumption quantities. *Journal of Consumer Research, 30*, 519–533.

Kautiainen, S., Kiovusilta, L., Lintonen, T., & Rimpela, A. (2005). Use of information and communication technology and prevalence of overweight and obesity among adolescents. *International Journal of Obesity, 29*, 925–933.

Keith, S. W., Redden, D. W., Katzmarzyk, P. T., et al. (2006). Putative contributors to the secular increase in obesity: exploring the roads less traveled. *International Journal of Obesity, 30*, 1585–1594.

Kloppenburg, J., Hendrickson, J., & Stevenson, G. W. (1996). Coming in to the foodshed. *Agriculture and Human Values, 13*, 33–42.

LaVeist, T. A., & Wallace, J. M. (2000). Health risk and inequitable distribution of liquor stores in African American neighborhoods. *Social Science and Medicine, 51*, 613–617.

Lee, S., Sobal, J. (2003). Socio-economic, dietary, activity, nutrition, and body weight transitions in South Korea. *Public Health Nutrition, 6*, 665–674.

Lopez, R. (2004). Urban sprawl and risk for being overweight or obese. *American Journal of Public Health, 94*, 1574–1579.

Lopez-Zetina, J., Lee, H., & Friis, R. (2006). The link between obesity and the built environment. Evidence from an ecological analysis of obesity and vehicle miles of travel in California. *Health & Place, 12*, 656–664.

Marston, S. A. (2000). The social construction of scale. *Progress in Human Geography, 24*, 219–242.

Morland, K., Wing, S., & Roux, A. D. (2002). The contextual effect of the local food environment on residents' diets: The Atherosclerosis risk in communities study. *American Journal of Public Health, 92*, 1761–1767.

Morland, K., Wing, S., Roux, D. A., & Poole, C. (2002). Neighborhood characteristics associated with the location of food stores and food service places. *American Journal of Preventive Medicine, 22*, 23–29.

Painter, J. E., Wansink, B., & Hieggelke, J. B. (2002). How visibility and convenience influence candy consumption. *Appetite, 38*, 237–238.

Pearce, J., Blakely, T., Witten, K., & Bartie, P. (2007). Neighborhood deprivation and access to fast-food retailing: A national study. *American Journal of Preventive Medicine, 32*, 375–382.

Pelto, G. H., & Pelto, P. J. (1983). Diet and delocalization: Dietary changes since 1750. In R. I. Rothberg & T. K. Raab (Eds.), *Hunger and history: The impact of changing food production and consumption patterns on Society* (pp. 309–330). Cambridge: Cambridge University Press.

Pirog, R., Van Pelt, T., Enshayan, K., & Cook, E. (2001). *Food, fuel, and freeways: An Iowa perspective on how far food travels, fuel usage, and greenhouse gas emissions.* Ames, IA: Leopold Center for Sustainable Agriculture, Iowa State University. Retrieved February 22, 2007, from http://www.leopold.iastate.edu/pubs/staff/ppp/index.htm

Pothukuchi, K. (2004). Inner city grocery retail: What planners can do. *Progressive Planning, 158*, 10–12.

Pothukuchi, K., & Kaufman, J. L. (1999). Placing the food system on the urban agenda: The role of municipal institutions in food system planning. *Agriculture and Human Values, 16*, 213–224.

Pothukuchi, K., & Kaufman J. L. (2000). The food system: A stranger to the planning field. *Journal of the American Planning Association, 66*, 113–124.

Saelens, B. E., Sallis, J. F., & Frank, L. D. (2003). Environmental correlates of walking and cycling: Findings from the transportation, urban design, and planning literatures. *Annals of Behavioral Medicine, 25*, 80–91.

Sallis, J. F., & Glanz, K. (2006). The role of built environments in physical activity, eating, and obesity in childhood. *Future of Children, 16*, 89–108.

Sallis, J. F., Nader, P. R., Rupp, J. W., Atkins, C. J., & Wilson, W. C. (1986). San Diego surveyed for heart-healthy foods and exercise facilities. *Public Health Reports, 101*, 216–219.

Schoggen, P. (1989). *Behavior settings.* Stanford, CA: Stanford University Press.

Scola, R. (1992). *Feeding the Victorian city: The food supply of Manchester, 1770–1870*. New York: Manchester University Press.

Sheppard, E., & McMaster, R. B. (2004). *Scale and geographic inquiry: Nature, society, and method*. Malden, MA: Blackwell.

Sobal, J. (1999). Food system globalization, eating transformations, and nutrition transitions. In R. Grew (Ed.), *Food in Global History*. Boulder, CO: Westview Press.

Sobal, J. (2001). Social and Cultural Influences on Obesity. In P. Bjorntorp (Ed.), *International Textbook of Obesity* (pp. 305–322). London: Wiley.

Sobal, J. (2004). Food and nutrition systems. In A. F. Smith (Ed.), *The Oxford Encyclopedia of Food and Drink in America* (pp. 495–498). New York: Oxford University Press.

Sobal, J., Khan, L. K., & Bisogni, C. (1998). A conceptual model of the food and nutrition system. *Social Science and Medicine, 47,* 853–863.

Sobal, J., & Lee, S. (2003). A food and nutrition system analysis of South Korea. *Journal of Community Nutrition, 5,* 209–217.

Sobal J, & Wansink B. (2007). Kitchenscapes, tablescapes, platescapes, and foodscapes: Influences of microscale built environments on food intake. *Environment and Behavior, 39,* 124–142.

Stroebele, N., & de Castro, J. M. (2004). Effect of ambience on food intake and food choice. *Nutrition, 20,* 821–838.

Swinburn, B., Egger, G., & Raza, F. (1999). Dissecting obesogenic environments: The development and application of a framework for identifying and prioritizing environmental interventions for obesity. *Preventive Medicine, 29,* 563–570.

Tansey, G., & Worsley, T. (1995). *The food system: A guide*. London: Earthscan.

Teitlebaum, A., & Goldman, R. F. (1972). Increasing energy costs of multiple clothing layers. *Journal of Applied Physiology, 32,* 743–744.

Thompson S. J., & Cowan, J. T. (1995). Durable food production and consumption in the world economy. In P. McMichael (Ed.), *Food and agrarian orders in the world economy* (pp. 35–52). Westport, CT: Praeger.

Wansink, B. (1996). Can package size accelerate usage volume? *Journal of Marketing, 60,* 1–14.

Wansink, B. (2004). Environmental factors that unknowingly influence the consumption and intake of consumers. *Annual Review of Nutrition, 24,* 455–479.

Wansink, B. (2006). *Mindless eating: Why we eat more than we think*. New York: Bantam.

Wansink, B. (2007), Food Marketing. In A. F. Smith (Ed.), *Oxford Companion to American Food and Drink* (pp. 230–231). New York: Oxford University Press.

Wansink, B., Cardello, A., & North, J. (2005). Fluid consumption and the potential role of canteen shape in minimizing dehydration. *Military Medicine, 170,* 871–873.

Wansink, B., & Cheney, M. M. (2005). Super bowls: Serving bowl size and food consumption. *Journal of the American Medical Association, 293,* 1727–1728.

Wansink, B., & Kim, J. (2005). Bad popcorn in big buckets: Portion size can influence intake as much as taste. *Journal of Nutrition Education and Behavior, 37,* 242–245.

Wansink, B., Painter, J. E., & Lee, Y. K. (2006). The office candy dish: Proximity's influence on estimated and actual consumption. *International Journal of Obesity, 30,* 871–875.

Wansink, B., & Sobal, J. (2007). Mindless eating: The 200 daily food decisions we overlook. *Environment and Behavior, 39,* 106–123.

Wansink, B., & Van Ittersum, K. (2003). Bottoms up! The influence of elongation on pouring and consumption volume. *Journal of Consumer Research, 30,* 455–463.

Wansink, B., & Van Ittersum, K. (2005). Shape of glass and amount of alcohol poured: Comparative study of effect of practice and concentration. *British Medical Journal, 331,* 1512–1514.

Wansink, B., Van Ittersum, K., & Painter, J. E. (2006). Ice Cream Illusions: Bowl Size, Spoon Size, and Serving Size. *American Journal of Preventive Medicine, 31,* 240–243.

Watkins, S. M. (1995). *Clothing: The portable environment*. Ames, IA: Iowa State University Press.

Wechsler, H., Basch, C. E., Zybert, P., Lantigua, R., & Shea, S. (1995). The availability of low-fat milk in an inner-city Latino community: implications for nutrition education. *American Journal of Public Health, 85,* 1690–1692.

Wells, N. M., Ashdown, S. P., Davies, E. H. S., Cowett, F. D., Yang, Y. (2007). Environment, design, and obesity:

Opportunities for Interdisciplinary collaborative research. *Environment and Behavior, 39,* 6–33.

White, M. (2007). Food access and obesity. *Obesity Reviews, 8*(Suppl. 1), 99–107.

Wilkins, J. W. (2005). Seeing beyond the package: Teaching about the food system through food product analysis. *Food, Culture & Society, 8,* 97–114.

Wrigley, N. (2002). 'Food deserts' in British cities: Policy context and research priorities. *Urban Studies, 39,* 2029–2130.

Zimring, C., Joseph, A., Nicoll, G. L., & Tsepas, S. (2005). Influences of building design and site design on physical activity: Research and intervention opportunities. *American Journal of Preventive Medicine, 28*(2, Suppl. 2), 186–193.

10 FROM PROTOCOLS TO POPULATIONS: ESTABLISHING A ROLE FOR ENERGY DENSITY OF FOOD IN THE OBESITY EPIDEMIC

Marion M. Hetherington and Barbara J. Rolls

Introduction

Most industrialized and many developing nations are facing a rapid rise in overweight and obesity that cannot be accounted for by a change in the gene pool, but must largely be due to changes in the food environment and our response to these changes. A predisposition to weight gain is common; humans are adapted to store energy as fat, presumably to counter food scarcity (Loos & Bouchard, 2003). The current food-permissive environment promotes food intake in many ways, including the widespread availability of a variety of energy-dense, highly palatable, inexpensive foods in large portions.

Restaurants and manufacturers, whose goal is to sell products, give consumers foods that they want: palatable, value for the money, and easy to prepare (Condrasky et al., 2007). Foods that are appealing and easy to overconsume are typically high in fat, sugar, and salt and low in fiber, vegetables, and fruit. These foods share a relatively high energy density (kilocalories per gram) and low nutrient density.

Demonstrating that energy-dense foods play a role in the obesity epidemic is challenging and requires a number of different approaches, including basic studies of the factors that influence food intake, clinical trials applying basic findings, and population-based studies documenting how these influences operate in natural settings. Unified hypotheses that integrate these various approaches and that suggest practical implications are needed for developing effective strategies to moderate energy intake and counter the obesity epidemic. This review will focus on recent studies examining what role the energy density of foods plays in the control of food intake, and how the mix of laboratory-, community-, and population-based approaches has led to practical solutions for moderating energy intake.

The Utility of Short-Term Experiments

Much of what is known about the controls of food intake has emerged from several decades of short-term, laboratory-based experiments. Such studies have allowed isolation and identification of the many factors that can affect intake during a meal. Rigorous, well-controlled studies that systematically vary a particular influence on intake can be used to assemble a unified understanding of a complex behavior such as eating.

For investigators in the field, the short-term paradigm has provided many robust phenomena that have served as platforms for longer-term studies. Results of these studies, in turn, have generally been consistent with all the major findings emerging from the well-controlled short-term studies. This congruity should not surprise us, because both short- and long-term studies reflect the experience and habits that determine food choice. Moreover, these studies engage the orogustatory, gastric, and postingestive controls that are normally recruited to determine spontaneous meal size. Thus, short-term laboratory-based protocols have repeatedly identified potentially influential components of the diet or the broader food context that affect energy intake.

Numerous dietary and situational manipulations have been devised to characterize critical influences on food intake (Hetherington, 2002, 2007). Since food intake tends to follow habitual, predictable patterns, experiments may reveal crucial food-related, situational, or individual-specific influences on intake, albeit within the constraints of a laboratory (Hetherington & Rolls, 1987; Rolls & Hetherington, 1990). When these influences have been established, it is then appropriate to extend the investigation into the longer term for further scrutiny. Before we explore how this research applies to the role of energy density in energy balance, it is important to understand the basic features of eating that can be usefully investigated in the laboratory.

Short-Term Controls of Food Intake

Food intake occurs in bouts, or "meals," so these have been the focus of most short-term experimental studies. The size of the meal is controlled, in part, by central mechanisms, which constantly monitor stored energy, as well as current energy and nutrient sources (Woods, 2005). In addition, human food intake is influenced by situational factors such as social context, as well as the availability and variety of foods (Hetherington, 2007). The decision to begin eating, the foods selected, and the amount then eaten will depend in part on the metabolism of previous meals (Levin, 2006) and, we would argue especially on the quality, variety, and presentation of food currently available for consumption.

The initiation of a meal, however, does not depend on energy deficit, and meal size only occasionally relates to the duration of energy depletion. For example, adults in the United Kingdom and the United States tend to eat their smallest meals after the longest period of energy deprivation (during sleep) and their largest meals at the end of the day, in anticipation of many hours of not eating (Weingarten, 1985). Human food intake may be best understood through the concepts of social facilitation, habit, palatability, and other nonphysiological factors. Nevertheless, consumers will regularly cite "hunger" as the main reason for initiating a meal; therefore deprivation, whether perceived or real (related to energy need), is associated with the decision to eat.

Many laboratory-based studies of intake have focused on the processes by which food intake is terminated. Meal termination, or satiation, occurs as a function of numerous, coordinated signals from the gastrointestinal tract in response to distension of the stomach and to the chemical properties of the food consumed (Cummings & Overduin, 2007). Satiation is assessed during *ad libitum* access to test foods by measuring both food and energy intake (Kral & Rolls, 2004). Therefore, a standard protocol for evaluating intake involves simply allowing study participants to eat as much as they like of a food or an array of foods.

This approach provides the means to assess the influence of a number of different food- or context-related variables on satiation and meal size, including changes in energy density, palatability, or variety. Numerous short-term studies have shown that meal size can be highly variable, subject to many different situational factors related to the food (palatability, volume, variety, etc.) or the context in which the food is provided (ease of access, cost, presence of other people, etc.). These short-term influences are largely uncoupled from specific energy deficits (Wiepkema, 1971; Lowe & Levine, 2005).

Another laboratory-based standard protocol for studying energy intake is to provide study participants with a compulsory food (a preload) and then determine how this preload affects subsequent intake. Studies utilizing preloads provide a method for assessing satiety, or the state that occurs following food consumption. The preloads may vary in volume, type of food, energy content, energy density, or macronutrient content. Systematically varying the amounts or types of nutrients in the preloads, for instance, provides a protocol for assessing the properties of foods that affect satiety, including, for example, energy density (Kral & Rolls, 2004).

Mammalian food intake tends to be poorly controlled from meal to meal (Mazlan et al., 2006) and not necessarily linked to energy expenditure (Kraly & Blass, 1982), so the potential for positive energy balance in a food-permissive environment is high. A great many features of the environment have been shown to increase intake, including providing large portion sizes (Rolls et al., 2002), providing a variety of foods (Rolls & Hetherington, 1989), eating while watching TV (Bellisle et al., 2004; Blass et al., 2006; Hetherington, Anderson, et al., 2006), and drinking alcohol before or with the meal (Caton et al., 2005, 2007).

Given that meal size can be increased by relatively minor changes to the environment (see Chapter 9), it is worth considering whether environmental changes can also be used to the advantage of consumers who wish to lose weight. Small systematic changes in eating can reduce total energy intake and may produce sustainable effects on body weight, since these small alterations will not necessarily produce compensatory behaviors. For example, because variety is known to stimulate food intake and to produce weight gain in lean participants (Stubbs et al., 2001), reducing variety is likely to result in a net reduction in energy intake (Hetherington, Foster, et al., 2006). Other studies find that eating in social contexts with friends promotes food intake, but eating alone tends to limit intake (de Castro, 1994; Hetherington, Anderson, et al., 2006; Shide & Rolls, 1991).

It is unrealistic, however, to translate these short-term findings on intake into the realm of long-term weight regulation, since advising consumers either to eat a less varied diet or to eat alone is neither sustainable nor healthy. Imposing a biologically based solution on the complex problem of feeding has typically failed in the long term. In contrast, a fundamental property of the diet, such as its energy density, influences meal size in the short term, total energy intake over several days, and dietary intake in the long term. The key questions are (1) will alterations in energy density to the diet be acceptable to the consumer? and (2) will this property of the diet, if manipulated, produce compensatory behaviors? If lower-energy-density foods are offered in place of high-energy-density foods, will the consumer simply eat more of the lower-energy-density foods and negate any net reduction in total energy intake? The following exploration of these questions will begin by defining energy density and will then review studies that have examined the impact of lowering energy density on energy intake in the acute and clinical context.

What Is Energy Density?

Energy density refers to the amount of energy provided by a given amount of food. Foods may be described as high, medium, or low in energy density, as determined by calculation of the energy delivered by a standard weight of food, such as a gram (g). For example, a high-energy-density food such as potato chips delivers 540 kilocalories in 100 grams, or 5.4 kcal/g, compared to 100 grams of a low-energy-density food such as strawberries, which provides 30 kilocalories, or 0.3 kcal/g. The fat content of the chips and the water content of the strawberries contribute to this disparity in energy density. Thus, every unit of potato chips provides 18 times as many calories as the equivalent unit of strawberries. The 18:1 ratio can be mitigated by lowering the energy density of potato chips. This lower energy density is typically achieved by lowering the fat content; the baked, low-fat version drops from 5.4 kcal/g to 3.9 kcal/g—and for fat-free, to 3.5 kcal/g. Even fat-free, however, a potato chip unit is still 12 times more energy-dense than a strawberry unit. Thus, simply lowering the fat content of an energy-dense food will not, in itself, necessarily create a low-energy-density product.

Incorporating water into a food lowers its energy density because water increases the weight but not the energy content of the food. Increasing intake of naturally water-rich foods will lower the energy density of the diet because water contains no energy (0 kcal/g). Similarly, increasing the consumption of foods high in fiber (1.5–2.5 kcal/g) will reduce dietary density, but the impact is much smaller than that of water because only limited amounts of fiber can be consumed. Thus, actively seeking out and increasing intake of foods with a high water or fiber content will lower dietary energy density.

The corollary is that reducing intake of energy-dense foods such as those high in fat will also reduce dietary density because fat has the highest energy density (9 kcal/g) of all macronutrients (alcohol has 7 kcal/g; protein has 4; carbohydrate has 4). A strategy that promotes intake of water-rich and high-fiber foods while reducing intake of high-fat foods should produce a net reduction in the energy density of the diet. If this strategy is to be effective for weight loss, a reduction in total energy intake resulting from lowering the energy density of the diet must not compromise food flavor and must not lead to compensatory eating. To gauge the effects of lowering energy density on satiety and satiation, a number of laboratory-based experiments have been conducted.

Energy density and preloading

The provision of preloads differing in energy density before a test meal has been used in a number of studies to assess the influence of energy density on satiety. An early study found that participants did *not* compensate during a test meal for differences in the energy density of a first course (preload) of soup or jello that varied in energy density but was matched for volume (Rolls et al., 1988). When the preloads were reduced in energy density, the total energy intake of the meal was significantly decreased. This evidence suggests that consuming low-energy-density foods at the start of a meal is a strategy that could be used to promote satiety while reducing total energy intake during a meal. Several more recent studies confirm this suggestion.

In one experiment, intake of a main course of pasta (700 grams, at 2 kcal/g) at lunch was compared across conditions in which participants consumed either no first course or a small (150-gram) or large (300-gram) first-course salad at three different energy densities (0.33, 0.67, and 1.33 kcal/g; Rolls et al., 2004). The large portion of the low-energy-density salad (100 kilocalories) reduced total energy intake (salad + pasta) by 12% compared with no salad. Total energy intake was greatest after the large, energy-dense salad (400 kilocalories). Note that reduction in pasta intake was related to salad size and not calories. Thus a large, low-calorie salad substantially reduced total intake. Poor planning of presenting a large calorically dense salad will enhance total intake.

These findings demonstrate that, for a given energy level of preload, the bigger the volume and the lower the energy density of the preload, the greater the decrease in intake of the more energy-dense pasta (Figure 10.1). In the applied setting, consumption of a preload high in energy density will simply add to the total energy of the meal, so practical solutions involving energy density emphasize the use of preloads low in both energy density and total energy, say under 150 kilocalories, in order to minimize the impact of a preload or starter on total energy intake.

FIGURE 10.1 Mean meal energy intake following intake of preload salads that differed in both weight and energy density. Significant differences in meal energy intake compared to consuming no salad are indicated by * ($p < 0.05$) and *** ($p < 0.0001$). (From Rolls et al., 2004, with permission from Elsevier.)

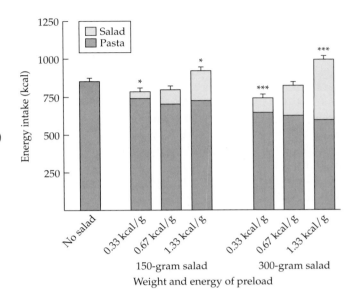

Several short-term, laboratory-based studies have found that consumption of other low-energy-density foods high in water content, such as soup, as a preload can substantially reduce energy intake at a meal (Kissileff, 1985; Himaya & Louis-Sylvestre, 1998; Rolls et al., 1990, 1999b). Note, however, that drinking water as a beverage does not have the same effect on satiety as incorporating it into a food to lower the energy density. One study found that cooking water into a casserole to make soup was more effective in increasing satiety and reducing subsequent energy intake than was consuming the same ingredients separately (Rolls et al., 1999b). The 100-kilocalorie reduction in lunch intake associated with the soup preload was not compensated for later in the day. Thus, a number of studies show that the energy density of a preload affects satiety and total energy intake in a meal. This finding offers a potential strategy for weight management because consuming a low-energy soup or salad at the start of a meal may reduce later intake.

Energy density and ad libitum intake

Studies have shown that lowering the energy density of the available foods also has robust effects on *ad libitum* consumption or satiation. In a study by Bell and colleagues (1998) in which energy density was manipulated, participants were served all of their meals for 2 days on three separate occasions. After eating a standard breakfast, they freely consumed lunch and dinner, which varied in energy density (low, medium, or high) along with compulsory side dishes. Energy density was varied by manipulation of the proportion of vegetables and pasta in the meals, so low-energy-density meals had a greater water and fiber content than did high-energy-density meals. The meals were rated as equally palatable, and the macronutrient composition was similar across energy density manipulations. Even with a 30% reduction in the energy density of the available foods, participants consumed a similar amount of food across conditions, with amounts varying by less than 50 grams. Therefore, the cumulative total energy intake for the low-energy-density condition was about 30% less than that for the high-energy-density condition.

Importantly, ratings of hunger, fullness, and prospective consumption did not differ by energy density (Bell et al., 1998). Despite differences in total energy intake between the diets, participants found the meals equally satisfying. In part, this result is likely due to the effects of eating to a constant weight of food to produce similar levels of fullness and satisfaction. Interestingly, the effect of energy density on food intake is similar in obese and lean participants (Bell & Rolls, 2001).

The effect of energy density on *ad libitum* intake has also been shown to persist over periods of 4 to 5 days without significant compensation for a reduction in energy intake. In one experiment, Duncan and colleagues (1983) provided lean and obese participants *ad libitum* access to either a low-energy-density (LED) or a high-energy-density (HED) diet for 5 days in a hospital setting. The LED diet contained fresh fruits and vegetables, whole grains, skim milk, and lean meats; the HED diet contained fattier meats, as well as high-fat and refined foods, including whole milk, fried foods, white bread, and high-fat, high-sugar desserts.

Because foods were freely available and intake was *ad libitum* in this study, one might expect LED participants to gradually increase the weight of food consumed from days 1 to 5 in an effort to achieve a higher total energy intake and perhaps to seek a higher level of satisfaction compared to the HED participants. Similarly, intake on the HED might decline over 5 days. Despite highly significant differences in average daily energy intake between the LED diet (1570 kilocalories) and the HED diet (3000 kilocalories), energy intake remained stable on both diets. The participants in the study did not compensate by increasing the weight of food consumed in the LED diet, nor did they reduce the weight of food eaten in the HED diet during the 5 days. However, participants reported higher ratings of fullness, even eating to the point of discomfort, on the HED diet. Although hunger was lower before lunch and dinner on the HED diet, ratings did not vary between the HED and LED diets in the evening and before breakfast.

In another experiment comparing obese and lean participants, energy intake was measured across a 4-day period (Rolls et al., 1999a). The palatability of foods was controlled, and the investigators manipulated either the energy density (4.4 and 6.7 kJ/g) or the fat content (16% and 36% of energy) of compulsory main-course foods representing about 50% of each individual's total energy intake. Intake of all self-selected foods at meals and snacks was then recorded following both energy density and fat manipulations. Overall, both lean and obese participants reduced energy intake of self-selected foods at meals by 16% (642

FIGURE 10.2 Effects of energy density (A) and fat content (B) of compulsory foods on mean (±SEM) energy intake over the 4 test days for 16 lean and 17 obese women. Within each weight group, mean *ad libitum* intakes of the side dishes labeled with different letters (a–d) are significantly different (*p* < 0.05). (After Rolls et al., 1999a, with permission from the American Society for Nutrition.)

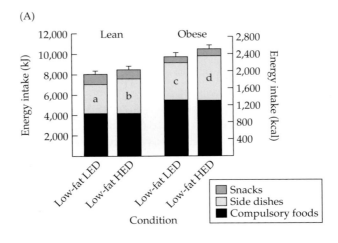

(A)

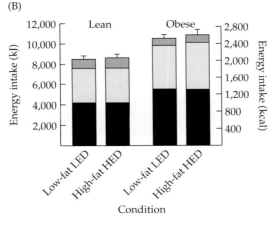

(B)

kilojoules; 153 kilocalories) when they were given the LED compared to the HED meals, but both groups failed to respond to differences in the fat content of the meals (Figure 10.2).

Clearly, both lean and obese individuals were influenced by the energy density of the compulsory component of the diet and not the fat content. Since there was no tendency to compensate for the reduction in energy intake over the 4-day period and ratings of hunger did not differ between the diets, this strategy of providing lower-energy-density meals to reduce intake could be used in weight loss programs (Rolls et al., 1999a).

Taken together, these studies suggest that consuming a LED diet for up to 5 days resulted in a net reduction in total energy intake with little effect on hunger ratings. The key question is whether LED diets can be developed that will control hunger and enhance satiety, achieving a level of compliance that will facilitate weight loss.

How does lowering energy density promote satiation and satiety?

The consumption of water-rich, high-fiber foods that are low in energy density is likely to activate a variety of processes that promote satiety and satiation. For example, eating such foods might prolong meal duration (Weinsier et al., 1982; Duncan et al., 1983) and therefore orosensory experience. In the study by Duncan and colleagues (1983), participants took longer to eat fewer calories on the LED diet compared to the HED diet. On average, participants spent 69 minutes per day eating on the LED diet and 52 minutes on the HED; and they chewed each meal for 17 minutes on the LED diet, compared to 12 minutes on the HED diet.

The fiber content of foods may facilitate satiation not only through orosensory effects but also through gastric distension, emptying, nutrient absorption rates, and gastrointestinal hormone release (Howarth et al., 2001). Foods with a high water content could promote satiety and satiation by enhancing gastric distension. Holt and colleagues (1995) calculated a satiety index for 38 common foods and found that although satiety was correlated with fiber content, an even stronger correlation coefficient was found for water content.

Meal size is determined by both orosensory positive feedback and postingestive negative feedback (Wiepkema, 1971; Smith, 1996, 2000). The satiating effects of LED foods may be achieved through maximizing positive orosensory exposure and optimizing negative feedback from the gut. If consumers are sensitive to energy content, however, even if volume is increased and orosensory exposure maximized they may compensate for energy content at the next meal(s). To examine these proposals, experiments have been conducted to investigate how the manipulation of energy content, volume, and orosensory experience affects energy intake within and beyond a meal.

Lowering the energy density of foods allows consumption of a greater volume of food for a defined energy intake. Manipulating the volume that is consumed influences the development of satiation and the expression of sensory-specific satiety. *Sensory-specific satiety* is defined as a decline in the rated pleasantness of the appearance, smell, texture, and taste of an eaten food relative to a tasted but uneaten food (Hetherington et al., 1989), as well as a reduced desire to eat more of that food relative to other foods (Rolls et al., 1981). Consuming a large volume of a milk-based drink (600 milliliters) produced greater changes in pleasantness than consuming a small volume (300 milliliters) with the same energy content (Figure 10.3). Doubling the energy content while keeping the volume the same (600 milliliters) had no additional effect on sensory-specific satiety (Bell et al., 2003). This finding suggests that consumers are more responsive to the duration of the sensory experience provided by large volumes than to the absolute energy content of the food.

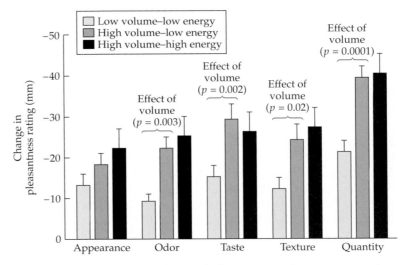

FIGURE 10.3 Changes in the rated pleasantness of appearance, odor, taste, texture, and prospective consumption of milk-based drinks following intake of different volumes of these drinks. These changes are calculated as the difference in rating before and after intake of the drink. Significant effects of the increase in volume of the drink are indicated below the bars; the increase in energy content had no significant effects. The three formulations of the milk-based drink were (1) low volume–low energy (300 milliliters, 500 kilocalories); (2) high volume–low energy (600, 500); (3) high volume–high energy (600, 1000). (After Bell et al., 2003, with kind permission from Elsevier.)

Consumers also respond to postingestive signals related to the volume consumed. Intragastric infusions of foods that bypass orosensory stimulation have been used to examine the role of negative feedback from the stomach on energy intake. Intragastric infusions of milk-based liquid preloads of differing volumes (0, 200, or 400 milliliters) or energy contents (0, 200, or 400 kilocalories) given 30 minutes before a buffet-style lunch revealed the importance of volume rather than energy content in suppressing appetite and food intake in both lean and obese women (Rolls & Roe, 2002). In this experiment the large (400-milliliter) infusion significantly reduced intake of lunch compared to a control condition in which the nasogastric tube was fitted but no nutrients were delivered. This effect was similar for the large-volume infusions at both 200 and 400 kilocalories.

Changes in the pleasantness and desire for a food as it is eaten (Hetherington, 1996) converge with negative feedback arising from the gut to affect satiation and the amount consumed. With repeated exposure to particular foods, consumers learn to associate specific orosensory features of a food with its postingestive consequences (Birch, 1986). Although the amount eaten is determined in part by such associative learning, this effect may be modified in response to changes in need state. Eating habits are established through repeated consumption of foods, and people learn to eat certain quantities of these foods, whether as part of a mixed meal or as a single-item portion. How learning affects the development of eating habits can most easily be observed in young children, who are building up experiences with foods varying in organoleptic properties, nutrient content, and energy density (see Chapter 6).

Establishing Eating Patterns

Infants and toddlers acquire liking for foods through associative conditioning, modeling, and social facilitation (Birch, 1986, 1999). Infants between 8 and 15 months of age are less likely than adults to be influenced by situational factors such as the presence of others (Pearcey & de Castro, 1997). Similarly preschoolers are not influenced by the portion size of food presented (Rolls et al., 2000).

Young children seem particularly sensitive to internal cues and are likely to adjust intake in response to prior ingestion. For instance, preschoolers are sensitive to the energy content of preloads given before *ad libitum* test meals (Birch & Deysher, 1986; Hetherington et al., 2000). They are able to adjust intake following a preload with a high degree of precision, but the ability to regulate accurately and immediately between meals declines with age (Cecil et al., 2005; Hetherington et al., 2000). This finding implies that smaller meals or less frequent eating occasions will follow larger meals in young children but that this association weakens with age. For example, 24-hour recall data collected from the mothers of more than 3000 infants and toddlers revealed that children who consumed fewer meals or snacks during the day consumed larger amounts than did children who ate more frequently (Fox et al., 2006). A significant inverse relationship between energy density and portion size was found in 6- to 11-month-olds; they adjusted their daily energy intake by consuming larger portions as the energy density of the diet decreased and reducing the amount consumed as energy density of the diet increased. However, Fox and colleagues (2006) found no such relationship in toddlers aged 12 to 24 months. Infants may learn to pair larger portion sizes with fewer eating occasions and smaller portions with greater eating frequency, but this pattern of eating declines with age.

Taken together, these findings suggest that the association of meal frequency, meal size, and energy density appears to be strongest in early infancy and may diminish over time. Older children (Birch et al., 1991) and adults tend to eat a certain weight of food (Kral & Rolls, 2004), and the amount eaten remains relatively constant despite variability in prior intake. If this is so, then although the amount of food eaten may be similar under different conditions, total energy intake will vary from meal to meal and from day to day depending on the energy density of the diet.

Therefore, if adults and, indeed, children (Leahy et al., 2007) are *offered* lower-energy-density foods, they will maintain the amount consumed, and total energy intake will be *lower* than when they are offered higher-energy-density foods. The reduction in total energy when consuming a diet reduced in energy density could facilitate a negative energy balance. Several long-term clinical trials have been conducted to assess the efficacy of adopting an LED diet to promote weight loss.

Implications of adopting a low-energy-density diet pattern for weight loss

Until recently, most weight loss diets focused on variations in the proportions of macronutrients. In particular, fat-reduced diets were found to be associated with reductions in energy intake and weight loss (Yu-Poth et al., 1999). Although the energy density was not measured, fat-reduced diets probably were also reduced in energy density. An example of a controlled investigation of fat reduction is a longitudinal study by Kendall and colleagues (1991) that involved obese participants consuming a low-fat diet for 11 weeks. This regimen produced significant weight loss compared to a control diet. The low-fat diet provided between 20% and 25% of energy as fat; the control diet, between 35% and 40%. Although participants could eat as much as they wanted from the two diets, the weight of food consumed per day was similar for each diet, and it did not vary over the 11 weeks of the study. Given the constancy in the weight of food consumed, daily energy intake was significantly less on the low-fat diet, and average weight loss was 2.5 kilograms, compared to 1.26 kilograms on the control diet (Kendall et al., 1991). The diets were rated equally palatable, although subjective appetite was not measured. This study supports the observation from shorter-term studies that consumers eat a constant weight of food. Clearly, when they do this in an environment where foods are low in energy density, the net result is likely to be a lower total energy intake and weight loss.

The impact of lowering the energy density of the diet on weight loss was specifically manipulated and assessed by Ello-Martin and colleagues (2007) in a yearlong trial comparing two strategies to reduce energy density. Participants in one group were counseled to reduce fat intake (RF); participants in the other group received the same advice and were also encouraged to increase intake of water- and fiber-rich foods, particularly fruits and vegetables (RF+FV). Both groups reduced reported fat intake to the same extent, but the RF+FV group ate more fruits and vegetables and reduced the energy density of the diet more.

After 1 year, participants who had completed the study in both groups (RF: 49 randomized – 13 dropped = 36 completed; RF+FV: 48 randomized – 13 dropped = 35 completed; $n = 71$) had significant decreases in body weight. Subjects in the RF+FV group, however, had a significantly different pattern of weight loss than did subjects in the RF group. On average, after 1 year the RF+FV group had lost 7.9 kilograms, and the RF group lost 6.4 kg. Participants rated diet satisfaction, ease of preparation, and cost as similar between the two diets. Diet records revealed that participants in the RF+FV group ate a significantly greater weight of food than did those in the RF group. Interestingly, daily hunger ratings were significantly lower on the RF+FV diet than on the RF diet, suggesting that the higher bulk associated with the RF+FV group more effectively reduced feelings of hunger.

These effects of consuming a diet low in energy density can persist beyond 1 year. For example, Greene and colleagues (2006) followed participants for an average of 2.2 years after starting the "EatRight" diet plan. EatRight is a physician-supported, 12-week program delivered by dietitians with a focus on increasing intake of LED foods such as fruits, vegetables, and whole grains and limiting intake of HED foods such as meat, cheese, fats, and sugar. The average weight loss achieved by this plan was 4.4 kilograms. During long-term follow-up, Greene and colleagues (2006) assessed the diets of those who had maintained weight loss or continued to lose weight compared to those who had gained weight. Gainers were defined as those who had gained more than 5% of their body weight since completing the program; maintainers, as those who had gained less than 5% of their body weight and had maintained weight loss below their program entry weight. Diet records revealed that both groups consumed the same amount of food, but that the energy density of the diets of maintainers was significantly lower (1.67 kcal/g) than that of gainers (1.98 kcal/g; Greene et al., 2006). Specifically, those who maintained weight loss at 2-year follow-up had diets that could be characterized as having a low-energy-density pattern with smaller portions of high-energy-density foods.

These studies illustrate how short-term, laboratory-based observations on food intake can be extended to longer-term practical applications that can be tested in clinical trials. They provide strong support for the capacity of LED diets to form a palatable, satisfying, and sustainable alternative to high-fat, HED Western diets. Most importantly, if adhered to, incorporating an LED diet plan appears to produce long-term benefits to weight management.

Implications for the general population

How do these findings from controlled research studies relate to the general population? Does energy density relate to weight status outside laboratory and clinical settings, and if so, under what conditions? The associations between energy density and weight status have been examined using dietary data collected from free-living individuals as part of the United States–based Continuing Survey of Food Intakes by Individuals (Tippett & Cypel, 1998). Information on food and beverage consumption was gathered from two multiple-pass 24-hour dietary recalls, collected between 1994 and 1996 on 7356 individuals on nonconsecutive days. This survey was initiated by the US Department of Agriculture, which used a thorough sampling strategy to ensure a nationally representative sample of free-living individuals.

Ledikwe and colleagues (2006a) examined whether energy density was associated with total energy intake, weight of food consumed, and body weight, and looked at the role of fruit, vegetable, and fat consumption on these variables. To classify diets as having low, medium, or high density, they applied sex-specific tertile cutoffs. Women eating an LED diet (<1.6 kcal/g) had significantly lower self-reported body mass index and body weight than did women eating an HED diet (>2.0 kcal/g). However, this relationship was not found for men. Nevertheless, the distribution of obesity prevalence was significantly lower in men with an LED diet (<1.7 kcal/g) than in men with an HED diet (>2.1 kcal/g), by 6% (Ledikwe et al., 2006a). This finding was mirrored in women but just failed to reach statistical significance.

When the diets of normal-weight, overweight, and obese individuals were compared, normal-weight individuals consumed diets with a significantly lower energy density (1.87 kcal/g) than did obese individuals (1.95 kcal/g). Individuals who consumed more than nine servings of fruits and vegetables per day consumed fewer calories as fat, and these individuals had the lowest-energy-density diets. Consumers with a relatively high-fat diet (>30% of energy) who ate fewer than five servings of fruits and vegetables per day had the highest prevalence of obesity.

In terms of nutrient quality, Ledikwe and colleagues (2006b) found that those consuming an LED diet had higher levels of vitamins—including A, C, B_6, folate, iron, calcium, and potassium—and consumed fewer caloric carbonated beverages and less fat than did those consuming an HED diet. The fact that low energy density was associated with a food choice pattern that included a large range of micronutrient-dense food further supports the health benefits of consuming a diet with high levels of fruits, vegetables, and whole grains. Using data collected under the NHANES III survey, Kant and Graubard (2005) categorized dietary energy density in three ways: (1) as kilocalories per gram, with all beverages included; (2) as kilocalories per gram, with only energy-yielding beverages; and (3) as kilocalories per gram, with no beverages. All three indicators of dietary energy density were inversely associated with fruit, vegetable, and micronutrient intakes; and two of the indicators were positively correlated with body mass index. HED diets are therefore characterized by poorer nutrient quality as a function of lower intakes of fruits and vegetables.

Promoting dietary patterns to lower the energy density of the diet through increased intake of fruits and vegetables is likely to provide considerable health benefits, but adoption of this kind of diet can be costly. Foods high in fiber, low in energy density, and rich in nutrients are relatively expensive. Aiming to achieve between 400 and 800 grams, or nine servings or more, per day of fruits and vegetables comes at a substantial cost; and in any case, few consumers achieve this target (e.g., only 16% of the Scottish adult population; Lean et al., 2003; National Center for Health Statistics 1999–2001).

Economists have calculated that foods high in energy density cost less than nutrient-rich, low-energy foods (Cawley, 2006). In a recent study of low-income women participating in the Special Supplemental Nutrition Program for Women, Infants, and Children (better known as WIC) in Los Angeles, vouchers were given to support the purchase of fresh fruits and vegetables. The results indicated an extremely high success rate, with uptake of about 90% at the two selected intervention sites (Herman et al., 2006). When cost was minimized as a barrier to food choice, the women in this study selected a wide variety of fresh fruits and vegetables, indicating that the foods were well accepted and liked. However, agricultural policies in Europe and the United States to subsidize overproduction of energy-dense foods ensures that fruits and vegetables will remain relatively expensive and out of the reach of less affluent families (see Chapter 11).

Interventions to promote the consumption of diets that are lower in energy density and higher in nutrient quality—with high levels of fruits, vegetables, and whole grains—may achieve several aims, including improvements in weight and nutritional status, and thereby enhance health. This may be of particular relevance to low-income families, who are at higher risk of obesity and whose diets are higher in energy density but lower in nutrient quality (Drewnowski & Specter, 2004; Mendoza et al., 2006).

Conclusion

Through different types of basic studies such as those investigating factors that influence food intake in controlled settings, those testing the application of these basic findings in clinical trials, and those examining population-based data in natural settings, energy density has been identified as a key dietary component influencing both energy intake and body weight. Such systematic studies of the role of energy density in the regulation of food intake and body weight are relatively recent and need to be replicated and extended.

Using the energy density of foods as a guide to food choices has been shown to enhance satiety and satiation and to lower energy intake. Increasing the intake of low-energy-density foods and limiting the intake of high-energy-density foods as part of a weight loss program has produced long-term benefits observed at 1- and 2-year follow-ups at different clinical sites. These controlled weight loss trials confirm the importance of energy density for energy balance. The role of energy density has also been observed through large-scale epidemiological studies of dietary patterns in the United States, indicating that normal weight is associated with a lower average daily energy density compared to the diets of obese individuals. Clearly the role of energy density extends beyond the laboratory and clinic to the real world.

Consumers are offered ready access to an enormous variety of relatively inexpensive, highly palatable convenience foods. This food environment often promotes overconsumption of high-energy-density foods. Energy density is a key contributor to the current obesity epidemic, and therefore part of the problem. Fortunately, energy density is also part of the solution because it provides a route through which body weight may be managed. Evidence suggests that adopting eating patterns to reduce energy density by increasing intake of fruits, vegetables, and whole grains produces sustainable effects on lowering body weight. Lowering energy density in this way also improves the nutrient quality of the diet, thereby increasing the potential to reduce body weight and to improve general health and well-being.

References Cited

Bell, E. A., Castellanos, V. H., Pelkman, C. L., Thorwart, M. L., & Rolls, B. J. (1998). Energy density of foods affects energy intake in normal-weight women. *American Journal of Clinical Nutrition, 67*, 412–420.

Bell, E. A., Roe, L. S., & Rolls, B. J. (2003). Sensory-specific satiety is affected more by volume than by energy content of a liquid food. *Physiology & Behavior, 78*, 593–600.

Bell, E. A., & Rolls, B. J. (2001). Energy density of foods affects energy intake across multiple levels of fat content in lean and obese women. *American Journal of Clinical Nutrition, 73*, 1010–1018.

Bellisle, F., Dalix, A. M., & Slama, G. (2004). Non-food related environmental stimuli induce increased meal intake in healthy women: comparison of television viewing versus listening to a recorded story in laboratory settings. *Appetite, 43*, 175–180.

Birch, L. L. (1986). The role of experience in children's food acceptance patterns. *Appetite, 7*, 323–331.

Birch, L. L. (1999). Development of food preferences. *Annual Review of Nutrition, 19*, 41–62.

Birch, L. L., & Deysher, M. (1986). Caloric compensation and sensory specific satiety: evidence for self regulation of food intake by young children. *Appetite, 7*, 323–331.

Birch, L. L., Johnson, S. L., Andersen, G., Peters, J. C., & Schulte, M. C. (1991). The variability of young children's energy intake. *New England Journal of Medicine, 324*, 232–235.

Blass, E., Anderson, D. R., Kirkorian, H. L., Pempek, T. A., Price, I., & Koleini, M. F. (2006). On the road to obesity: Television viewing increases intake of high-density foods. *Physiology & Behavior, 88*, 597–604.

Caton, S. J., Bate, L., & Hetherington, M. M. (2007). Acute effects of an alcoholic drink on food intake: Aperitif versus co-ingestion. *Physiology & Behavior, 90*, 368–375.

Caton, S. J., Marks, J. E., & Hetherington, M. M. (2005). Pleasure and alcohol: the effects of manipulating pleasantness on the acute effects of alcohol on food intake. *Physiology & Behavior, 84*, 371–377.

Cawley, J. (2006). Markets and childhood obesity policy. *The Future of Children, 16*, 69–88.

Cecil, J. E., Palmer, C., Wrieden, W., Murrie, I., Bolton-Smith, C., Watt, P., et al. (2005).

Energy intakes of children after preloads: adjustment not compensation. *American Journal of Clinical Nutrition, 82*, 302–308.

Condrasky, M., Ledikwe, J. H., Flood, J. E., & Rolls, B. J. (2007). Chefs' opinions of restaurant portion sizes. *Obesity, 15*, 2086–2094.

Cummings, D. E., & Overduin, J. (2007). Gastrointestinal regulation of food intake. *Journal of Clinical Investigation, 117*, 13–23.

de Castro, J. M. (1994). Family and friends produce greater social facilitation of food intake than other companions. *Physiology & Behavior, 56*, 445–455.

Drewnowski, A., & Specter, S. E. (2004). Poverty and obesity: the role of energy density and energy costs. *American Journal of Clinical Nutrition, 79*, 6–16.

Duncan, K. H., Bacon, J. A., & Weinsier, R. L. (1983). The effects of high and low energy density diets on satiety, energy intake, and eating time of obese and nonobese subjects. *American Journal of Clinical Nutrition, 37*, 763–767.

Ello-Martin, J. A., Roe, L. S., Ledikwe, J. H., Beach, A. M., & Rolls, B. J. (2007). Dietary energy density in the treatment of obesity: a year-long trial comparing two weight-loss diets. *American Journal of Clinical Nutrition, 85*, 1465–1477.

Fox, M. K., Reidy, K., Karwe, V., & Ziegler, P. (2006). Average portions of foods commonly eaten by infants and toddlers in the United States. *Journal of the American Dietetic Association, 106*(1, Suppl. 1), S66–S76.

Greene, L. F., Malpede, C. Z., Henson, C. S., Hubbert, K. A., Heimburger, D. C., & Ard, J. D. (2006). Weight maintenance 2 years after participation in a weight loss program promoting low-energy density foods. *Obesity, 14*, 1795–1801.

Herman, D. R., Harrison, G. G., & Jenks, E. (2006). Choices made by low-income women provided with an economic supplement for fresh fruit and vegetable purchase. *Journal of the American Dietetic Association, 106*, 740–744.

Hetherington, M. M. (1996). Sensory-specific satiety and its importance in meal termination. *Neuroscience & Biobehavioural Reviews, 20*, 113–117.

Hetherington, M. M. (2002). The physiological-psychological dichotomy in the study of food intake. *Proceedings of the Nutrition Society, 61*, 497–507.

Hetherington, M. M. (2007). Cues to overeat: psychological factors influencing over-consumption. *Proceedings of the Nutrition Society, 66*, 113–123.

Hetherington, M. M., Anderson, A. S., Norton, G. N., & Newson, L. (2006). Situational effects on meal intake: A comparison of eating alone and eating with others. *Physiology & Behavior, 88*, 498–505.

Hetherington, M. M., Foster, R., Newman, T., Anderson, A. S., & Norton, G. N. M. (2006). Understanding variety: Tasting different foods delays satiation. *Physiology & Behavior, 87*, 263–271.

Hetherington, M., & Rolls, B. J. (1987). Methods to study human eating behavior. In N. Rowland & F. Toates (Eds.), *Methods and Techniques to Study Feeding and Drinking Behavior* (pp. 77–109). Amsterdam: Elsevier.

Hetherington, M., Rolls, B. J., & Burley, V. J. (1989). The time course of sensory-specific satiety. *Appetite, 12*, 57–68.

Hetherington, M. M., Wood, C., & Lyburn, S. C. (2000). Response to energy dilution in the short term: evidence of nutritional wisdom in young children? *Nutritional Neuroscience, 3*, 321–329.

Himaya, A., & Louis-Sylvestre, J. (1998). The effect of soup on satiation. *Appetite, 30*, 199–210.

Holt, S. H., Miller, J. C., Petocz, P., & Farmakalidis, E. (1995). A satiety index of common foods. *European Journal of Clinical Nutrition, 49*, 675–690.

Howarth, N. C., Saltzman, E., & Roberts, S. B. (2001). Dietary fiber and weight regulation. *Nutrition Reviews, 59*, 129–139.

Jebb, S. A., Siervo, M., Fruhbeck, G., Goldberg, G. R., Murgatroyd, P. R., & Prentice, A. M. (2006). Variability of appetite control mechanisms in response to 9 weeks of progressive overfeeding in humans. *International Journal of Obesity, 30*, 1160–1162.

Kant, A. K., Graubard, B. I. (2005). Energy density of diets reported by American adults: association with food group intake, nutrient intake, and body weight. *International Journal of Obesity, 29*, 950–956.

Kendall, A., Levitsky, D. A., Strupp, B. J., & Lissner, L. (1991). Weight loss on a low-fat diet: consequence of the imprecision of the control of food intake in humans. *American Journal of Clinical Nutrition, 53*, 1124–1129.

Kissileff, H. R. (1985). Effects of physical state (liquid-solid) of foods on food intake: procedural and substantive contributions. *American Journal of Clinical Nutrition, 42*, S956–S965.

Kral, T. V., & Rolls, B. J. (2004). Energy density and portion size: their independent and combined effects on energy intake. *Physiology & Behavior, 82*, 131–138.

Kraly, F. S., & Blass, E. M. (1976). Mechanisms for enhanced feeding in the cold in rats. *Journal of Comparative and Physiological Psychology, 90*, 714–726.

Leahy, K. E., Birch, L. L., & Rolls, B. J. *Will a reduction in the energy density of an entrée decrease children's energy intake?* Manuscript submitted for publication.

Lean, M. E., Anderson, A. S., Morrison, C., & Currall, J. (2003) Evaluation of a dietary targets monitor. *European Journal of Clinical Nutrition, 57*, 667–673.

Ledikwe, J. H., Blanck, H. M., Khan, K. L., Serdula, M. K., Seymour, J. D., Tohill, B. C., et al. (2006a). Dietary energy density is associated with energy intake and weight status in US adults. *American Journal of Clinical Nutrition, 83*, 1362–1368.

Ledikwe, J. H., Blanck, H. M., Khan, K. L., Serdula, M. K., Seymour, J. D., Tohill, B. C., et al. (2006b). Low-energy-density diets are associated with high diet quality in adults in the United States. *Journal of the American Dietetic Association, 106*, 1172–1180.

Levin, B. E. (2006). Metabolic sensing neurons and the control of energy homeostasis. *Physiology & Behavior, 89*, 486–489.

Loos, R. J., & Bouchard, C. (2003). Obesity—is it a genetic disorder? *Journal of Internal Medicine, 254*, 401–425.

Lowe, M. R., & Levine, A. S. (2005). Eating motives and the controversy over dieting: eating less than needed versus less than wanted. *Obesity Research, 13*, 797–806.

Mazlan, N., Horgan, G., & Stubbs, R. J. (2006). Energy density and weight of food effect short-term caloric compensation in men. *Physiology & Behavior, 87*, 679–686.

Mendoza, J. A., Drewnowski, A., Cheadle, A., & Christakis, D. A. (2006). Dietary energy density is associated with selected predictors of obesity in U.S. Children. *Journal of Nutrition, 136*, 1318–1322.

National Center for Health Statistics. National Health and Nutrition Examination Survey 1999–2001. Retrieved from http://www.cdc.gov/nchs/nhanes.htm

Pearcey, S. M., & de Castro, J. M. (1997). Food intake and meal patterns of one year old infants. *Appetite, 29,* 201–212.

Rolls, B. J., Bell, E. A., Castellanos, V. H., Chow, M., Pelkman, C. L., Thorwart, M. L. (1999a). Energy density but not fat content of foods affected energy intake in lean and obese women. *American Journal of Clinical Nutrition, 69,* 863–871.

Rolls, B. J., Bell, E. A., & Thorwart, M. L. (1999b). Water incorporated into a food but not served with a food decreases energy intake in lean women. *American Journal of Clinical Nutrition, 70,* 448–455.

Rolls, B. J., Engell, D. M., & Birch, L. L. (2000c). Serving portion size influences 5 year-old but not 3 year-old children's food intakes. *Journal of the American Dietetic Association, 100,* 232–234.

Rolls, B. J., Federoff, I. C., Guthrie, J F., & Laster, L. J. (1990). Foods with different satiating effects in humans. *Appetite, 15,* 115–126.

Rolls, B. J., & Hetherington, M. (1989). The role of variety in eating and body weight. In R. Shepherd (Ed.), *Psychobiology of Human Eating and Nutritional Behavior* (pp. 58–84). Sussex, England: Wiley.

Rolls, B. J., & Hetherington, M. (1990). A behavioral scientist's perspective on the study of diet and behavior. In G. H. Anderson (Ed.), *Diet and Behavior: Multidisciplinary Approaches* (pp. 209–219). London: Springer-Verlag.

Rolls, B. J., Hetherington, M., & Burley, V. J. (1988). Sensory stimulation and energy density in the development of satiety. *Physiology & Behavior, 44,* 727–733.

Rolls, B. J., Morris, E. L., & Roe, L. S. (2002). Portion size of food affects energy intake in normal-weight and overweight men and women. *American Journal of Clinical Nutrition, 76,* 1207–1213.

Rolls, B. J., & Roe, L. S. (2002). Effect of the volume of liquid food infused intragastrically on satiety in women. *Physiology & Behavior, 76,* 623–631.

Rolls, B. J., Roe, L. S., & Meengs, J. S. (2004). Salad and satiety: energy density and portion size of a first course salad affect energy intake at lunch. *Journal of the American Dietetic Association, 104,* 1570–1576.

Rolls, B. J., Rolls, E. T., Rowe, E., & Sweeney, K. (1981). Sensory specific satiety in man. *Physiology & Behavior, 27,* 137–142.

Shide, D. J., & Rolls, B. J. (1991). Social facilitation of caloric intake in humans by friends but not by strangers [Abstract]. *International Journal of Obesity, 15,* 8.

Smith, G. P. (1996). The direct and indirect controls of meal size. *Neuroscience & Biobehavioral Reviews, 20,* 41–46.

Smith, G. P. (2000). The controls of eating: a shift from nutritional homeostasis to behavioral neuroscience. *Nutrition, 16,* 814–820.

Stubbs, R. J., Johnstone, A. M., Mazlan, N., Mbaiwa, S. E., & Ferris, S. (2001). Effect of altering the variety of sensorially distinct foods, of the same macronutrient content, on food intake and body weight in men. *European Journal of Clinical Nutrition, 55,* 19–28.

Stubbs, R. J., & Tolkamp, B. J. (2006). Control of energy balance in relation to energy intake and energy expenditure in animals and man: an ecological perspective. *British Journal of Nutrition, 95,* 657–676.

Tippet, K. S., & Cypel, Y. S. (1998). *Design and operation: The Continuing Survey of Food Intakes by Individuals and the Diet and Health Knowledge Survey, 1994–96.* Washington, DC: US Department of Agriculture, Agricultural Research Service.

Weingarten, H. P. (1985). Stimulus control of eating: implications for a two-factor theory of hunger. *Appetite, 6,* 387–401.

Weinsier, R. L., Johnston, M. H., Doleys, D. M., & Bacon, J. A. (1982). Dietary management of obesity: evaluation of the time-energy displacement diet in terms of its efficacy and nutritional adequacy for long-term weight control. *British Journal of Nutrition, 47,* 367–379.

Wiepkema, P. R. (1971). Behavioural factors in the regulation of food intake. *Proceedings of the Nutrition Society, 30,* 142–149.

Woods, S. C. (2005). Signals that influence food intake and body weight. *Physiology & Behavior, 15,* 709–716.

Yu-Poth, S., Zhao, G., Etherton, T., Naglak, M., Jonnalagadda, S., & Kris-Etherton, P. M. (1999). Effects of the National Cholesterol Education Program's Step I and Step II dietary intervention programs on cardiovascular disease risk factors: a meta-analysis. *American Journal of Clinical Nutrition, 69,* 632–646.

11 PROPOSED MODIFICATIONS TO THE FOOD STAMP PROGRAM: LIKELY EFFECTS AND THEIR POLICY IMPLICATIONS

Conner C. Mullally, Julian M. Alston, Daniel A. Sumner, Marilyn S. Townsend, and Stephen A. Vosti

Introduction

The links among poverty, policy, and nutritional outcomes are complex. The growing numbers of people who are categorized as obese and overweight are drawn from all socioeconomic, ethnic, and demographic groups, but not uniformly. Several writers have observed that low-income women—including those receiving food stamps—are more likely than the rich to be obese and overweight (Gibson, 2003; Townsend et al., 2001). This observation leads to two questions. First, has the current Food Stamp Program contributed to the problems of growing obesity among the poor in the United States? Second, could the Food Stamp Program be redesigned such that it would contribute positively toward improving diet quality and ultimately reducing or reversing the trend among recipient groups to become more obese and overweight? This chapter uses the tools of economics to explore these questions, focusing mainly on the second. Specifically, the discussion examines how proposed changes to the US Food Stamp Program (FSP) would be likely to affect obesity.

When the Food Stamp Program was first established during the Great Depression as a pilot project, its primary purpose was to stabilize agricultural prices by stimulating the consumption of surplus farm commodities. This primary purpose worked in tandem with the secondary purpose of alleviating hunger by providing additional calories to recipients who had too little to eat (US Department of Agriculture, 1996). In the twenty-first century, however, the Food Stamp Program is no longer seen as a significant element of farm program policies per se. Its primary purpose today is to alleviate the nutritional consequences of poverty, in an era when food and nutrition policy makers are concerned about the consequences of both rich and poor consumers having more than enough calories available for consumption.

The next section of this chapter briefly reports the trends in obesity, poverty, and food consumption patterns, and identifies the key policy issues. The discussion then turns to the current Food Stamp Program and specific changes that have been proposed to encourage more healthful diets among recipients. Next a simple model of consumer choice is presented, to illustrate how the optimizing decisions of consumers are relevant in predicting the consumption and nutritional consequences of policy changes. Discussion of this model is followed by a theoretical analysis of how the food industry might respond to changes in demand by FSP participants, and thus the marketwide economic implications. A quantitative counterpart to this analysis then speculates on the likely short- and long-run marketwide impacts, working on the basis of knowledge of the relevant markets and drawing on some related studies. Finally, the chapter considers the likely nutritional consequences of consumer and market response to the proposed changes in the list of allowable foods, with particular emphasis on the poor.

The Problem of Rising Obesity in the United States: Trends and Linkages

Excessive body weight has been cited by many as *the* key health problem in the United States today (e.g., Townsend, 2006). The prevalence of obesity in the United States doubled between 1971 and 2000 (Zhang and Wang, 2004), and the percentage of children and adolescents who are overweight also increased dramatically, from 5% in 1976 to 17% in 2003 (Ogden et al., 2006). The growing prevalence of obesity has offset some of the gains from healthy changes in Amer-

Table 11.1
Aggregate US Medical Spending Attributable to Overweight and Obesity, by Insurance in 1998

Insurance category	Medical spending in 1998 (billions of 1998 US $)	
	Attributable to overweight and obesity	Attributable to obesity
Out-of-pocket	12.8	6.9
Private	28.1	16.1
Medicaid	14.1	10.7
Medicare	23.5	13.8
Total	78.5	47.5

Source: Finkelstein et al., 2003. Figures based on data from the National Health Accounts (NHA) collected by the US Department of Health and Human Services.

ican behavior, such as dramatic reductions in smoking and better control of blood pressure, and it will continue to do so if current trends continue (Cutler et al., 2007). Obese and overweight Americans generate large additional direct and indirect health care expenses, estimated to be $78.5 billion in 1998 alone (Finkelstein et al., 2003, Raebel et al., 2004; Pronk et al., 1999). Table 11.1 presents estimates of these private and public costs.

High and rising social costs of obesity may call for policy action, but determining the appropriate policy action is not easy, in part because the prevalence of obesity varies among socioeconomic, demographic, and ethnic groups (Figure 11.1). Among adults, for example, women are more likely to be obese than

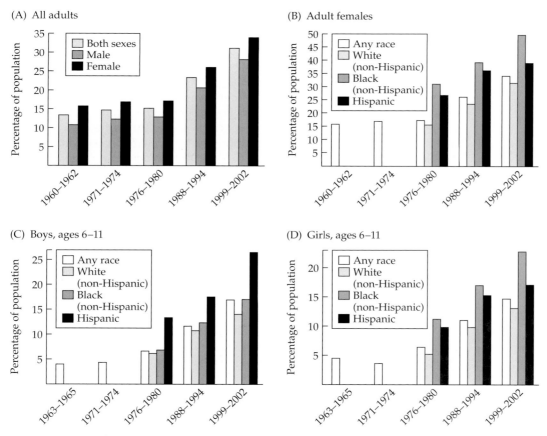

FIGURE 11.1 Obesity and overweight in the United States, by age, race, and gender. (A) All adults. (B) Adult females. (C) Boys, ages 6–11. (D) Girls, ages 6–11. (Data from NHANES, www.cdc.gov/nchs/about/major/nhanes/datatblelink.htm.)

men. African American females of all ages are much more likely to be obese or overweight than their white and Hispanic counterparts. Relative to blacks and whites, Hispanic males are consistently more likely to be overweight as children, and also more likely to be obese as adults.

This heterogeneity in obesity patterns among demographic and other groups complicates in several ways the search for policy actions to address the problem. First, obesity policies may have different nutritional effects on and different economic consequences for different groups, perhaps especially for the poor. Second, obesity itself may have differential economic impacts across groups, and it may be particularly burdensome to the poor if they are more likely to be obese or less able to bear the economic burden of weight-related health problems. Thus, the choice of obesity policies may require balancing their distributional consequences against their effects on economic efficiency. A first step, then, is to identify the relationship between poverty and obesity and, if a relationship exists, how it has changed over time.

Poverty and obesity

Data on poverty in the United States suggest that individuals who are significantly more likely to be obese or overweight are also more likely to be poor. Figure 11.2 displays poverty trends according to gender, age, and ethnicity. The trends in income poverty largely reflect what is evident in the data from the National Health and Nutrition Examination Survey (NHANES): individuals who are below the poverty line are also more likely to be women or of minority status. Figure 11.2A compares poverty rates for men and women of all ages; women have always been more likely to be in poverty, and this gap in poverty has varied between 2 and 4 percentage points since 1966. Beginning in 1974, the data are broken down by ethnicity (see Figures 11.2B and C); blacks are the group most likely to be in poverty in each year—with a few exceptions in the mid 1990s—followed by Hispanics, Asians and Pacific Islanders, and whites.

Poor households are often "food-insecure" (Bartfeld & Dunifon, 2005), and food insecurity has been linked to obesity in adults (Townsend et al., 2001) and overweight in children (Alaimo et al., 2001).[1] But the link between poverty and obesity may be weakening over time. Jolliffe (2006) reports that the historical trend of higher prevalence of overweight (BMI >25) among low-income adults (income <130% of the poverty line) in the United States disappeared by 2001–2002, although distribution-sensitive measures of overweight clearly indicated an increased presence of the poor in the tail of the overweight distribu-

---

[1]The basis here is the USDA definition of *food security*: access by all people at all times to enough food for an active, healthy life. Data are collected annually in the Current Population Survey Food Security Supplement (CPS-FSS). By definition, food-insecure households are those responding affirmatively to three or more questions indicating concerns about the quality or quantity of food available to the household.

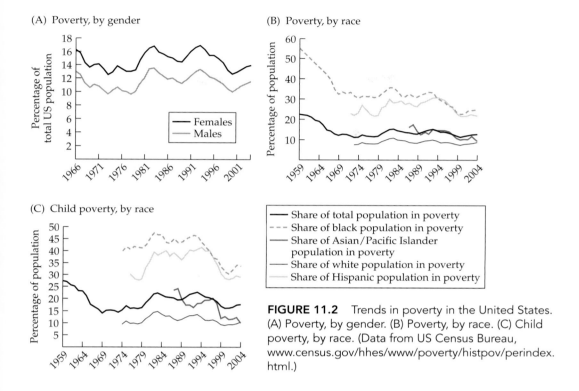

FIGURE 11.2 Trends in poverty in the United States. (A) Poverty, by gender. (B) Poverty, by race. (C) Child poverty, by race. (Data from US Census Bureau, www.census.gov/hhes/www/poverty/histpov/perindex. html.)

tion. Among children, those from low-income households are more likely to be overweight relative to those from wealthier households; the severity of over-weight is also greater for low-income children.

To slow or reverse obesity trends, policy action must result in reduced caloric intake over the long term.[2] But the links between different forms of policy action and caloric intake are not easy to identify. Food purchase decisions are deter-mined by individuals' preferences for different foods; these preferences are influ-enced not only by nutritional information, but also by prices, income, and prod-uct characteristics such as taste. The result is that people consume an array of foods and beverages, some of which might be equally satisfying to consumers yet contain differing amounts of calories and nutrients. To be successful, then, policy action must be able to target specific types of foods and beverages that contribute to improved diet quality. This policy action must overcome con-sumers' demonstrated preferences for energy-dense foods and beverages, and it must do so in low-income communities.

---

[2]See Chapter 10 for the role of increased ingestion of lower-energy-density foods, such as veg-etables and fruits, in reducing caloric intake.

The US Food Stamp Program and Proposed Changes

One federal food assistance program available to policy makers seeking to improve diets while combating weight problems among low-income Americans is the Food Stamp Program (FSP). The first FSP was initiated in 1939 and was intended to create a mechanism for linking farm surpluses with undernourished urban populations; it ended in the spring of 1943 when these two conditions (surpluses and undernourishment) were perceived no longer to exist. Approximately 20 million people were reached, and nearly $262 million was spent. The program was reborn in pilot form in 1961 under President Kennedy. The scope of the program was increased, but the concept of special stamps for surplus foods was eliminated.

The Food Stamp Act of 1964 made the FSP a permanent fixture in US agricultural and food security programs. Key provisions required participants to purchase food with food stamps, and allowed food stamps to be used for almost any food (alcoholic beverages and imported foods were excluded). The program was amended (e.g., in the Food Stamp Act of 1977) and greatly expanded in the 1970s to become a truly national program (US Department of Agriculture, 2007a). Cost increases led to cutbacks in the early 1980s that were achieved by, among other things, changes in eligibility requirements. By the mid 1980s, the FSP had begun to expand again; benefits were increased and changes were made to facilitate demonstration of eligibility. Electronic benefit transfer (EBT) cards were introduced in 1984.

In 1993, the Mickey Leland Childhood Hunger Relief Act greatly expanded the FSP and further eased some eligibility requirements, especially for families with dependent children. Welfare reform in the 1990s, among other things, reduced FSP benefits to able-bodied adults, established new time and value limits to FSP benefits, and eliminated eligibility for most illegal aliens. Some of these limitations were relaxed with reauthorization of the FSP in the context of the Food Security and Rural Investment Act of 2002; FSP participation has expanded greatly since then, in part as a consequence of the restoration of eligibility for aliens who have been in the United States at least 5 years (US Department of Agriculture, 2007a).

When the Food Stamp Program was first established, its primary purpose was to stimulate the consumption of surplus farm commodities; providing additional calories to recipients who had too little to eat was a secondary purpose (USDA, 1996). Over time, what was initially a secondary purpose has evolved into the main, if not sole, purpose of the program; and the program has grown from a minor part of the USDA's budget to one of the largest elements.

Table 11.2 sets out participation rates, benefits, and total costs of the FSP for selected years. In 2005, over 25 million people participated in the FSP and received average benefits of approximately $93 per person per month (amounting to about $1,100 per annum). Total cost of the program in 2005 was approximately $31 billion, accounting for 37.9% of the USDA's $81.7 billion budget.

Table 11.2

Average Participation, Benefits, and Costs for the Food Stamp Program, Selected Years

Fiscal year	Average number of participants (thousands of persons)	Benefits per person per month (current US $)	Total benefits per year (millions of current US $)	Total costs per year (millions of current US $)
1970	4,340	10.55	549.7	576.9
1980	21,082	34.47	8,720.9	9,206.5
1990	20,049	58.96	14,185.9	15,490.4
2000	17,194	72.62	14,983.3	17,054.0
2005	25,674	92.72	28,567.3	31,129.8

Source: Data from www.fns.usda.gov/pd/fssummar.htm

Rates of participation and average household benefits vary significantly across states. States with the largest share of population enrolled in the FSP in 2005 were concentrated in the South, where enrollment rates ranged from 13% of the total population for Mississippi to nearly 18% of the total population for Louisiana. Texas, California, and New York had the largest absolute numbers of participants in 2005, with roughly 2.4, 2.0, and 1.7 million individuals enrolled, respectively. New Hampshire had the smallest share of population enrolled in the FSP, with 4%; and Wyoming had the smallest number of residents participating in the program, with a total of 24,636.[3] Average monthly benefits per participating household also varied across states: Louisiana and Mississippi topped the list with approximately $250 per household per month in 2005; New Hampshire and Vermont were at the bottom of that list, with approximately $167 per household per month.

Generally, households with incomes at or below 130% of the poverty line are eligible for food stamps, and about 50% of eligible individuals have participated (Cunnyngham, 2004).[4] Of the roughly 25 million FSP participants in 2005, just over half were children under the age of 17 (two-thirds of whom were between the ages of 5 and 17 years), about 17% were elderly, and 23% were disabled nonelderly individuals; 45.5% of all participants lived in households headed by

---

[3]These figures are based on population projections from the US Census Bureau (www.census.gov/popest/states/NST-ann-est.html) and average monthly FSP enrollment data from the US Department of Agriculture (www.fns.usda.gov/oane/menu/Published/FSP/FSPPartState.htm).

[4]Although participation rates in the Food Stamp Program will have implications for the efficacy of the proposed changes considered here, estimating the effects of FSP changes on enrollment in the Food Stamp Program are beyond the scope of this chapter. See Currie and Grogger, 2001, for a review of the literature on that topic.

Table 11.3
Average Income, Benefits, and Household Size for Food Stamp Program Participants, 2005

Participant group	Gross monthly countable income[a] (current US $)	Net monthly countable income[b] (current US $)	Monthly food stamp benefit (current US $)	Household size
Total participant population	648	319	209	2.3
Households with children	768	397	300	3.3
Households comprising elderly individuals	690	359	87	1.3
Households comprising disabled nonelderly individuals	802	445	145	2.0
Other households	205	60	146	1.1

Source: Data from Barrett, 2006.

[a]Gross monthly countable household income is used to determine eligibility for FSP benefits. It includes most kinds of cash income and excludes in-kind benefits.

[b]Net monthly countable income is used to determine benefit levels under the FSP. It is the net of deductions permitted under FSP rules; see Barrett, 2006, for a list of allowed deductions.

white adults, 31.3% lived in households headed by African American adults, and 13% lived in households headed by Hispanic adults. Nearly 94% of all participants were United States–born citizens; only 3.1% were noncitizens.

Table 11.3 reports average gross and net incomes (adjusted according to FSP benefit calculation rules), monthly benefits, and household size for the approximately 11 million US households that participated in the FSP in 2005. Note that average benefits were approximately $200 per household per month, and that families with children received approximately 1.5 times that amount. Table 11.3 also provides a snapshot of the demographic composition of FSP participants and the flow of benefits to particular sociodemographic groups.

Intended and unintended consequences of the Food Stamp Program

Over the years, the FSP has benefited millions of low-income adults and children, as well as the food industry.[5] The FSP has had several different impacts on the welfare of participants, the most obvious being increased expenditures on food. Studies of the effects of the FSP on food expenditures suggest that the marginal propensity to spend for food stamps is in the range of 0.17 to 0.47, meaning that every dollar of food stamp benefits generated between 17 and 47 cents of additional expenditures on food (Fox et al., 2004). In other words, receiving a dollar in food stamps frees up a dollar in cash that was previously spent on food; between 53 and 83 cents of this additional dollar is spent on things other than food. However, few studies have examined the distribution of FSP benefits across healthful versus unhealthful foods (the FSP changes being considered here). (Note 15 gives the definitions of *healthful* and *unhealthful* used in this chapter.)

The FSP has probably had a positive impact on food security, but determining the effect empirically has been difficult (Wilde and Nord, 2005). Several analysts have measured the impact of the FSP on food security by comparing mean levels of food security among FSP participants and eligible nonparticipants.[6] Studies generally find positive effects of FSP participation on the overall *household* availability of food energy and protein. Fewer survey data and hence fewer empirical studies are available to explore the effects of FSP participation on diet composition or quality (e.g., the availability of carbohydrates, fats, vitamins, and minerals), but the studies that do exist suggest that households of FSP participants generally have greater amounts of nutrients available for consumption. At the *individual* level, however, several studies suggest that FSP participation has had little or no effect on food consumption, although a consensus in the literature has yet to emerge (Fox et al., 2004).[7]

FSP participation may also generate a variety of unintended consequences. Kennedy and colleagues (1995) found that FSP participants eat less healthful diets than do eligible nonparticipants and higher-income nonparticipants.[8] This difference was especially pronounced for the fruit and food variety components of the Healthy Eating Index (HEI) measure for female FSP participants. As one consequence of these diets, FSP participants are more likely to suffer from iron deficiencies and anemia than higher-income and eligible nonparticipants (Fox and Cole, 2004).

Overall, the empirical literature has yielded mixed findings on the effects of participation in the FSP on body weight. Studies based on longitudinal data (e.g.,

---

[5]Though the exact benefits of the FSP to the food industry are difficult to assess, Hanson and colleagues (2002) estimated that a $5 billion cut in the FSP would result in the loss of 7500 jobs in the farm and food-processing sectors, and an overall loss of $437 million in income to the US economy as a whole.

[6]In empirical analysis of the impact of food stamps on food security, food security is typically measured by the USDA definition (see note 1) or by data collected in other household surveys.

[7]The discrepancy between household nutrient availability and individual intake may have several causes, including unequal consumption of foods by individuals out of household supplies, consumption by guests, and waste.

[8]Here, diet quality was measured by Healthy Eating Index (HEI) scores. The HEI was created by the USDA in 1995 to measure conformity with the *Dietary Guidelines for Americans*; for details, see www.cnpp.usda.gov/Publications/HEI/healthyeatingindex2005factsheet.pdf

FIGURE 11.3 Trends in predicted BMI for white, non-Hispanic females: FSP participants and nonparticipants. Predicted BMI levels were calculated using the coefficients from a logit regression of BMI on a set of explanatory variables; for this graph, an age of 40 was assumed. The regressions were estimated using the NHANES data set. (Data from ver Ploeg et al., 2006, and NHANES.)

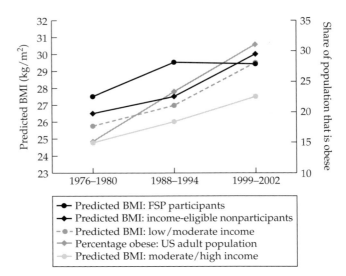

Predicted BMI: FSP participants
Predicted BMI: income-eligible nonparticipants
Predicted BMI: low/moderate income
Percentage obese: US adult population
Predicted BMI: moderate/high income

Gibson, 2006) suggest that there is a positive relationship between participation in the FSP and obesity for adult women, whereas no such correlation exists for men. However, these studies assume that the impact of FSP participation on body weight has been constant over time; more recent data suggest that this is not the case. As Figure 11.3 shows, the rate of obesity among US adult females has continued to increase, while expected body mass index (BMI) among female FSP participants has declined in the most recent round of the NHANES survey. The NHANES data also suggest that obesity rates among male FSP participants are still lower than those of eligible nonparticipants. For some socioeconomic groups, FSP participation may now be associated with lower expected body weight (ver Ploeg et al., 2006).

Although the list of *allowable* foods in the FSP has not changed significantly in the past 40 years, the list and characteristics of *available* foods surely have; and the same is likely true for foods actually purchased using food stamps. Detailed historical data on food stamp expenditures by food type are not available, but the information that is available suggests that today's FSP participants spend their food budgets differently, relative to FSP households in previous years.

Table 11.4 presents the share of food stamps spent on different food groups for households sampled in the National Food Stamp Program Survey (NFSPS) of 1995. Although we can only speculate on how FSP participants in previous years may have spent their food stamp allotments, it seems reasonable to presume that the 11% share of food stamps allocated to sweets and soft drinks, or the 14.5% share devoted to processed grain products, is much higher than in years past.

Modifications to lists of foods allowed under the FSP may cause FSP participants to consume different combinations of foods, improve diet quality, reduce

Table 11.4
Foods Most Commonly Purchased with Food Stamps, 1995

Food type	Example(s)	Share (%)[a]
Whole grains as final product	Whole-grain/high-fiber flour, meal, rice, pasta	0.4
Other grains as final product	White flour	2.2
Whole-grain/high-fiber products	Whole-wheat bread, whole-grain breakfast cereals	2.6
Other grain products	Sugar-frosted cornflakes, white bread, cakes, cookies, grain mixtures	14.5
Fruit	Apples, oranges, and so on	7.9
High-nutrient vegetables	Broccoli	3.8
Other vegetables	Potatoes	7.8
Beans and legumes	Dry beans, peas, lentils	0.9
Low-cost red meat, pork, and luncheon meats	Hamburger, bologna, bacon, sausage	13.7
High-cost red meat and variety meats	Lean cuts of beef	6.7
Poultry and eggs	Chicken	6.6
Dairy products	Milk, yogurt, cheese	12.5
Seafood	Fish, shellfish	3.1
Sugars, sweets, fats, and oils	Sweet and savory snacks (e.g., candy, potato chips), white sugar, shortening, vegetable oil	5.4
Soft drinks	Cola	5.6

Note: The data do not include restaurant meals or meals eaten outside the home, and do not clearly distinguish ready-to-eat foods purchased at the grocery store (e.g., a roasted chicken dinner) from other foods. All of these may comprise a large share of expenditures, and have important nutritional characteristics.

[a]Numbers in the "Share" column were taken from Cohen et al., 1999, and based on data from the National Food Stamp Program Survey conducted in 1995. The numbers represent the share of expenditures on different commodity groups made by surveyed households participating in the FSP, as estimated from 7-day food intake recall data; shares do not add up to 100% because a few categories were excluded here.

overall caloric intake, and ultimately help reduce obesity among participants. However, the lack of detailed data on food consumption by participants and nonparticipants, and on the links between FSP participation and obesity, limits what can be said about the expected effects of any such changes.

Currently, ready-to-eat hot meals and alcohol are the only foods and beverages for which foods stamps cannot be redeemed. In the 1930s and 1940s, it made sense to include virtually all foods in the list of products that could be purchased using food stamps. The objective was to be certain that recipients received sufficient calories for growth (children) or maintenance of body weight (adults). Food was expensive, and households spent large proportions of their income on it. Food ingredients were the major purchases because consumers prepared meals "from scratch." Ready-to-eat hot foods or meals were generally not available for purchase in markets.

Circumstances have changed. Thanks mainly to dramatic increases in productivity in agriculture and the food industry, the prices of most foods have fallen substantially in the past 40 years (Alston, Sumner, et al., 2006) and incomes generally have risen such that the proportion of income spent on food has declined. Consumers now generally spend a much higher proportion of income on services associated with food than they did in the past. More meals are consumed away from home, and even for meals consumed at home, a higher proportion of food preparation is done elsewhere; the same is true for FSP participants, who have less time available for preparing foods at home than used to be the case (Mancino & Newman, 2007). Supermarkets now sell predominantly prepared foods, ready-to-eat items, and even complete meals. These newer food items are often more energy-dense (more caloric) than the home-prepared versions (Kuchler et al., 2005; see also Chapter 9).

Proposed changes to the Food Stamp Program

These new circumstances (cheaper and different types of foods, changes in food supply chains, and higher incomes) and the associated trends (different lifestyles, altered consumption patterns, and increases in obesity) have not made the FSP redundant, but they suggest that it might be appropriate to modify the program to better achieve its original purpose of providing food assistance, and to add the new objective of improving dietary quality for the poor, especially children in poor households. More specifically, the existing FSP could be redesigned to promote the consumption of foods like fruits and vegetables, low-fat dairy and meat products, and dried beans and legumes, as a strategy for improving the participants' dietary quality and reducing total calories consumed (Guthrie et al., 2007).

In the popular press, much of the discussion about changes to the FSP in response to obesity trends has focused on reducing the monthly allotment of stamps given to participating households (e.g., Besharov, 2002). Some believe that reducing benefits would harm the poor (ver Ploeg et al., 2006), and hence such action should be avoided. Others have suggested improving the quality of the diets of FSP participants (e.g., Center on Hunger and Poverty, 2003), but few have offered specific suggestions for accomplishing this goal.[9]

This chapter addresses the likely effects of specific changes to the foods allowable under the FSP on food purchases and nutrition outcomes of FSP participants and nonparticipants.[10] The goal of these changes would be to improve

---

[9]The state of Minnesota requested federal permission to prohibit candy and soft drink purchases using food stamps, but that request was denied, in part because of difficulties identifying precisely which foods would and would not be prohibited (Guthrie et al., 2007).

[10]There are other options for increasing the consumption of healthful foods—e.g., targeted food stamps for fresh fruits and vegetables. Most of the analysis in this chapter, however, deals exclusively with restricting the list of allowable foods under the FSP.

Table 11.5

General Characteristics of the Current and the Proposed Redesigned Food Stamp Program

Characteristic	Current	Proposed /redesigned
Nutrition purpose	Increased calories	Improved diet quality, supporting US dietary guidelines (fruits, vegetables, foods low in saturated fat, high-fiber foods)
Allowable foods	All food items sold in markets/ food outlets participating in the FSP. No restrictions. Examples: energy-dense, low-nutrient foods such as potato chips, candy, doughnuts, etc.	Emphasizing fresh fruits and vegetables, low-fat dairy products, high-fiber (low-sugar) cereals, and whole-grain products—foods emphasized in the US dietary guidelines
Allowable beverages	All nonalcoholic beverages, including soft drinks, fruit punch, etc	Only those beverages meeting a predetermined nutrition standard—beverages emphasized in the US dietary guidelines
Excluded food/beverages	Alcohol and tobacco	Alcohol, tobacco, and energy-dense (high-fat or high-sugar) foods and beverages not meeting the US dietary guidelines
Primary program goal	Support farmers, stabilize commodity prices	Improve diet quality, especially of children in low-income households
Secondary program goal	Provide calories to food-insecure households	Ultimately improve health and reduce risk of obesity

Source: After Townsend, 2006.

Note: The US dietary guidelines refers to the Dietary Guidelines for Americans (2005) at http://www.cnpp.usda.gov/DietaryGuidelines.htm and Healthy People 2010 at http://www.healthypeople.gov/

diet quality, particularly for children participating in the FSP, and ultimately to reduce obesity. Table 11.5 presents the general characteristics of the current FSP and a set of changes to it proposed by Townsend (2006). Table 11.6 lists a more specific set of suggestions regarding foods that would and would not be allowed under the revised FSP. Such specificity is needed to begin to examine the likely responses by producers to increased demand for some more healthful foods (e.g., fruits and vegetables), especially in the short term.

The suggestions laid out in Table 11.6 can be placed into context by juxtaposition with the expenditure shares listed in Table 11.4. FSP participants who were surveyed as part of the NFSPS spent 14.5% of their food stamp benefits on processed grain products such as cakes and sugar cereals, many of which would

Table 11.6
Specific Foods Allowed in the Food Stamp Program for 12 Food Types

Food type	Current FSP	Proposed revised FSP
Grains	White bread, rice, pasta, hot and cold cereals	Whole-grain bread, rice, pasta, hot and cold cereals
	Cakes, cookies, and muffins made with white flour[a]	
	Whole-grain[b] bread, rice, pasta, hot and cold cereals	
Dairy products	All milks, cottage cheese, yogurts	Nonfat, 1% and 2% milks, cottage cheese, yogurts
	Cream, cream cheese	
	Cheese	Cheese
Fruit	All forms (fresh, canned, frozen, dried)	All forms (fresh, canned, frozen, dried)
	100% fruit juice	100% fruit juice
	Juice drinks	
Vegetables	All forms (fresh, canned, frozen, dried)	All forms (fresh, canned, frozen, dried)
	100% juice	100% juice
Beans and legumes	All beans and legumes	All beans and legumes
	Peanut butter	Peanut butter
Nuts and seeds	All, including nut butters	Raw and dry-roasted nuts, seeds
Meats	All	Low-fat cuts of meats (chicken, turkey, lean ground beef, turkey hot dogs, roasts)
Fish	All, including breaded and fried	Fresh, frozen, canned
Eggs	All	All
Snacks	Savory snacks (e.g., potato chips, corn chips, crackers)	None
	Sweet snacks (e.g., hard candy, chocolate, candy bars)	
Mixed prepared foods	Pizza	Only those foods meeting US dietary guidelines for fat, saturated fat, and whole grain
	Lasagna	
	Frozen dinners	
Other beverages	Water	Water
	Soft drinks	
	Fruit juice drinks, punch	
	Sport drinks	

Note: The US dietary guidelines refers to the Dietary Guidelines for Americans (2005) at http://www.cnpp.usda.gov/DietaryGuidelines.htm and Healthy People 2010 at http://www.healthypeople.gov/
[a]Also referred to as unbleached flour or wheat flour.
[b]These grain products contain some or all whole-grain flour.

not be allowed under a redesigned FSP; only processed whole-grain products would be included in the new list of allowable foods. The 11% share of FSP benefits spent on sweets and soft drinks would be driven to zero because food stamps would not be redeemed for these products under the suggestions outlined in Table 11.6. Dairy products and inexpensive meats, which account for a combined 26% share of purchases made with food stamps, would be restricted to low-fat products.

The current Food Stamp Program makes it possible to consume a diet dominated by energy-dense foods and beverages. A less energy-dense diet lower in fats and sugars would include more foods that are nutritionally more dense and energetically less dense, such as fruits and vegetables. Assuming that people consume a constant weight of food each day, eating foods with lower energy density (fewer calories per unit weight) should reduce overall energy intake and (over time) the prevalence of overweight and obesity. Short-term experimental studies consistently find that decreasing the energy density of the diet enhances satiation, resulting in a lower energy intake (Darmon et al., 2004; Devitt et al., 2004; Kral and Rolls, 2004; Rolls et al., 2005; see also Chapters 10 and 14). The predominance of laboratory evidence supports the hypothesis that energy density is related to obesity (as suggested in Drewnowski et al., 2004). The high palatability of energy-dense foods also actively contributes to their passive overconsumption (see Chapter 4).

However, empirical analyses of large observational data sets have not yielded consistent or conclusive evidence of the relationship between energy density and adiposity, although they have found a positive association with calorie intake (Yao et al., 2003; Alexy et al., 2004). Given the absence of prevention trials that evaluate the impact of energy density on adiposity, the limited number and inconclusive findings from large-scale empirical studies (evaluating the impact on adiposity), and the lack of secular trend data, it is not possible to come to a firm conclusion regarding the role of the energy density of the diet on adiposity.

Challenges in determining implications of proposed changes to the Food Stamp Program

How might the suggested changes to the FSP affect the foods purchased by the average FSP participant? The first challenge in addressing this question is predicting the responses of program participants while other factors are held constant. An important question is the extent to which changes in the foods that are eligible for purchase using food stamps will alter the consumption choices made by consumers, rather than just providing different methods of payment for the same consumption bundle. Yet harder to predict are the aggregate market outcomes, allowing for induced changes in food prices and food production. These topics are discussed briefly next and in more depth later in the chapter.

Changing the list of allowable foods and beverages will affect consumption choices among FSP participants, which will be reflected as changes in total market demand. The consequences will depend on how those changes in demand are absorbed—between adjustments in prices and quantities consumed—which in turn will depend on how the food industry responds in terms of production and supply. The confluence of these effects would be reflected in price changes for both the more healthful foods promoted under the new FSP rules, and the low-nutrient, energy-dense foods that would be disallowed if the policy changes were implemented, which would feed back into the purchase decisions of consumers, as well as the long-term adjustments of food producers. Hence, even if we know the initial demand response by FSP participants, the ultimate responses to FSP changes will depend on complex interactions between the supply and demand for foods, the effects of these interactions on food prices, and the effects of price changes on food purchases.

The tools of economics can help simplify this process into tractable parts and predict responses to changes in the FSP. The proposed analysis is somewhat limited by the fact that this policy intervention has yet to be attempted. In the absence of any historical policy variation that would make it possible to statistically estimate the impact of changes to the Food Stamp Program, analytical models based on conventional economic theories of consumer and producer behavior are presented here. These models reveal what can reasonably be expected by way of direct and indirect effects of the proposed changes to the FSP.

Finally, but most importantly, the ultimate consequences of these proposed changes for nutritional outcomes are even more difficult to predict, because they depend not only on changes in the amounts of allowable foods in the revised FSP that are purchased and consumed, but also on the amounts of nonallowed foods consumed and on the rates of energy expenditures. To be effective in addressing obesity, the revised list of allowable FSP foods must improve diet quality *and* reduce overall caloric intake; these two objectives are often linked, but achieving either of them should not be considered automatic. The remainder of this chapter examines why these objectives are not a foregone conclusion, and, using stylized facts about demand for a supply of particular types of foods, suggests what the likely results of a revised FSP might be, for both FSP participants and other consumers.

Likely Responses of Consumers to Proposed Changes to the FSP

In fiscal year 2004, 34.3% of the 10 million households participating in the FSP were headed by single adults with children.[11] These households were poorer than other food stamp recipients, and overwhelmingly headed by females (Poikolainen, 2005); thus they might be expected to be more likely to struggle with weight-related health concerns. Forty-two percent of FSP households consisted of a single person. These two demographic groups are the first to be examined in the following analysis of food stamps and consumer behavior.[12]

A simple model of consumer response to food stamps

Before discussing a model of the choices made by an individual while enrolled in the FSP, let us look at the basics of the standard economic model of consumer behavior. The standard economic model of rational consumer choice assumes that consumers seek to maximize their satisfaction, or "utility," subject to constraints in the form of time, money, information, and other resources. Although all individuals are assumed to prefer more consumption, as well as greater variety in the goods they enjoy, the model recognizes that individuals also have unique preferences with respect to consumption of goods; a given bundle of goods will not necessarily yield the same total satisfaction for two distinct individuals. Consequently, two people with identical incomes and facing the same set of prices may make very different choices.

An individual is said to be consuming optimally if no other bundle of goods that she could consume would make her better off (i.e., raise her total utility), given her budget constraint and market prices. Although we can never actually observe an individual's utility level, assuming that people do the best they can (i.e., maximize utility) within certain constraints allows economists to predict how people will respond to changes in the decision-making environment.[13] It is also assumed that individuals are "price takers;" that is, no single person is able to affect prices. Instead, prices are the result of choices made by all consumers and businesses, as well as available resources.

An individual who is eligible to enroll in the FSP faces two decisions: whether to participate in the FSP and, if she decides to enroll, which combination of food and nonfood items to consume. Figure 11.4 represents this scenario graphically. In this simple model, two commodities are available for purchase: food (*f*) and an aggregate commodity meant to represent all other goods (*x*).[14] The con-

---

[11]All decision making with respect to household expenditures is assumed here to be made by persons 18 or older, although the presence of children will certainly have an influence on household consumption patterns (e.g., see Chapter 12). This assumption may be problematic with respect to earnings by older teenagers. However, previous analyses of behavior by households receiving food stamps have found that adjusting this cutoff age to 16 generates no change in the substantive conclusions of empirical work (e.g., Bruenig and Dasgupta, 2005).

[12]Households that include multiple adults may behave differently in response to changes in the FSP. See Bruenig and Dasgupta, 2005, for empirical evidence on differences in expenditure patterns between single-adult and multiple-adult households.

[13]For a more detailed description of utility theory and its foundations, see Varian, 2005.

[14]Note that the focus here is the decisions made by the household member in charge of food purchases—that is, choices made by the adult head of the household. Although child welfare is not represented explicitly, the utility gained from purchases of food and other goods will reflect the emphasis placed on child welfare by the household head.

FIGURE 11.4 Effects of the current Food Stamp Program on consumption. See text for explanation.

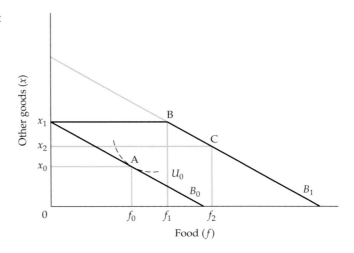

sumer's preferences are represented by indifference curves, exemplified by the curve labeled U_0. These curves connect bundles of f and x that yield the same level of utility, and higher levels of utility are gained as the consumer moves to curves that are farther from the point where the two axes intersect; that is, utility increases as the individual consumes more of either good. The slope of U_0 measures the rate at which the consumer can trade other goods for food and still remain at the same level of utility; that is, the slope indicates the rate at which the consumer can trade off between the two goods while remaining "indifferent," since her level of utility has not changed. The convex shape of the curve reflects the fact that the consumer prefers variety in consumption; the more other goods she has, the more willing she is to trade them for food, and vice versa.

This consumer's budget constraint prior to enrolling in the FSP is given by the solid diagonal line labeled B_0. If she does not enroll in the FSP, she will select the bundle (f_0, x_0) corresponding to point A; given her budget constraint and preferences, this is the best she can do. If she enrolls and is given food stamps, her budget constraint is shifted out in parallel by the amount of the food stamp allocation (the shift is parallel because the prices of food and other goods have not changed). The new budget constraint is represented by the solid diagonal line labeled B_1 up to point B but is discontinuous (i.e., "kinked" rather than "smooth") at that point, reflecting that food stamps cannot be used to purchase nonfood items. The newly chosen consumption bundle will depend on the consumer's preferences regarding food and nonfood items. If the allocation of food stamps is large relative to her preferred consumption of food versus other goods, she may select the bundle (f_1, x_1) corresponding to point B, in which all of her cash income is spent on nonfood items. If, on the other hand, she has stronger preferences for food, then she may select the bundle (f_2, x_2) corresponding to point C, in which she spends all of her food stamps and some additional cash on food.

Evaluating a revised Food Stamp Program

The proposed changes to the FSP would strategically alter the list of foods that FSP participants could purchase with their food stamps. Figure 11.5 depicts this situation—this time focusing on choices between "healthful" foods (foods meeting the US dietary guidelines) and "unhealthful" foods.[15] Figure 11.5A essentially replicates Figure 11.4, representing the choice between food and nonfood items; Figure 11.5B represents the choice between healthful food and unhealthful food. Suppose that if the consumer described in the previous section does not enroll in the FSP, she selects the bundle (f_0, x_0) corresponding to point A on budget line B_0 in Figure 11.5A. The food budget (corresponding to f_0, the total amount spent on food) is allocated in Figure 11.5B between healthful food and unhealthful food, and the consumer might choose the bundle (h_0, u_0) at point A in Figure 11.5B.

If the consumer enrolls in the FSP and is given food stamps that may be used to purchase *any* kind of food, in Figure 11.5A the budget constraint shifts out in parallel from B_0 to B_1. Suppose that, as in the typical case (e.g., see Fraker, 1990), the consumer ends up spending some cash as well as food stamps on food, and the new consumption bundle is (f_1, x_1) at point B in Figure 11.5A. In Figure 11.5B, then, the food budget constraint shifts in parallel from f_0 to f_1 and

---

[15]For the purposes of this chapter, *healthful* foods are those foods meeting the requirements of the US dietary guidelines. *Unhealthful* foods are foods that are likely to be calorie-dense and nutrient-poor, and hence are not included on the list of allowable foods in the revised FSP.

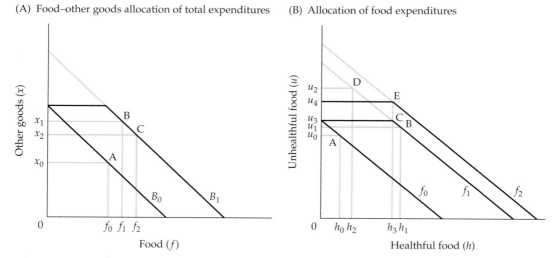

(A) Food–other goods allocation of total expenditures   (B) Allocation of food expenditures

FIGURE 11.5   Effects of a revised Food Stamp Program. See text for explanation.

extends all the way to both axes because the food stamps may be applied to either kind of food. The new optimal consumption bundle could be (h_1, u_1) at point B in Figure 11.5B and would contain more of both healthful and unhealthful foods, compared to the bundle in the absence of the FSP, (h_0, u_0) at point A. Of course, the exact location of the new optimal point may differ from what has been presented here. However, if the consumer enjoys eating both healthful and unhealthful food, giving her food stamps that may be spent on either type of food will result in an increase in the consumption of both healthful and unhealthful food.

Now suppose that food stamps may be used to purchase *only* healthful foods. Under this revised FSP, holding total expenditure on other goods constant, the revised budget constraint in Figure 11.5B is formed by the solid diagonal line labeled f_1 up to u_3 (point C) but becomes discontinuous at that point. In this case, as drawn, the consumer can still afford the bundle (h_1, u_1). Consumers like this, who are participating in the FSP and already spending more than the value of their food stamps on healthful food under the current program, will not be affected by the change.

A simple example can clarify this conclusion. Suppose that the consumer is currently receiving $50 per month in food stamps, and she bolsters her monthly food budget with $50 in cash. Furthermore, suppose she is currently spending $60 a month in combined cash and food stamps on healthful foods. Now imagine that the rules of the FSP are changed so that she may purchase only healthful foods with her $50 benefit. Obviously there is no need for her to change her eating habits. She may devote a greater share of food stamps to the purchase of healthful foods than she did previously, but there is no reason for her actual consumption of healthful foods to change. In this sense the constraint imposed on her decision making by the revised list of allowable foods is *not binding*; that is, it does not force her to choose differently from how she would if the program did not change.

Alternatively, suppose that with the current food stamps the consumer would have chosen the bundle (h_2, u_2) at point D in Figure 11.5B, with a smaller expenditure on healthful food than the total value of the food stamps. In this case, with the switch to revised food stamps, the constraint is binding and the consumer would choose the bundle (h_3, u_3) at point C in Figure 11.5B, spending the entire food stamp allocation on healthful food and the entire cash budget for food on unhealthful food.

However, unlike the case in which the constraint was not binding, in this situation it is no longer reasonable to assume that total expenditure on food will remain unaffected. The underlying reasoning can be explained with an example. Suppose that, under the current FSP rules, the consumer is spending $70 a month in cash and food stamps on unhealthful food, $30 in cash and food stamps on healthful food, and $1,000 on other items, while receiving $50 in food stamps. This is her optimal bundle—that is, the combination of goods that maximizes her utility, given her preferences, her budget constraint, and her food stamp benefit. Now imagine that food stamps may be spent only on healthful foods. Since she was only spending $30 a month on healthful foods, the constraint imposed by the rule change will be binding, and her purchases of healthful food will increase by $20. However, she will try to come as close to her original optimal bundle as possible, requiring her to spend some of her budget for nonfood items on unhealthful food, and thus increasing her overall food budget.

A change of this nature is illustrated in Figure 11.5A by a movement *along* the budget constraint resulting in a new consumption bundle of (f_2, x_2) and a concomitant *shift* in the food budget constraint from f_1 to f_2 in Figure 11.5B. The final food consumption choice will still be constrained to the bundle (h_3, u_4) at point E in Figure 11.5B, with the same quantity of healthful food being purchased but an increased quantity of unhealthful food being purchased and financed at the expense of the consumption of other goods. As a consequence of being given restricted food stamps rather than generic food stamps, the consumer benefits less; the constraint imposed by the revised list of allowable foods is binding, forcing her to make different choices from those that she could make in the absence of the rule change. However, she consumes more "healthful" food and, most likely, less (but still some) unhealthful food.

In summary, under most conditions the theoretical analysis indicates that if the current FSP were replaced with the proposed revised FSP, the consumption of healthful foods by some recipients would increase. However, the effects on total food purchases and on the purchases of unhealthful food by recipients are less clear. Some recipients might not change their eating habits, if already consuming more healthful food than the value of their food stamp allotment permits. Some recipients might increase their consumption of healthful food using food stamps, but at the same time might reduce their consumption of other goods to avoid reducing their consumption of less healthful food items. These issues turn on the extent to which the constraint to spend food stamps only on healthful food is binding on consumption choices, as well as other characteristics of the recipients.

Implications for consumption choices

How likely is it that the constraint on food consumption generated by the food stamp benefit will be binding for single-adult households, and thus lead to higher consumption of healthful foods than under the current FSP? With the current rules, nearly all households fall into the "unconstrained" category: observed food expenditures exceed food stamp benefits. In his review of the food stamp literature, Fraker (1990) reports that between 5% and 15% of beneficiary households purchase food solely through the use of food stamps, although it is not known what proportion of these are single- versus multiple-adult households.

The proportion of constrained households would undoubtedly increase if the list of allowable foods were revised, since making these changes would effectively tighten the constraint on household consumption. For example, suppose the revised FSP focused on promoting the consumption of fruits and vegetables. Blisard and colleagues (2004) report that households with income levels below 130% of the poverty line in 2000 spent about $24.41 per month on fruits and vegetables, of which $14.82 was used to purchase *fresh* fruits and vegetables; households with a greater number of members older than 45 years of age spent significantly more on these foods, but no other significant effects of household age structure were observed. The $24.41 figure represented 10.4% of the average monthly FSP benefit for FSP households with children and 15.4% of the average monthly FSP benefit for all participating households in 2000 (Cunnyngham, 2001).[16] These data suggest that a large fraction of households participating in the FSP would find themselves constrained following the suggested revisions to the list of allowable foods, and would change consumption behavior as a result.

Empirical evidence in support of this conclusion is scant because nothing on the scale of reforming the FSP with the purpose of improving nutrition has been attempted. However, Herman and colleagues (2008) present evidence from a pilot project in Los Angeles suggesting that individuals may increase their consumption of healthful foods when given proper incentives. In that study, WIC[17]participants who received vouchers redeemable for fresh fruits and vegetables significantly increased their consumption of fruits and vegetables relative to a control group, at least in some instances.[18]

Herman's conclusions do not tell us what effect the vouchers may have had on purchases of other types of foods, or what the effect on fruit and vegetable expenditures was at the margin (i.e., the impact of an additional dollar in vouchers on fruit and vegetable purchases). There is no way to rule out the possibility that providing a dollar of vouchers for healthful foods will lead consumers to reorganize spending in a way that also increases purchases of unhealthful foods; as indicated in the preceding analysis, this is a very real possibility that would lead to improvements in diet quality *and* to increases in caloric intake. It is also difficult to infer the actual impact on individual consumption of fruits and vegetables; changes in consumption were measured at the household level, as is typically the case in studies of food purchase behavior. Finally, it is difficult to distill practical policy implications from studies that provide incentives to consumers that if applied at the scale of the market may require much larger outlays of government funds than current program budgets would allow.

---

[16]Comparing the expenditures estimated by Blisard and colleagues to 2004 average monthly FSP benefits (in constant 2000 US dollars) yields approximately the same results (Barrett, 2006).

[17]*WIC* is the better-known name for the USDA's Special Supplemental Nutrition Program for Women, Infants, and Children.

[18]Results varied by intervention site and by how changes in consumption were measured. At one site, participants demonstrated a significant increase in consumption of both fruits and vegetables measured separately, relative to members of the control group. At the other site, participants significantly increased vegetable consumption relative to the control group, but there was no discernible increase in fruit consumption.

The conclusion that participants will likely increase their consumption of healthful foods assumes that participation in the FSP will not be affected. If other costs of participation in the FSP remain unchanged (time spent filling out paperwork, social stigma, etc.), shortening the list of foods that may be purchased using food stamps seems more likely to discourage participation than to increase enrollment. Holding other program characteristics constant, revising the list of allowable foods to include fewer items will likely make FSP participation less appealing. Households that previously found the rewards of participating just barely sufficient to cover the costs (i.e., households at the participatory margin) will no longer find enrolling in the FSP worthwhile.

This conclusion may seem counterintuitive, in that one may think that a program designed to lead to better health and nutrition ought to encourage participation in the FSP. However, individuals participating in the FSP already have the option of consuming more fruits and vegetables; if they believed that consuming more fruits and vegetables would make them happier, they would already be doing so. This is one of the main points of the analytical and graphical analysis presented in the preceding discussion: by further limiting the choices of participants, revising the list of allowable foods necessarily makes enrolling in the FSP less appealing. For individuals on the razor's edge of enrolling or not enrolling, such a change would probably push them toward exiting the FSP or not enrolling in the first place.[19]

In addition, questions remain as to how effective the proposed changes will be in reaching the targeted demographic group (i.e., low-income households, particularly those with children). The low rate of participation in the FSP by eligible households indicates that a large proportion of poor households will not be directly affected by changes to the list of allowable foods. We know that women in households enrolled in the FSP are more likely to be obese (Gibson, 2003), although, as stated earlier, this relationship appears to be weakening (ver Ploeg et al., 2006). However, in Gibson's sample of low-income women from the National Longitudinal Survey of Youth, 19.8% of women *not* participating in the FSP were obese; households headed by these females would not directly benefit from the revised FSP, and they would be unlikely to enroll in the program if the list of allowable foods were revised. Indeed, given the likely effects of the revised FSP on the prices of healthful and unhealthful foods (examined in the next section), these nonparticipating households might consume even greater amounts of unhealthful foods, although, as we will see, any price effects are likely to be modest.

---

[19]This conclusion assumes that preferences for different foods are constant, which is reasonable for the analysis of the policy change being considered. An alterative proposal might include an element of nutrition education as well, in which case the policy package might entail changes in preferences along with changes in the Food Stamp Program.

Potential Market Responses to Changes in the FSP: Theoretical Relationships

The preceding analysis of choice at the level of individual consumers assumed constant prices for food and other goods. If effective, however, the proposed changes to the FSP would generate increases in demand for the foods included on the revised list of what may be purchased with food stamps, as well as decreases in demand for goods that were formerly included on this list but are now excluded. These changes in demand may be accommodated by changes in production or in prices, or some of both, with the balance depending on the nature of the industry in question and the length of run (the period of time allowed for the industry to adjust to the changes). To the extent that increases in demand for more healthful foods cause their prices to rise, and decreases in demand for less healthful foods cause their prices to drop, the second-round or indirect effects of the policy through induced price changes will be to counteract the first-round, or direct, effects. Consequently, the ability of policy makers to bring about meaningful changes in eating habits among FSP participants will hinge in part on the behavior of farmers, grocery retailers, and other links in the agricultural supply chain.

Conceptual single-market model of supply and demand for agricultural commodities

A convenient way of breaking down the response of an industry to price changes is to characterize it in terms of short-run, intermediate-run, and long-run supply response to price changes. In the short run, firms would be expected to be constrained by previous decisions, and largely unable to respond to price changes; this is likely to be the case even if producers are made aware ahead of time of any potential changes to the FSP, given the sometimes long lags between planting and harvesting in agriculture, the lack of international trade in some crops, and other sources of inflexibility. In the intermediate run, the industry will be better able to adjust, as resources flow in and out, depending on the direction of price changes. Some resources (e.g., appropriate lands for cultivating specific crops) will still be limited, however, and the supply curve will slope upward as a result. In the very long run, if all inputs are variable and not limited, the supply curve will be horizontal, and increases in demand will not affect prices.

These ideas and their implications are illustrated in Figure 11.6, which contains a conventional competitive market model of supply and demand for an agricultural commodity, A. In the very short run, total supply of the commodity is fixed, determined by prior decisions. In Figure 11.6, the vertical line labeled $S_{A,SR}$ represents the total supply of commodity A in the very short run and shows that the quantity supplied is the same regardless of the price, in this case at $Q_{A,0}$. An example would be a perishable fresh vegetable, like lettuce, that cannot be

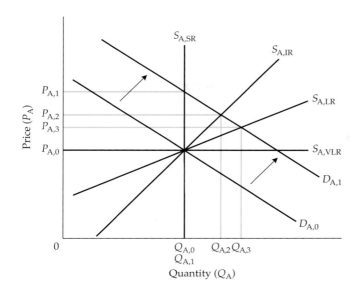

FIGURE 11.6 Price effects of a demand shift in a particular food commodity, A, in different time frames: short run (SR), intermediate run (IR), long run (LR), and very long run (VLR). D, demand; P, price; Q, quantity; S, supply. See text for explanation.

imported from other areas and whose potential supply is fixed during the harvest period (e.g., see Sexton and Zhang, 1996). The output price, $P_{A,0}$ is determined by consumers' willingness to pay for that quantity, $Q_{A,0}$. This equilibrium price is taken from the aggregate demand across all consumers for the commodity, represented by the curve $D_{A,0}$. Now suppose that demand for commodity A increases from $D_{A,0}$ to $D_{A,1}$ as a result of a change in the Food Stamp Program. In the short run, this increase in demand will result in an increase in price from $P_{A,0}$ to $P_{A,1}$, but there will not be any change in aggregate consumption or production, which stays constant at $Q_{A,1} = Q_{A,0}$, though there will likely be a change in the composition of the group of consumers after the price increase.

In the intermediate run, which allows greater time to respond to changes in incentives, supply is more responsive to price, as represented by the upward-sloping curve labeled $S_{A,IR}$. The upward slope reflects the fact that in this length of run it is possible, but increasingly expensive, to expand production; and thus progressively higher prices call forth progressively greater quantities supplied. Hence, when demand for commodity A increases from $D_{A,0}$ to $D_{A,1}$, the effects include both an increase in price from $P_{A,0}$ to $P_{A,2}$ and an increase in consumption and production from $Q_{A,0}$ to $Q_{A,2}$. The intermediate-run equilibrium after the demand shift is thus at the point where intermediate-run supply and demand cross in Figure 11.6, and quantity supplied at price $P_{A,2}$ is equal to quantity demanded at the same price, $Q_{A,2}$.

In the long run, supply is even more responsive to price (or more elastic), as represented by the curve labeled $S_{A,LR}$, and the long-run equilibrium after the demand shift is thus at $(P_{A,3}, Q_{A,3})$, where long-run supply and demand cross in

Figure 11.6. Thus, with increasing length of run (or more time for producers to respond), the demand response is met more by increases in quantity consumed and less by increases in prices paid by consumers. In the extreme case, which applies for some commodities—such as intensive livestock (poultry, hogs) and smaller-scale crops that use comparatively small amounts of the relevant types of land and other resources, including most fruit and vegetable crops—the very-long-run supply is perfectly elastic, such that any demand increase is entirely met by changes in quantity, with no increase in price (this case is represented by the horizontal supply curve, $S_{A,VLR}$).[20]

In many cases over the relevant length of run for policy analysis, supply will be less than perfectly elastic and each change in demand will be accommodated by a combination of changes in prices and quantities.[21] This is perhaps especially so for demand decreases because agricultural supply response is asymmetrical. That is, supply may be more elastic with respect to output price increases than to output price decreases, because of the presence of specialized capital (e.g., automatic milking machines on dairy farms) or immobile capital (e.g., a grain silo), and the resulting asset fixity in agriculture.[22] This notion of asymmetry is supported by the literature on empirical supply analysis (Mundlak, 2001).

On the other hand, when the commodity is traded internationally, there is another dimension for absorbing changes in US demand—either by reducing exports or by increasing imports—and this added dimension reduces the potential for demand changes to cause price changes, even in the very short run. To complicate things further, however, trade barriers (e.g., tariffs and quotas) and other policies modify the transmission of price signals through the market mechanism, as does the food industry and other intermediaries that are involved between farmers and final consumers (e.g., see Wohlgenant, 2001).

Some multimarket complications

The single-market analysis in this section ignores some key features of the question. First, the proposed policy, if effective, will directly affect the demand for

---

[20]The elasticity of supply (or demand) measures the percentage change in quantity supplied (demanded) in response to a 1% increase in price. Economists use these unit-free measures of responsiveness to characterize supply functions ranging from totally inelastic (an elasticity of zero) corresponding to a vertical supply curve, to perfectly elastic (an elasticity of infinity) corresponding to a horizontal supply curve.

[21]More generally, we can think of an infinite series of supply curves fanning out from a vertical, short-run supply curve, with each curve representing industry response to price changes when adjustment periods of different lengths are allowed (Cassells, 1933).

[22]The term *asset fixity* refers to the situation in which the value of additional output from an asset is less than the acquisition cost of the asset and greater than its salvage value. The asset is said to be "stuck" in its current use; since the value of marginal output is less than the acquisition cost, there is no incentive to acquire more of the asset, and there is no incentive to scrap the asset while the value of marginal outputs exceeds the salvage value (Johnson, 1956).

all food commodities at the same time: it will increase the demand for all foods on the revised FSP list of included foods, and it will decrease the demand for all other foods (whether included on the current FSP list or not). In addition, the resulting price changes for any individual food commodity will have cross-commodity effects on demand for other food commodities related in consumption as substitutes or complements,[23] and they will have cross-commodity effects on the supply of commodities related in production. The discussion that follows assumes away the cross-commodity impacts on the supply side, which are likely to be comparatively minor, in order to focus attention on the cross-commodity impacts on the demand side, which may be important.

The cross-commodity story can be illustrated by combination of the intermediate-run analysis for commodity A from Figure 11.6 with a corresponding analysis for another commodity, B, which (let's assume) is a substitute in consumption for commodity A. For some purposes A could be thought of as representing all of the foods included in the revised FSP list and B as representing all other foods, but for other purposes we may be interested in more individualized comparisons.

Figure 11.7A represents the market for commodity A (a healthful food); Figure 11.7B, the market for commodity B (an unhealthful food). The demand curves,

---

[23]Goods are *substitutes* in consumption if an increase in the price of one good has a positive effect on consumption of the other, and a decrease in the price of one good negatively affects consumption of the other. Goods are *complements* in consumption if the opposite relationship holds.

(A) The market for healthful food

(B) The market for unhealthful food

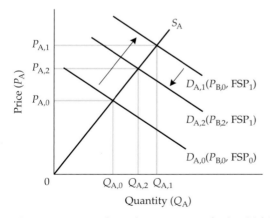
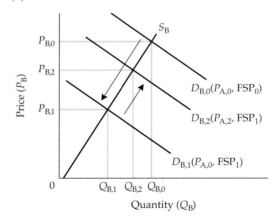

FIGURE 11.7   Multimarket responses for healthful (A) and unhealthful (B) foods to changes in the Food Stamp Program (FSP). *D*, demand; *P*, price; *Q*, quantity; *S*, supply.

quantities, and prices of goods are labeled with corresponding subscripts A and B. Now suppose that, as a result of a change in the Food Stamp Program (from FSP_0 to FSP_1), demand for commodity A increases from $D_{A,0}$ to $D_{A,1}$, and demand for B decreases from $D_{B,0}$ to $D_{B,1}$. Holding other factors constant, these demand shifts would cause an increase in price of A from $P_{A,0}$ to $P_{A,1}$ and a decrease in price of B from $P_{B,0}$ to $P_{B,1}$. Because the two commodities are substitutes in consumption, however, the increase in price of A would cause a second-round increase in demand for B, and the decrease in price of B would cause a second-round decrease in demand for A—in each case offsetting the direct effects of the initial demand shifts.

The ultimate picture will depend on the relative magnitudes of the direct effects (through the proposed FSP changes) and indirect effects (through the induced price changes) on demands for the two goods. A reasonable conjecture is that the net effects are to increase demand for A and reduce demand for B, but by less in each case than the direct effect alone would imply. In Figure 11.7, the final equilibrium demands reflecting all these effects are depicted as $D_{A,2}$ and $D_{B,2}$. The corresponding quantities and prices for good A are $Q_{A,2}$ and $P_{A,2}$, both greater than their initial values; and the corresponding quantities and prices for good B are $Q_{B,2}$ and $P_{B,2}$, both less than their initial values.

In this more complete analysis, allowing for both direct and indirect effects, the program changes will have encouraged participants to consume more of the healthful food (A) and less of the unhealthful food (B). However, the induced price changes will have caused *non*participants to consume less of the healthful food (A) and *more* of the unhealthful food (B). The relative importance of these effects for the different groups of consumers will depend on the relative sizes of the own- and cross-price elasticities (or slopes) of the supply and demand functions. These issues are explicitly explored in the technical appendix to this chapter for a range of plausible values for demand and supply elasticities for FSP participants and eligible nonparticipants.

Implications of the analysis

Several observations relevant to the current topic can be gleaned from the analysis in this section. Assuming that the changes to the FSP do indeed generate increases in demand for healthful foods, the immediate result will likely be increases in prices and a muted consumption response. In the extreme short run, FSP recipients may increase their consumption of healthful foods, but entirely at the expense of reduced consumption of the same foods by other consumers, such that total consumption of these foods is unchanged. Over time, however, as the industry adjusts progressively and makes quantity changes in response to the changed incentives in the intermediate- and longer-run scenarios, the price-increasing effects will be increasingly muted. The consequences for the healthfulness of the diets of participants and nonparticipants will therefore evolve, because they depend on the relative magnitudes of the demand shifts and induced price changes, among other things.

The speed with which the supply curves "fan out" as depicted here will vary substantially across commodity types, as dictated by product and market characteristics. The nature of supply response to price, and the amount of time it takes for full adjustment to a new long-run equilibrium varies systematically among agricultural commodities, reflecting differences in the biology and technology of production. For example, the supply of annual crops will be far more responsive in the short run to price changes than will perennial tree crops or livestock; the latter are characterized by very slow adjustment and long lags in supply response, as demonstrated in the empirical literature on commodity supply (e.g., French & Matthews, 1971; Chavas & Klemme, 1986; Alston et al., 1995).

Systematic differences may also be found in other factors that influence price effects of demand changes, including the extent to which products are traded or processed between farmers and final consumers, and the roles of policies. The following section will examine these differences in production and market conditions on a commodity-by-commodity basis, and then return to the issue of the likely ways in which the proposed FSP changes will affect FSP participants and eligible nonparticipants.

Potential Market Response to Changes in the FSP: Quantitative Speculation

The simple model presented in the preceding discussion, and in its equivalent algebraic form in the technical appendix to this chapter, is conceptually useful but has some empirical limitations. For a start, it skips over the important link between changes in policies affecting demands for foods at retail and changes in wholesale or farm markets for food commodities, which is the emphasis here. Even if we can measure the implied demand shifts for the different categories of foods, to go from there to commodity markets is a big and difficult step. A practical empirical counterpart would have to include separate equations for many different food commodities reflecting their different demand and supply elasticities; roles of government policies, international trade, and the food industry; these roles may be different roles in the original versus the revised FSP (e.g., see Abbott, 1999; and Jetter et al., 2006). Relevant information for identifying parameters of such an empirical model is not immediately available. Rather than build such a model, this discussion will conjecture about the potential impacts, commodity by commodity, according to knowledge of the nature of their markets and other relevant factors, and drawing on some related work in previous studies.

Stylized facts for the main commodities

GRAINS   Whole grains and high-fiber cereals are two of the product categories included on the proposed list of allowable foods. If FSP participants were to substantially increase their consumption of these products, the result would be an increase in demand for the grain that is used to produce these foods, a greater use of processing capacity, and additional demand for the other inputs that go into making these products (labor, energy, materials, and so on). However, there are good reasons to conclude that any change in demand generated by reforming the FSP would have little impact on grain prices.

Wheat comprises the vast majority of grain consumption in the United States, accounting for 71% of food grains available for consumption in 2003. In general, it takes less raw grain to produce a whole-grain product than a similar refined product; whole-grain products use most of the kernel, whereas refined products lose much of the bran in processing. In 2004, the US Department of Agriculture estimated that for every 1% increase in domestic production of whole-wheat flours in that year, 50,000 to 70,000 *fewer* acres of wheat would have been harvested in the United States in 2005 (Buzby et al., 2005). This estimate implies that a shift toward greater consumption of whole grains is likely to have a *downward* effect on the demand for wheat products in the United States.

The role of the United States globally as a producer and exporter of major grain crops lends further support to the expectation that any change in the FSP will not significantly affect grain prices. The United States is among the world's largest exporters of wheat, corn, soy, and rice (Vocke et al., 2005). In the case of rice, for example, 40% of the US crop is exported (US Department of Agriculture, 2006a); if increases in demand for whole-grain products increased the domestic demand for brown or unmilled rice, it is highly likely that this demand would be met by reduced exports, with minimal effects on domestic or export prices. Similarly for the other major grains, the existence of substantial US exports means that the effective supply to the domestic market is highly elastic for moderate changes in quantities, such that changes in demand would have only modest effects on prices. Thus, any changes in demand arising from reform of the FSP should have minimal effects on grain prices.

DAIRY PRODUCTS   It is more complex to predict the marketwide consequences of a shift in demand toward low-fat dairy products and away from higher-fat dairy products because of (1) the joint nature of production of fat and nonfat solids in milk and in products made from milk, (2) the slower dynamics of supply response in livestock production, and (3) the complications of US and international dairy policy.

Raw milk, which is the primary input into all dairy foods, comprises milk fat and nonfat solids in roughly fixed proportions. Different dairy products contain different proportions of fat and nonfat solids, and they are produced jointly, such that the overall mix of products contains the same mixture of fat and nonfat solids as the raw milk that was used to produce them.[24] For example, separat-

---

[24]In modeling the impacts on the US market of a movement toward freer trade in dairy products, Alston, Balagtas, Brunke, and Sumner (2006) explicitly represented milk and dairy products in terms of the constituents of fat and nonfat solids.

ing cream from raw milk yields fat for the production of butter, as well as non-fat milk that can then be dried and used in low-fat products (Balagtas et al., 2003). Butter is also made from cream left over from cheese and fluid milk production (US Department of Agriculture, 2004). The essential conservation of the total amount of fat and nonfat solids means that if someone consumes less milk fat by switching to skim milk, someone else will consume more milk fat, in the form of cream, butter, cheese, or other dairy products. The additional milk fat left over from skim milk production has value and will therefore not be thrown away by dairy product producers; it will be placed on the market for consumption in some form.

Estimates of supply response in the literature indicate that the dairy industry would take time to adjust production of milk fully to any sustained demand increase (e.g., see Chavas & Klemme, 1986; or Howard & Shumway, 1988). This implies that in the short run, dairy prices would change in response to a demand shift, muting the consumption response. But the extent of these effects would be mitigated by the extensive government intervention in the market and the role of international trade in the main manufactured dairy products.[25]

Combining an outward shift in demand for low-fat dairy products with a similarly sized inward shift in demand for high-fat dairy foods would imply changes in the overall product mix, perhaps with a change in the domestic versus international market allocation of products (to increase the amount of fat being exported), with unclear effects at the farm level. In this case, as with grains, international trade plays an important role in accommodating changes in domestic demand and consumption, muting any induced changes in prices and production of milk. However, even if the effects on the farm production of raw milk are not substantial, there might well be some significant effects on the relative prices of fat and nonfat solids as components of milk and thus of the relative prices of dairy products with higher and lower fat content: making more healthful (lower-fat) dairy foods more expensive and less healthful (higher-fat) dairy foods less expensive.

SWEETENERS　In terms of raw inputs, since about the mid 1990s caloric sweetener consumption in the United States has been divided roughly evenly between cane/beet sugar and high-fructose corn syrup (HFCS), which averaged 44% and 42%, respectively, of total caloric sweetener consumption between 1995 and 2006. The remaining 14% was composed of glucose and dextrose (also derived from

---

[25]Dairy farmers receive direct price support from the federal government. The Commodity Credit Corporation, an office of the US Department of Agriculture, purchases unlimited amounts of butter, nonfat dry milk, and cheese at announced prices, if the products are offered to it. Dairy product prices in most states are also affected by federal milk marketing orders, which set minimum milk prices according to end use and local market conditions. These regulations are in addition to federal export promotion through the Dairy Export Incentive Program, import restrictions, and state government interventions in dairy markets. In some cases, tracing the impact of these distortions on consumer prices is difficult.

corn), honey, and other edible syrups. The United States imported approximately 20% of the sugar available for consumption and processing in the United States in 2005, but imports are managed under a system of tariff-rate quotas. Although the United States is a large producer of HFCS, trade is a negligible component of the production and consumption of HFCS, with combined imports and exports averaging just under 4% of total domestic availability from 2000 to 2005 (US Department of Agriculture, 2006b).

The immediate impact of the proposed changes to the FSP would likely be a decrease in demand for sweeteners, with some corresponding decrease in prices for sweetened products. These lower prices could lead to higher consumption of sweetened products by households not participating in the FSP, while mitigating the drop in demand among households using food stamps. At the same time, they will induce responses by growers and processors, who have a number of options for adjusting in response to price changes resulting from any induced changes in demand for sweeteners; and these responses could be expected to limit the size and duration of the price changes.

Adjustments that could help growers and processors to accommodate the reduced demand for sweeteners include reduced US production of HFCS (produced from corn, which would readily be diverted to other uses such as feed grains and biofuels), reduced US imports of sugar (under tariff-rate quotas, which act essentially as import quotas), and reduced US production of sugar for human consumption (sugarcane and sugar beet can be used for other products, such as biofuels, and farm production of sugar can adjust as well). For growers, this adjustment period should be relatively short, given that corn, sugarcane, and sugar beets are annual crops. Processors may have greater difficulty making adjustments, especially with respect to HFCS; HFCS is by far the dominant product derived from the wet milling of corn. All this implies that modest changes in prices for sweeteners generated by the proposed reforms of the FSP might persist over the short to medium term of a few years.

FATS AND OILS   Although fats and oils are not referred to specifically in the suggested changes to the FSP, the revised list of allowable foods would presumably be designed to reflect the US dietary guidelines in this regard (i.e., that fats and oils should be consumed in moderation, and should emphasize polyunsaturated and monounsaturated fats, rather than saturated and trans fats).

Unsaturated fats are consumed largely in the form of vegetable oil, trans fats as shortening or margarine, and saturated fats as components of animal products such as meat and butter. The suggested changes to the FSP would probably cause participating households to substitute away from products like butter and shortening in favor of vegetable oils. The aggregate effect on vegetable oil consumption is not certain, however, and depends on the size of the substitution toward unsaturated fats compared with the decrease in overall consumption of fatty foods. Any price effects of increases in demand for vegetable oil could also be offset by falling demand for shortening; the latter uses vegetable oil as its primary input. In any case, the fact that the United States is a major exporter of oilseed products suggests that price impacts stemming from FSP reforms will be minimal (US Department of Agriculture, 2005a). Though short-run effects on the vegetable oil market could include price changes that would influence the behavior of FSP participants and nonparticipants alike, the inter-mediate- to long-run price effects would probably be small.

MEATS   Adoption of the revised list of foods that may be purchased using food stamps would encourage greater consumption of low-fat cuts of poultry, eggs, and lean cuts of red meat; fattier cuts of red meat would no longer be included on the list of allowable foods. These changes would cause shifts in demand implying higher prices for lean cuts of meat and eggs on the one hand, and lower prices for fatty cuts of beef and pork on the other, depending on the extent to which quantities could adjust to accommodate the increased demand. As is the case with the dairy industry analyzed earlier, adjustments in the supply of meats and poultry are affected by the biological lags inherent in changing the size and characteristics of a herd or a flock, which imply more pronounced price effects in the short run. In the case of poultry meat, exports are important, domestic production response is likely to be relatively rapid, and longer-run supply is comparatively elastic, so price effects would be muted. Trade is a minimal com-ponent of the egg market, so higher prices might persist a little longer, until the poultry industry has time to increase the size of the breeder flock, but not more than a few years (e.g., see Chavas & Johnson, 1982).

Likely impacts on the markets for beef and pork are more ambiguous because demand would increase for lean cuts while falling for fattier cuts—in this respect similar to the pattern for milk and dairy products. The dynamic nature of herd size adjustment implies that the beef and pork industries cannot immediately adjust to demand shocks by altering the total number of animals. In the case of pork, the United States is a significant exporter, with net exports of pork increas-ing fivefold since 2000 (US Department of Agriculture, 2006c). This increase implies that export markets could absorb much of an excess domestic supply in the event of a decrease in pork prices, and that exports could be redirected to the US market if demand were to increase.

In the case of beef, the price effects of changes to the FSP are less likely to be mitigated through international trade, partly because the trade is more com-plex—with border trade in cattle as well as beef, bilateral trade in different cat-egories of beef, and the United States acting as both a major exporter of higher-quality beef and a major importer of lower-quality beef. The bulk of US imports consist of grass-fed beef that is processed into hamburger. Greater imports could thus alleviate price increases for lean ground beef resulting from an increase in demand for lean beef, but less so for other lean beef products. For fattier cuts, the suggested changes to the FSP could generate decreases in prices that might not be eliminated by increases in exports.

Although beef exports from the United States have grown steadily since the 1980s, concerns over bovine spongiform encephalopathy (BSE) have led many countries to ban shipments of American beef (US Department of Agriculture, 2007b). In the short to medium run, then, lower prices for fattier beef would probably weaken the downward shift in demand among FSP participants, while stimulating demand among nonparticipants. In the long term, however, the industry would likely adjust its product mix and the balance of imports and exports to accommodate the changes in demand without very substantial impacts on relative prices, such that the second-round impacts of the policy, through induced price changes, would be muted.

FRUITS, NUTS, AND VEGETABLES   The proposed changes in the FSP would result in increases in demand for fresh and processed fruits, nuts, and vegetables, implying increases in demand for all commodities in this category. The United States is a large importer and exporter of most of these goods, partly reflecting their perishable nature and seasonal availability. Thus, the impacts of any outward shift in US demand will hinge in part on the response of foreign producers. Most fruits and vegetables are consumed in both fresh and processed (and thus storable) form, which may also mitigate price response to demand shocks. Most commodities in this broad category do not benefit from significant government support. One important exception is the orange industry, which is protected from import competition by barriers to imported orange juice.[26]

The nature of supply response differs very substantially for commodities within this category, between annual crops (most vegetables) and perennial crops (most fruits and nuts). Perennial crops have lags of several years between tree or vine planting and the realization of output, so the supply response to price in the short run is limited. In contrast to fruits and nuts, most vegetables are annual crops for which supply response will be far more flexible, although production will still be seasonal.

International trade mitigates price effects of changes in domestic demand, and in many cases eliminates them. However, the United States (or in some cases California) is responsible for a significant share of the global production for many specialty crops, and an increase in demand in the short run is likely to result in increases in both quantities consumed and prices for a long list of commodities such as table grapes, apples and pears, citrus fruits, dried plums, other stone fruit, strawberries, almonds, pistachios, walnuts, and avocados (results from studies of the returns to generic promotion have quantified these relationships, as documented in Kaiser et al., 2005). Different results may apply for tropical

---

[26]Alston and Pardey (2007) discuss the evolving patterns of productivity, prices, and production for US specialty crops. Alston (2007) discusses the pattern of government subsidies and policy-induced price distortions in US agricultural commodity markets, which are generally small for most commodities (notable exceptions are rice, sugar, cotton, and dairy products) and negligible for most fruits and vegetables.

fruits, such as bananas, papayas, mangoes, and pineapples, which are less extensively produced in the United States.

Some vegetables are well suited to a relatively quick adjustment to any demand shock brought about by reforming the FSP. Tomatoes, potatoes, and sweet corn comprise the largest share of vegetables consumed per capita by weight (Lucier et al., 2006); the vast majority of tomatoes and potatoes are grown under contract for food processors; all three crops are picked with mechanical harvesters; and all are suitable for cultivation under a wide variety of agronomic conditions. As a result, once farmer/processor contractual arrangements have been established, these crops can readily expand production if any reforms to the FSP result in increased demand.

For some vegetables grown for the fresh market, however, factors will work in concert to cause per-unit production costs to increase as area dedicated to particular vegetables increases, especially in the short run and especially for products that make intensive use of labor, and for those that require specialized equipment, specialized crop production knowledge, or (scarce) land with very specific agroecological conditions (e.g., LeStrange et al., 1996).

For example, crops like lettuce and asparagus must be picked by hand, greatly increasing harvesting costs vis-à-vis other vegetables. In addition, although land is available for increasing fresh vegetable production, no land that can be profitably cultivated in vegetable production zones is currently idle. Therefore, sustained increases in vegetable prices are required to make it profitable to bid land away from other uses and expand vegetable production. Moreover, competition for land *among* specific vegetables grown for the fresh market already exists, and this competition is particularly keen during the winter months, when the amount of suitable land for vegetable production is greatly reduced. Therefore, the proposed changes in the FSP will likely lead to sustained increases in per-unit production costs and consumer prices for *all* vegetables with these or similar production requirements.

Related previous work

Though no author has explicitly analyzed the potential supply response of the food industry if FSP participants changed their eating habits, Young and Kantor (1999) and Jetter, Chalfant, and Sumner (2006) estimated the adjustments that would have to be made by US agriculture if all Americans were to consume the amounts of fruits and vegetables prescribed by the federal government's dietary guidelines, and Johansson and colleagues (2006) estimated changes in US agricultural production and returns if Americans achieved healthier body weights.

Young and Kantor (1999) compared consumption data from the US Department of Agriculture with the *Dietary Guidelines for Americans*, and calculated the changes in output needed to meet the estimated shortfalls in consumption. Cropland adjustments were calculated from the average annual fruit and vegetable output over 1991 to 1995, divided by planted acreage, which yielded average productivity, and from the estimated shortfall in current production divided by this average productivity. The authors concluded that meeting the consumption increase necessary to fulfill the guidelines would require a 3- to 4-million-acre increase in cropland area planted with fruits, and a 2- to 3-million-acre increase in the area planted with vegetables. To put this number in national perspective, the US Department of Agriculture estimates that there were 442 million acres of harvested cropland in the US in 2002 (US Department of Agriculture, 2005b); meeting the dietary requirements of the population at large would require a relatively minor portion of total sown area in the United States, and an even smaller portion could meet the needs of the share of the population enrolled in the FSP. Young and Kantor did not estimate adjustments that would be needed for other inputs.

Jetter, Chalfant, and Sumner (2006), building on the results of Young and Kantor, estimated the adjustments that would be implied for US fruit and vegetable farmers under several different demand scenarios, for both land and labor. Jetter, Chalfant, and Sumner constructed an equilibrium displacement model of the agricultural economy wherein a market in equilibrium (i.e., equal supply and demand for all goods) was subjected to a shock in the form of an increase in demand for fruits and vegetables. Behavioral responses in the model were determined largely by supply and demand elasticities, which were gleaned from the literature. Supply elasticities were specified for annual and perennial crops, and demand elasticities were specific to different income groups. Jetter, Chalfant, and Sumner estimated that it would be sufficient to divert approximately 1% of the 218 million acres dedicated to field crops (such as alfalfa, rice, wheat, field corn, and cotton) to supply the increase in fruit and vegetable consumption if the entire US population adopted the dietary-guidelines recommendation of nine servings per day of fruits and vegetables (three to four fruit servings, and four to five vegetable servings). Despite the size of the demand increase in the nine-servings-a-day scenario, the adjustments needed in the allocation of planted cropland are not especially large.

Johannsson and colleagues (2006) estimate changes in production and returns to US agriculture if the American public were to achieve the "Healthy People 2010" goals outlined by the US Department of Health and Human Services. Two of the goals of this initiative are an increase in the percentage of Americans who are of healthy body weight to 60%, and a decrease in the share of the population that is obese to no more than 15%. Using a simulation model, the authors estimated the impacts on US agriculture of meeting these goals under two different scenarios: in one, decreases in body weight are achieved without adjusting activity levels; in the other, reduced consumption is combined with increased activity. Changes in prices and production were reported relative to baseline USDA forecasts for the year 2010, with the estimated losses to US agriculture ranging from 2.4% to 6.7% of net revenues. Simulated decreases in production were modest and concentrated among fattier products like meats and dairy products, whereas wheat and rice production increase; changes in fruit and vegetable production were not estimated. Given that the authors were computing the effects of a change in demand among all overweight Americans, analogous impacts due to reforms of the FSP would be much smaller. The results of Johannson et al. suggest that, if changing the list of commodities that may be purchased using food stamps results in significantly lower caloric intake among overweight and obese FSP participants, US agriculture is more than capable of adjusting to these changes in demand.

There is little doubt that the food industry can meet any swings in demand caused by reforming the FSP. The possibility remains, however, that short-run supplies for certain commodities are highly inelastic. As a result, we may see little initial increase in consumption of certain healthful foods following changes to the list of allowable foods, even if the proposed reforms generate the desired outward shift in demand. Therefore, if the reforms are implemented and do not appear to have much effect on FSP participant behavior in the short run, we should not necessarily conclude that they have failed. The full impact of the proposed changes should not be evaluated until agriculture and the other links in the food supply chain have had sufficient time to adjust production.

Middlemen, competition, and other factors

Though we can only speculate as to how long this adjustment will take, the food industry has shown a willingness to adapt to consumer demand for more healthful products. ConAgra has responded to greater demand for whole-grain products by introducing a new type of whole-wheat flour called Ultragrain that, when processed, has a taste and texture similar to more refined grain products (Buzby et al., 2005). Vegetable oil has virtually replaced solid saturated animal fats in American cooking, and reduced-fat milk now comprises the majority of milk purchased by American consumers; these changes would not have been possible if agriculture were unresponsive to consumer demand (Duxbury and Welch, 1999).

Agriculture and food processors have worked together to create innovations such as baby carrots, bagged salads, and fresh cut fruit (Duxbury & Welch, 1999; Lucier et al., 2006). Kentucky Fried Chicken, Taco Bell, and Starbucks have all announced that they will eliminate trans fats from their foods (Harris, 2007). The food industry may have played a role in promoting unhealthy eating habits, and it may sometimes act only in the face of intense public pressure. But it has also demonstrated that it is responsive to the demand for more healthful products; if there is money to be made by providing more healthful diets, profit-seeking firms will do their best to earn it. What is less certain is the timing of any supply response to changes in eating habits on the part of FSP participants.

Likely Nutrition Consequences of Proposed Changes to the FSP

Given the changes in food prices that are likely to be brought about by the proposed modifications to the FSP, and the implications of these changes for food purchases by the poor, what inferences can be drawn about the likely nutrition outcomes for low-income consumers? This section addresses the issue for FSP participants and eligible nonparticipants.

For at least some FSP participants, diet quality is expected to improve. Frequency of fruit and vegetable consumption will likely rise, and the overall caloric density of meals will likely decline. The result could be reductions in total caloric intake for FSP participants (the key factor in determining weight gain and obesity), and even small reductions in caloric intake sustained over time will reduce body weight. However, the effects of FSP changes on total caloric intake cannot be easily predicted, in part because even relatively small reallocations of expenditures (even for the poor) between nonfood and unhealthful food items would be sufficient to overcome the potential effects of likely improvements in diet quality on reducing total caloric intake.

For eligible nonparticipants the effects are somewhat easier to predict. In the short to medium term, this group will face increasing prices for most healthful foods and decreased prices for most unhealthful foods. Consequently, their diets will likely deteriorate in quality, and overall caloric density will likely increase; both of these responses will probably increase both weight gain and the incidence of obesity among the approximately 25 million poor who, for one reason or another, choose not to participate in the FSP program.

Furthermore, there is no *a priori* reason to believe that changing the list of foods that may be purchased using food stamps will increase participation in the FSP; the more likely outcome is that participation will decrease or remain unchanged. By restricting what may be purchased using food stamps, revising the list of allowable foods will necessarily restrict choices, while possibly increasing the costs of participation (e.g., through greater time spent figuring out what may be purchased using stamps). The FSP will become less appealing for current participants as well as potential future enrollees, and participation rates will either fall or stagnate as a result.

Therefore, although the aggregate effects cannot be precisely estimated now, there seems little reason to be optimistic. Diet quality among FSP participants (adults and children) may improve, and ultimately obesity may decline, if the new set of allowable foods is implemented. However, the number of FSP participants will likely decline because of new restrictions on allowable foods. Obesity among eligible *non*participants may eventually increase because the diet quality of the noneligible (i.e., the nonpoor) population may deteriorate as a consequence of changes in the relative prices of healthful and unhealthful foods, at least in the short term, although these effects are likely to be modest.

Regardless of the size of price effects, redesigning the list of allowable foods appears to be a poorly targeted intervention with respect to combating obesity among the poor. It ignores a large portion of those below the poverty line—that is, those who do not participate in the FSP—and it provides incentives that may swell the number of eligible nonparticipants. It restricts the choices of FSP participants, regardless of whether they are struggling with obesity. Finally, the administrative costs associated with implementing the revised FSP would probably be higher than those of the current FSP because of the monitoring and periodic updating of allowable foods that would be required in view of the many thousands of new food products introduced annually into the US food market. Although the magnitude of these costs cannot be estimated prior to implementation of the new policy, they will increase the share of the FSP budget allocated to administration at the expense of the benefits distributed to participating households.

Conclusion

This chapter began with an illustration of the differences in proportions of Americans who are obese or overweight according to age, ethnicity, sex, and poverty. These various correlates confound one another, such that inferring particular causal connections is not a straightforward matter. Nevertheless, it is clear that many of the poor are also obese, and increasingly so, so food policies directed at the poor may have implications for obesity that should be considered as part of the policy design. The particular policy considered in this chapter is the Food Stamp Program, which is earmarked for low-income households and has hitherto allowed participants to spend food stamps on foods that may have little nutritional value, apart from the provision of calories, and that have very likely contributed to decreases in diet quality and ultimately to increases in obesity among FSP participants.

The discussion of the Food Stamp Program and proposed FSP changes that would restrict the foods allowed to be purchased using food stamps to a shorter list of "healthful" foods included a look at the potential nutritional outcomes from dietary changes that could result from such a change. Key points from this discussion and analysis are that the FSP has been effective in increasing food expenditures and in reducing food insecurity among participant households, but the final effects on body weight have been difficult to identify. Moreover, little evidence is available for assessing the effects of changes in the types of allowable foods, because the guidelines for FSP foods have not changed radically in the past 40 years, but the number, types, and characteristics of available foods have changed dramatically during this same period of time. Finally, because the aggregate effects on *all* poor families are what interest policy makers, it is important to consider the effects of proposed changes to the FSP on the roughly 25 million eligible (i.e., poor) individuals (and households) who choose *not* to participate in the program, as well as the effects on the comparable number of individuals (and households) who do participate.

The theoretical analysis of consumer response to proposed changes in the FSP began with a conventional analysis showing how consumers may respond to food stamps compared with a cash grant worth the same amount of money. The same analysis is also relevant for food stamps applied to a revised list of allowable foods. In short, this model illustrates the following points:

- A consumer will enroll in the Food Stamp Program if the gross benefits from enhanced consumption exceed the costs of enrolling and participating.

- The gross benefits of participating will be less than the benefits of an equivalent cash grant if the consumption bundle is affected by the form of the subsidy (cash versus food stamps).

- The consumption bundle will not be affected by the form of the subsidy if the total value of consumption of the subsidized good (in this case, food) in the presence of the subsidy exceeds the total value of the subsidy (i.e., if the consumer is spending some of her own money on the subsidized good in the presence of the subsidy).

- Whether the form of the subsidy affects consumption choices will depend on the preferences of the consumer and other determinants of presubsidy consumption choices.

These predictions are borne out strongly by data for single-adult households, but they do not hold up as well for multiple-adult households.

The same kinds of implications follow with respect to a shift from the current FSP to a revised FSP emphasizing more healthful foods. Different consumers may be affected in different ways, depending on their costs of participation and the extent to which the constraint on the use of food stamps will influence their consumption choices. For poorer people, for whom food stamps may represent a large share of total food expenditures—especially those who are consuming a relatively large share of less healthful foods—the change in policy is more likely to affect consumption choices. Even so, the extent to which such changes will result in changes in consumption choices among FSP recipient households is uncertain.

Enrolling in the Food Stamp Program has both costs and benefits. Navigating the FSP bureaucracy is one of the costs of participation; receiving a food stamp allotment is the obvious benefit. Whether a consumer chooses to enroll in the Food Stamp Program depends on whether the additional utility is worth more to her than the additional costs of enrolling and participating, including any transaction costs and costs of stigmatization. Some consumers may find it uneconomic to enroll in the program; some may enroll and consume as though they had received an equivalent cash grant; others may enroll but consume more food than if they had received a cash grant. Regardless of how food expenditure decisions are made by the household, placing restrictions on food stamp purchases will make participation less appealing. As a result, a decline in participation rates seems likely, but it is difficult to predict the magnitude of this effect.

Combining the model of individual consumer choice based on prices, with a conceptual model of the aggregate market supply and demand for food commodities, in which prices are endogenous, showed that, to the extent that prices are affected by policy-induced shifts in demand patterns for FSP participants, the ultimate consumption choices of both participants and nonparticipants will be subject to second-round effects. Key determinants of the ultimate outcome include:

- **Size and direction of initial demand shifts.** The policy change will increase the demand for commodities used in production of the foods included on the revised FSP list and decrease the demand for all other food commodities.

- **Cross-commodity impacts in a multimarket structure.** Directly induced price changes resulting from the policy change induce shifts in supply or demand for other goods that are substitutes or complements in production or consumption, such that the ultimate outcome in terms of prices and quantities consumed involves a simultaneous multimarket equilibrium.

- **Elasticities of supply and demand, and length of run.** The outcomes are determined by elasticities that differ among commodities and that increase in size as more time is allowed for adjustments. There may be systematic differences in these elasticities between so-called "healthy" foods (especially California specialty crops) and "unhealthy" foods.

- **International trade.** To the extent that commodities are traded internationally, the effective supply in the US market is much more elastic than otherwise, implying a much smaller potential for price changes in response to changes in the FSP rules. Farm program policies in many industries involve interventions that mean that international prices are not fully transmitted to the domestic market and, as a result, the role of international trade is modified. Some of these policies themselves mean that prices paid by consumers or received by farmers are not responsive to shifts in domestic demand.

- **Role of food industry.** The food industry mediates between consumers and producers in ways that will tend to dampen the market response to policy-induced changes in demand by FSP participants.

An illustrative example indicated that the proposed change in FSP rules would be expected to result in some increases in consumption of "healthy" foods and decreases in consumption of "unhealthy" foods by some FSP participants; such improvements in diet quality could, eventually, lead to reductions in obesity. At the same time, however, the induced changes in prices would result in decreases in consumption of "healthy" foods and increases in consumption of "unhealthy" foods by other consumers. For all consumers, the extent of the unintended and undesired effects depends on the extent of the induced price changes.

Speculation about the consequent implications for nutritional outcomes for different groups, including the poor, identified the key determinants of these outcomes, but indications of the directions, let alone magnitudes of the effects on a number of important variables, are not yet clear.

This mixture of directions of effects and their uncertain magnitudes means that we cannot be certain of the overall consequences of the proposed change in terms of improving diet quality among the poor or others, or for other nutritional or social purposes that the FSP may be supposed to achieve. Predicting the effects on obesity trends is even more challenging, in part because of the likely long time lags between changes in diet quality and changes in body weights. This outcome reflects a fundamental problem with the concept.

An important lesson from economics is that, if policy has more than one objective, more than one policy instrument should be used. The Food Stamp Program was initially supposed to assist Americans who were too poor to feed themselves, and this is still a central purpose. It is probably unreasonable to use the same policy instrument to achieve a second objective: a healthful diet. Therefore, although a redesigned FSP may lead to more healthful diets and reductions in obesity for some FSP participants, in the aggregate the revised FSP alone is likely to be ineffective or inefficient, so complementary policy instruments will be required.

Finally, an array of complementary policies—for example, increased funding to promote the FSP, or increased spending on research on fresh fruits and vegetables to reduce the retail prices and enhance the quality of these products, or nutritional education programs—could make the redesigned FSP more effective. However, such policy options could be pursued independently of changes to the FSP, and hence should be evaluated on their own merits.

Technical Appendix:
A Simple Mathematical Model of Multimarket Implications of the Proposed Changes to the Food Stamp Program

An algebraic counterpart of the model represented in Figure 11.7 can be used to make the arguments more concrete and, if information on the key parameters can be obtained, to quantify the main effects. The equations of the model include supply and demand equations for each of the two categories of goods (healthful and less healthful foods). For the present purposes, it is of interest to disaggregate each demand into demand by FSP participants and demand by nonparticipants. Thus the model is given by the following equations:

$$H_f = h_f(P_h, P_u, A_f)$$
$$U_f = u_f(P_h, P_u, A_f)$$
$$H_n = h_n(P_h, P_u)$$
$$U_n = u_n(P_h, P_u)$$
$$H = h(P_h)$$
$$U = u(P_u)$$
$$H = H_f + H_n$$
$$U = U_f + U_n$$

(11.1)

where H and U denote the quantities of healthful and unhealthful foods, respectively; P_h and P_u denote the corresponding prices; subscripts f and n denote demand by FSP participants and nonparticipants, respectively; and A denotes demand shifters resulting from changes in the FSP rules (these demand shifters are included only in the market for participants, reflecting an implicit assumption, for now, that participation rates are not affected by the program rules). The first four equations represent the demands by participants and nonparticipants for healthful and unhealthful food, the next two equations represent the supply equations for healthful and unhealthful food, and the last two equations are market-clearing quantity identities.

Taking logarithmic differentials, the equations of the model can be expressed in terms of proportional changes and elasticities of supply and demand as follows:

$$d\ln H_f = \eta_{hh}^f d\ln P_h + \eta_{hu}^f d\ln P_u + \alpha_h$$

$$d\ln U_f = \eta_{uh}^n d\ln P_h + \eta_{uu}^f d\ln P_u + \alpha_u$$

$$d\ln H_n = \eta_{hh}^n d\ln P_h + \eta_{hu}^n d\ln P_u$$

$$d\ln H_n = \eta_{uh}^n d\ln P_h + \eta_{uu}^n d\ln P_u$$

$$d\ln H = \varepsilon_h d\ln P_h$$

$$d\ln U = \varepsilon_u d\ln P_u \tag{11.2}$$

$$d\ln H = \left(\frac{H_f}{H}\right) d\ln H_f + \left(1 - \frac{H_f}{H}\right) d\ln H_n$$

$$d\ln U = \left(\frac{U_f}{U}\right) d\ln H_f + \left(1 - \frac{U_f}{U}\right) d\ln H_n$$

These eight equations can be solved for the four quantities consumed, two quantities supplied, and two prices as functions of the two parameters representing the proportional shocks to demand generated by the changes in the FSP rules (α_h, α_u), the elasticities of supply $(\varepsilon_h, \varepsilon_u)$ and demand $(\eta_{hh}, \eta_{hu}, \eta_{uh}, \text{ and } \eta_{uu})$, and the initial consumption mix.

Assuming, for simplicity, that the elasticities of demand are identical between participants and nonparticipants, the solution for prices is this:

$$d\ln P_h = (\varepsilon_u - \eta_{uu})\left(\frac{H_f}{H}\right)\frac{\alpha_h}{D} + \eta_{hu}\left(\frac{U_f}{U}\right)\frac{\alpha_u}{D}$$

$$d\ln P_u = (\varepsilon_h - \eta_{hh})\left(\frac{U_f}{U}\right)\frac{\alpha_u}{D} + \eta_{uh}\left(\frac{H_f}{H}\right)\frac{\alpha_h}{D} \tag{11.3}$$

$$D = (\varepsilon_h - \eta_{hh})(\varepsilon_u - \eta_{uu}) - \eta_{hu}\eta_{uh}$$

Substitution of these results into equations (11.2) yields the corresponding quantities.

The solution to the model will be influenced by the fact that the two demand shift parameters, α_h and α_u, are not independent. In the extreme case where expenditure on food is constant, any increase in expenditure for "healthy" food must be offset by an equal corresponding decrease in expenditure on "unhealthy" food. This consequence of the budget constraint is reflected in the elasticities of demand. The implication is that $s_u \alpha_u = -(1-s_u)\alpha_h$, where s_u is the share of the FSP participants' budget that is spent on less healthful food. Substituting this result into equation (11.3) and eliminating α_u yields:

$$d \ln P_h = \left[(\varepsilon_u - \eta_{uu}) \left(\frac{H_f}{H} \right) \; \eta_{hu} \left(\frac{U_f}{U} \right) \left(\frac{1-s_u}{s_u} \right) \right] \frac{\alpha_h}{D}$$

$$d \ln P_u = -\left[(\varepsilon_h - \eta_{hh}) \left(\frac{U_f}{U} \right) \left(\frac{1-s_u}{s_u} \right) - \eta_{uh} \left(\frac{H_f}{H} \right) \right] \frac{\alpha_h}{D} \qquad (11.4)$$

$$D = (\varepsilon_h - \eta_{hh})(\varepsilon_u - \eta_{uu}) - \eta_{hu}\eta_{uh}$$

The law of demand states that changes in demand for a commodity and changes in its price are inversely related; e.g., demand for healthful food will decrease as its price increases. Thus, the own-price elasticities of demand will be negative numbers (i.e., $\eta_{hh} < 0$, $\eta_{uu} < 0$). Under most reasonable assumptions the cross-price elasticities will be positive numbers (i.e., $\eta_{hu} > 0$, $\eta_{uh} > 0$); for example, as the price of less healthful food increases, the demand for healthful food will increase as consumers substitute away from the more expensive foods. Further, conditions for market stability imply that $D > 0$. Therefore, as a result of the change in policy that causes FSP participants to switch toward more healthful food, the price of healthful food will certainly rise and the price of less healthful food will fall (i.e., $d \ln P_h > 0$ and $d \ln P_n < 0$) as long as the supply functions slope up (i.e., $0 < \varepsilon_h < \infty$; $0 < \varepsilon_u < \infty$). Substituting these results into the demand equations shows that FSP participants' consumption of healthful food will increase and their consumption of less healthful food will decrease, but the converse will be true for nonparticipants.

Further, applying particular values for the parameters implies the magnitudes of these changes in prices and consumption. Table 11.7 (see p. 364) contains a summary of model results for different values of the initial demand shock (α_h), the own-price elasticity of healthful food (η_{hh}), and the own-price elasticity of less healthful food (η_{uu}). Although the empirical literature on consumer and firm behavior contains a wide range of elasticity estimates, the values employed in Table 11.7 represent a range that can reasonably be expected to bracket the true parameter values for the model presented here.[27]

In each case, the initial increase in demand for healthful food among FSP participants is blunted by the resulting increase in prices. The degree to which this is true depends on the sensitivity of consumers to price changes, as represented by the own-price elasticities of demand, η_{hh} and η_{uu}. If other parameters are held constant, greater increases in consumption of healthful foods among FSP participants are associated with lowering the own-price elasticity of demand for healthful foods, or raising the own-price elasticity of demand for less healthful foods. For nonparticipating households, higher values of η_{hh} result in smaller decreases in the consumption of healthful foods following the initial demand shock, along with larger increases in the consumption of less healthful foods.

Acknowledgments

We acknowledge helpful assistance by Abigail Okrent and Grant Aaron. This project was supported by the National Research Initiative of the Cooperative State Research, Education and Extension Service, USDA, Grant #2006-55215-16720. We also gratefully acknowledge financial support from the University of California Agricultural Issues Center; the Center for Natural Resources Policy Analysis at the University of California, Davis; the USDA Economic Research Service, and the Giannini Foundation of Agricultural Economics. The opinions expressed in this paper are not necessarily those of the supporting agencies.

---

[27]For example, Durham and Eales (2006) surveyed the literature on demand for fresh fruits. The ranges of elasticity estimates they found were bounded by –1.32 and –0.21, with an average of –0.60. Huang and Lin (2000) estimate a comprehensive set of demand elasticities using data from the 1987–1988 Nationwide Food Consumption Survey. Barring a few exceptions, their results are in line with the range of elasticities employed in the model presented here.

Table 11.7
Sensitivity Analysis of the Multimarket Numerical Model

Parameter values			Price effects (% change)	
Elasticity of demand for healthful food (η_{hh})	Elasticity of demand for unhealthful food (η_{uu})	Initial demand shift (α_h)	Healthful food $(d \ln P_h)$	Unhealthful food $(d \ln P_u)$
−0.5	−0.5	1.0	0.25	−0.25
		5.0	1.25	−1.25
		10.0	2.50	−2.50
	−1.0	1.0	0.27	−0.18
		5.0	1.36	−0.91
		10.0	2.73	−1.82
	−1.5	1.0	0.29	−0.14
		5.0	1.43	−0.71
		10.0	2.86	−1.43
−1.0	−0.5	1.0	0.18	−0.27
		5.0	0.91	−1.36
		10.0	1.82	−2.73
	−1.0	1.0	0.20	−0.20
		5.0	1.00	−1.00
		10.0	2.00	−2.00
	−1.5	1.0	0.21	−0.16
		5.0	1.05	−0.79
		10.0	2.11	−1.58
−1.5	−0.5	1.0	0.14	−0.29
		5.0	0.71	−1.43
		10.0	1.43	−2.86
	−1.0	1.0	0.16	−0.21
		5.0	0.79	−1.05
		10.0	1.58	−2.11
	−1.5	1.0	0.17	−0.17
		5.0	0.83	−0.83
		10.0	1.67	−1.67

Note: These results were found by adjustment of the values of the parameters in equations (11.2) and (11.3). Other model parameters are held constant at the following values: $\varepsilon_u = 1.0$, $\varepsilon_h = 1.0$, $\eta_{hu} = 0.5$, $\eta_{uh} = 0.5$, $U_f = 0.5U$, $H_f = 0.5H$, $s_u = 0.5$.

Table 11.7
Continued

| Consumption effects (% change) | | | |
| Food stamp participants | | Nonparticipants | |
Healthful food ($d \ln H_f$)	Unhealthful food ($d \ln U_f$)	Healthful food ($d \ln H_n$)	Unhealthful food ($d \ln U_n$)
0.75	−0.75	−0.25	0.25
3.75	−3.75	−1.25	1.25
7.50	−7.50	−2.50	2.50
0.77	−0.68	−0.23	0.32
3.86	−3.41	−1.14	1.59
7.73	−6.82	−2.27	3.18
0.79	−0.64	−0.21	0.36
3.93	−3.21	−1.07	1.79
7.86	−6.43	−2.14	3.57
0.68	−0.77	−0.32	0.23
3.41	−3.86	−1.59	1.14
6.82	−7.73	−3.18	2.27
0.70	−0.70	−0.30	0.30
3.50	−3.50	−1.50	1.50
7.00	−7.00	−3.00	3.00
0.71	−0.66	−0.29	0.34
3.55	−3.29	−1.45	1.71
7.11	−6.58	−2.89	3.42
0.64	−0.79	−0.36	0.21
3.21	−3.93	−1.79	1.07
6.43	−7.86	−3.57	2.14
0.66	−0.71	−0.34	0.29
3.29	−3.55	−1.71	1.45
6.58	−7.11	−3.42	2.89
0.67	−0.67	−0.33	0.33
3.33	−3.33	−1.67	1.67
6.67	−6.67	−3.33	3.33

References Cited

Abbott, P. (1999). Agricultural Commodity Production and Trade: A Trade Economist's View on Filling U.S. Food Supply Gaps. *Food Policy, 24,* 181–195.

Alaimo, K., Olson, C. M., & Frongillo, E. A. (2001). Low Family Income and Food Insufficiency in Relation to Overweight in US Children: Is There a Paradox? *Archives of Pediatrics and Adolescent Medicine, 155,* 1161–1168.

Alexy, U., Sichert-Hellert, W., Kersting, M., & Schultze-Pawlitschko, V. (2004). Pattern of Long-term Fat Intake and BMI During Childhood and Adolescence: Results of the DONALD Study. *International Journal of Obesity Related Metabolic Disorders, 28,* 1203–1209.

Alston, J. M. (2007). Benefits and Beneficiaries from U.S. Farm Subsidies. In B. L. Gardner & D. A. Sumner (Eds.), *Agricultural Policy for 2007 Farm Bill and Beyond.* Retrieved on July 1, 2007 from http://www.aei.org/research/farmbill/publications/pageID.1476,projectID.28/default.asp

Alston, J. M., Balagtas, J. V., Brunke, H., & Sumner, D. A. (2006). Supply and Demand for Commodity Components: Implications of Free Trade versus the AUSFTA for the U.S. Dairy Industry. *Australian Journal of Agricultural and Resource Economics, 50,* 131–152.

Alston, J. M., Carman, H. F., Christian, J., Dorfman, J. H., Murua, J.-R., & Sexton, R. J. (1995). Optimal Reserve and Export Policies for the California Almond Industry: Theory, Econometrics and Simulations (Giannini Foundation Monograph Series no. 42). Oakland, CA: Giannini Foundation of Agricultural Economics.

Alston, J. M., & Pardey, P. G. (2007). *Public Funding for Research into Specialty Crops* (Staff Paper Series P07–09). Retrieved May 1, 2007, from University of Minnesota, Department of Applied Economics at: http://agecon.lib.umn.edu/cgi-bin/pdf_view.pl?paperid=26207&ftype=.pdf

Alston, J. M., Sumner, D. A., & Vosti, S. A. (2006). Are Agricultural Policies Making Us Fat? Likely Links between Agricultural Policies and Human Nutrition and Obesity, and Their Policy Implications.

Review of Agricultural Economics, 28, 313–322.

Balagtas, J. V., Huchinson, F. M., Krochta, J. M., & Sumner, D. A. (2003). Anticipating Market Effects of New Uses for Whey and Evaluating Returns to Research and Development. *Journal of Dairy Science, 86,* 1662–1672.

Barrett, A. (2006). *Characteristics of Food Stamp Households: Fiscal Year 2005* (USDA, FNS Report No. FSP-06-CHAR). Alexandria, VA: US Department of Agriculture, Food and Nutrition Service.

Bartfeld, J., & Dunifon, R. (2005). *State-Level Predictors of Food Insecurity and Hunger among Households with Children* (Contractor and Cooperator Report No. 13). Washington, DC: US Department of Agriculture, Food Assistance and Nutrition Program.

Besharov, D. J. (2002, December 1). We're Feeding the Poor as if They're Starving. *The Washington Post,* p. B1. Retrieved May 6, 2007, from http://www.welfareacademy.org/pubs/overfeedingthepoor.pdf

Blisard, N., Stewart, H., & Jolliffe, D. (2004). *Low-Income Households' Expenditures on Fruits and Vegetables* (Agricultural Economic Report Number 833). Washington, DC: US Department of Agriculture, Economic Research Service.

Bruenig, R., & Dasgupta, I. (2005). "Do Intrahousehold Effects Generate the Cash-Out Puzzle?" *American Journal of Agricultural Economics, 87,* 552–568.

Buzby, J., Farah, H., & Vocke, G. (2005). Will 2005 be the Year of Whole Grain? *Amber Waves, 3,* 14–17.

Cassells, J. M. (1933). The Nature of Statistical Supply Curves. *Journal of Farm Economics, 15,* 378–387.

Center on Hunger and Poverty. (2003). *The Paradox of Hunger and Obesity in America.* Waltham, MA: Brandeis University, Heller School for Social Policy and Management.

Chavas, J. P., & Johnson, S. R. (1982). Supply Dynamics: The Case of U.S. Broilers and Turkeys. *American Journal of Agricultural Economics, 64,* 558–563.

Chavas, J., & Klemme, R. M. (1986). Aggregate Milk Supply Response and Investment Behavior on U.S. Dairy Farms. *American Journal of Agricultural Economics, 68,* 55–66.

Cohen, B., Ohls, J., Andrews, M., Ponza, M., Moreno, L., Zambrowski, A. et al. (1999). *Food Stamp Participants' Food Security and Nutrient Availability*. Washington, DC: US Department of Agriculture, Food and Nutrition Service.

Cunnyngham, K. (2001). *Characteristics of Food Stamp Households: Fiscal year 2000* (USDA, FNS Report No. FSP-01-CHAR). Alexandria, VA: US Department of Agriculture, Food and Nutrition Service.

Cunnyngham, K. (2004). *Trends in Food Stamp Program Participation Rates, 1976–2002*. Retrieved August 8, 2006, from http://www.fns.usda.gov/oane/MENU/Published/FSP/FSPPartNational.htm

Currie, J., & Grogger, J. (2001). Explaining Recent Declines in Food Stamp Program Participation. In W. Gale & J. Rothenbert-Pack (Eds.), *Brookings-Wharton Papers on Urban Affairs 2001* (pp. 203–229). Washington, DC: Brookings Press.

Cutler, D., Glaeser, E., & Rosen, A. (2007). *Is the U.S Population Behaving Healthier?* (Working Paper 13013). National Bureau of Economic Research. Retrieved August 1, 2007, from http://www.nber.org/papers/w13013

Darmon, N., Briend, A., & Drewnowski, A. (2004). Energy-dense Diets are Associated with Lower Diet Costs: a Community Study of French Adults. *Public Health Nutrition, 7*, 21–27.

Devitt, A. A., & Mattes, R. D. (2004). Effects of Food Unit Size and Energy Density on Intake in Humans. *Appetite, 42*, 213–20.

Drewnowski A., Almiron-Roig, E., Marmonier, C., & Lluch, A. (2004). Dietary Energy Density and Body Weight: Is There a Relationship? *Nutrition Reviews, 62*, 403–413.

Durham, C., & Eales, J. (2006). *Demand Elasticities for Fresh Fruit at the Retail Level*. Retrieved September 5, 2006, from http://www.ftc.gov/be/seminardocs/061012DurhamEales.pdf.

Duxbury, J. M., & Welch, R. M. (1999). Agriculture and Dietary Guidelines. *Food Policy, 24*, 197–209.

Finkelstein, E. A., Fiebelkorn, I. C., & Wang, G. (2003). National Medical Spending Attributable to Overweight and Obesity: How Much, and Who's Paying? *Health Affairs, 22*, 219–226.

Fox, M. K., & Cole, N. (2004). *Nutrition and Health Characteristics of Low-Income Populations: Volume I, Food Stamp Program Participants and Non-participants* (Agriculture Information Bulletin Number 796). Washington, DC: US Department of Agriculture, Economic Research Service, Retrieved July 1, 2006, from http://www.ers.usda.gov/Publications/AIB796/

Fox, M. K., Hamilton, W., & Lin, B. (2004). *Effects of Food Assistance and Nutrition Programs on Nutrition and Health, Volume 4, Executive Summary of the Literature Review* (Food Assistance and Nutrition Research Report Number 19-4). Washington, DC: US Department of Agriculture, Economic Research Service.

Fraker, T. M. (1990). *The Effect of Food Stamps on Food Consumption: A Review of the Literature*. Washington, DC: Mathematica Policy Research, Inc.

French, B. C., & Matthews, J. (1971). A Supply Response Model for Perennial Crops. *American Journal of Agricultural Economics, 53*, 478–490.

Gibson, D. (2003). Food Stamp Program Participation is Positively Related to Obesity in Low Income Women. *Journal of Nutrition, 133*, 2117–2118.

Gibson, D. (2006). Long-Term Food Stamp Program Participation Is Positively Related to Simultaneous Overweight in Young Daughters and Obesity in Mothers. *Journal of Nutrition, 136*, 1081–1085.

Guthrie, J. F., Frazao, E., Andrews M., & Smallwood, D. (2007). Improving Food Choices—Can Food Stamps Do More? US Department of Agriculture, Economic Research Service, *Amber Waves, 5*, 22–28. Retrieved January 2, 2008, from http://www.ers.usda.gov/AmberWaves/April07/PDF/Improving.pdf

Hanson, K., Golan, E., Vogel, S., & Olmsted, J. (2002). *Tracing the Impact of Food Assistance Programs on Agriculture and Consumers* (Food Assistance and Nutrition Research Report Number 18). Retrieved July 20, 2007, from US Department of Agriculture, Economic Research Service Web site: http://www.ers.usda.gov/Publications/FANRR18

Harris, C. (2007, January 7). Good-bye, Trans Fats at Starbucks. *The Seattle Post-Intelligencer*. Retrieved February 28, 2007, from http://seattlepi.nwsource.com/business/298154_starbuckstransfat03.html

Herman, D. R., Harrison, G. G., Afifi, A. A., et al. (2008). Effect of a targeted subsidy on intake of fruits and vegetables among low-income women in the Special Supplemental Nutrition Program for Women, Infants, and Children. *American Journal of Public Health, 98,* 98–105.

Howard, W. H., & Shumway, C. R. (1988). Dynamic Adjustment in the U.S. Dairy Industry. *American Journal of Agricultural Economics, 70,* 837–847.

Huang, K., & Lin, B. (2000). *Estimation of Food Demand and Nutrient Elasticities from Household Survey Data* (Technical Bulletin Number 1887). Washington, DC: US Department of Agriculture, Economic Research Service.

Jetter, K. M., Chalfant, J. A., & Sumner, D. A. (2006). *Does 7 to 9 a day pay? The Economic Benefits to Fruit and Vegetable Industries Should People Consume the U.S. Department of Agriculture Recommendations.* Retrieved August 10, 2006, from the University of California at Davis, Agricultural Issues Center Web site: http://aic.ucdavis.edu/research1/F_&_V_ajae.pdf

Johansson, R. C., Mancino, L., & Cooper, J. (2006). The Big Picture: Obesity, Consumption, and Food Production. *Agribusiness, 22,* 491–503.

Johnson, G. L. (1956). Supply Functions-Some Facts and Notions. In E. O. Heady, H. G. Diesslin, H. R. Jensen, & G. L. Johnson (Eds.) *Agricultural Adjustment Problems in a Growing Economy.* Ames, IA: Iowa State University Press.

Jolliffe, D. (2006, August). *The Income Gradient and Distribution-Sensitive Measures of Overweight in the U.S.* Paper presented at the International Association of Agricultural Economists Conference, Gold Coast, Australia.

Kaiser, H., Alston, J., Crespi, J., & Sexton, R. (2004). *Commodity Promotion Programs in California, Economic Evaluation and Legal Issues.* New York: Peter Lang Publishing.

Kennedy, E. T., Ohls, J., Carlson, S., & Fleming, K. (1995). The Healthy Eating Index: Design and Applications. *Journal of the American Dietetic Association, 95,* 1103–1109.

Kral, T., & Rolls, B. (2004). Energy Density and Portion Size: Their Independent and Combined Effects on Energy Intake. *Physiology and Behavior, 82,* 131–138.

Kuchler, F., Golan, E., Variyam, J. N., & Crutchfield, S. R. (2005). Obesity Policy and the Law of Unintended Consequences. *Amber Waves, 3,* 28–33.

LeStrange, M., Mayberry, K. S., Koike, S. T., & Valencia, J. (1996). *Broccoli Production in California* (Division of Agriculture and Natural Resources, Publication 7211). Oakland, CA: University of California.

Lucier, G., S. Pollack, M. Ali, & A. Perez. (2006). *Fruit and Vegetable Backgrounder* (Outlook Report No. VGS-313-01). Washington, DC: US Department of Agriculture. Retrieved February 1, 2007, from the USDA Economic Research Service Web site: http://www.ers.usda.gov/Publications/vgs/apr06/VGS31301

Mancino, L., & Newman, C. (2007, May). *Who Has Time To Cook? How Family Resources Influence Food Preparation* (Economic Research Report No. 40). Washington, DC: US Department of Agriculture, Economic Research Service.

Mundlak, Y. (2001). Production and Supply. In B. L. Gardner and G. C. Rausser (eds.), *Handbook of Agricultural Economics, Vol. 1: Agricultural Production.* New York: North-Holland Elsevier.

National Health and Nutrition Examination Survey (NHANES). (2004).Table 70. *Overweight.* Table 69. *Overweight, obesity, and healthy weight among persons 20 years of age and over, according to sex, race, and Hispanic origin: United States, 1960–62, 1971–74, 1976–80, 1988–94, and 1999–2002.* Retrieved June 1, 2006, from National Center for Health Statistics, Center for Disease Control web site: www.cdc.gov/nchs/about/major/nhanes/datatblelink.htm

Ogden, C. L., Flegal, K. M., Carroll, M. D., & Johnson, C. L. (2006). Prevalence of Overweight and Obesity in the United States, 1999–2004. *Journal of the American Medical Association, 295,* 1549–1555.

Poikolainen, A. (2005). *Characteristics of Food Stamp Households: Fiscal Year 2004* (USDA, FNS Report No. FSP-05-CHAR). Washington, DC: US Department of Agriculture, Food and Nutrition Service.

Pronk, N., Tan, A., & O'Connor, P. (1999). Obesity, Fitness, Willingness to Communicate and Health Care Costs. *Medicine & Science in Sports & Exercise, 31,* 1535–1543.

Raebel, M., Malone, D., Conner, D., Xu, S., Porter, J., & Lanty, F. (2004). Health Services Use and Health Care Costs of Obese and Nonobese Individuals. *Archives of Internal Medicine, 164,* 2135-2140.

Rolls, B. J., Roe, L. S., Beach, A. M., & Kris-Etherton, P. M. (2005). Provision of Foods Differing in Energy Density Affects Long-Term Weight Loss. *Obesity Research, 13*, 1052–1060.

Sexton, R. J., & Zhang, M. (1996). A Model of Price Determination for Fresh Produce with Application to California Iceberg Lettuce. *American Journal of Agricultural Economics, 78*, 924–934.

Townsend, M. S. (2006). Obesity in Low Income Communities: Prevalence, Effects, a Place to Begin. *Journal of the American Dietetic Association, 106*, 34–37.

Townsend, M. S., Peerson, J., Love, B., Achterberg, C., & Murphy, S. P. (2001). Food Insecurity is Positively Related to Overweight in Women. *Journal of Nutrition, 131*, 1738–1745.

US Census Bureau. (2005). Current Population Survey and Annual Social and Economic Supplement.

US Department of Agriculture. (1996). *Nutrition and Food Security in the Food Stamp Program*. D. Hall & M. Stavrianos (Eds.). Alexandria, VA: US Department of Agriculture, Food and Consumer Services.

US Department of Agriculture. (2004). *Dairy: Trade*. Retrieved October 10, 2006, from Economic Research Service at: http://www.ers.usda.gov/Briefing/Dairy/Trade.htm

US Department of Agriculture. (2005a). *Soybeans and Oilcrops: Trade*. Retrieved November 1, 2006, from Economic Research Service at: http://www.ers.usda.gov/Briefing/SoybeansOilcrops/trade.htm

US Department of Agriculture. (2005b). *Land Use, Value, and Management: Major Uses of Land*. Retrieved November 1, 2006, from Economic Research Service at: http://www.ers.usda.gov/Briefing/LandUse/majorlandusechapter.htm

US Department of Agriculture. (2006a). *Rice Briefing Room*. Retrieved November 1, 2006, from Economic Research Service at: http://www.ers.usda.gov/Briefing/Rice

US Department of Agriculture. (2006b). *U.S. Consumption of Caloric Sweeteners: Table 49*. Retrieved November 1, 2006, from Economic Research Service at: http://www.ers.usda.gov/Briefing/Sugar/data.htm

US Department of Agriculture. (2006c). *Hogs: Trade*. Retrieved November 1, 2006, from Economic Research Service at: http://www.ers.usda.gov/Briefing/Hogs/Trade.htm

US Department of Agriculture. (2007a). *Food Stamp Program: A Short History of the Food Stamp Program*. Retrieved January 2, 2008 from Economic Research Service at: http://www.fns.usda.gov/fsp/rules/Legislation/history.htm

US Department of Agriculture. (2007b). *Cattle: Trade*. Retrieved March 1, 2007 from Economic Research Service at: http://www.ers.usda.gov/Briefing/Cattle/Trade.htm

Varian, H. (2005). *Intermediate Microeconomics: A Modern Approach*. New York: Norton.

Vocke, G., Allen, E. W., & Ali, M. (2005). Wheat Backgrounder (USDA. WHS-05k-01). Retrieved July 29, 2006, from Economic Research Service at: http://www.ers.usda.gov/publications/whs/dec05/whs05k01

ver Ploeg, M., Mancino, L., & Lin, B. (2006). Food Stamps and Obesity: Ironic Twist or Complex Puzzle? *Amber Waves, 4(1)*, 32–37.

Wilde, P., & Nord, M. (2005). The Effect of Food Stamps on Food Security: A Panel Data Approach. *Review of Agricultural Economics, 27*, 425–432.

Wohlgenant, M. K. (2001). Marketing Margins: Empirical Analysis. In B. L. Gardner & G. C. Rausser (Eds.), *The Handbook of Agricultural Economics* (Vol. 1B, chap. 16). Amsterdam: Elsevier.

Yao, M., McCrory, M. A., Ma, G., Tucker, K. L., Gao, S., Fuss, P., et al. (2003). Relative Influence of Diet and Physical Activity on Body Composition in Urban Chinese Adults. *American Journal of Clinical Nutrition, 77*, 1409–1416.

Young, C. E., & Kantor, L. S. (1999). *Moving Toward the Food Guide Pyramid: Implications for U.S. Agriculture* (USDA Economic Report No. 779). Retrieved August 5, 2006, from Economic Research Service at: http://www.ers.usda.gov/publications/aer779

Zhang, Q., & Wang, Y. (2004). Trends in the Association Between Obesity and Socioeconomic Status in U.S. Adults: 1971–2000. *Obesity Research, 12*, 1622–1632.

12 ENVIRONMENTAL FOOD MESSAGES AND CHILDHOOD OBESITY

Shauna Harrison, Darcy A. Thompson,
and Dina L. G. Borzekowski

Introduction

Although electronic and technological changes of the last few decades have proven advantageous in many regards (improved transportation, greater access to information about new products, new forms of entertainment, etc.), these developments have also conferred negative outcomes. Among them is the increased prevalence of overweight and obesity among US children and adolescents—a public health issue that is of great concern. Sedentary behavior, coupled with heightened, efficient, and targeted advertising; greater exposure to low-nutrient, high-density foods; and subsequent consumption of such foods, has increased the vulnerability of children and adolescents to obesity.

This chapter examines increased overweight and obesity among children and adolescents in relation to media use. The discussion begins with a look at overweight and obesity rates among youth and then turns to the various factors that contribute to these current rates. Next the theoretical structures and underlying mechanisms that identify the routes from media to diet-related outcomes are considered. Finally, current and potential interventions to mitigate the media's impact are discussed. In short, the discussion draws on and synthesizes information about the relationship(s) between media use and weight and determines how to alter the media's influence on increasing youth obesity rates.

Overweight and Obesity among Children and Adolescents

In the last three decades, overweight and obesity rates among US children (2–19 years of age) have tripled from about 5% in the late 1970s to almost 35% for boys and 32% for girls in 2005 (Ogden et al., 2006). Moreover, 18% of US boys and 16% of US girls are considered obese (BMI ≥ ninety-fifth percentile;

Ogden et al., 2006). The trend is disturbing because higher-than-average weight during childhood—in addition to having immediate physical, emotional, and social effects—strongly predicts the likelihood of adult obesity with its attendant increased morbidity and mortality, as well as social, emotional, and employment consequences (Must et al., 1992; Dietz, 1998; Maffeis & Tato, 2001).

Associated with observed increases in BMI are changing patterns in children's food and beverage consumption (St. Onge et al., 2003). Today children eat more processed fast foods and drink more sugary soft drinks than did generations past (St. Onge et al., 2003; Nielsen et al., 2002). Indeed, 75% of adolescents eat energy-dense, nutrition-poor meals at fast-food restaurants on a weekly basis (French et al., 2001). Because portion size and consumption have increased in the past few decades, these eating habits are associated with increased intake and storage of energy and fat (Nielsen & Popkin, 2003; French et al., 2001; Paeratakul et al., 2003). Children's diets exceed the recommended requirements of saturated fatty acids, trans fatty acids, sodium, and calories; but they are deficient in vitamin E, calcium, magnesium, potassium, and fiber, producing the paradox of chronic overweight and undernutrition (US Department of Health and Human Services & US Department of Agriculture, 2005).

This condition is exacerbated by contemporary lifestyles, in which children are more sedentary than in past generations. In general, today's children do not engage in physical activity on a regular basis. There is growing concern that time in front of screen media is displacing time that could be spent expending energy in physical play and exercise. Because an imbalance between caloric intake and energy expenditure leads to weight gain, poor food choices and increased sedentary behavior are key components of the obesity problem. Behaviors for both eating and physical activity take shape very early in life and are influenced by a multitude of factors, on an individual level as well as societal and environmental levels (Campbell et al., 2007; Dubois & Girard, 2006; Nader et al., 2006; Gable et al., 2007; Dubois et al, 2007; Kelder et al., 1994).

Contributing Factors

Considering an ecological perspective, the Institute of Medicine (IOM) recognizes that multiple spheres influence children's eating behaviors. On an individual level, contributing factors include biology (such as hunger, appetite, and satiety), sensory stimulation (taste, smell, and visual appearance of food), gastrointestinal signals, and chemical signals, as well as genetic factors (affecting either weight status or eating behaviors), developmental stages, psychological and psychosocial factors (e.g., food preferences, gender, concern about health and nutrition, nutrition knowledge, stress and depression, dieting and portion size), consumer socialization and behavior (e.g., requests made to parents, brand awareness), and lifestyle factors (e.g., time, convenience, and cost of food; McGinnis et al., 2006). Finally, there are macrosystem influences.

Several spheres affect the relationship between children's media use and food intake. Individual-level differences are striking. When two children are exposed to the same food commercial, one child may ignore the message while the other child immediately begins to nag his parents for the advertised product.

Family and neighborhood influences can affect the amount of media that a child engages in, as well as (un)nutritious food that a child consumes. For example, parental television preferences and habits directly influence a child's viewing patterns (St. Peters, 1991). The home environment, such as the number of televisions in the home, directly affects the access a child has to the media and therefore the number of hours viewed (Saelens et al., 2002). Family eating habits affect a child's consumption. Meals eaten in front of the television are associated with higher caloric intake and less fruit and vegetable intake (Coon et al., 2001).

The role of the neighborhood is also important. Parental perception of neighborhood safety is associated with TV viewing; the safer the neighborhood is, the less a child watches TV (Burdette & Whitaker, 2005). In addition, the wealthier a neighborhood is, the more likely a family is to have access to supermarkets that sell nutritious foods (Morland et al., 2002). In addition, families and communities differ with regard to physical activity. Some families and communities encourage their children to participate in physical activities after school; others roll in video equipment, exposing children to television and DVDs within the day care setting (Christakis et al., 2006).

On a broader, macrosystem level, national practices and policies affect media and food consumption by children. These represent the most distal sphere, but they have an important impact on the sociocultural, marketing, and economic systems that shape food production, distribution, and consumption (McGinnis et al., 2006). As we will describe later in this chapter, the amount and content of media are increasingly becoming areas of concern for policy makers at more macro levels.

Media Use by Children and Adolescents

Greater availability of different media technologies has increased both actual utilization time and exposure to previously inaccessible content. For example, in previous decades children grew up in households with just one television, which offered an average of just four channels and had no remote-control gadgets (Woodard, 2000). Today, US school-aged children and adolescents (8–18 years old) live in households that average 3.5 TVs, 2.9 VCR/DVD players, 2.1 video game consoles, 3.6 CD or tape players, 3.3 radios, and 1.5 computers (Roberts, et al., 2005). One-fourth of these children live in homes with five or more TVs, and eight in ten have either cable or satellite TV, with 55% having premium channels (Roberts et al., 2005).

Many media can be found in children's bedrooms. Slightly more than two-thirds (68%) of children have TVs in their bedrooms; 50% of children report personal ownership of a VCR/DVD player, another 50% say they have their own video game players, and 33% have their own computers. Even the youngest children have extensive media access; 36% of children younger than age 6 have TVs in their bedrooms (Rideout, Vandewater, & Wartella, 2003). Household and family organization have also been affected by media, including changes in spatial living (room arrangement with the TV as the central piece; Bryce & Leichter, 1983) to timing of daily events (bedtimes, mealtimes, homework periods, etc.) to better accommodate media utilization (Lull, 1990).

Given the essentially unlimited access to the mass media, it is hardly surprising that exposure amounts have increased dramatically. According to Roberts and colleagues (2005), the average 8- to 18-year-old spends about 6.5 hours per day using media. Video media (including broadcast and cable television, videocassettes, and DVDs) account for almost 4 hours; music (via radio, CDs, tapes, or MP3s) occupies about 1.75 hours; and non-school-related computer use and video game playing consume 60 and 50 minutes, respectively (Roberts et al., 2005). *Media multitasking* is a new term that describes typical media use by young people. About 26% of the time that young people use one medium, they are simultaneously using a second one (Roberts et al., 2005). For example, while a teenager is watching a television program, she may also be surfing the Internet for new music (Figure 12.1; Roberts et al., 2005). If media use is considered individually, exposure time is actually equivalent to about 8.5 hours a day (Rideout et al., 2003).

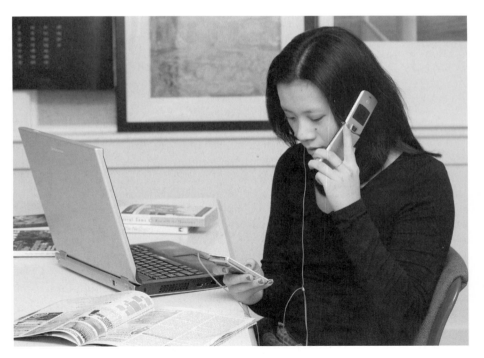

FIGURE 12.1 This typical teenager is using multiple media (textbooks, telephone, digital music player, computer, Internet, etc.) simultaneously.

Despite recommendations to the contrary, even very young children have high levels of media exposure. For many, media use starts during the very first year of life. Children under 1 year of age, on average, watch an hour of TV daily (Thompson & Christakis, 2005). For children under 6 years old, 92% watch TV, 88% screen videos and/or DVDs, 92% listen to music, and 48% use a computer (Rideout et al., 2003). These younger children average nearly 2 hours daily watching screen media, essentially the same amount of time they spend playing outside. The daily amount of time that children spend using screen media is almost three times the amount that they spend reading or being read to. Indeed, a remarkable number of very young children actively seek out media: 77% turn on the television themselves, 67% ask for particular shows, 62% use the remote control, and 71% ask for their favorite videos or DVDs (Rideout et al., 2003). In short, excessive media use begins at a young age and continues through childhood and adolescence. Moreover, as with other early experiences, these early viewing patterns strongly predict future media habits (Certain & Kahn, 2002).

The Marketing of Unhealthful Choices

Though media use statistics are stunning in their own right, particular concern has been raised regarding how access and use relate to increased prevalence of overweight and obesity in children. Various causal relationships have been explored, with recent attention focusing increasingly on the linkage(s) between media food messages and obesity (Hawkes, 2004; Hastings et al., 2003; Christakis, 2006; McGinnis et al., 2006; Koplan et al., 2005).

Marketing and advertisements are the most pervasive form of media messaging; industries spend billions of dollars promoting their products through multiple media channels. The US food industry is the second largest advertiser in the American economy, the first being the automotive industry. Approximately 12.5% of consumer spending goes toward food products, and repeat-purchase and brand loyalty greatly affect selection decisions (Gallo, 1999). In recent years children—teenagers especially—have become targets for advertisers because they often spend their own dollars and influence their household's food purchases. As future adult consumers, children are considered "consumers in training." It is estimated that adolescents spend annually about $140 billion of their own money, and children 12 years and under influence another $200 billion of household purchases (sometimes called "nag factor" or "pester power"; McNeal, 1998; Story & French, 2004; Strasburger, 2001).

A more stratified analysis of US food product advertising budgets shows that breakfast cereals account for $792 million, soft drinks $549 million, and snacks $330 million, respectively. Although these figures are for all advertising and not necessarily for advertisements geared at children, all of these products are frequently consumed by children (Gallo, 1999). As far as total expenditures on youth-focused media advertising go, exact figures are unknown, but estimates reach $1 billion (McNeal, 1998). In addition, other youth-focused promotions (premiums, sampling, coupons, contests, and sweepstakes) account for $4.5 billion in spending; targeted print and broadcast publicity, event marketing, and school relations account for another $2 billion; and $3 billion more is spent on specially designed packaging for children (McNeal, 1998). Message saturation through various channels is the most effective means of product promotion. Television represents the largest single source of media messaging for children about food, and food is actually the most frequently advertised product category on US children's television (Gallo, 1999; Gamble & Cotunga, 1999). With the amount of television that children watch, it is estimated that children may see one food-related commercial every 5 minutes, and up to 3 hours of food commercials per week (Kotz & Story, 1994).

Besides the obvious television food commercials, the food industry now increasingly uses product placement to promote its products. In one well-known example, Reese's Pieces were incorporated into the story line of the 1982 hit movie *E.T.* Especially in the new and popular genre of reality television, food products are common and are highlighted. In addition to television programming, product placement occurs in radio, music videos, comic strips, plays, and songs (Gupta & Gould, 1997). Individual companies spend anywhere from $50,000 to $100,000 for each such placement.

Children also see food branding and marketing on their toys. Toy manufacturers have teamed up with food companies to incorporate and promote brand awareness and preferences (Story & French, 2004). For instance, in addition to the small toys found in the McDonald's Happy Meals, parents can go online and purchase the McDonald's McKids Restaurant Play Tent (bearing the McDonald's logo) or the Coca-Cola version of the card game Uno.

The newest "branded environment" is the Internet. Web sites feature food products through "advergaming," where games, puzzles, contests, quizzes, and downloads have food product labels and logos. Consider the new and popular phenomenon of Neopets. First launched in 1999, the free Neopets Web site allows users (of which it has over 70 million) to become virtual pet owners. Users create and take care of Neopets; to do this, users earn "neopoints" by playing games or completing tasks, often through repeat visits to commercial Web sites and games. As an example, people can feed their Neopets by earning points playing a General Mills Cocoa Puffs word game.

Once separate from the consumer world, schools now deliver direct and indirect messages about food products and corporations. To increase sales, as well as foster product loyalty, advertisers see schoolchildren as captive, attentive audiences. Facing budget cuts and financial difficulties, the schools themselves are easily enticed by the potential extra dollars afforded to them through commercial activities (Consumers Union Education Services, 1995). In fact, the current fight against soda and snack machines in schools is resisted the most by school principals who need the funds to meet their budgets.

The commercial activities found within schools include product sales, direct advertising, indirect advertising, and market research. Reportedly, food sales (including soft-drink purchases and short-term fund-raising sales) are the most common form of commercial activity in school systems (US General Accounting Office, 2000). According to the 2000 School Health Policies and Programs Study (CDC, 2000), across the United States 43% of elementary, 74% of middle/junior high, and 98% of senior high schools offer students some opportunity to purchase branded foods or beverages (either vending machines or school stores; CDC, 2000). School fund-raisers provide another venue for branded products to enter the school environment. Some 82% of schools, through various organizations, teams, clubs, and associations, sell food products as a way to raise additional funds (CDC, 2000). Of these, 76% sell chocolate candy; 63%, nonchocolate candy; and 37%, soft drinks, sports drinks, or fruit drinks (CDC, 2000).

Direct advertisement is often seen via contracts between schools and food companies. Beverage companies contract with almost half of US schools to allow drink sales on school campuses. As part of this negotiated contract (usually done on a school district level), 92% of the schools receive a percentage of completed sales. Almost 38% of these schools permit product advertisements within school buildings and 28% on school grounds (CDC, 2000). Soft-drink and corporate names appear on school scoreboards, gym banners, textbook covers, and screen savers. Even school print and online media deliver advertisements and promotions for food products.

Indirect advertising includes corporate-sponsored educational materials. For example, corporations or specific trade associations may provide science or geography kits to middle or high school children. In addition, corporations may sponsor incentive programs that reward schoolchildren of elementary school age for reading. Without fail, these kits or programs prominently feature the corporation or association's name and/or logo.

Pathway to Consumption—From Television to the Stomach: A Causal Framework

To examine the relationship of media use to messaging and childhood obesity, it is necessary to identify the hypothesized causal framework and then consider its various components. As the IOM conceptualizes it, the relationship between marketing and the actual health outcomes of children can be best understood from an ecological perspective, under which there are many interactions between other influential factors in a child's physical, social, emotional, and economic environments (McGinnis et al., 2006).

Marketing—which can be defined as an "organizational function and a set of processes for creating, communicating, and delivering value to customers

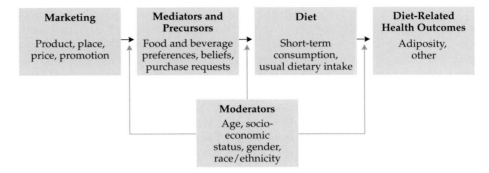

FIGURE 12.2 The causal framework used by the Institute of Medicine to organize the systematic evidence review that considers the relationship between children's media use and obesity. (From McGinnis et al., 2006; with permission from the National Academies Press, 2006, National Academy of Sciences.)

and for managing customer relationships in ways that benefit an organization and its stakeholders" (American Marketing Association, n.d.)—is hypothesized to have direct and indirect effects on diet and diet-related behavior in children. The IOM, after examining and synthesizing the evidence that addresses this relationship between media use and obesity, has organized the current research and its hypotheses by using the causal framework shown in Figure 12.2.

The framework includes marketing, mediators and precursors, diet, diet-related health outcomes, and moderators. *Marketing*, the first element identified in the framework, and thus the initiating factor, includes the four Ps of advertising: product, place, price, and promotion. Product has to do with what is being advertised, place is where it is being advertised, price concerns how much the item costs, and promotion is the way in which a product is advertised (McGinnis et al., 2006). Dietary *mediators and precursors*, the second element, include the factors that are directly influenced by marketing and that, subsequently, may affect diet. This category could include preferences for particular foods, requests made to parents as a result of marketing messages, and/or beliefs and perceptions about products (McGinnis et al, 2006). Marketing affects diet via these mediating influences.

The third element, *diet*, consists of the regular distribution and amount of food consumed. The IOM acknowledges that an individual's actual food consumption patterns and intake are most often measured as short-term patterns (e.g., the number of pieces of candy consumed in a day), which may or may not influence long-term outcomes (McGinnis et al., 2006). *Diet-related health outcomes* are the fourth element in the framework and could be measured in terms of body mass index, adiposity tissue, or various other conventional measures of overweight. Finally, *moderators* influence the causal pathway and alter outcomes; moderator variables include age, gender, socioeconomic status, and race or ethnicity (McGinnis et al., 2006).

Research on the Relationship between Media Use and Weight

Given the ubiquity of food messages in all the aforementioned environments, the next questions are, "what are the messages that children see?" and "what is the influence of these messages?" Through a range of methodologies, researchers are investigating the larger as well as the nuanced aspects of the relationship between food message exposure and childhood obesity.

In 2005, Harrison and Marske explored the types and nutritional content of foods advertised to children by analyzing the advertisements shown during the most popular television shows for viewers aged 6 to 11 years (as determined by Nielsen Media Research; Harrison & Marske, 2005). On average, 10.7 food advertisements were shown hourly, and the majority of advertised foods were of low nutritional value. There was an unequal distribution of food types for the general audience and child-audience advertisements, with the categories of "candy/sweets/soft drinks" and "convenience foods" the two most frequently advertised for child audiences (44% and 34% of advertisements, respectively; Harrison & Marske, 2005). At the same time, foods of high nutritional value were practically invisible: 2% of the advertisements were for fruits and/or vegetables; 2% for meats, poultry, or fish; and 4% for dairy products (Harrison & Marske, 2005).

Food advertisements emphasize taste over nutritional content; hardly ever is there mention of health or the value of eating healthful foods in the majority of these advertisements. About 90% of advertisements lacked health-related messages; in the few that said something related to health, the message concerned the fact that the product was made with natural ingredients (Harrison & Marske, 2005). Note also that almost 60% of the advertised foods were consumed as snacks—greater than the percentages of advertised foods consumed for breakfast, lunch, and dinner combined.

Foods typically found in commercials directed at child audiences were especially high in sugar. If an individual consumed a 2000-kilocalorie-per-day diet consisting of the foods portrayed in the child-audience advertisements, the recommended daily allowance (RDA) for fiber, vitamin A, calcium, and iron would be insufficient, and the individual would consume 2547 milligrams of sodium (106% of the RDA) and 171 grams (684 kilocalories) of sugar. Foods advertised to child audiences contained on average 34% of their calories in sugar—well above recommended levels. In addition, the advertised general-audience foods on average contained 1.3 times the recommended daily value (RDV) of fat intake (Table 12.1). Consuming a diet of primarily advertised food products would lead to severely malnourished yet overweight children (Harrison & Marske, 2005).

The extent of food advertising and the content of the food advertised during television programming geared toward toddlers and preschool children has been recently demonstrated by Connor (2006), who analyzed early-weekday-morning programming of three child-oriented television stations (PBS, Disney,

Table 12.1

The Nutrients and Percentages of Recommended Daily Values for a 2000-Calorie-a-Day Diet, Considering Advertised Foods

Nutrient (measure)	All advertisements		General-audience advertisements		Child-audience advertisements		t-test	p
	Amount	RDV (%)	Amount	RDV (%)	Amount	RDV (%)		
Total fat (g)	79	122	87	134	63	97	−3.64	0.001
Saturated fat (g)	26	131	26	130	18	90	−5.09	0.001
Cholesterol (mg)	157	52	199	66	90	30	−5.84	0.001
Sodium (mg)	3197	133	3576	149	2547	106	−3.96	0.001
Carbohydrate (g)	245	82	208	69	305	102	8.98	0.001
Fiber (g)	9	36	9	36	9	36	−0.81	0.49
Sugars (g)	114	—	78	—	171	—	10.11	0.001
Protein (g)	61	—	78	—	45	—	−6.05	0.001
Vitamin A	—	78	—	104	—	36	−4.85	0.001
Vitamin C	—	78	—	69	—	99	2.29	0.02
Calcium	—	78	—	87	—	63	−2.01	0.03
Iron	—	61	—	61	—	63	0.16	0.71

Source: After Harrison and Marske, 2005, with permission from the American Public Health Association.

Note: RDV = recommended daily value. Percentages are rounded and presented in whole numbers to reflect the format used on the nutrition facts label.

and Nickelodeon). The stations used different approaches, with 60% of PBS's advertising for food products or companies—compared to 35% of Disney and 21% of Nickelodeon's advertisements (Connor, 2006). On average, 1.3 food advertisements were shown per half hour. Fast foods dominated the food-related advertisements (100% for Disney, 59% for PBS, and 46% for Nickelodeon; Connor, 2006).

Various techniques and strategies are used by marketers to capture young viewers' attention. The majority of advertisements try to associate the food product with an entertaining message; 82% of child-oriented food advertisements convey a "fun" message, followed by 43% that tell an "action" story. Focus on "taste" appears in only 25% of the advertisements. Fast-food advertisers rely heavily on their licensed characters (e.g., Ronald McDonald, Chuck E. Cheese) and animation. Rarely does the food product actually appear in child-oriented food advertisements. In fact, less than half of all food messages and only 20% of the fast-food advertisements actually showed their food products (Connor, 2006). Quite intentionally, marketers promote the emotional and social benefits that presumably accrue when the food product is purchased and consumed.

International studies offer similar findings. A 2005 New Zealand study examined 155 hours of children's television and then compared the findings to earlier national data from 1997 and Australian data from 2002. Hourly food advertisements had increased from 8 to almost 13, and the percentage of all food advertisements had increased to 42% in 2005, from 29% in 1997 (Wilson et al., 2005). Indeed, 70% of food advertisements were for foods considered to be "counter to improved nutrition," and only 5% were for foods "favoring improved nutrition" (Wilson et al., 2005). In addition, the hour immediately after school (3:30–4:30 PM) had more advertisements for high-fat/sugar-rich snack foods than did the later times (4:30–6:30 PM). Given the observed density and the total amount, researchers postulated that from ages 3 to 16, children would be exposed to an astonishing 113,000 food advertisements (Wilson et al., 2005).

A recent Turkish study analyzed the advertisements appearing with children's television programming and, through survey research, assessed children's food consumption during television watching and their purchasing requests while grocery shopping. During the weekend morning hours, children saw approximately 35 minutes of advertisements (for a yearly total of 1890 minutes) including about 350 food advertisements per weekend (close to 19,000 per year). Almost 45% of the advertisements were food-related, with 28% for candy/chocolate, 24% for chips, 13% for milk products, and 12% for breakfast cereals (Arnas, 2004).

In addition, the children in this sample (ages 3–8 years) averaged 19 hours per week watching television (about 143 minutes per weekday and 202 minutes per weekend day; Arnas, 2004). Almost 90% ate a snack while watching TV, and over a third of the preferred food items were considered unhealthful—for example, soft drinks, chips, chocolate, and candy (Arnas, 2004). Younger children were more likely to pay attention to the advertisements and request advertised products, compared to older children. Requests aligned with featured items; the most common requests were for candy/chocolate (59%), ice cream (51%), biscuits/cakes (37%), fruit juice (36%), soda (34%), and milk products (27%; Arnas, 2004).

Research drawn from experimental studies suggests that it may take only one or two exposures to short commercials (10–30 seconds each) to influence children's food preferences (Borzekowski & Robinson, 2001). Such short-term impact was observed in a randomized controlled experiment done with 2- to 6-year-olds in northern California. Children in this study were randomized to view a cartoon video with or without embedded commercials, after which they were asked to identify their preferences for products. Children who viewed the video with advertisements were much more likely to select the advertised products than were children in the control group. This ability to entice children to choose products after such short exposure affords great power to marketing companies to affect young viewers. Experimental research also shows a dose–response effect to commercials. Seeing a commercial twice compared to just once resulted in greater preference for a product (Borzekowski & Robinson, 2001). With just a small number of exceptions, advertisements are repeated multiple times, even appearing several times during a single broadcast. Given the amount of television that children regularly watch, the influence of repeated commercials is presumed to be high.

Correlational Data: The Association between Media Use and Obesity

Conscious of the amount and content of media that children watch, several studies have examined the associations of media exposure, diet, and diet-related outcomes. The latter refers to the causal pathway discussed earlier. These correlational data may help us understand how food messages in the media relate to diet choice and to subsequent ingestion and obesity.

The relationship between television viewing and total energy intake was investigated by Wiecha and colleagues (2006), who found that even modest increases of television viewing were associated with an average daily energy increase of 167 calories. This additional caloric intake was attained through increased consumption of "foods commonly advertised on television" (Wiecha et al., 2006). Thus, the media influence both specific consumption patterns and, consequently, total caloric intake. Regression analysis showed a reliable positive relationship between airtime dedicated to commonly advertised foods (identified as baked sweet snacks, candy, fast-food main courses, fried potatoes, salty snacks, and sugar-sweetened beverages) and change in energy intake. Thus, television viewing can powerfully affect the selection of food products and caloric consumption, both of which contribute to overweight and obesity among children.

Individuals who view a lot of TV show decreased consumption of healthful foods in addition to increased consumption of unhealthful foods. Boynton-Jarrett and colleagues (2003) examined the association between increased television viewing and negative health behaviors, focusing on children's intake of healthful foods (fruits and vegetables; Boynton-Jarrett et al., 2003). From baseline data collected in the fall of 1995, they found a decrease of 0.16 serving per day in fruits and vegetables for every hour increase of television watched per day. The follow-up data collected in the spring of 1997 showed an additional decrease of 0.14 serving per day of fruits and vegetables for every additional hour increase in television viewing (even after adjustment for anthropometric, demographic, baseline dietary variables, and physical activity; Boynton-Jarrett et al., 2003).

On average, children watching 3 hours per day of television or more consumed 2.25 fewer fruits and vegetables per week compared to those who watched minimal amounts of television (Boynton-Jarrett et al., 2003). This finding is noteworthy, given that the children in this study on average did not consume the recommended five fruit and vegetable servings per day (the average was 4.23 servings per day). With few positive messages featuring fruits and vegetables, the intense marketing of unhealthful food products is a leading candidate for children's misconceptions about which foods are nutritious and should be consumed (Harrison, 2005; Connor, 2006; Wilson et al., 2005; Arnas, 2004; Boynton-Jarrett et al., 2003).

In addition, TV viewing has been found to be associated with the diet-related outcomes of overweight and obesity. In a well-designed study, Dietz and Gortmaker (1985) suggested a causal relationship between television viewing and overweight/obesity. Children (ages 6–11 years) and adolescents (ages 12–17 years) who watched more television had a greater prevalence of obesity and superobesity (defined as triceps skinfolds $\geq 85^{th}$ percentile for obesity, and $\geq 95^{th}$ percentile for superobesity) than did other children ($p < 0.05$). Evaluating two cycles of the National Health Examination Survey (NHES), the prevalence of obesity increased by 1.2% to 2.9%, and the prevalence of superobesity increased by 1.2% to 1.4% for each additional hour of TV viewed, suggesting a dose–response relationship.

Studying the mechanisms thought to explain the association of television viewing and obesity among children, researchers have examined consumption patterns during television viewing. An ethnically diverse sample of children consumed food most often during television viewing (including watching shows, movies, videotapes) than during any of the other specified time or activity (Matheson et al., 2004). Notably, the weekday and weekend consumption patterns were different. On weekdays, about a fifth of total energy was taken in with the television on, and on weekend days that proportion increased to more than a fourth of total energy intake (Matheson et al., 2004).

Children ate snacks more often during weekday than during weekend television viewing. Not surprising for a sample of school-aged children, there was a significant increase in both breakfast and lunch consumption during television viewing on the weekends compared to weekdays (Matheson et al., 2004). These researchers also found significant decreases in vegetable consumption during television viewing versus other times and activities (Matheson et al., 2004). Finally, among the younger schoolchildren, researchers observed a significant correlation between body mass index and percentage of energy from fat consumed during television viewing (Matheson et al., 2004).

Also examining consumption during TV viewing, Blass and colleagues used a within-subjects design to evaluate, among undergraduate students, the consumption of two high-density foods (pizza, and macaroni and cheese) during a 30-minute TV viewing session. They found that those viewing TV consumed 36% more calories of pizza and 71% more calories of macaroni and cheese in comparison to those listening to classical music. Eating patterns also varied: those viewing TV took seconds of pizza more quickly and ate macaroni and cheese faster (Blass et al., 2006).

Theories that Help Explain the Relationship between Media Use and Obesity

Several theories—notably Bandura's *social cognitive theory* (Bandura 1977, 1986, 2001, Glanz et al., 2002), Fishbein and Ajzen's *theory of planned behavior* (Glanz et al., 2002; Ajzen, 1991) and Gerbner's *cultivation theory*—help explain the framework and causal pathway dynamics between media use and obesity (Hammer-meister et al., 2005; Signorielli & Stapes, 1997).

Bandura's social cognitive theory asserts that the individual, the environment, and one's behavior continuously interact and influence each other bi-directionally—a concept known as *reciprocal determinism* (Bandura, 1977; Glanz et al., 2002). A primary construct of social cognitive theory is self-efficacy; to change behavior, individuals must have confidence that they can engage successfully in a given behavior (Glanz et al., 2002).

Also central to social cognitive theory is the concept of *modeling*. Individuals can learn from observing others (either in person or through screen media), noting the ways people behave and the rewards and punishments they receive (Bandura 1986, 2001). In a direct pathway, a communication system such as television can "promote changes by informing, enabling, motivating and guiding" individuals; in an indirect pathway (or a socially mediated pathway), the influences of mass media "link [individuals] to social networks and community settings" (Bandura, 2001, p.285). This provides natural incentives and personalized guidance for desired change (Bandura, 2001). In addition, social cognitive theory suggests that humans' unique capability for symbolization helps drive comprehension of the environment (Bandura, 2001). This "symbolizing capability" combines with one's "self-regulatory capability," which posits that self-regulation of motivation and action involves both proactive control and reactive control. Media offer a rich symbolic environment, and people turn to and make sense of this environment through vicarious experiences.

To understand the impact of the media, according to Bandura, one must consider the following four processes (Robinson & Borzekowski, 2006):

1. **Attentional processes**—factors that determine what an individual observes, including cognitive skills, preconceptions, value preferences, salience, and attractiveness.

2. **Cognitive representational processes**, involving retention, recall, and reconstruction.

3. **Behavioral production processes**—translating conceptions into action.

4. **Motivational processes**, consisting of direct, vicarious, and self-produced motivators.

These processes serve as determinants of diffusion and, thus Bandura sees media's influence as a "dual link" (operating on behavior directly, as well as through the social norms connection; Bandura, 2001).

Fishbein and Ajzen's theory of planned behavior (TPB; discussed in Chapter 8) states that the most important determinant of behavior is one's intention to do a behavior—that is, whether it is likely that he or she plans to engage in the behavior. Intention is affected by one's attitudes, subjective norms, and perceived behavioral control regarding the behavior (Glanz et al., 2002; Ajzen, 1991). Attitudes toward a behavior are shaped by "behavioral beliefs" and "evaluations of behavioral outcomes," subjective norms by "normative beliefs" and "motivation to comply" and perceived behavioral control by "control beliefs" and "perceived power" (Glanz et al., 2002). This latter construct of perceived behavioral control is what distinguishes the theory of planned behavior from the theory of reasoned action (TRA), the earlier model proposed by Fishbein and Ajzen (see Chapter 8). TPB accounts for one's perception of the environmental factors affecting the individual's ability to accomplish the behavior (Glanz et al., 2002). Perceived behavioral control is particularly pertinent in discussions of children and their diets because children often lack control of their environment or their choices.

Finally, Gerbner's cultivation theory suggests that media use is powerful and can alter one's perception of reality and, subsequently, one's actions. This theory can explain gradual, long-term shifts among different generations (Signorielli & Staples, 1997). Gerbner and colleagues found that heavy television viewing leads individuals to believe that the televised world is real; with greater media exposure comes greater concordance between constructed realities and individuals' perceived realities (Gerbner et al., 1994).

Cultivation analysis uses two approaches to examine the images, portrayals, and values presented in media and then looks at the way viewers perceive the messages, in comparison to their real-world experience. The first approach is *message system analysis,* which monitors the messages conveyed through media, including the under- and overrepresentations of gender, age, ethnicity, and occupation of the characters portrayed on television (Glanz et al., 2002). The second approach involves understanding the constructs of *mainstreaming* and *resonance.* *Mainstreaming* is the process by which heavy exposure cultivates common beliefs among viewers that resemble what they see in the media. *Resonance* occurs when viewers' reality may, in fact, be similar to what they see on television, thus amplifying the cultivation effect.

Cultivation theorists divide audiences into "light viewers" and "heavy viewers" according to how much they see media in a given day or week. Besides media exposure levels, these groups differ demographically and socially (including variables such as gender, income, education, occupation, race, time use, and social isolation or integration; Gerbner et al., 1994). Signorielli and Staples (1997) assert that viewing patterns begin in childhood (often before the child learns to walk or talk) and that patterns are modeled after parents. Interestingly, many children (regardless of their media exposure levels) look like "heavy viewers" because much of the information that children receive about the world comes not from their own experiences, but rather from the world portrayed on television (Signorell & Staples, 1997). Children receive a tremendous amount of food information through media advertising and programs. The contrived reality regarding food and eating is not healthy and can contribute to problems of overweight and obesity among children.

The three theories—social cognitive theory, theory of planned behavior, and cultivation theory—are useful in understanding why a relationship exists between media use and obesity. Besides helping to clarify the relationship, these theories can assist in altering the negative impact of media use. In fact, researchers and educators can turn to these theories to design and evaluate interventions that affect media use habits and improve the eating habits of children and adolescents.[1]

Interventions: How and Where Can We Alter the Trajectory?

Given the proposed pathway, growing evidence, and explanatory theories, how can we alter the problematic relationship between exposure to food messages and obesity among children? One obvious intervention is to decrease children's media use. More than 5 years ago, the American Academy of Pediatrics (AAP) formally recommended that children older than 2 years spend no more than 1 to 2 hours per day with screen media (American Academy of Pediatrics, 2001).

Dennison, Russo, Burdick, and Jenkins (2004) designed and evaluated a randomized control trial to reduce viewing time among New York preschoolers. Through interactive educational sessions in the child care setting, the intervention, which occurred over 39 weeks, provided materials and activities to foster discussion between parents and children at home. Activities included coming up with alternatives to television viewing, teaching social skills by turning off the TV during mealtime, and making "no TV" signs (Dennison et al., 2004).

At baseline, both the intervention and the control groups were similar in the number of hours per week of television that they watched: 12.8 and 13.5, respectively. After the intervention, there were significant differences in viewing patterns for weekday and Sunday viewing. Those in the intervention group decreased viewing, on average, 3.1 hours per week; those in the control had an average increase of 1.6 hours per week (Dennison et al., 2004). Saturday viewing differed, but not significantly. Growth did not differ significantly, although the intervention group (but not the control group) showed a decreased-BMI trend (Dennison et al., 2004).

Considering the AAP recommendation that pediatricians and other health care providers encourage parents to reduce their children's media use time, researchers conducted a small pilot study to examine whether an intervention delivered through primary-care facilities can reduce media use among low-income, minority children. The control group received a brief counseling session and AAP brochures about the problems associated with excessive media use; the intervention group received control group materials and a behavioral exercise. This exercise consisted of parents and children discussing the children's current media use and then creating a "media budget" (Ford et al., 2002). The intervention group also received an electronic time manager to help them mon-

---

[1]Described here are some of the more commonly used theories and models on which health communication studies draw. Well-regarded research and intervention work tends to be more theoretically based.

itor and control the media budget (Ford et al., 2002). Those in the intervention group reported decreases in television use and increases in some types of physical activity. Because this was a small pilot study, the researchers suggest further investigations to assess the potential effects of interventions delivered through health care settings.

Another intervention worked with elementary school children within the school setting (Robinson & Borzekowski, 2006). In this study, media use was reduced either nonselectively (regardless of content or context) or selectively (with regard to content or context). Nonselective strategies included budgeting viewing time and limiting physical access; selective strategies included limiting viewing time to certain hours or days, limiting content, and limiting viewing to particular circumstances. The curriculum, based on Bandura's social cognitive theory, consisted of 18 sessions with the following goals and lessons (Robinson & Borzekowski, 2006):

1. **Raising TV awareness**, to increase the awareness of roles of television, videotapes, and video games in the children's lives; inform the children of consequences of overuse; and promote positive attitudes about reducing viewing time.

2. **Turning off the TV**, to learn strategies, invent and practice skills, experience positive outcomes, and gain mastery in reducing television, videotape, and video game usage.

3. **Staying in control**, to learn additional skills, enhance perceived self-efficacy regarding these skills, and maintain motivation to reduce usage of the aforementioned media.

The control group had no new activities introduced except for the study assessments. Results showed significant reduction in weekday television viewing (from 1.8 to 1.1 hours per day on average) and in weekday and Saturday video game playing (from 0.3 to 0.2 hour per day and from 0.6 to 0.3 hour per day, respectively) for the intervention group compared to the control group. In addition, researchers observed significant differences in the reduction of television viewing for household members in the intervention versus the control group. In the intervention group, for example, mothers or female guardians watched an average of 10.5 hours per week at baseline and 8.8 hours per week after intervention. Boys in general, children who spent little time unsupervised by an adult, and children who watched more television at baseline were all found to respond more to the intervention and were, therefore, deemed moderators (Robinson & Borzekowski, 2006). This intervention was very effective not only for the schoolchildren, but also for their respective households—and this extended effect may be attributed to the strong theoretical framework shaping the intervention curriculum. Children were also afforded the ability to take control of their own media use. These foundations may inform future interventions for reducing children's media use.

Finally, a randomized, controlled school-based trial by Robinson (1999) from September 1996 to April 1997 evaluated the effects of TV, video, and video game reduction on BMI, physical activity, and dietary intake in third- and fourth-graders. Children in the intervention group participated in an 18-lesson, 6-month, in-school curriculum aimed at reducing television, videotape, and video game use. The intervention was based on Bandura's social cognitive theory and was taught by schoolteachers trained by research staff. Lessons included self-monitoring and self-reporting of use, followed by a TV turnoff period, followed by a TV budget period. Newsletters were used to motivate parents to help their children.

Results showed that the intervention group significantly decreased their TV viewing compared to controls, reducing viewing by about a third from baseline. Robinson also found a relative decrease in the BMI for children in the intervention group (from 18.38 to 18.67 kg/m^2) versus the control group (from 18.10 to 18.81 kg/m^2). However, there were no notable differences in their physical activity or intake of high-fat foods (Robinson, 1999).

Barriers and Solutions: Considering Top-Down Approaches

Although individual behavior change is ultimately the avenue for reducing the amount of television time and exposure to messages about low-nutrition foods, the manner in which such change is achieved may be better solved through policy and industry initiatives. This, however, is a source of great debate. Should the government step in to create policies dictating what can and cannot be advertised to children via the media? What about messages that appear in children's schools? Should food industry and marketing companies be punished or rewarded for the messages they convey? How does influencing the creation and communication of food messages relate to rights regarding free speech? When considering legislative action on any level (school, community, local, state, national), it is necessary to address these controversial questions and issues.

At the school level, various approaches can be and have been attempted. Because many children receive their lunch (and often breakfast) through schools, school food service becomes a decisive point for potential legislative action. Under consideration are the types of foods served, how they are prepared, what and how they are promoted, and the degree to which "competitive foods" are tolerated. Undeniably, the foods that a school cafeteria serves (whether sold or subsidized by child nutrition programs) affect children's actual nutrient intake. However, they also send messages to children about what foods are valued for their nutritional content and, in so doing, can promote good choices and behaviors.

The National School Lunch Program (NSLP), once the primary provider of middle and high school students' nutritional intake during the school day, now constitutes a smaller portion of what is consumed (McGinnis et al., 2006; Koplan et al., 2005). The NSLP meals offered in participating schools provide about one-third of the RDA of protein, calcium, iron, vitamin A, vitamin C, and calories

(Koplan et al., 2005); and they meet specific guidelines for calories from fat (≤30%) and saturated fat (≤10%). To receive cash subsidies and donated commodities from the USDA, participating schools must maintain these requirements, but they can select which foods to serve to meet these requirements (Koplan et al., 2005).

"Competitive foods," which are any foods sold outside of the school meal program (e.g., chips, candy, and cookies), do not have to meet any of these requirements. No federal guidelines exist with regard to the nutritional makeup of the competitive foods sold in cafeterias, vending machines, fund-raisers, or other school vending points (although a set of comprehensive recommendations is being developed by the Institute of Medicine under the direction of Congress; Koplan et al., 2005). Federal guidelines on such issues do exist in some European countries. For example, France has banned all vending machines from schools, and the United Kingdom has laws controlling the content of vending machines (Ungoed-Thomas, 2005).

Local, district, and state governments can implement their own legislative action. For example, the Los Angeles Unified School District (California) has instituted policies mandating that fund-raising activities not involve food-related products, prohibiting the sale of foods of minimal nutritional value (FMNV) in vending machines at certain times, and eliminating contracts with branded fast-food companies (McGinnis et al., 2006). Some local school districts have met success in establishing nutrition standards for competitive foods, including the Austin Independent School District (Texas), Grand Forks Public Schools (North Dakota), Mercedes Independent School District (Texas), and Old Orchard Beach School Department (Maine; USDA, 2005). Districts that have influenced food and beverage contracts include Fairfax County Public Schools (Virginia), Fayette County Public Schools (Kentucky), Richland One School District (South Carolina), and Vista Unified School District (California; US Department of Agriculture, 2005).

On a statewide level, 17 states have moved to implement nutritional standards for school meals that are stricter than those of the USDA. Twenty-two states have set nutritional standards for competitive foods; and 26 states limit access (time and location) to competitive foods sold outside of the school meal programs (Trust for America's Health, 2007). Such actions may include limiting or eliminating the selling of soda, requiring healthful choices at school functions, including more fruits and vegetables in school meals, turning off vending machines at certain times of the day, and banning competitive foods or FMNV in elementary schools. These are only a few actions that address the availability of the unhealthful options that are frequently advertised to children and adolescents. If deemed appropriate, several of these actions could be implemented on a national level.

Recent claims brought against the McDonald's Corporation by two obese children prompted the introduction of the Personal Responsibility in Food Consumption Act in both 2004 and 2005 (HR 554, 109th Cong., 1st sess., 2005). While this Act passed in the House of Representatives, it failed to achieve Senate approval. This act attempted to protect the producers, distributors, or sellers of food from potential lawsuits, such as the one against McDonald's (Koplan et al., 2005; McGinnis et al., 2006). As stated, the bill sought "to prevent legislative and regulatory functions from being usurped by civil liability actions brought or continued against food manufacturers, marketers, distributors, advertisers, sellers and trade associations for claims of injury relations to a person's weight gain, obesity, or any health condition associated with weight gain or obesity." Essentially, this bill would diffuse liability from the food and marketing industry, placing full responsibility on consumers.

For advertising and marketing, the Federal Trade Commission (FTC) is the chief regulator of claims communicated about food products. Since its early years as a regulating agency, the FTC has set out to prevent deceptive practices in commerce. Related to food advertisements, the FTC enforces statues to prevent false advertisements, where misleading information might encourage the purchase of foods or beverages. Advertisements directed at children are evaluated even more stringently by the FTC than are advertisements intended for adults. This is because children are considered more vulnerable to advertising because of their cognitive limitations (McGinnis et al., 2006).

The FTC (1978) proposed legislation to protect children from advertisements that extended beyond their comprehension, and from advertisements that were detrimental to dental health. This legislation was later thrown out because of intense criticism by the advertising, food, and toy industries claiming violation of their First Amendment rights (McGinnis et al., 2006; Story, 2004). Restrictions on speech and expression are hot-button topics, bringing attention and controversy over the need for special regulation of "commercial speech" (McGinnis et al., 2006). The Central Hudson test was ultimately created by the US Supreme Court to determine the level of regulation that the government could take with advertisements. This test essentially grants commercial entities their First Amendment rights on the assumption that the advertisement "must concern lawful activity and not be misleading." It is unclear whether the Central Hudson test will hold up in different venues, including school settings and the Internet.

Federal policies relating to children and food advertising do exist in Europe. Sweden and Norway restrict advertising to children during children's programming. France has legislation requiring all food companies that advertise junk food to donate a portion of their advertising budget to obesity prevention programs (Garde, 2006). The United Kingdom has banned all advertising of food items high in fat, salt, and sugar during and around programs aimed at children under 16 years (Ofcom, 2006). In addition, the European Union has legislation, albeit somewhat limited, restricting advertising to children (Garde, 2006). In addition, there is a push in Europe to create stronger regulations governing food advertising to children (Casert, 2005).

In the United States, although laws relating to food marketing are currently quite limited, there is nevertheless a precedent for stronger legislation related to the advertising activities of other industries. A variety of laws exist on the state level that pertain to alcohol advertising, including laws that limit the alcohol industry's ability to target minors—in some states including laws regarding the use of children in advertisements or the placement of advertisements where children may be exposed to them (Center on Alcohol Marketing and Youth, 2003). In addition, federal laws restrict the tobacco industry from advertising cigarettes on television and the radio (Federal Trade Commission, 2001).

Encouraged instead of public policy is the option of self-regulation. Originally created in 1974, the Children's Advertising Review Unit (CARU) seeks to promote responsible children's advertising in conjunction with the Better Business Bureau and the National Advertising Review Council (Better Business Bureau, 2000). CARU reviews and evaluates child-directed media and attempts to invoke change through voluntary cooperation based on a philosophy with six main principles. CARU states (Better Business Bureau, 2000) that every advertiser should:

1. Account for the knowledge, sophistication, and maturity levels of the audience to which their message is primarily directed;

2. Exercise care not to exploit unfairly the imaginative quality of children;

3. Communicate information in a truthful and accurate manner and in language understandable to young children with full recognition that the child may learn practices from advertising which can affect his or her health and well-being;

4. Address itself to positive and beneficial social behavior;

5. Incorporate minority and other groups in advertisements in order to present positive and pro-social roles and role models whenever possible; and

6. Contribute to [the] parent–child relationship in a constructive manner.

CARU seeks to help self-regulation among all media, considering product presentation and claims; sales pressure; disclosures and disclaimers; comparative claims; endorsement by program or editorial characters; premiums, kids' clubs, promotions, and sweepstakes; and even product safety (Better Business Bureau, 2000). Specifically, attention is given to food marketing and products in the section on product presentation and claims. The section starts with the following statement: "Children look at, listen to, and remember many different elements in advertising. Therefore advertisers need to examine the total advertising message to be certain the net communication will not mislead or misinform children" (Better Business Bureau, 2000, p. 4). The eighth guideline states, "Representation of food products should be made so as to encourage sound use of the product with a view toward health development of the child and development of good nutritional practices. Advertisements representing mealtime should clearly and adequately depict the role of the product within the framework of a balanced diet. Snack foods should be represented as such, and not as substitutes for meals." (p.4) Other guidelines pertain to food product advertisements, recommending that messages not mislead children about a product's benefits, and not urge children to pester their parents or others to buy products (National Advertising Review Council, 2004). CARU also gives special consideration and attention to online content, especially with regard to Web sites attempting to sell or collect data from minor children (Better Business Bureau, 2000).

CARU operates under a policy of voluntary cooperation; thus, when an advertisement counters one of the guidelines, CARU simply suggests that the advertiser modify or discontinue the advertisement (National Advertising Review Council, 2004). Critics argue that CARU cannot appropriately monitor the overwhelming number of messages reaching children, nor does it have the command to have more powerful food and marketing companies adhere to its vague and subjective guidelines (Kelley, 2005). Other criticisms point to CARU's inability to act in a timely manner; to rigorously enforce breaches of the guidelines, reviews, and decisions that occur after their dissemination; and to keep up with a rapidly changing industry (Kelley, 2005). CARU's intentions and the concept of self-regulation are undeniably good; however, the actual way that they play out may be in need of modification. Guidelines and codes of conduct differ from legally binding policies and, therefore, do not necessarily motivate advertisers or corporations that lack a strong interest in the public good to adopt such interest.

Personal freedom is highly valued in US society, but with regard to children who lack adults' capacity for mature cognitive reasoning, regulation of "commercial speech" may be the only way to effectively discontinue the delivery and spread of misleading and unhealthy messages reaching children. With the ubiquity of environmental food messages, completely shielding children seems unlikely. Perhaps eliminating messages from certain media and settings (e.g., children's Web sites, schools), while controversial, is the most effective manner of regulating. Likewise, controlling the types of advertised food products that are sold and the ease with which children can purchase them may also be useful in directing children to make healthier decisions. Interventions and self-regulations appear to be important avenues for change, but formal policies and regulations may be more effective in influencing children's behaviors.

Conclusion

It is hard to deny the existence of a relationship between media use and diet-related outcomes (namely, overweight and obesity), especially given the breadth of research dedicated to establishing and teasing apart these ties. What have proven less obvious are the appropriate and efficient ways of altering the pathway and poor outcomes. At the conclusion of its extensive report, the Institute of Medicine's Committee on Food Marketing and the Diets of Children and

Youth offers ten important recommendations (Table 12.2). These recommendations involve multiple influential industries and stakeholders that have successfully resisted efforts to improve (i.e., make healthy) children's food messages in ways that might mitigate obesity. Simple behavioral or purely policy interventions have proven ineffective. An honest, integrative collaborative effort engaging government, industry, schools, parents, and children is necessary for deliberate, effective action.

Table 12.2

Ten Important Recommendations by the Institute of Medicine's Committee on Food Marketing and the Diets of Children and Youth

Recommendation 1 Food and beverage companies should use their creativity, resources, and full range of marketing practices to promote and support more healthful diets for children and youth.

Recommendation 2 Full service restaurant chains, family restaurants, and quick-serve restaurants should use their creativity, resources, and full range of marketing practices to promote healthful meals for children and youth.

Recommendation 3 Food, beverage, restaurant, retail, and marketing industry trade associations should assume transforming leadership roles in harnessing industry creativity, resources, and marketing on behalf of healthful diets for children and youth.

Recommendation 4 The food, beverage, restaurant, and marketing industries should work with government scientific, public health, and consumer groups to establish and enforce the highest standards for the marketing of foods, beverages, and meals to children and youth.

Recommendation 5 The media and entertainment industry should direct its extensive power to promote healthful foods and beverages for children and youth.

Recommendation 6 Government, in partnership with the private sector, should create a long-term, multifaceted, and financially sustained social marketing program supporting parents, caregivers, and families in promoting healthful diets for children and youth.

Recommendation 7 State and local educational authorities, with support from parents, health authorities, and other stakeholders, should educate about and promote healthful diets for children and youth in all aspects of the school environment.

Recommendation 8 Government at all levels should marshal the full range of public policy levers to foster the development and promotion of healthful diets for children and youth.

Recommendation 9 The nation's formidable research capacity should be substantially better directed to sustained, multidisciplinary work on how marketing influences the food and beverage choices of children and youth.

Recommendation 10 The Secretary of the US Department of Health and Human Services (DHHS) should designate a responsible agency, with adequate and appropriate resources, to formally monitor and report regularly on the progress of the various entities and activities related to the recommendations included in this report.

Source: After McGinnis et al., 2006, with permission from the National Academies Press.

Children's intellectual and emotional vulnerability puts them at a disadvantaged position in today's ruthless media environment. As emphasized in this chapter, childhood obesity is a serious and growing public health issue. The fact that overweight and obesity are starting at progressively earlier ages bodes poorly for increasingly greater complications throughout the life span. Unlike most other epidemics, which can be controlled medically or through public health initiatives, obesity thrives in a medium fed by policies that do not protect the child from misleading, compelling advertising. Providing a healthier environment that protects children and thereby enables them to make informed, nonbiased decisions is vital.

The argument that this protection comes at the expense of "commercial speech" or personal freedoms is fatuous. Indeed, given the special case of children, interventions and regulations are warranted and welcome. Modern-day technologies and advancements have created this pathway from the television to the stomach. At this point, a concerted effort is needed to redirect children toward healthier behaviors and outcomes. Protection against cigarette advertising provides a strong moral and pragmatic example; public health officials, researchers, and educators would be well advised to learn lessons from the tobacco controversy to improve and enhance the health of children and adolescents.

References Cited

Ajzen, I. (1991). The theory of planned behavior. *Organizational Behavior and Human Decision Processes, 50*, 179–211.

American Academy of Pediatrics. Children, adolescents, and television. (2001) *Pediatrics 107*, 423–426.

American Marketing Association. (n.d.). *AMA Adopts New Definition of Marketing*. Retrieved May 25, 2007, from http://www.marketingpower.com/content21257.php

Arnas, Y. (2004). The effects of television food advertisement on children's food purchasing requests. *Pediatrics International, 48*, 138–145.

Bandura, A. (1977). *Social Learning Theory*. Englewood Cliffs, NJ: Prentice-Hall.

Bandura, A. (1986). *Social Foundations of Thought and Action: A Social Cognitive Theory*. Englewood Cliffs, NJ: Prentice-Hall

Bandura, A. (2001). Social Cognitive Theory of Self-Regulation. *Organizational Behavior and Human Decision Processes, 50*, 248–287.

Better Business Bureau, Children's Advertising Review Unit. (2000). *Self-regulatory Guidelines for Children's Advertising*. Revised February, 2000. Accessed November 2006 at: http://www.ftc.gov/privacy/safeharbor/caruselfreg.pdf

Blass, E. M., Anderson, D. A., Kirkorian, H. L., Pempek, T. A., Price, I., & Koleini, M. F. (2006). On the road to obesity: Television viewing increases intake of high-density foods. *Physiology & Behavior, 88*, 597–604.

Borzekowski, D. L. G., & Robinson, T. N. (2001). The 30-second effect: An experiment revealing the impact of television commercials on food preferences of preschoolers. *Journal of the American Dietetic Association, 101*, 42–46.

Boynton-Jarrett, R., Thomas, T. N., Peterson, K. E., Wiecha, J., Sobol, A. M., & Gortmaker, S. L. (2003). Impact of television viewing patterns on fruit and vegetable consumption among adolescents. *Pediatrics, 112*, 1321–1326.

Bryce, J. W., & Leichter, H. J. (1983). The Family and television. *Journal of Family Issues, 4*, 309–327.

Burdette, H. L., & Whitaker, R. C. (2005). A national study of neighborhood safety, outdoor play, television viewing, and obesity in preschool children. *Pediatrics, 116*, 657–662.

Campbell, K. J., Crawford, D. A., Salmon, J., Carver, A., Garnett, S. P., & Baur, L. A. (2007). Associations between the home food environment and obesity-promoting eating behaviors in adolescence. *Obesity, 15,* 719–730.

Casert, R. (2005). Europe takes aim at obesity: EU wants to keep junk food advertising away from children. *CBS News Online.* Retrieved June 1, 2007, from http://www. cbsnews.com/stories/2005/01/20/health /main668194.shtml

Centers for Disease Control, National Center for Chronic Disease Prevention and Health Promotion. (2000). *School Health Policies and Programs Study Fact Sheet.* Retrieved November 2006, from http://www.cdc. gov/HealthyYouth/shpps/index.htm

Center on Alcohol Marketing and Youth, Georgetown University. (2003). *State Alcohol Advertising Laws: Current Status and Model Policies.* Retrieved June 1, 2007, from the Center on Alcohol Marketing and Youth Web site: http://camy.org/research/ files/statelaws0403.pdf

Certain, L. K., & Kahn, R. S. (2002). Prevalence, correlates, and trajectory of television viewing among infants and toddlers. *Pediatrics, 109,* 634–642.

Christakis, D. A. (2006). The hidden and potent effects of television advertising. *Journal of the American Medical Association, 295,* 1698–1699.

Christakis, D. A, Garrison, M. M., & Zimmerman, F. J. (2006). Television viewing in child care programs: A National Survey. *Communication Reports, 19,* 111–120.

Connor, S. M. (2006). Food-related advertising on preschool television: Building brand recognition in young viewers. *Pediatrics, 118,* 1478–1485.

Consumers Union Education Services. (1995). *Captive Kids: Commercial Pressures at School.* Yonkers, NY: Author.

Coon, K. A., Goldberg, J., Rogers, B. L., & Tucker, K. L. (2001). Relationships between use of television during meals and children's food consumption patterns. *Pediatrics, 107,* E7.

Dietz, W. H., & Gortmaker, S. L. (1985). Do we fatten our children at the television set? Obesity and television viewing in children and adolescents. *Pediatrics, 75,* 807–812.

Dietz, W. H., & Gortmaker, S. L. (2001). Preventing obesity in children and adolescents. *Annual Review of Public Health, 22,* 337–353.

Dennison, B. A., Russo, T. J., Burdick, P. A., & Jenkins, P. L. (2004). An intervention to reduce television viewing by preschool children. *Archives of Pediatrics and Adolescent Medicine, 158,* 170–176.

Dubois, L., Farmer, A., Girard, M., Peterson, K., & Tatone-Tokuda, F. (2007). Problem eating behaviors related to social factors and body weight in preschool children: A longitudinal study. *International Journal of Behavioral Nutrition and Physical Activity, 4,* 9.

Dubois, L., & Girard, M. (2006). Early determinants of overweight at 4.5 years in a population-based longitudinal study. *International Journal of Obesity, 30,* 610–617.

Federal Trade Commission. (2001). *Advertising practices: Frequently Asked Advertising Questions: A Guide for Small Business.* Retrieved June 1, 2007, from http://www. ftc.gov/bcp/conline/pubs/buspubs/ ad-faqs.shtm

Ford, B. S., McDonald, T. E., Owens, A. S., & Robinson, T. N. (2002). Primary care interventions to reduce television viewing in African-American children. *American Journal of Preventive Medicine, 22,* 106–109.

French, S. A., Story, M., Neumark-Sztainer, D., Fulkerson, J. A., & Hannan, P. (2001). Fast food restaurant use among adolescents: associations with nutrient intake, food choices and behavioral and psychosocial variables. *International Journal of Obesity and Related Metabolic Disorders, 25,* 1823–1833.

Gable, S., Chang, Y., & Krull, J. L. (2007). Television watching and frequency of family meals are predictive of overweight onset and persistence in a national sample of school-aged children. *Journal of American Dietetic Association, 107,* 53–61.

Gallo, A. E. (1999). Food advertising in the United States. In E. Frazao (Ed.), *America's eating habit: Changes and consequences* (pp. 173–180). Washington, DC: US Department of Agriculture, Economic Research Service.

Gamble, M. & Cotugna, N. A. (1999). Quarter century of TV food advertising targeted at children. *American Journal of Health Behavior, 23,* 261–267.

Garde, A. (2006). *The regulation of food advertising and obesity prevention in Europe: What role for the European Union.* EUI Law Working Paper No. 2006/16. Available at: http://ssrn.com/abstract=910877

Gerbner, G., Gross, L., Morgan, M., & Signorelli, N. (1994). Growing up with television: The cultivation perspective. In J. Bryant & D. Zillmann (Eds.), *Media Effects: Advances in Theory and Research*. Mahwah, NJ: Erlbaum.

Glanz, K., Rimer, B. K., Lewis, F. M. (2002). *Health Behavior and Health Education* (3rd ed.). San Francisco, CA: Jossey-Bass.

Gupta, P. B., & Gould, S. J. (1997). Consumers' perceptions of the ethics and acceptability of product placement in movies: product category and individual differences. *Journal of Current Issues and Research in Advertising, 19*, 37–50.

Hammermeister, J., Brock, B., Winterstein, D., & Page, R. (2005). Life without TV? Cultivation theory and psychosocial health characteristics of television-free individuals and their television-viewing counterparts. *Health Communication, 17*, 253–264.

Harrison, K. (2005). Is "Fat-Free" good for me? A panel study of television viewing and children's nutritional knowledge and reasoning. *Health Communication, 17*, 117–132.

Harrison, K., & Marske, A. L. (2005). Nutritional content of foods advertised during television programs children watch most. *American Journal of Public Health, 95*, 1568–1574.

Hastings, G., Stead, M., McDermott, L., Forsyth, A., MacKintosh, A., Rayner, M., et al. (2003). *Review of the research on the effects of food promotion to children*. Glasgow, Scotland: University of Strethclyde, Centre for Social Marketing.

Hawkes, C. (2004). *Marketing food to children: The global regulatory environment*. Geneva: World Health Organization.

Kelder, S. H., Perry, C. L., Klepp, K. I., & Lytle, L. L. (1994). Longitudinal tracking of adolescent smoking, physical activity, and food choice behaviors. *American Journal of Public Health, 84*, 1121–1126.

Kelley, B. (2005). *Industry Controls over Food Marketing to Children: Are They Effective?* Boston: Public Health Advocacy Institute.

Koplan, J., Liverman, C., & Kraak, V. (Eds.). (2005). *Preventing Childhood Obesity: Health in Balance*. Washington, DC: Institute of Medicine, National Academy of Sciences.

Kotz, K. & Story, M. (1994). Food advertisements during children's Saturday morning television programming: Are they consistent with dietary recommendations?

Journal of the American Dietetic Association. 94, 1296–1300.

Lull, J. T. (1990). *Inside Family Viewing: Ethnographic Research on Television's Audiences*. London: Routledge.

Maffeis, C., & Tato, L. (2001). Long-term effects of childhood obesity on morbidity and mortality. *Hormone Research, 55*, 42–45.

Matheson, D. M., Killen, J. D., Wang, Y., & Robinson, T. N. (2004). Children's food consumption during television viewing. *American Journal of Clinical Nutrition, 79*, 1088–1094.

McGinnis, J. M., Gootman, J. A., & Kraak, V. I. (Eds.); Committee on Food Marketing and the Diets of Children and Youth. (2006). *Food Marketing to Children and Youth: Threat or Opportunity?* Washington, DC: The National Academies Press.

McNeal, J. (1998). Tapping the three kids' markets. *American Demographics, 20*, 37–41.

Morland, K., Wing, S., Roux, A. D., & Poole, C. (2002). Neighborhood characteristics associated with the location of food stores and food service places. *American Journal of Preventive Medicine, 22*, 23–29.

Must, A., Jacques, P. F., Dallal, G. E., Bajema, C. J., Dietz, W. H. (1992). Long-term morbidity and mortality of overweight adolescents. A follow-up of the Harvard Growth Study of 1922 to 1935. *New England Journal of Medicine, 327*, 1350–1355.

Nader, P. R., O'Brien, M., Houts, R., Bradley, R., Belsky, J., Crosnoe, R., et al. (2006). Identifying risk for obesity in early childhood. *Pediatrics, 118*, e594–e601.

National Advertising Review Council. (May, 2004). *White Paper Guidance for Food Advertising Self-Regulation*. Retrieved October, 2006, from http://www. narcpartners.org/reports/whitepaper.asp

Nielsen, S. J., & Popkin, B. M. (2003). Patterns and trends in food portion sizes, 1977–1998. *Journal of the American Medical Association, 289*, 450–453.

Nielsen, S. J., Siega-Riz, A. M., & Popkin, B. M. (2002). Trends in food locations and sources among adolescents and young adults. *Preventive Medicine, 35*, 107–113.

Ofcom (2006, November). *New restrictions on the television advertising of food and drink products to children*. Retrieved July 23, 2007, from http://www.ofcom.org.uk/ media/news/2006/11/nr_20061117

Ogden, C. L., Carroll, M. D., Curtin, L. R., McDowell, M. A., Tabak, C. J., & Flegal, K.

M. (2006). Prevalence of overweight and obesity in the United States, 1999–2004. *Journal of the American Medical Association, 295,* 1549–1555.

Paeratakul, S., Ferdinand, D. P., Champagne, C. M., Ryan, D. H., & Bray, G. A. (2003). Fast-food consumption among U.S. adults and children: dietary and nutrient intake profile. *Journal of the American Dietetic Association, 103,* 1332–1338.

Rideout, V. J., Vandewater, E. A., & Wartella, E. A. (2003). *Zero to Six: Electronic Media in the Lives of Infants, Toddlers, and Preschoolers.* Menlo Park, CA: Henry J. Kaiser Family Foundation.

Roberts, D. (2000). Media and youth: Access, exposure, and privatization. *Journal of Adolescent Health, 27S,* 8–14.

Roberts, D., Foehr U. G., Rideout V. (2005). Generation M: Media in the Lives of 8–18 Year olds. A Kaiser Family Foundation Study. Menlo Park, CA:The Henry J. Kaiser Family Foundation.

Robinson, T. N. (1999). Reducing children's television viewing to prevent obesity: a randomized controlled trial. *Journal of the American Medical Association, 282,* 1561–1567.

Robinson, T. N., & Borzekowski, D. L. G. (2006). Effects of the SMART classroom curriculum to reduce child and family screen time. *Journal of Communication, 56,* 1–26.

Saelens, B. E., Sallis, J. F., Nader, P. R., Broyles, S. L., Berry, C. C., & Taras, H. L. (2002). Home environmental influences on children's television watching from early to middle childhood. *Journal of Developmental and Behavioral Pediatrics, 23,* 127–132.

Signorelli, N., & Staples, J. (1997). Television and children's conceptions of nutrition. *Health Communication, 9,* 289–301.

St-Onge, M. P., Keller, K. L., & Heymsfield, S. B. (2003). Changes in childhood food consumption patterns: A cause for concern in light of increasing body weights. *American Journal of Clinical Nutrition, 78,* 1068–1073.

Story, M., & French, S. (2004). Food advertising and marketing directed at children and adolescents in the U.S. *International Journal of Behavioral Nutrition and Physical Activity, 1,* 3.

St. Peters, M. (1991). Television and families: what do young children watch with their parents? *Child, 62,* 1409–1423.

Strasburger, V. C. (2001). Children and TV advertising: nowhere to run, nowhere to hide. *Journal of Developmental and Behavioral Pediatrics, 22,* 185–187.

Thompson, D. A., & Christakis, D. A. (2005). The association between television viewing and irregular sleep schedules among children less than 3 years of age. *Pediatrics, 116,* 851–856.

Trust for America's Health. (November, 2007). *F as in Fat: How Obesity Policies are Failing America.* Retrieved January 31, 2008, from http://healthyamericans.org/reports/obesity2007/Obesity2007Report.pdf.

Ungoed-Thomas, J. (2005, September 25). School's out for junk vending. *The Sunday Times.* Retrieved June 1, 2007, from http://www.timesonline.co.uk/tol/news/uk/article570570.ece

US Department of Agriculture, Food and Nutrition Services. (2005, January). *Making it Happen: School Nutrition Success Stories.* Retrieved November 29, 2006, from http://www.fns.usda.gov/tn/Resources/makingithappen.html

US Department of Health and Human Services and US Department of Agriculture. (2005). *Dietary Guidelines for Americans, 2005.* Retrieved November 30, 2006, from http://www.health.gov/dietaryguidelines/dga2005/document/pdf/DGA2005.pdf

US General Accounting Office. (September, 2000). Public Education: commercial activities in school. Report to congressional requesters (GAO/HEHS-00-156). Washington, DC: US General Accounting Office.

Wiecha, J. L., Peterson, K. E., Ludwig, D. S., Kim, J., Sobol, A., & Gortmaker, S. L. (2006). When Children Eat What They Watch: Impact of Television Viewing on Dietary Intake in Youth. *Archive of Pediatrics and Adolescent Medicine, 160,* 436–442.

Wilson, N., Signal, L., Nicholls, S., & Thomson, G. (2005). Marketing fat and sugar to children on New Zealand television. *Preventive Medicine, 42,* 96–101.

Woodard, E. (2000). *Media in the Home. The Fifth Annual Survey of Parents and Children.* Philadelphia: University of Pennsylvania, Annenberg Public Policy Center.

13 A FRAMEWORK FOR THE TREATMENT OF OBESITY: EARLY SUPPORT

*Cecilia Bergh, Matthew Sabin, Julian Shield, Göran Hellers,
Modjtaba Zandian, Karolina Palmberg, Barbro Olofsson,
Kerstin Lindeberg, Mikael Björnström, and Per Södersten*

> *What a curious attitude scientists have—"we still don't know
> that; but it is knowable and it is only a matter of time before we
> get to know it!" As if that went without saying.*
> — Wittgenstein, 1980

Introduction

Although obesity is a growing problem and many of its medical consequences are becoming manifest even in children (Drake et al., 2002), most methods of treating obese children and adults are only marginally successful (Norris et al., 2005; Padwal & Majumdar, 2007; Summerbell et al., 2003). Several assumptions underlie these methods. For example, recent studies in neuroscience and molecular genetics have led Spiegel and colleagues (2005) to suggest that obesity is a "hypothalamic disease" and a "complex genetic disease," and Nath and colleagues (2006) to suggest that "understanding . . . abnormal regulation of energy metabolism through to dysfunction of molecular mechanisms—will pave the ways for development of new treatment strategies". These assumptions bring Wittgenstein's quote to mind. They express the belief (hope) that it is only a matter of time before the problem of obesity is solved. But the limited success of presently used approaches to curb obesity could reflect the possibility that the underlying assumptions are only partially correct. The second part of Wittgenstein's quote should encourage us to consider this possibility. The discussion that follows briefly reviews and evaluates some contemporary assumptions concerning the cause of obesity and the proper approach to its treatment. The chapter then provides an alternative framework and reports preliminary results of treating extremely obese adolescents and obese patients with binge-eating disorder using a method based on this framework.

The Energy Intake–Energy Expenditure Mismatch

Diet and body weight

The relationship between diet and health has long been studied (Oddy, 2003). For example, Keys and colleagues (1963) reported that the incidence of coronary heart disease markedly decreased during periods of reduced intake of food—fat in particular. These observations stimulated interest in the relationship between fat intake and health, including body weight, and provided the basis for the recommendations that fat intake should be reduced. However, recent large-scale trials offer little support for the possibility that intake of low-fat diets reduces body weight more than marginally in the intermediate term; indeed, weight rebound is the decided norm (Howard et al., 2006).

Interestingly, although the body mass index (BMI; measured in kilograms per square meter) has increased recently in, for example, men in Great Britain (Figure 13.1A), self-reported daily energy intake displays the opposite trend (Figure 13.1B; DEFRA, 2001). However, self-reported data on food consumption must be viewed with caution; it is well known that consumption is understated, sometimes by as much as 25% (Swan, 2004). For example, American men and women reported consuming 2347 and 1658 kilocalories a day, respectively, in 1994 to 1996 (Cutlet et al., 2003); and the corresponding numbers for British men and women in 1991 were virtually the same—2313 and 1632 kilocalories per day, respectively (Swan, 2004). This is less than the caloric requirement for maintaining a normal body weight.

For an analysis of changes in consumption over time, however, underreporting may not represent a problem, if it can be assumed to be constant (Cutlet et al., 2003). The decreasing trend in intake (see Figure 13.1B) is therefore likely to represent a real time-dependent decrease in the consumption of food. And even if the data do not take into consideration snacking between meals, which contributes significantly to overall caloric intake (Cutler et al., 2003), it is still estimated that the total caloric intake in men in Great Britain has decreased during the last 20 years (Swan, 2004).

Thus, although BMI has increased during the last 30 years, probably reflecting increasing adiposity, there has been a parallel decrease in the reported daily intake of carbohydrate, fat, and protein (Figure 13.1C and D). The reason for the mismatch between intake and expenditure of energy is unknown, but it challenges the assumption that body weight is physiologically regulated. Alternatively, it calls the validity of the BMI for defining obesity into question, or it reveals a basic lack of understanding about the relationship between intake and BMI.

Diet interventions

Attempts to reduce BMI by means of diets containing reduced carbohydrate, fat, or protein have been minimally successful. Such diets typically yield weight losses

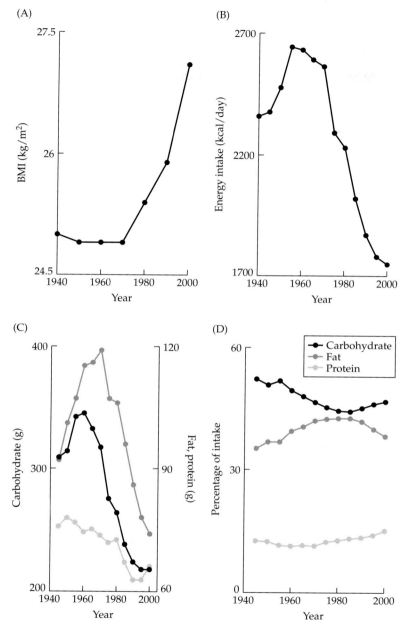

FIGURE 13.1 Body mass index (A), total energy intake (B), and intake of carbohydrate, fat, and protein expressed as total intake (C) and percentage of total intake (D) from 1940 to 2000. (Data from Floud, 1998; the National Health Service, 2004; and the Department of the Environment, Food and Rural Affairs, 2001; reproduced with permission.)

of between 2.1 and 3.2 kilograms within a year in adults who have an average BMI of 35 (Dansinger et al., 2005). A diet reduced in fat content yielded an average weight loss of 2.2 kilograms within a year in a sample of 20,000 women aged 50 to 79 years who had an average BMI of 29.1. However, this effect was reduced to 0.4 kilogram during a 7.5-year period of follow-up (Howard et al., 2006). Reducing carbohydrate intake may prove more helpful, although the long-term health effects have not been extensively studied (Adam-Perrot et al., 2006).

Interestingly, weight loss recorded among participants on a low-carbohydrate diet was found to be related to a reduction in caloric intake, not specifically to reduced carbohydrate intake and it was recently pointed out that the amount of food eaten rather than the type of diet is the important factor for reducing body weight (Dansinger & Schaefer, 2006). When implemented into clinical practice, currently used weight loss diets, while having some effects on health—for example, reduced risk of cardiovascular disease—have very small, generally unsustainable effects on body weight. No evidence suggests that one diet is more effective than another (Malik & Hu, 2007).

Summary of the intake–expenditure mismatch

It seems unlikely that a change in the intake of a single nutrient—for example, carbohydrate or fat—can explain more than a small part of the variation in the BMI, which is a likely reason that dietary interventions have rather small, transient effects on the BMI. Despite the publicity (and subsequent denouement) of some diets that constrain intake of a single macronutrient, there is no evidence that dieting consistently affects body weight.

The Hypothalamus and Eating Behavior

Homeostasis

Most neuroscience research on eating behavior and body weight, including obesity, rests on the assumption that energy balance is homeostatically controlled so that constancy is maintained across a range of conditions. For example, following food restriction and weight loss, overeating occurs until the original body weight is reattained. The converse holds when obesity is induced through forced feeding. This topic is continually being revisited, and there are many excellent recent reviews (e.g., Beck, 2006). The theory of homeostatic regulation of body weight dates back to the first half of the twentieth century and was summarized as a hypothalamic theory of motivation by Stellar in 1954. Stellar hypothesized that eating (and other types of motivated behavior as well) is a function of the activity of excitatory and inhibitory, anatomically separate "centers" in the hypothalamus (Stellar, 1954). The theory remains essentially the same today, with the exception that excitation and inhibition of eating are now thought to be chemically mediated and, at least to some extent, anatomically overlapping. It is also recognized that the neural network engaged in eating is distributed beyond hypothalamic "centers" to brainstem and limbic areas (Grill & Kaplan, 2002).

The instability of body weight in rats and humans in the face of an energy-dense food cornucopia makes it unlikely that body weight is controlled, so much as simply attained. Yet the homeostatic view is maintained. For example, Murphy and Bloom (2006) argue that "energy balance is a homeostatic system" but suggest that it is unlikely that the recent increase in obesity is caused by a deficit in this system. Their alternative is that "the regulatory system is unable to cope with the current context of cheap–high energy foodstuffs." However, the recent increase in the BMI is not the only example that human body weight is not maintained at a stable level.

Historically, at least through the late nineteenth century, body weight has been quite variable, dictated mainly by the economic and social factors of the times, with periods of decreases and increases long before the present, conspicuous increase (Floud, 1998). This historical view suggests a flexibility in eating strategies, with its consequent changes in body weight, that has allowed individuals to cope with periods of plenty and little, albeit often at a cost to health (Fogel et al., in press; Oddy, 2003).

Feedback from adipocytes to the brain

The hypothalamic homeostatic theory predicts that when energy intake is reduced for some time, fat is depleted and hormonal signals from adipocytes are down-regulated. The brain senses the change and adapts by up-regulating neurotransmitters, often peptides that are thought to stimulate food intake. One of the best studied of these so-called *orexigenic* peptides is neuropeptide Y (NPY), which is controlled by leptin, an *anorexigenic* peptide secreted by adipocytes. In line with the hypothesis, many studies have shown that NPY stimulates food intake and leptin inhibits it (Beck, 2006; see Chapter 3).

The physiological importance of the endocrine part of this theory has not been convincingly demonstrated. For example, to cause a reduction of body weight, leptin must be given in doses that increase plasma levels of leptin tenfold above normal levels (Rosenbaum et al., 2005). Moreover, doses of NPY that typically stimulate food intake in, for example, rats are also very high and have never been validated against endogenous levels under physiological circumstances (O'Shea et al., 1997). Thus, although there is some coherence in support of roles for NPY and leptin in feeding control, the defining and necessary criterion of the physiological level has not yet been met. Other difficulties will be addressed in the discussion that follows.

Although protocols for testing the details of ingestive behavior in experimental animals have been available for many years (Toates & Rowland, 1987), the amount of food eaten per time unit remains a commonly used indirect measure of eating behavior (Keen-Rhinehart & Bartness, 2007). Emphasis on this lone measure is surprising because it has been recognized for close to a century that eating, like other motivated behaviors, consists of two phases: *appetitive* (the search for a particular object, or commodity) and *consummatory* (the terminal *fixed* act elicited by that object; Craig, 1918; Sherrington, 1906).

The appetitive and consummatory phases can be studied separately. For example, infusing a solution of sucrose directly into the mouth of a rat circumvents the need for appetitive ingestive behavior, making it possible to measure consummatory ingestive behavior selectively. If, by contrast, the rat has to work for or search out the sucrose solution before ingestion, the amount consumed is a function of both appetitive and consummatory ingestive behaviors. As will be seen, these measures provide very different profiles of eating behavior.

In tests selective for consummatory ingestive behavior, NPY and leptin exert effects on sucrose intake that are opposite those found in tests measuring both appetitive and consummatory responses (Ammar et al., 2000). For example, when ingesting sucrose from a drinking spout located inside a test cage, rats ingest less when leptin is infused into the cerebral ventricles (Figure 13.2A). In contrast, when they receive sucrose via intraoral infusion, intracerebroventricular infusion of leptin stimulates intake (Figure 13.2B). The same paradoxical effect is obtained with intracerebroventricular NPY. More is drunk from the spout, and, paradoxically, less is received from intraoral infusions when NPY is received in the ventricles (see Figure 13.2). In short, whereas NPY stimulates intake in conventional tests, it inhibits intake in a test selectively measuring consummatory ingestive behavior. Conversely, leptin reduces intake in the conventional test, but it markedly stimulates consummatory ingestive behavior, causing a 50% increase in intake of sucrose infused intraorally.

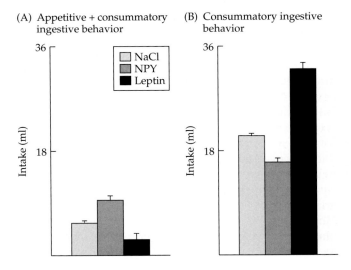

FIGURE 13.2   Intake of a 1-molar solution of sucrose available from a bottle (A) or infused intraorally at a rate of 0.5 milliliters per minute (B) in male rats. (Data from Ammar et al., 2000, reproduced with permission.)

These findings demonstrate that classification of peptides, and perhaps also of neural networks, as orexigenic and anorexigenic requires further elaboration. This distinction is especially important if one conceptualizes overeating as an addictive state. The line demarcating appetitive from consummatory may shift with chronic overeating, making the individual more vulnerable to subtle cue changes that might have otherwise been ignored when at normal weight and eating normal meals at a normal rate.

Implementing the hypothalamic theory clinically

The test described in the preceding section (see Figure 13.2) was motivated by the clinical observation that although patients with anorexia nervosa do not eat enough to sustain body weight—indeed, some die from undernutrition—they routinely display behavior in anticipation of a meal that might correspond to appetitive ingestive behavior in rats. Videotape recordings showed that anorexic patients spent more time on food preparation activities, such as cutting, moving, breaking, and mixing food before eating, than did a control group; and of course they ingested less food than did control subjects (Tappe et al., 1998). This observation was interpreted as a means by which the patient could delay eating, but this sense of purpose may not be necessary. "Playing" with the food may reflect enhancement of appetitive ingestive behavior at the expense of consuming the food.

Anorexic patients, of course, have depleted fat stores and, correspondingly, low levels of leptin in the blood; as a consequence, the level of NPY is elevated in the cerebrospinal fluid (Gendall et al., 1999). Interestingly, evidence suggests that the synthesis of NPY is also up-regulated in the brain in anorexia nervosa (Goldstone et al., 2002). These endocrine changes are consequences of the starved condition of the patients, and they are reversed upon weight restoration (Gendall et al., 1999). The endocrine scenario in anorexia nervosa is inconsistent with the idea that there are hypothalamic (and extrahypothalamic) homeostatic mechanisms that, in the case of starvation, excite eating behavior in order to maintain constant body weight. However, the same scenario is consistent with the experimental maneuvers described in Figure 13.2. Hence, we suggest that the high level of NPY in the brain of anorexic patients is an endocrine adaptation that allows the search for food (i.e., display of appetitive ingestive behavior) at the expense of eating food (i.e., display of consummatory ingestive behavior).

This hypothesis has been confirmed by recent studies on the hamster, a hoarding species. Food deprivation and subsequent replenishment of food or treatment with NPY cause an increase not in eating but in hoarding and other measures of appetitive ingestive behavior (Keen-Rhinehart & Bartness, 2007). The conclusion that NPY is an "orexigen" is based on observations of rats infused with very high doses of NPY into the brain and provided with food during a limited period of time (Beck, 2006). When this conclusion is implemented beyond the rat in a conventional test, it fails. For example, although NPY can stimulate short-term food intake in the hamster, there is no effect on 24-hour intake, and merely reducing the temperature during testing turns NPY into an inhibitor of eating (Paul et al., 2005).

Benoit and colleagues (2005) reported that the stimulatory effect of NPY on carbohydrate intake (NPY is considered particularly potent in stimulating the intake of this macronutrient; Beck, 2006) may be an artifact of the way rats are trained during testing. There was no effect of NPY in rats that had become thoroughly accustomed to the testing situation (Benoit et al., 2005). Together these findings argue against the idea that NPY is always an orexigen. They support the alternative idea that, in starvation, NPY selectively stimulates appetitive behavior and, at the same time, inhibits consummatory ingestive behavior (Ammar et al., 2000; Södersten et al., 2006a,b). Stated differently, NPY, and perhaps other peptides, assumes different roles dependent on physiological context (Södersten et al., 2006a). This physiological ambiguity should restrain the therapeutic use of such peptides.

The problem with leptin resistance

As the previous discussion has indicated, the reciprocal relationship between leptin and NPY interpreted within the hypothalamic homeostatic framework fails to explain the behavior of starved humans. But what about obesity? When rats eat palatable foods (cafeteria feeding), there is a gradual increase in the level of leptin in the blood and, as a neuroendocrine concomitant, a decrease in the synthesis of NPY in the brain (Beck, 2006). However, the brain eventually adapts, and when the rat is obese, the synthesis of NPY in the brain is back to the normal level (Beck, 2006). Obese rats do not respond to treatment with leptin by eating less food; leptin "insensitivity" develops in parallel with the development of obesity and an adjustment in the synthesis of NPY by the brain (Beck, 2006). Thus, as a corollary to the hypothalamic theory, leptin "insensitivity" is thought to develop in parallel with the development of obesity and an adjustment in the synthesis of NPY by the brain (Beck, 2006). This corollary is clearly circular and brings to mind the explanation of why opium induces sleep that was offered by Molière's doctor: "It is because opium has a soporific nature." As Bernard (1865/1927) pointed out long ago, a label is not an explanation.

The concept of leptin insensitivity makes it even more difficult to understand when leptin is a physiological inhibitor of feeding. Perhaps never. Recall that doses of leptin that are well beyond the physiological range are necessary to reduce intake. In addition, endogenous leptin is not effective during cafeteria feeding, because in this situation the rats gradually become leptin-insensitive—indeed, obese. During obesity development, leptin is apparently never able to stop rats from eating. In fact, with weight gain, a positive feedback cycle might ensue with leptin facilitating rather than inhibiting cafeteria feeding and, hence, obesity (Zhang & Scarpace, 2006).

Behavioral changes during cafeteria feeding do not accord with the idea that leptin restricts body weight gain. However, the same changes are consistent with the finding that leptin stimulates consummatory ingestive behavior in circumstances that require minimal effort to obtain food (Ammar et al., 2000). Interestingly, humans also overconsume food when it is easily available (Cutler et al., 2003; Wansink, 2004), although it remains to be demonstrated whether leptin has a role in this situation. Together these findings raise the interesting possibility that, rather than inhibiting hunger (and therefore feeding), leptin may be acting on the mediators of sensory-specific satiety that cause omnivores to switch from one food to the next (see the Epilogue).

Especially in the obese, palatable foods may circumvent certain homeostatic systems that might govern feeding. The possibility must be considered and evaluated that leptin may stimulate intake when eating does not demand substantial appetitive behavior (Ruffin et al., 2004). It follows that leptin may enhance intake in today's ambience, in which food is easily and conveniently available, with many commercial inducements and conditioned reminders. Such enhancement is consistent with the rightward shift of the consummatory appetitive divide, thereby making eating in the obese more vulnerable to cues that might otherwise be ignored. The idea that leptin might recruit different neural networks that determine behavioral strategy to deplete or replenish energy stores was first suggested by Fulton and colleagues (2000). Hence, in obesity leptin might further reduce physical activity and increase eating (Franks et al., 2007). Although not studied to our knowledge, such a mechanism might be favorably "looked upon" by hibernators that eat to the point of obesity and beyond.

The leptin–NPY neuroendocrinology of obese rats (for a full description, see the excellent review by Beck, 2006) is also inconsistent with that of obese humans. Unlike in obese rats (Beck, 2006), high leptin levels in humans reduce NPY synthesis in the brain (Goldstone et al., 2002). The brains of obese humans are not insensitive to leptin. This observation begs the question, If leptin is an inhibitor of food intake and NPY is an "orexigen," why do the obese eat too much food? The hypothalamic theory of body weight regulation cannot answer this question.

Summary of the hypothalamus and eating behavior

de Castro and Plunkett (2002) have made the point that food intake in humans living in normal environments is not controlled in the precise manner predicted by homeostatic models, particularly of the one-factor genre. Instead, human eating behavior is affected by "uncompensated" factors—that is, factors that escape homeostatic control (de Castro & Plunkett, 2002). Not surprisingly, then, drugs that have been used within the homeostatic framework and have often targeted only one "compensated" factor have very small effects on the body weight of obese patients (Despres et al., 2005; Padwal & Majumdar, 2007; Pi-Sunyer et al., 2006; Van Gaal et al., 2005). An analysis of the neural networks mediating eating behavior should consider the possibility that the effect of a peptide, as well as other neurotransmitters, varies depending on physiological state (Södersten et al., 2006b). Thus, a new approach is called for to complement the deterministic physiological model of the control of eating behavior in humans. Behavioral methods of treating disordered eating, including overeating in the obese, must be attuned to the factors that co-opt physiological control.

Obesity Surgery: Relapse in 30 Minutes

Surgery is effective

The most effective treatment of radical obesity is surgical intervention (Näslund & Kral, 2006). Currently, to qualify, the patient's BMI must equal or exceed 35 kg/m^2. There are three types of obesity surgery: one that limits the capacity of the stomach, one that reduces the absorption of ingested food, and one that combines these two methods (Näslund & Kral, 2006). Each procedure causes marked weight loss and alleviates the medical consequences of obesity—for example, diabetes—even before weight loss (Näslund & Kral, 2006). In the long term, there can be no question of the health-promoting effect of gastric surgery for obesity, ranging from a decrease in mortality to improvement in lifestyle (Sjöström et al., 2004).

Because currently used surgical treatments for obesity are irreversible, the function of mechanisms normally engaged during eating cannot be assessed after surgery. It has been suggested that the reduction of diabetic symptoms after surgery is partly mediated by alterations in gastrointestinal hormone secretion (Näslund & Kral, 2006), which, of course, exerts ingestive control (see Chapter 3), while also affecting pancreatic endocrine function directly (Vilsboll & Holst, 2004). For example, surgical gastric bypass decreases the BMI more than surgically restricting gastric capacity. This distinction may reflect differences in the hormonal consequences of the operation (Korner et al., 2006). If differences in hormone secretions were causally related to differences in BMI reduction after the operation, the endocrine consequences of surgery would be expected also to cause changes in eating behavior. Reversible obesity surgery, such as implanting an adjustable gastric band (Forsell & Hellers, 1997), provides an opportunity to examine whether changes in eating after the operation persist after gastric restriction has been reversed.

Reversible effect of gastric banding on eating behavior

One study focused on eating in nine Swedish women who had been treated with gastric banding for obesity. They averaged 27 years of age at the time of the operation, and each had made several unsuccessful attempts to lose weight. A silicone gastric band was tied around the upper part of the stomach about 15 centimeters from the cardia. The volume of the pouch between cardia and band was 5 to 7 milliliters. The band was connected to a nasogastric tube that was exteriorized and connected to a subcutaneous port anchored to the lower part of the sternum, thereby making the band accessible from the outside. The band was filled with 5 to 7 milliliters of a radiology-contrast medium during surgery, and it was adjusted at monthly intervals thereafter. For further details on the surgery and the postoperative procedures, see Forsell and Hellers, 1997.

The women ate regular food (manufactured by Findus in Bjuv, Sweden; amounting to 580 kilojoules, or 140 kilocalories; and consisting of 5.5 grams of protein, 6 grams of fat, and 16 grams of carbohydrate per 100 grams of food), measured using a Mandometer in a procedure that will be described later in the chapter. This procedure includes rating of satiety at regular intervals postoperatively. The women were tested twice, with a week between the tests, before gastric banding. They were monitored postoperatively at monthly intervals, and the band was adjusted; that is, fluid was either infused or withdrawn. They were retested about 15 months after surgery. Then, 1 to 3 days later, they were tested again, about 30 minutes after the gastric band was evacuated, thereby allowing the complete stomach to participate. The band was then refilled, and the women were tested with the band filled a week later—that is, with stomach contracted. Following this test, the band was again evacuated, and 1 to 3 days later the patients were studied again. The procedures were approved by the ethics committee of the Karolinska Institute.

Figure 13.3 shows that the BMI of these women was markedly reduced (about 35%) 1 year after the operation, presumably because of chronic feeding reduc-

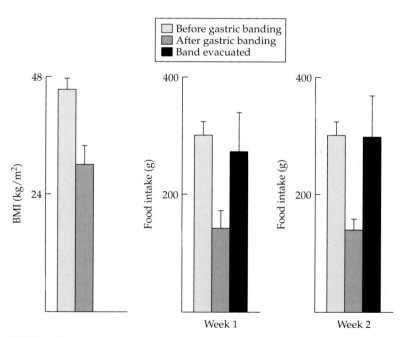

FIGURE 13.3   Body mass index in nine women before and 15 months after gastric banding. The women were tested twice for eating behavior and satiety before and after gastric banding, with a week between the tests. The gastric band was evacuated 1 to 3 days after the test, and filled for each of the two tests after gastric banding.

tion. This finding is supported by reduced food intake (about 50%) in both tests with the band filled. Figure 13.3 also shows that the diminished food intake was immediately reversed when the stomach was returned to full capacity (Week 1). Refilling the band reduced intake in a test 1 week later to the same level as the week before, and evacuating the band once more increased intake to the same level as before the gastric banding 15 months earlier (Week 2). Interestingly, the perception of satiety was similar under the three conditions (data not shown), demonstrating that the surgical effects did not cause fundamental change in either the patients' eating or the perception of small and large meals. This is of particular meaning in the light of "constant" satiety ratings after both tests. That is, satiety reflects meal completion, and not the amount consumed. This finding is reminiscent of studies by Rolls that examined the effects of eating meals of different sizes, which showed that satiety ratings were stable within an individual regardless of meal size. See the epilogue for a more complete discussion.

Summary of obesity surgery

Restraining gastric capacity for 15 months markedly affected the amount of food eaten by obese women and, consequently, their BMI. However, the effect on food intake was reversed immediately with gastric relief. The conditions that curtail meal size when the gastric band is constricted reflect minimized gastric capacity and not a fundamental reorganization of central control mechanisms. Food intake adapts to rapid changes in gastric capacity. Inhibitory neural control of eating does not develop as a result of peripheral constraints even over a relatively long period of time. The time to imprint the feeding system surgically, with all of its concomitant changes, has passed. Other strategies are called for. In short, although surgical interventions are effective in reducing body weight in obese patients, their cost (about 20,000 US dollars in 2007), surgical risk, and other negatives make it unlikely that these methods can be used for population-based treatment of obesity (Padwal & Majumdar, 2007).

An Alternative Framework

A framework is not a detailed hypothesis or set of hypotheses; rather, it is a suggested point of view for an attack on a scientific problem, often suggesting testable hypotheses. Biological frameworks differ from frameworks in physics and chemistry because of the nature of evolution. Biological systems do not have rigid laws, as physics has. Evolution produces mechanisms, and often sub-mechanisms, so that there are few "rules" in biology which do not have occasional exceptions.

A good framework is one that sounds reasonably plausible relative to available scientific data and that turns out to be largely correct. It is unlikely to be correct in all the details.

A framework often contains unstated (and often unrecognized) assumptions.

— Crick and Koch, 2003

Because of the demonstrated null to modest success of presently used methods to treat obesity (with the exception of surgery) and the sometimes questionable assumptions on which the methods are based (identified at the start of the chapter), a new framework should be useful. Here the term *framework* is used as suggested by Crick and Koch (2003).

This situation is similar to one that arose several years ago in an examination of methods used at that time to treat anorexia nervosa and other eating disorders. These methods were also marginally effective, being based on assumptions that did not take into consideration either the physiology of starvation or the biology of the brain (Södersten et al., 2006a,b). To paraphrase Crick and Koch (2003), a point of view was developed to attack the problem of anorexia nervosa. Two suggestions were made: first, that disordered eating emerges because starvation recruits a brain substrate for reward; second, that anorexic behavior is maintained through conditioning to the situations in which the reward was originally provided (Bergh & Södersten, 1996).

This framework was plausible, given the data available from animal studies. Food deprivation enhances dopamine release in the terminal region of the mesolimbic dopamine neurons in the ventral striatum. The mesolimbic dopamine system is engaged in behavioral events perceived as rewarding (see Chapter 4). Moreover, norepinephrine neurons of the locus coeruleus are activated indirectly via the enhanced secretion of corticotropin-releasing factor in a state of food deprivation. The cell bodies of the locus coeruleus, which project to mid- and forebrain structures, are engaged when attentional mechanisms are activated and constitute a neural substrate required for learning (reviewed by Zandian et al., 2007). This framework suggested testable clinical hypotheses. First, patients with anorexia nervosa and other eating disorders should be able to relearn how to eat. Second, because starvation induces increased physical activity and reduced body temperature (Wang et al., 2006), anorexic hyperactivity should be reduced if the patients are kept warm, as was first suggested by Gull in 1874.

The effect of combining these interventions was evaluated in a randomized, controlled trial against a control group that received no treatment (Bergh et al., 2002). The randomized, controlled trial is considered to be the gold standard to determine the effectiveness of clinical interventions because it parallels the proper procedure of basic science (Smith, 2006). Relatively few exclusion criteria were used; patients with unspecified eating disorders and those who were in need of acute medical attention did not participate. Both anorexic ($n = 19$) and bulimic ($n = 13$) patients were included. The anorexics were younger (median 16 years old; range 10–33) than the bulimics (median 19 years old; range 15–54). The duration of the illness (2 years; range 0–21) and the number of previous treatments (3; range 1–15) were similar between the anorexic and bulimic groups and not used as exclusion criteria. The median BMI of the anorexic patients was 15 (10.8–17.5); that of the bulimic patients was in the normal range (21.6; 17.9–31.8), with the exception of one obese patient. Symptoms of depression, anxiety, and obsession are seen in all eating-disorder patients, including the patients in this study, who also scored high on an eating-disorder inventory.

These patient characteristics are similar to those of patients participating in many other studies, with the exception that many fewer exclusion criteria were adopted for this study. In addition, anorexia and bulimia were considered to be two phases of the same disorder. Most commonly, anorexic and bulimic patients are kept separate when the effect of treatment is evaluated. The hope in using few exclusion criteria was to demonstrate that the principles of treatment were applicable to at least two feeding disorders with partially overlapping characteristics.

A successful outcome was characterized by the following criteria: (1) BMI should return to normal and be sustained in the anorexic patients. (2) Bulimics should stop binge-eating for at least 3 months. (3) Eating behavior, psychiatric profile, and laboratory tests should become normal. Patients should be able to state (4) that food and body weight were no longer problems and (5) that they had to return to school or professional activities. To be in remission, a patient had to meet all these criteria. These are strict remission criteria, which are generally not met in most outcome studies on patients with eating disorders (Södersten et al., 2006b).

Figure 13.4 shows that treatment significantly affected the number of patients going into remission. Half of the treated patients went into remission within

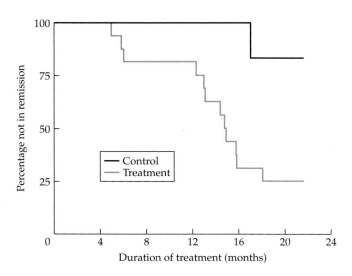

FIGURE 13.4 Outcome of treatment versus no treatment of patients with anorexia or bulimia nervosa. Each group contained 16 patients. (Data from Bergh et al., 2002, reproduced with permission.)

an average of 14 months, but only one of these treated patients went into remission spontaneously.

Because relapse is a serious problem once patients with eating disorders have been treated to the point of remission (Walsh et al., 2006), patients are followed for 5 years after treatment. Fewer than 10% of the patients relapse during this period of follow-up (Bergh et al., 2002).

These results show that the treatment had a major effect. To paraphrase Crick and Koch (2003) once more, this framework for anorexia nervosa has, so far, turned out to be largely correct, although of course it is unlikely to be correct in all details. For example, it is not known which, if any, of the interventions that were used is more important than any other.

A treatment of obesity

"A framework often contains unstated (and often unrecognized) assumptions" (Crick and Koch, 2003). An assumption that emerged from the framework for anorexia is that obesity is at the opposite extreme of the same continuum as anorexia. In line with this view, it was recently pointed out that, from a metabolic perspective, "caloric restriction [i.e., starvation] and metabolic syndrome [i.e., obesity] lie at the opposite ends of the same spectrum and so involve an overlapping set of regulators" (Guarente, 2006). Starvation and obesity are also at different ends of the same continuum from a behavioral perspective. Thus, whereas anorexic patients display reduced consummatory ingestive behavior and increased appetitive ingestive behavior (Tappe et al., 1998; discussed earlier), obese subjects behave in the opposite way. That is, compared to normal-weight subjects, they eat more if the food is easily available but less if eating demands an effort (Sclafani & Springer, 1976; Schachter, 1971).

The tests of this hypothesis were perhaps somewhat unusual. Presented with a choice between nuts with or without shells, obese subjects readily ingested nuts with no shells but ignored the nuts if it was necessary to remove the shells before eating them. By contrast, the presence or absence of the shell was irrelevant for normal-weight subjects, who were less likely to eat nuts without shells and more likely to eat nuts with shells than were obese subjects (Schachter, 1971). Furthermore, obese subjects were less likely to eat Chinese food with chopsticks, a more demanding task, than with silverware; whereas normal-weight subjects were more likely to try the chopsticks (Schachter, 1971). These interesting early studies have recently been extended by several observations that convenient access to food facilitates eating (Wansink, 2004), and a recent theory suggests that "reductions in the time costs of food" are a main cause of obesity (Cutler et al., 2003).

On the basis of these observations, it should be possible to treat obesity using procedures conceptually similar to those used for the treatment of anorexia nervosa. Whereas anorexics are encouraged to increase their eating rate, obese subjects are encouraged to slow down their eating.

A core intervention in anorexia treatment is changing the patient's eating pattern. Therefore, it was predicted that the pattern of eating behavior, and not the patient's psychological state, is what had to be addressed. Anorexic patients with BMIs as low as <14 kg/m^2 ($n = 27$) and up to 17.5 ($n = 18$), with psychological symptoms that differed markedly from normal on a standardized self rating scale (Svanborg & Åsberg, 1994), were studied (Zandian et al., 2007). The hypothesis was verified: relearning how to eat normalized both the BMI and the psychological symptoms in both groups of anorexics studied, including those with extraordinary low BMIs (Zandian et al., in press).

These findings predicted that gaining *control of obese individuals' meal patterns*, as in anorexics, would alleviate their symptoms. A radical additional prediction was that the critical variable was not the type of food eaten so much as the meal patterns.

Normal human eating behavior

Humans show a big variation in the amount of food they consume from day to day (Figure 13.5). Under normal conditions, many individuals control their eating, protecting against eating too little rather than eating too much. Because this pattern of behavior is practiced for long periods of time, such individuals are at greater risk of becoming overweight (Periwal & Chow, 2006). In addition, considering that food intake in humans in everyday life is affected by a variety of factors, most of which are not compensated for by homeostatic controls (de Castro & Plunkett, 2002; Cutler et al., 2003; Wansink, 2004), humans were hypothesized to require external support to reduce body weight. Curtailing the peaks and troughs of the daily variation in food intake (Periwal & Chow, 2006) might protect against eating too much and, in the long term, against obesity and its return.

A pilot study on obese adolescents

PATIENTS   Seven girls (median age 15.5 years; range 11–17) were recruited from the Childhood Obesity Clinic in Bristol, England. Their median BMI was 39.1 kg/m^2 (34.4–50.5), and they were considered resistant to standard therapy such as diet intervention and programs for physical activity. Six children had at least one obese parent, three had at least one absent parent, four had at least one parent who was being treated either for alcoholism or a psychiatric illness, and two were not attending school. Extensive social problems were universal within the group. The patients were not dysmorphic and had no underlying endocrine or metabolic cause for their obesity. Together, the extreme obesity and the social situation of these patients made them poor candidates for successful interventions, as their records indicated.

One patient, a 13-year-old with a BMI of 50.5, has a heterozygous mutation of the melanocortin-4 receptor (MC4R) gene (Farooqi et al., 2003). Insufficiency of this receptor in humans is thought to be "the most common monogenetic *cause*

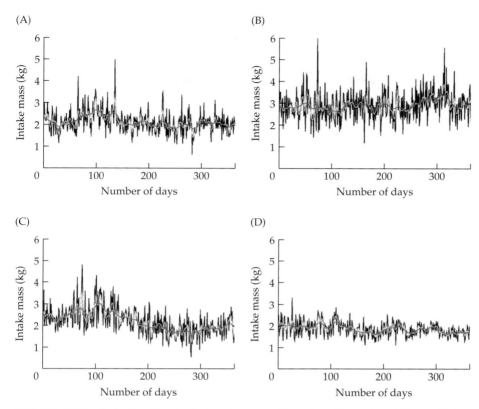

FIGURE 13.5 Daily food intake in four humans. (Data from Periwal and Chow, 2006, reproduced with permission.)

of severe obesity" (Farooqi et al., 2003, italics added), and humans with this deficiency are considered unable to regulate their eating behavior because a neural satiety mechanism has been disrupted (Cone, 2005). The possibility that the morbid obesity of this patient might be reduced by a change in eating habit was particularly interesting.

APPARATUS, QUESTIONNAIRES, AND PROCEDURE   The patients were trained to eat using the Mandometer, a scale that is connected to a computer. A plate of food is placed on the scale, and the computer stores the weight loss of the plate during feeding to yield a curve of eating rate. At regular intervals, a rating scale appears on the computer screen. The patient indicates her experience of fullness on the monitor, which is also stored. This process yields a curve of satiety development. A screening test at admission identified a target rate of food intake for each patient, which was programmed into the computer and used to train normal eating patterns. A linear depiction of eating rate was displayed on the computer screen and the patient was asked to adjust her eating to this function. Such adjustment was possible because the patient could see her own eating rate appear on the screen during the meal. The following values were used for the training curve: breakfast, 125 to 250 grams eaten within 6 to 10 minutes; morning and afternoon snacks, 100 to 120 grams eaten within 5 to 10 minutes; and lunch and dinner, 290 to 400 grams eaten within 12 to 15 minutes.

A sigmoid curve, starting at 0 and ending at 10, for training meal-associated satiety (Bergh et al., 2002) was displayed on the monitor at 1-minute intervals at all meals, and the patient rated her level of fullness by pressing on a touch screen. Healthy volunteers ate 300 to 350 grams within 10 to 15 minutes and rated their satiety at about 5 to 6 under these conditions (Bergh et al., 2002). In this protocol it is important not to modify patients' diets but rather to allow them to choose a wide variety of food and drink. The reason is that the patients said that they often felt hungry when on diets and they felt ashamed of being both overweight and hungry. Patients were able to use the Mandometer in their home settings with each dinner because the device is lightweight, is easy to carry, and runs on rechargeable batteries.

Patients also filled in the Eating Disorder Inventory, a self-rating questionnaire for eating-disorder symptoms (Garner, 1991), and the Comprehensive Psychopathological Rating Scale Self-Rating Scale for Affective Syndromes (CPRS-SA; Svanborg & Åsberg, 1994). The CPRS-SA measures obsessive-compulsive behaviors, anxiety, and depression. Body weight and height were determined at monthly to bimonthly visits. The patients were also tested using the training system without the normal eating guide to evaluate change in rate and amount eaten.

RESULTS   On average, patients initially ate a large amount of food (median 413 grams; range 219–775) at a high rate (median 40 grams per minute; range 20–50) when unassisted by training. These measures were reduced significantly—food intake to a median of 290 grams (168–344; $p = 0.043$), eating rate to a median of 20 grams per minute (13–29; $p = 0.028$; Wilcoxon test)—within on average 62 days (42–185) of treatment and before any change in BMI could be observed. The perception of satiety was low in three patients, but it normalized rapidly and was normal in the other patients (data not shown).

Two patients failed to comply with the treatment. One had lost weight at the time of dropout (BMI = –1.3 after 142 days of treatment), and one had gained weight (BMI = 2.4 after 364 days of treatment). The five other patients had remained in the study for a mean of 617 days (482–651) when treatment was terminated. Figure 13.6 shows that there was a significant change in BMI accrual before and during treatment.

Three patients (Patients 7, 8, and 10; Figure 13.7) had improved BMI; their BMIs decreased by 2.3, 3.4, and 8.8 kg/m² , respectively. At follow-up 7 months after treatment, their BMIs had increased only slightly—by 0.4, 0.5, and 0.9 kg/m² , respectively—and remained low at follow-up 1 year after treatment in two patients—having changed by –0.5 and 1.7 kg/m² , respectively—compared

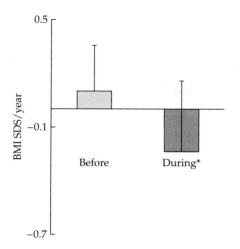

FIGURE 13.6   Change in BMI before and during treatment in five obese children. Standard deviation scores (SDSs) were generated from the 1990 British growth data using LMS curves generated by the Child Growth Foundation (Cole et al., 1998) and converted to change per year. The BMI development before treatment was based on a mean of 330 (318–384) days. *p = 0.024, paired t-test.

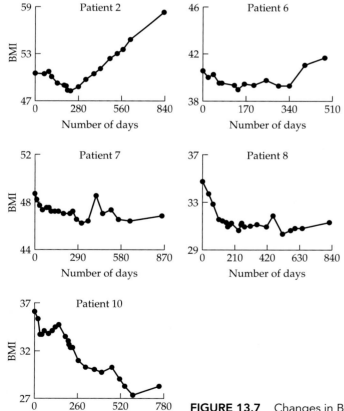

FIGURE 13.7   Changes in BMI in five obese adolescent patients during treatment.

to the value at the end of treatment. The third patient had also lost weight 1 year after treatment, but she had been treated with orlistat outside the study protocol during one month, so her data were not considered.

None of the patients showed signs of having an eating disorder, as indicated by normal scores on the Eating Disorder Inventory (data not shown), and the three patients who managed to reduce their body weight also had normal levels of psychiatric symptoms on the CPRS-SA rating scale (data not shown).

The two other patients (Patients 2 and 6; Figure 13.7) also improved their BMIs initially. The level of psychiatric symptoms was initially high in these patients but decreased as they lost weight. However, maternal suicidal intent led to an increase in psychiatric symptoms and BMI in one of these patients (Patient 6), who was prescribed antidepressant medication.

Interestingly, the patient who has an MC4R gene mutation and had an extremely high BMI (50.5) at the start of the study (Patient 2) initially reported that she could not feel satiety. At that time she consumed a very large test meal (600 grams) at a very high rate (50 grams per minute). By contrast, after 62 days of treatment she reported being able to feel full for the first time ever, and she consumed a normal test meal (312 grams) at a normal rate (16 grams per minute). Unfortunately, paternal interference in compliance with treatment led to weight regain and an increase in psychiatric symptoms.

DISCUSSION   All patients in this preliminary study had been previously treated without success using standard lifestyle modification. All had major social problems, reflecting their living in dysfunctional settings. The prognosis for these adolescent girls was bleak. Yet five of the seven, including one who dropped out of the program, lost weight during training; and three maintained this improvement for one-half to a full year after treatment. Two other patients also improved their BMIs initially, but increased complexities in their already complicated home situations may have compromised their ability to lose additional weight.

Although these results must be viewed with caution, it is interesting that body weight was affected at all, because the patients were morbidly obese and had proven resistant to treatment. All of these patients would have met the exclusion criteria commonly used in studies on the effect of pharmacological interventions to combat obesity (e.g., Despres et al., 2005; van Gaal et al., 2005). Yet the effect obtained in three patients was as large as, or larger than, that reported in previous pharmacological studies (e.g., Despres et al., 2005; van Gaal et al., 2005).

When first tested, six of the seven patients either ate an abnormally large meal or ate at an abnormally high rate. Only one participant (BMI = 34.7) ate a normal-sized meal (330 grams) at a normal rate (20 grams per minute). More interestingly, eating rate normalized in all patients before an effect on BMI was observed (within, on average, 2 months of treatment). Patients were intentionally not required to modify their diet. These pilot results generate the hypothesis that normal eating behavior may be a prerequisite for losing weight and more important than a change in diet.

The melanocortin system in the hypothalamus and brainstem is thought to play a role in satiety and body weight regulation, and "haploinsufficiency of the MC4R in humans is the most common monogenetic cause of severe obesity" (Farooqi et al., 2003). In line with this hypothesis, the patient with the MC4R gene mutation in the present study had a very high BMI (50 kg/m^2) and ate a very large meal (600 grams) at a very high rate (50 grams per minute) when first tested. She also reported being unable to perceive satiety. However, and more interesting, as she learned to eat a normal-sized meal at a normal rate, she reported feeling fullness for the first time, and she lost weight. Perhaps equally interesting, she experienced simultaneous relief from psychiatric symptoms. Unfortunately, because of parental interference, she was unable to comply with the study protocol for more than about 330 days, and at that time she relapsed into weight gain and developed psychiatric symptoms again.

Although the data from this patient must be interpreted with caution, they raise the possibility that normal eating behavior and the perception of satiety are possible in the absence of functional MC4Rs. As a corollary hypothesis, we suggest that obese patients with genetic "disorders" may be more dependent on external support for the control of body weight than are patients without such "disorders." The term *disorders* is in quotation marks here because under normal human conditions—that is, marked variations in the availability of food as discussed earlier—it has been suggested that mutation of the MC4R is a "thrifty" genotype (Cone, 2000) rather than a disorder.

Weight reduction in patients with binge-eating disorder

In 1959, Stunkard pointed out that about 15% of patients who are obese have a pattern of eating behavior characterized by loss of control and overeating of large quantities of food, which is referred to as *binge-eating disorder (BED)*. Behaviorally, BED patients are similar to bulimic patients, but they do not vomit and, as a consequence, they are obese. Behavioral methods are often ineffective in reducing body weight in BED patients (Stunkard & Alison, 2003), but pharmacological treatment, although often associated with unpleasant side effects, can be effective (Appolinario et al., 2003). Obesity surgery can also be effective, but BED can persist after surgery (Latner et al., 2004). The present framework predicts that reversal of disordered eating is important for reducing body weight in obese patients. The results of a preliminary study of BED patients verify this derived hypothesis.

PATIENTS   Eighteen female BED patients (median 34 years old, range 22–61; median BMI 36, range 25–46.3) were treated with the Mandometer procedure described earlier. No exclusion criteria were adopted.

RESULTS   Three of the patients are still in treatment. The other patients were treated to the point of remission in a median of 9 months (3–15). Three of the

FIGURE 13.8 Loss of body weight in 11 adult women with binge-eating disorder from admission to remission, and at a 1-year follow-up.

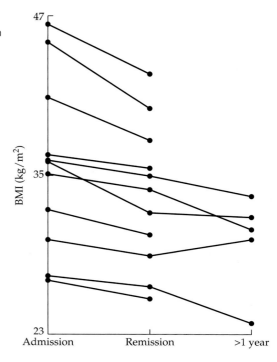

four women who had been treated surgically lost weight, decreasing BMI from 44.2 to 40.2, 27.6 to 24.6, and 25.4 to 23.6, respectively; the fourth patient gained weight, increasing BMI from 28 to 30.3.

Figure 13.8 shows that all other patients lost weight. Four have maintained their reduced weight for at least 2 years (2, 3, 3, and 5 years, respectively). Another patient lost only a little weight, which she had regained by the 1-year follow-up. The rest of the patients have not yet had extensive follow-up.

DISCUSSION These results from BED patients offer further early support for the hypothesis that control of eating behavior is an important intervention in the management of obesity, although the method described here has not yet brought body weight down to the normal level in more than one patient (BMI = 23.8 at the bottom right in Figure 13.8). The fact that the BED patients had a highly variable BMI at admission, varying as much as from a minimum of 25 to a maximum of 46.3, offers further support for this hypothesis.

Summary

This chapter is founded on the confluence of three factors concerning obesity:

1. The failure of even contemporary homeostatic approaches to feeding to gain any traction on what is rapidly becoming a leading worldwide public health issue in nonpoor societies.

2. The abject failure of all diets, since their inception almost a century ago, to effect body weight loss during the intermediate or long term. Weight that is lost through dieting is reinstated after a leveling-off period. For some, this cycle of weight loss and reinstatement is repeated many times over.

3. The success of the approach to feeding disorders (namely, the disorders of anorexia nervosa and bulimia—both disorders of insufficient intake and retention) on the opposite end of the spectrum described here is encouraging.

Together, these considerations have given rise to a framework to counteract obesity. Because success in the most difficult instance predicts success in less difficult cases, the new framework was tested in seven women with a mean BMI of 39.1. Six of the seven reduced both meal size and eating rate through the feedback procedure, and three of the six either held their weight loss or even extended it when the treatment phase terminated. These early data, along with the data from very obese patients with binge-eating disorder, are of interest because the prognoses for patients of this stature were dim in the extreme. Because this is the first preliminary report of this approach, there is room for improvement either by combining eating changes with appropriate exercise regimes and/or by introducing variants in Mandometer usage. Because the approach is simple and far less expensive than other forms of dieting, it should become readily available in the public sector.[1]

Acknowledgments

We thank the National Health Service, the Information Centre, and the Department of the Environment, Food and Rural Affairs for permission to reproduce the data in Figure 13.1. Professor Carson Chow kindly permitted us to reproduce Figure 13.5, and the American Physiological Society granted us permission to reproduce Figures 13.2 and 13.5. We thank the National Academy of Sciences for permission to reproduce Figure 13.4. We also thank Professor Stafford Lightman for help in initiating the study on obese adolescents and the patients for participating. Professor Elliott Blass, highly interactive editor of this book, questioned all of the obscurities that we produced in the earlier versions of this paper and made writing challenging, rewarding, and endlessly entertaining.

---

[1]A randomized, controlled trial using a Mandometer in 100 obese adolescents, some carrying an MC4R mutation currently conducted through the Bristol obesity clinic, should further inform these preliminary findings.

References Cited

Adam-Perrot, A., Clifton, P., Brouns, F. (2006). Low-carbohydrate diets: nutritional and physiological aspects. *Obesity Reviews, 7,* 49–58.

Ammar, A. A., Sederholm, F., Saito, T. R., Scheurink, A. J., Johnson, A. E., & Södersten, P. (2000). NPY- leptin: opposing effects on appetitive and consummatory ingestive behavior and sexual behavior. *American Journal of Physiology – Regulatory, Integrative and Comparative Physiology, 278,* R1627–R1633.

Appolinario, J. C., Bacaltchuk, J., Sichieri, R., Claudino, A. M., Godoy-Matos, A., Morgan, C., et al. (2003). A randomized, double-blind, placebo-controlled study of sibutramine in the treatment of binge-eating disorder. *Archives of General Psychiatry, 60,* 1109–1116.

Beck, B. (2006). Neuropeptide Y in normal eating and in genetic and dietary-induced obesity. *Philosophical Transactions of the Royal Society of London B, 361,* 1159–1185.

Benoit, S. C., Clegg, D. J., Woods, S. C., & Seeley, R. J. (2005). The role of previous exposure in the appetitive and consummatory effects of orexigenic neuropeptide. *Peptides, 26,* 751–757.

Bergh, C., Brodin, U., Lindberg, G., & Södersten, P. (2002). Randomized controlled trial of a treatment for anorexia and bulimia nervosa. *Proceedings of the National Academy of Sciences, USA, 99,* 9486–9491.

Bergh, C., & Södersten P. (1996). Anorexia nervosa, self-starvation and the reward of stress. *Nature Medicine, 2,* 21–22.

Bernard, C. (1927). *An introduction to the study of experimental medicine* (H. C. Greene, Trans.). New York: Dover Publications. (Reprinted from original work published 1865.)

Cole, T. J., Freeman, J. B., & Preece, M. A. (1998). British 1990 growth reference centiles for weight, height, body mass index and head circumference fitted by maximum penalized likelihood. *Statistics in Medicine, 17,* 407–429.

Cone, R. D. (2000). Haploinsufficiency of the melanocortin-4 receptor: part of a thrifty genotype? *Journal of Clinical Investigation, 106,* 185–187.

Cone, R. D. (2005). Anatomy and regulation of the central melanocortin system. *Nature Neuroscience, 8,* 571–578.

Craig, W. (1918). Appetites and aversions as constituents of instinct. *Biological Bulletin, 34,* 91–107.

Crick, F., & Koch, C. (2003). A framework for consciousness. *Nature Neuroscience, 6,* 119–126.

Cutler, D. M., Glaeser E. L., & Shapiro J. M. (2003). Why have Americans become more obese? *Journal of Economic Perspectives, 17,* 93–118.

Dansinger, M. L., Gleason, J. A., Griffith, J. L., Selker, H. P., & Schaefer, E. J. (2005). Comparison of the Atkins, Ornish, Weight Watchers, and Zone Diets for weight loss and heart disease risk reduction: a randomized trial. *Journal of the American Medical Association, 293,* 43–53.

Dansinger, M. L., & Schaefer, E. J. (2006). Low-fat diets and weight change. *Journal of the American Medical Association, 295,* 94–95.

de Castro, J. M., & Plunkett, S. A. (2002). General model of intake regulation. *Neuroscience and Biobehavioral Reviews, 26,* 581–595.

Department of the Environment, Food and Rural Affairs. (2001). National Food Survey. http://statistics.defra.gov.uk/esg/publications/nfs/datasets/nutshist.xls

Despres, J. P., Golay, A., & Sjöström, L., (2005). Rimonabant in Obesity-Lipids Study Group. Effects of rimonabant on metabolic risk factors in overweight patients with dyslipidemia. *New England Journal of Medicine, 353,* 2121–2134.

Drake, A. J., Smith, A., Betts, P. R., Crowne, E. C., & Shield, J. P. (2002). Type 2 diabetes in obese white children. *Archives of disease in childhood, 86,* 207–208.

Farooqi, I. S., Keogh, J. M., Yeo, G. S. H., Lank, E. J., Cheetham, T., & O'Rahilly, S. (2003). Clinical Spectrum of Obesity and Mutations in the Melanocortin 4 Receptor Gene. *New England Journal of Medicine, 348,* 1085–1095.

Floud, R. (1998). Height, weight and body mass of the British population since 1820. *Historical paper No. 108.* Cambridge, MA: National Bureau of Economic Research. Retrieved December 30, 2007, from

http://papers.ssrn.com/sol3/displayab
stractsearch.cfm

Fogel, R., Floud, R., & Harris, B. (in press). *Our Changing Bodies: 300 Years of Technophysico Evolution*. Cambridge: Cambridge University Press.

Forsell, P., & Hellers, G. (1997). The Swedish Adjustable Gastric Banding (SAGB) for morbid obesity: 9 year experience and a 4-year follow-up of patients operated with a new adjustable band. *Obesity Surgery, 7*, 345–351.

Franks, P. W., Loos, R. J., Brage, S., O'Rahilly, S., Wareham, N. J., & Ekelund, U. (2007). Physical activity energy expenditure may mediate the relationship between plasma leptin levels and worsening insulin resistance independently of adiposity. *Journal of Applied Physiology, 102,* 1921–1926.

Fulton, S., Woodside, B., & Shizgal, P. (2000). Modulation of brain reward circuitry by leptin. *Science, 287*, 125–128.

Garner, D. M. (1991). *Eating Disorder Inventory-2*. Odessa, FL: Psychological Assessment Resources.

Gendall, K. A., Kaye, W. H., Altemus, M., McConaha, C. W., & La Via, M. C. (1999). Leptin, neuropeptide Y, and peptide YY in long-term recovered eating disorder patients. *Biological Psychiatry, 46,* 292–299.

Goldstone, A. P., Unmehopa, U. A., Bloom, S. R., & Swaab, D. F. (2002). Hypothalamic NPY and agouti related protein are increased in human illness but not in Prader–Willi syndrome and other obese subjects. *Journal of Clinical Endocrinology and Metabolism, 87*, 927–937.

Grill, H. J., & Kaplan, J. M. (2002). The neuroanatomical axis for control of energy balance. *Frontiers in Neuroendocrinology, 23,* 2–40.

Guarente, L. (2006). Sirtuins as potential targets for metabolic syndrome. *Nature, 444,* 868–874.

Gull, W. W. (1874). Anorexia nervosa (apepsia hysterica, anorexia hysterica). *Transaction of the Clinical Society, London, 7*, 22–28.

Howard, B. V., Manson, J. E., Stefanick, M. L., Beresford, S. A., Frank, G., Jones, B., et al. (2006). Low-fat dietary pattern and weight change over 7 years: the Women's Health Initiative Dietary Modification Trial. *Journal of the American Medical Association, 295*, 39–49.

Keen-Rhinehart, E., & Bartness, T. J. (2007). NPY Y1 receptor is involved in ghrelin- and fasting induced increases in foraging, food hoarding and intake. *American Journal of Physiology – Regulatory, Integrative and Comparative Physiology, 292*, R1728–R1737.

Keys, A., Longstreet Taylor, H., Blackburn, H., Brozek, J., Naderson, J. T., & Simonson, E. (1963). Coronary heart disease among Minnesota business and professional men followed fifteen years. *Circulation, 28,* 381–395.

Korner, J., Inabnet, W., Conwell, I. M., Taveras, C., Daud, A., Olivero-Rivera, L., et al. (2006). Differential effects of gastric bypass and banding on circulating gut hormone and leptin levels. *Obesity, 14*, 1553–1561.

Latner, J. D., Wetzler, S., Goodman, E. R., & Glinski, J. (2004). Gastric bypass in a low-income, inner-city population: eating disturbances and weight loss. *Obesity Research, 12*, 956–961.

Malik, V. S., & Hu, F. B. (2007). Popular weight-loss diets: from evidence to practice. *Nature Clinical Practice – Cardiovascular Medicine, 4*, 34–41.

Murphy, K. G., & Bloom, S. R. (2006). Gut hormones and the regulation of energy homeostasis. *Nature, 444*, 854–859.

Näslund, E., & Kral, J. G. (2006). Impact of gastric bypass surgery on gut hormones and glucose homeostasis in type 2 diabetes. *Diabetes, 55*, S92–S97.

Nath, D., Heemels, M.-T., & Anson, L. (2006). Obesity and diabetes. *Nature, 444*, 839.

National Health Service. (2004). *The Information Centre*. Retrieved December 30, 2007, from www.ic.nhs.uk/webfiles/pub lications/hlthsvyeng2004upd/HealthSurv eyForEnglandTrendTables161205_XLS.xls

Norris, S. L., Zhang, X., Avenell, A., Gregg, E., Schmid, C. H., & Lau, J. (2005). Long-term non-pharmacological weight loss interventions for adults with prediabetes. *Cochrane Database of Systematic Reviews, 2*, Article CD005270.

Oddy, D. J. (2003). *From Plain Fare to Fusion Food. British diets from 1890 to the 1990*. Woodbridge, Suffolk: Boydell Press.

O'Shea, D., Morgan, D. G., Meeran, K., Edwards, C. M., Turton, M. D., Choi, S. J., et al. (1997). Neuropeptide Y induced feeding in the rat is mediated by a novel receptor. *Endocrinology, 138*, 196–202.

Padwal, R. S., & Majumdar, S. R. (2007). Drug treatments for obesity: orlistat, sibutramine, and rimonabant. *Lancet, 369,* 71–77.

Paul, M. J., Freeman, D. A., Park, J. H., & Dark, J. (2005). Neuropeptide Y induces torpor-like hypothermia in Siberian hamsters. *Brain Research, 1055,* 83–92.

Periwal, V., & Chow, C. V. (2006). Patterns in food intake correlate with body mass index. *American Journal of Physiology – Endocrinology and Metabolism, 291,* E929–E936.

Pi-Sunyer, F. X., Aronne, L. J., Heshmati, H. M., Devin, J., & Rosenstock, J.; RIO-North America Study Group. (2006). Effect of rimonabant, a cannabinoid-1 receptor blocker, on weight and cardiometabolic risk factors in overweight or obese patients: RIO- North America: a randomized controlled trial. *Journal of the American Medical Association, 295,* 761–775.

Rosenbaum, M., Goldsmith, R., Bloomfield, D., Magnano, A., Weimer, L., Heymsfield, S., et al. (2005). Low-dose leptin reverses skeletal muscle, autonomic, and neuroendocrine adaptations to maintenance of reduced weight. *Journal of Clinical Investigation, 115,* 3579–3586.

Ruffin, M. P., Adage, T., Kuipers, F., Strubbe, J. H., Scheurink, A. J., & van Dijk, G. (2004). Feeding and temperature responses to intravenous leptin infusion are differential predictors of obesity in rats. *American Journal of Physiology – Regulatory, Integrative and Comparative Physiology, 286,* R756–R763.

Schachter, S. (1971). Some extraordinary facts about obese humans and rats. *American Psychologist, 26,* 129–144.

Sclafani, A., & Springer, D. (1976). Dietary obesity in adult rats: similarities to hypothalamic and human obesity syndromes. *Physiology & Behavior, 17,* 461–471.

Sherrington, C. H. (1906). *The Integrative Action of the Nervous System.* New York: Charles Scribner's Sons.

Sjöström, L., Lindroos, A. K., Peltonen, M., Torgerson, J., Bouchard, C., Carlsson, B., et al.; Swedish Obese Subjects Study Scientific Group. (2004). Lifestyle, diabetes, and cardiovascular risk factors 10 years after bariatric surgery. *New England Journal of Medicine, 351,* 2683–2693.

Smith, R. (2006). *The Trouble with Medical Journals.* London: Royal Society of Medicine Press.

Södersten, P., Bergh, C., & Zandian, M. (2006a). Understanding eating disorders. *Hormones and Behavior, 50,* 572–578.

Södersten, P., Bergh, C., & Zandian, M. (2006b). The psychoneuroendocrinology of anorexia nervosa. *Psychoneuroendocrinology, 31,* 1149–1153.

Spiegel, A., Nabel, E., Volkow, N., Landis, S., & Li, T.-K. (2005). Obesity and the brain. *Nature Neuroscience, 8,* 552–553.

Stellar, E. (1954). The physiology of motivation. *Psychological Review, 61,* 5–22.

Stunkard, A. J. (1959). Eating patterns and obesity. *Psychiatric Quarterly, 33,* 284–292.

Stunkard, A. J., & Alison, A. J. (2003). Binge eating disorder: disorder or marker. *International Journal of Eating Disorders, 34,* S107–S116.

Summerbell, C. D., Ashton, V., Campbell, K. J., Edmunds, L., Kelly, S., & Waters, E. (2003). Interventions for treating obesity in children. *Cochrane Database System Reviews, 3,* Article CD001872.

Svanborg, P., & Åsberg, M. (1994). A new self-rating scale for depression and anxiety states based on the Comprehensive Psychopathological Rating Scale. *Acta Psychiatrica Scandinavica, 89,* 21–28.

Swan, G. (2004). Findings from the latest national diet and nutrition survey. *British Journal of Nutrition, 63,* 505–512.

Tappe, K. A., Gerberg, S. E., Shide, D. J., Andersen, A. E., & Rolls, B. J. (1998). Videotape assessment of changes in aberrant meal-time behaviors in anorexia nervosa after treatment. *Appetite, 30,* 171–184.

Toates, F. M., & Rowland, N. E. (1987). *Feeding and Drinking.* Amsterdam: Elsevier.

Van Gaal, L. F., Rissanen, A. M., Scheen, A. J., Ziegler, O., & Rössner, S.; RIO-Europe Study Group. (2005). Effects of the cannabinoid-1 receptor blocker rimonabant on weight reduction and cardiovascular risk factors in overweight patients: 1-year experience from the RIO-Europe study. *Lancet, 365,* 1389–1397.

Vilsboll, T., & Holst, J. J. (2004). Incretins, insulin secretion and Type 2 diabetes mellitus. *Diabetologia, 47,* 357–366.

Walsh, B. T., Kaplan, A. S., Attia, E., Olmsted, M., Parides, M., Carter, J. C., et al. (2006). Fluoxetine after weight restoration in anorexia nervosa: a randomized controlled trial. *Journal of the American Medical Association, 295,* 2605–2612.

Wang, T., Hung, C. C., & Randall, D. J. (2006). The comparative physiology of food deprivation: from feast to famine. *Annual Review of Physiology, 68,* 223–251.

Wansink, B. (2004). Environmental factors that increase the food intake and consumption volume of unknowing consumers. *Annual Review of Nutrition, 24,* 455–479.

Wittgenstein, L. (1980). *Culture and Value* (P. Winch, Trans.). G. H. von Wright (Ed.) (p. 40). Oxford: Blackwell.

Zandian, M., Ioakimidis, I., Bergh, C., & Södersten, P. (2007). Cause and treatment of anorexia nervosa. *Physiology & Behavior, 92,* 283–290.

Zhang, Y., & Scarpace, P. J. (2006). The role of leptin in leptin resistance and obesity. *Physiology & Behavior, 88,* 249–256.

EPILOGUE

Elliott M. Blass

Introduction

As editor of this multidisciplinary text, and as its first reader, I feel it appropriate to integrate the chapters and, for better or worse, provide my perspective of where the fields of obesity research, treatment, and prevention now stand, and where they might be headed. To that end, I make several general points.

First, the concept of obesity was raised in the preface: is obesity an attribute like height that varies along a continuum, or is excess weight a disease? We do not have a categorical term for very tall people. Yet the statement "obesity is a behavioral disorder" appears over and over, even in articles that eschew the derogatory treatment of obese people. Actually, *overweight* and *obesity* are classifications formulated by the insurance industry over 75 years ago to indicate the probability of morbidity or early mortality and to adjust rates accordingly (in fact, their data linking obesity to morbidity pre-dated the twentieth century).

The proper analogy here is smoking. A person who smokes is not necessarily sick by any medical criterion but is addicted to tobacco. Should smoking behavior continue, the odds of dying *because of smoking* are considerably increased. So, to the question, "Is an overweight or obese person sick at the time of treatment initiation?" the statistical answer is, probably not. However: (1) *health status must be absolutely evaluated by a physician at the decision point*; and (2) even if one is judged to be in good health, the odds ratios are greater that *overweight and especially obese people will develop an illness that is obesity related and provoked.*

Not to distinguish between present and potential future illness colors the perception of a person as sick, as opposed to occupying one end of a body mass continuum. Embracing this distinction makes for more humane health care delivery, thereby lowering the barrier for seeking consultation and support. Moreover, the decision to treat becomes more pointed when evaluators do not automatically see their clients' behaviors as disordered. If "perceptual neutrality" is established from the outset, say by providing the criteria for treatment, then recommendations of diet and/or exercise have the persuasive thrust of a differential diagnosis.

If obese people, as a group, are not classified as having a behavioral disorder, their perception of self will not automatically be that of a sick person. Failure to make this distinction has fueled the pattern of repeated and failed dieting because of the belief that "fat cannot be fit." There is merit to the case for "fat and fit," thereby questioning the need for extensive dieting that works in the short run but only very rarely is sustained. The controversy burns, with little sign of abatement. *Filiault*'s[1] take on it (see Chapter 8) is splendid: "It may be favorable to be both fit *and* trim."

Second, as *Bovbjerg* documents in Chapter 2, obesity is a long-standing public health issue that has spawned a multibillion-dollar industry. The amount of money involved not only in products that encourage slimness and weight loss but also in products that encourage overeating of energy-dense foods—with both product types often coming from different branches of the same megacorporation—has prompted Campos and others to express concern about vulnerability to hucksterism. Campos et al. (2006) and Eckel (2005; Eckel et al., 2006), among others, have argued that dieting does not improve morbidity or early mortality, but fitness does. In fact, a considerable literature draws the distinction between exercising as part of a diet program to facilitate weight loss and exercising as integral to a lifestyle.

In this context, the goal of changing physical activity is to diminish the consequences of being unfit, or having conditions such as cardiovascular disease or diabetes (Andersen et al., 1999; Dunn et al., 1999; Pratt, 1999, for two of the influential early reports and commentary on efficacy of lifestyle changes on metabolic and cardiovascular indices in the absence of weight loss). Regardless of the reasons for increasing physical activity, it is likely to be beneficial when supervised by a trainer and built up gradually. The long-term benefits of successful dieting, coupled with appropriate changes in lifestyle, must continue to be evaluated empirically and will be discussed extensively below.

Profiting off the vulnerable is not new. Today's concerns, however, are heightened by the scope and organization of advertising, marketing, and media,[2] along with the unparalleled influence of the fashion industries as arbiters of not only what to wear but also (especially) what size we should be.[3] There is some hope and encouragement, however. The influence of investing hundreds of millions of dollars in advertising foods of low nutritional value (FLNV) may start to

---

[1]In this epilogue, authors' names are italicized when their chapters in this book are referred to.

[2]I have found the online publication *Advertising Age*, www.adage.com, to be revealing and informative.

[3]There are about 75 monthly fashion periodicals in the United States alone, and the number of advertising pages continues to grow.

diminish with the reconsideration of Kellogg and, more recently, other top FLNV producers concerning advertising in media that are directed toward children[4] [*Harrison et al.* (Chapter 12)].

That said, however, the actions of normal-weight people who take in more calories than they expend are theirs alone. This is not to diminish the impact of social, societal, and mercantile forces that encourage the figures of supermodels but simultaneously prod consumers to eat more FLNV. These persuasive outside forces must be neutralized so that individuals are better able to reach healthier decisions before obesity onset. My own reading of the preceding chapters—as well as of literatures addressed to image-making, fast-food, and other like industries; and of literatures addressed to addiction, diet, and exercise—makes it clear to me that actions that can be taken at individual, group, community, and political levels to induce and sustain better and healthier decisions have at their core, the *necessity of working with and providing mutual support to others.*

Third, difficulties in effecting change abound at all levels and should never be underestimated. Indeed they are illuminated by lessons from Big Tobacco. Tobacco advertising budgets, which once ran to the hundreds of millions of dollars, targeted very specific audiences, including children who had not yet become smokers. Eventually Big Tobacco was forced to discontinue TV ads. After tobacco companies were obliged to release the damning results of their own studies on the harmful effects of smoking, which had been hidden for obvious reasons, tobacco was heavily taxed; and cigarettes now (August 2007) run about $5.50 a pack. Two things are noteworthy about this tawdry episode in the present context. First, when tobacco stocks went into freefall, it was the USDA that infused huge dollar amounts to stop it (US Department of Agriculture, 2007). In the present context, the USDA cannot be counted on to act primarily on behalf of the public welfare. Its base is agriculture, and it acts to protect agricultural interests, even when they might conflict with the public weal.

Increased tax, negative publicity, and the advent of "smoke-free" public spaces have reduced the incidence of smoking, although not by as much as one would suppose of a toxic product. Sadly, the largest increase of tobacco use is now among the young, who, undeterred, are starting the habit. To the extent that no good can come of smoking and that it increases the likelihood of a painful death, we start to appreciate the challenge of improving health decisions on a large scale. Given the biological imperative of eating, it is much more difficult to resist the temptation to selectively avoid particular foods. We have a long way to go. In fact, the public has sometimes ignored market decisions that could have

---

[4]The victory over Kellogg, which reduces advertising of FLNV by preventing such ads on shows in which half of the audience is 16 years of age or younger, is important. It must be remembered, however, that the plaintiffs received only a fraction of what they had sued for, that FLNV advertising can be directed to "family shows" that are watched by children. Most European countries have far more stringent restrictions. It comes as no surprise that there is considerable organized mercantile and political resistance in the United States to changes in advertising policies.

benefited customers. Recently General Mills, after the loss of some $30 million, pulled the less sweet, lower-calorie version of Kix cereal off the market. In this case a food manufacturer did the "right thing" in developing, producing, marketing, and distributing a more healthful product, but the public did not seize the moment.

Despite decades of research on the control of food intake, and the clinical efforts to contain overeating, we remain under a weight of obesity that has only increased in complexity and cost. The elements that may potentially combat the problem may be knit into an effective strategy based on the diverse literatures in this text. I will now identify, review, and evaluate these literatures and others, and I will express a more concise sense of where we now stand and where we might be heading.

Genetic Dispositions

Only the smallest number of morbid obesity conditions, such as Prader–Willi syndrome, can be attributed to single-gene causes. Analyses of genetic relationships, however, show strong obesity linkages among family members. Contemporary genetics and molecular analyses may provide products or treatments that can prevent or help treat obesity. We are not there yet. In addition, once such a product was created and tested, it would be a mistake to market it in a way that ignored the behavioral principles reviewed in various chapters herein, and their successors. Although they hold future promise, *genetic changes do not account for the explosion of the obesity phenotype* during the recent past, and the topic will not be addressed further.

Developmental Considerations

In Chapter 6, *Lumeng* raised a number of important themes of focal and general import that can be recruited toward a systematic defense against obesity development. One such theme is *responsibility toward others*: it is a given that parents are responsible for infant feeding and care—responsibilities that extend beyond weaning, even to when children leave home. The first opportunity for acting responsibly to prevent obesity is for women to target the lower end of their normal-weight distribution at the time of conception and during the first trimester of pregnancy. The second opportunity is for new mothers to engage in *breast-feeding*. Breast-fed infants, in addition to having received immunological benefits, weigh less at weaning and, importantly, have tasted the flavors of the mother's foods that filter into her milk. As *Lumeng* has demonstrated, two developmental obesity factors that leap forward in time are infant/child weight and diet variety that diminishes the constraints of neophobia to allow sampling more healthful foods—fruits and vegetables in particular. Maternal overweight or obesity at conception increases the likelihood of childhood obesity, possibly by curtailing the length of breast-feeding (Baker et al., 2007).

Developing Food Preferences

Classical conditioning is readily attained in newborns. As will be discussed in greater detail, food preferences are strongly influenced by prior flavor experiences, even prenatal ones (Mennella & Beauchamp, 1999; Pedersen & Blass, 1982; Schaal et al., 1995; Smotherman & Robinson, 1985), and by the postnatal social milieu. For the moment, recall the Rozin and Schiller (1980) report, discussed by *Lumeng* (see Chapter 6), of preference development for piquant foods by children in Mexican villages where young children are offered spicy chili that is being eaten by their family at the moment. Eventually, over the course of many meals and decisive rejections, the children accept the food to great cheers and congratulations, and the preference continues.

The chimpanzee report by Rozin and Kennel (1983) is also of considerable interest. Food was restricted for a number of months to a bitter, quinine-laced food, which the chimp was obliged to eat. When provided with a choice between the adulterated food and the bland standard diet, the former was rejected even though it had been the food that had sustained the animal. Later the well-fed chimp's beloved handler arrived eating the adulterated food, which the chimp readily accepted within the context of the social interactions during a meal. Now, the bitter food was accepted and, through ongoing social interactions that overwhelmed the bitter taste, became defined as "normative." Our own personal experiences with coffee, for example, confirm social facilitation as an everyday widespread occurrence. These profound social effects should be exploited by systematic expansion of the diets of infants and toddlers *to broaden their eating base* by feeding them a greater variety of foods, especially in the fruit and vegetable categories. Expanding the eating base helps protect against childhood obesity. Unfortunately, the time frame is limited because children are not very wont to accept new foods beyond 4 years of age.

Despite the extraordinary wealth of the United States, American children who attend public schools are served USDA-sponsored school meals that are minimally edible on the whole, and are at or below threshold nutritional value. Reflecting low palatability, the meals are increasingly rejected as children routinely purchase FLNV in the cafeteria itself, and at school-supported kiosks. A number of schools are on the verge of losing USDA-sponsored lunch and breakfast programs because of low purchase rates of the USDA-supported meals. As *Lumeng* and *Harrison et al.* report (see Chapters 6 and 12), schools have resisted removing FLNV from the school campus because the income that they generate allows badly stretched, restricted budgets to be met and underfunded programs to be saved.

A recent USDA-funded test program (Buzby et al., 2003) in which fruits were distributed gratis by parents, teachers, staff, and students in the hallways and various places on school grounds was successful because it reached all students, many of whom reported liking the fruits. Equally impressive, children in a number of the test schools reduced their intake of energy-dense foods at school, especially at breakfast. To my knowledge this report has languished, and its important findings have not been implemented on a national scale. These are exactly the types of empirically proven programs that provide agency to the participants and should be encouraged at a community level. I will return to these themes.

Social Determinants of Food Preference and Intake

I think it fair to say that conditioning processes cast the strongest influences over food selection and volume intake. Neophobia helps protect against sampling new foods, and sampled foods that cause sickness are shunned by both rats and humans—indeed, by all species that have been studied. Protection against negative consequences in omnivores is intuitive and immediately transparent. This powerful device can also be harnessed to help with weight loss and maintenance.

Positive affective conditioning has been studied recently in rats and humans, as reviewed by *Yeomans* in Chapter 7. The available literature highlights a number of findings. First, preferences can be formed and intake of neutral foods increased if they are associated with high-energy postingestive consequences. Preferences based on postingestive *nutritional effects* are much more difficult to obtain. Palatable, high-density foods tempt us in at least two ways. First, we universally seek sweet and fatty foods for their taste and flavor. Second, we eat more of these foods because of their ingestive history. These processes are separable neurologically. Whereas taste and flavor afferents exert direct control over brainstem mechanisms that integrate motor patterns of chewing and swallowing, acquired controls operate indirectly through the rostral portions of the brain that heighten positive affect and ramp up the intensity of urges and appetites. In principle, they are available through behavioral means to neutralize postabsorptive linkages to ingestion, thereby neutralizing feed-forward devices for overeating.

Other experiential, social events also gain control over food intake and ultimately body weight. A small taste of a delicious food whets our appetite as demonstrated in the research literature, and is known to us experientially. In Chapter 4, *Wise* teaches us about this fundamental attribute of motivational systems: a free "taste" of a drug strongly sustains drug-taking behavior and breaks the resistance of addicts who have been "clean" for a period of time. The studies of Hermann and colleagues (Hermann et al., 2003) and of de Castro (1994) have shown that unknowing "messages" sent by tablemates proximally influence the amount of food eaten. We eat more with friends and less with strangers. Hermann and colleagues have identified two "unknowing strategies" that, when clearly conveyed, constrain meal size. In the minimalist strategy, we peg our intake to that of the minimal eater. The other strategy links us to the person who eats the largest meal. Meals under this strategy fall short of the target. By identifying "normative intake," both strategies actually rein in eating. Participants who received ambiguous messages ate substantially larger meals (Leone et al., 2007). In principle, responsiveness to normalized standards can be turned to advantage through explicit support and "contractual" arrangements with family, peers, and friends.

In a remarkable study, Christakis and Fowler (2007) demonstrated that "normative standards" of eating—indeed, body weight—can be established *at a distance* by "critical" friends or relatives. Thus, even when a close friend who now lives in a distant city becomes obese, the "target" friend will more likely become obese too. To the extent that our behaviors are influenced by peers, the normative studies by Hermann, Polivy, and colleagues that show very strong proximal social influences on intake, and by Christakis and Fowler (2007), alert us to the possibility that the power of friends and siblings, whether at table or at a distance, can be harnessed to correct or avoid behaviors that we will later regret.

Rozin's reports of social factors overwhelming intensely unpalatable tastes, and the studies by Hermann, Christakis, and others on proximal and distal social determinants, combined with *Yeomans'* review of learning influences (see Chapter 7), demonstrate that social and associative factors determine palatability perception so that foods taste better for reasons that are independent of the individual's physiology or physical needs. Thus, eating a standard fast-food meal after a movie, just a few hours after dinner, with some overweight friends actually runs counter to our needs because, first, we do not need the extra calories (overweight and obese individuals, by definition, are in positive energy balance) and second, despite the caloric surfeit of fast foods, they are nutritionally deficient.

Thus, our experiences with and the circumstances of the meal might "make a food taste better" and can certainly diminish inhibitory signals arising from stomach and gut. Our feeding history becomes translated into hunger, despite positive balance, so that larger meals are eaten and changes in motivation, cognition, and perception diminish satiety and enhance palatability. In principle, recruiting experiential determinants of meal size and body weight to selectively reduce energy intake should prove useful in formulating weight loss strategies. Unfortunately, obese people are further trapped by their heightened hedonic experience from a given taste or flavor than are normal-weight individuals, as revealed by *Snyder and Bartoshuk's* remarkable set of findings (see Chapter 5).

Control of meal size

Both *Smith* (Chapter 1) and *Moran* (Chapter 3) have addressed some outcomes of decades of research on the controls of feeding behavior. The controls are impressive and express a harmony among mechanical (gastric distension), chemical (increased effective osmotic pressure), nutritional, and hormonal factors that coalesce to slow down a meal and bring it to a close. Moreover, as *Hetherington and Rolls* demonstrate in Chapter 10, gastric fill, independent of energy load, can also determine intake, so diluting meals can contribute to caloric reduction. Gastric distension interacts with the other controls of meal termination. Thus, a hypertonic load is more effective than an isotonic load.

The harmony, in principle, is expressed against a proximal background of energy expended since the last meal, through either length of time since having eaten or amount of energy burned off through work, exercise, or other forms of muscular activity, as discussed by *Filiault* in Chapter 8. Feeding is also moderated by long-term signals. The recent discoveries of ghrelin, leptin, and other signals that give impetus to the affective states of hunger and satiation in meal control hold promise for a harvest of new breakthroughs in our understanding of feeding, some of which may help to moderate human intake.

We are not yet there, however. The large portions of varied, appealing, energy-dense foods of contemporary Western feeding styles readily overturn short-term controls. Some perspective on overeating can be gained through evolutionary considerations that place a premium on seizing the safe moment to eat safe, bountiful, and energy-dense foods. Given that, historically, our primate and hominid forebears traversed great distances, and given the checks and balances of natural selection,[5] there was probably little pressure to defend against overweight.

Following the logic of maximizing intake in the face of (presumed) scarcity, competition, and danger, local inhibitory afferents should be relaxed when a large volume of safe, palatable, and varied food is available in a safe location. Cultural forces have also favored overeating. Traditionally obesity has been a sign of wealth, of being able to afford and have prepared vast quantities of food. There were probably few social or health costs to this practice because of the short life expectancies during the Victorian eras. Thus, historically, overeating has been prevalent among the wealthy. Today, however, overeating is distributed throughout the population, especially among poorer people for whom low-priced, tasty, and filling fast foods are affordable (see *Bovbjerg*'s related discussion in Chapter 2).

The first bite or two of a palatable meal or of small delicacies (the amuse-bouche of the French) increase hunger, delay satiety sensations, and extend meals. Satiety ratings at the ends of meals of vastly differing sizes were fairly constant, implying that *satiety sensations are defined by a meal's end as opposed to a meal's end being dictated by satiety sensations.*

Citing the report of Ammar and colleagues (2000), in Chapter 13 *Bergh et al.* raise another warning flag on the limits of our understanding of hormonal and neurohumoral controls of ingestion. Food was infused into the mouths of intact rats, which could either swallow or reject the infused food. The behavior obtained was *opposite* that predicted by studies in which rats either had to work for food or approach, chew, and move the food to the back of the mouth for the purposes of swallowing. In particular, *leptin enhanced food intake, and ghrelin reduced it*. These findings of opposite outcomes of hormonal and neurotransmit-

---

[5]Although this line of reasoning is plausible from today's distant perspective, it does *not* address the actual evolutionary determinants, which must be empirically documented. See Speakman, 2004, on this important issue.

ter determinants on what might be considered a consummatory facet of behavior highlight how early we are in our understanding of feeding determinants.

To the point of the current issue, the conceptual boundaries between appetitive and consummatory facets of feeding in normal-weight, overweight, and obese individuals may shift in ways that lead to opposite drug effects. For example, ghrelin might stimulate feeding in normal-weight and obese individuals who had to *work* for the food, while *at the same time inhibiting feeding in an obese eater* whose plate was heaped with food. It is not too early to propose that the line between *appetitive* and *consummatory* in this example may shift from moving food from front to back for swallowing purposes, to moving food from table to mouth. If this were true, then weight reduction through ghrelin or leptin would have to be under constrained circumstances because untoward opposite effects might be obtained.

All this notwithstanding, the animal and human literatures on food intake as documented by *Smith* and *Moran* (Chapters 1 and 3) have demonstrated body weight stability in all species studied, allowing for seasonal and reproductive cycles. In a sense the field has been blindsided by the burgeoning waistlines in Western societies, the United States in particular. Although some have clung to the idea that regulatory systems work and that obesity is storage of but a fraction of total long-term intake (Seely & Woods, 2003), the fact is that a national and rapidly worldwide condition exists that, for obese individuals, is a source of discomfort, objective underachievement, and threat of morbidity and early mortality, as described by *Bovbjerg* in Chapter 2. It is hardly surprising that many industries that generate massive dieting and treatment revenues, without improving the situation, have arisen in response.

Thus, obesity remains a problem. What, if anything, can be done about it? In the remainder of this essay I address the issue in four ways. First, I evaluate research on dieting. Second, I highlight common approaches to fitness and weight loss of successful dieters. Third, I present a new pragmatic conceptualization of obesity as an addiction. Fourth, within this framework I merge lessons in addiction treatment with the material in this text to provide guidelines on individual, group, and policy levels that might relieve current and prevent further obesity expansion.

Diet assessments

Prominently displayed diet books weigh down the shelves of bookstores as their authors make the talk show rounds. Dozens appear annually. Some even guarantee short-term 20-pound losses. Unfortunately, these diets almost never work in the long run; most of the weight returns within a year or so, and all of it within about 2 years. There is a paradox of great concern over weight and appearances, sacrifices made through dieting and exercise, cycles of weight loss, and return to starting weight; and after a while, the determination reappears and through advertising and word of mouth, "this year's" diet book is purchased and the cycle reborn.

The extensive literature on clinical trials has repeatedly demonstrated that diets work, pretty equally in fact, during the initial weight loss component. Weight *loss* may be helped by exercise, although that remains under debate. There is general agreement that exercise helps in weight *maintenance*. My impression of dieting resonates with that provided by the influential psychotherapist Jerome Frank (1971) in writing about psychotherapy. Frank's analogy was that judging the success of psychotherapy was akin to judging the success of a revival meeting. If the criterion is "a good time was had," then the meeting is deemed a success. Using the criterion of the number of people who approached the nave, then success is considerably more modest. When judged by the number of people whose religious behavior was changed in the long run, the meeting was hardly at all successful. The diet analogy is obvious. Why maintaining the lower weight that the dieter worked so hard to achieve is so difficult is not known, but lack of compliance is a bane in all of medicine, especially in branches that seek behavioral change.

DIET AND PHARMACOLOGY   At present, only one drug, sibutramine, has been approved by the FDA for long-term use in treating obesity. A second agent, orlistat, has been recently approved for over-the-counter sale. Reviewing some of the research on these agents is illuminating. Sibutramine acts centrally by affecting transporter molecules of serotonin and norepinephrine, which remain available longer in the synapse. When administered alone, sibutramine's effects are modest, although they improve in individuals whose intake has been reduced by 600 kilocalories per day. At the end of the weight loss phase, when drug therapy is discontinued, lost weight is regained within a year or so. Further research by the STORM (Sibutramine Trial of Obesity Reduction and Maintenance) study group, a consortium of European laboratories funded in part by BASF, the manufacturer of sibutramine, is revealing.

James and colleagues (2000), reporting in the prestigious journal *Lancet*, studied individuals who had lost 5% of their body weight during a 6-month period of taking 10 milligrams daily of sibutramine and reducing daily food intake by 600 kilocalories. They reported that only 467 of 605 people (77%) started and completed the 6-month run-up period. Of the 352 people who continued the program for the additional 18 months, 204 (58%) completed it; and of those, 89 (44%) hit the target goal of maintaining 80% of the loss. The assignment was made double-blind, and this protocol was followed until a patient in the sibutramine group had regained 1 kilogram of the lost weight, at which point the dose was increased to 15 milligrams daily. Additional gain of 1 kilogram triggered a dose of 20 milligrams daily. Of the 204 patients who completed the 18-month weight maintenance portion of the trial, 183 were at the highest dose allowed by the protocol. Although the authors claimed that maintenance was successful, Frank's admonition comes to mind. True, 43% of those who completed the 2-year trial hit the target goal. However, only 25% (89/352) of those who started maintenance succeeded. If the potential sibutramine assignments are reasonably considered to be 454 (0.75 × 605), the success rate of the drug drops to 20%.

All of these figures are correspondingly higher by a factor of three than the figures for control subjects who received the drug in only the first portion of the study, but still a 20% hit rate does not dazzle. Perspective on the odds of success can be evaluated against the probability of dropping out of the study. During the original 6-month run-up, 138 of all 605 treated participants either dropped out or did not meet the modest 5% weight loss (about 5.2 kilograms). Then, during the 18-month treatment phase, an additional 148 left the study. By the end of the study only 89 participants remained. So, from the perspective of remaining in the study till the end, only 89 were "left standing" whereas 286 had fallen by the way. We will not even discuss the side effects of the drug, or the fact that the dose had to be increased by a factor of two for the vast majority of the participants in order to maintain target weight. The lesson is clear. Careful scrutiny of the claim that a majority of the 77% who lost weight kept the weight off reveals that, in fact, only 20% of those who started the diet achieved criterion.

Another representative study is also informative. This one, by Wadden and colleagues (2005), assessed the interactive effects of supervised dieting along with sibutramine. Participants in the drug-alone group lost about 6 kilograms, as did those who received therapy alone. To their credit, the authors reported that drug therapy participants who kept careful daily records of their food intake lost 18 kilograms during the treatment period, whereas those who did not keep records lost only 6 kilograms—the same amount as the control group receiving therapy alone. The investigators did not elaborate on this finding, nor did they report the food intake of any participant. One might argue that self-reports of feeding are not accurate. Although this is a concern, there should not be differential effects in double-blind studies. If the available data are not reported, then neither practitioner nor consumer can know the mechanism of action.

The orlistat story is more grim because, under the brand name *alli*, it is sold as an over-the-counter medication, and it is now being widely advertised in fashion and teen magazines as an integral part of thoughtful dieting. Orlistat reduces the amount of fat that is absorbed from the gastrointestinal tract by about 30%. The rest of the fat is absorbed and enters the metabolic process. The nonabsorbed fat is excreted. The effect of orlistat during the weight loss phase of the clinical trials was modest, slightly exceeding that of controls. In studies that evaluated orlistat in weight maintenance, Hill and colleagues (2000) reported that orlistat-treated participants in this "double-blind" study preserved over 50% of their weight loss at the end of the year, whereas controls retained about a third. The text figures were impressive. However, as McCarthy (2000) pointed out, given the modest starting weight losses, the difference between the two groups at the end of the maintenance year was just about a kilogram. As indicated, this loss in weight comes at a price of gastric distress, and even bowel incontinence, as reported by the authors. In addition, well over half of the participants dropped out of the study because of the drug's side effects.[6]

As is customary in pharmaceutical clinical trials, all three of these studies were funded by the drug manufacturer, and the primary investigators of the US studies had received consulting and speaker honoraria from the company.[7] Moreover, the *manufacturer's scientific staff reviewed the data with the US investigators in some of the studies, at which point the investigators conducted the data analyses and wrote the report.* I am not for a moment accusing the authors of explicit or deliberate wrongdoing. The circumstances under which the research was conducted, however, which are representative of pharmacological clinical trials, invite a less than fully objective scrutiny, as discussed by Nestle (2002).

In a series of studies justly famous in the experimental-psychology literature, Robert Rosenthal (Rosenthal & Fode, 1963) directly evaluated the impact of suggestion on experimental outcome to reveal the vulnerability of scientific accuracy. He was concerned about the possible bias that could be conveyed to undergraduate research assistants by the laboratory director, or by graduate students. Harvard undergraduates who were receiving course credit for independent study simply recorded the number of daily running-wheel revolutions of normal, untreated rats divided into two groups: A and B. The experimental manipulation consisted of casually hinting to one group of undergraduates that rats in Group A should run more each day. The other group received the same hint, but favoring Group B rats. The undergraduates dutifully recorded the number of daily revolutions (from a counter) of the *same rats in the same wheels*, to discover that Group A rats "ran more" for Group A undergraduates and Group B rats "ran more" for Group B undergraduates. The students, of course, were stunned by these findings, because they were completely unaware of the expected outcomes that had been subtly revealed to them and thought they had been scrupulous in their data collection.

Rosenthal's lessons must be taken seriously by drug/diet researchers and by the journals that publish studies on drug efficacy. In my view, clinical research can continue to be funded by the product manufacturer, but the influence must not go beyond writing the check. Scientists conducting the study must remain "blind" until data collection and analyses have been completed. Study safety committees need to track whether participants, individually or as a group, are vulnerable to untoward side effects during data collection, and act accordingly.

---

[6]The alli story has become the darling of the advertising industry (see AdAge, July 2007). Smith, Kline & French (SKF) purchased the rights to orlistat for the bargain price of $100 million, and through a brilliant ad campaign (another $150 million) that used "honest" advertising acknowledging the difficulties that one might encounter with alli, the entire investment was realized within months of hitting the market. There was one oversight, however; the recommended dose on the package is 60 milligrams three times a day before meals. In fact, however, this dose was *not* effective in clinical trials. But clients are told that if 60 does not work, they should increase the dose to 120.

[7]It was not made clear whether the STORM group received fees from the sponsor.

Safety committees are already in place and have enhanced the quality of the research enterprise. Sponsor scientists should not be able to access the data set until the manuscript has been submitted for scientific review, if that is what the authors have decided. Original data should remain in the possession of the primary investigator, although as research sponsors, the manufacturers are certainly entitled to a copy of both raw and summarized data, as well as the statistical analyses that were performed. Without these safeguards, unknowing errors of omission or commission should be expected.

The quest for an effective pharmacological agent for treating obesity continues, as well it should. A potentially effective agent is rimonabant, a cannabinoid-1 (CB_1) receptor blocker. The drug's history is of interest. Use of cannabinoids, such as marijuana, has been associated with increased appetite for millennia. The drug has been scrutinized in laboratories for the past 25 years. Its orexic effects have been replicated in a dose-dependent manner in rats and humans. Rats that have received the active compound in marijuana work more for food than when not in the drugged state. Moreover, according to Thorton-Jones and colleagues (2005), CB_1 but not CB_2 receptor blockers curb intake following deprivation (see Kirkham and Tucci, 2006, for a superb review of this literature).

CB_1 receptors are found in the medial forebrain bundle, interdigitated with opioid receptors. Interestingly, like opioid receptors, CB_1 receptors are found in the stomach and intestine, among other places. Moreover, cannabinoid and endorphin systems function similarly. Their activation induces analgesia, they are rewarding in the sense of supporting working for stimulation of the central nervous system, and they induce feeding, especially the ingestion of sweets (Mechoulam et al., 2006).

On the whole, the few rimonabant clinical trials have been successful, although not without raising a number of flags (Despere's et al., 2005). Participants who had received drug treatment, in fact, ate substantially less than did control participants, and although a fairly large number of the drug-receiving participants dropped out of the study, the rate of attrition was no higher than among control participants. The reasons may differ, however. Controls often state that they leave because their efforts have not met with weight loss and they are no longer motivated to continue. People who receive the drug often drop out because of unpleasant and unwanted side effects. There were quite a few, as one would suspect from the distribution of gastric CB_1 receptors.

As the following discussion will make clear, diet drugs are not necessary for successful weight loss. Once the drug is stopped, weight comes back at the same rate as in controls. Patients habituate to drugs, but the dose can be pushed only so far. Moreover, thousands of individuals have successfully shed 30 kilograms or more and have kept a substantial portion of the lost weight off for over 5 years. Almost none of these subjects used drugs to facilitate weight loss. It is worth seeking commonalities among these people to help guide the efforts of others who may try to lose weight effectively (i.e., for the long term).

Elements of successful weight loss

Some weight loss enterprises are run by snake oil salesmen, who sprout like mushrooms after the rain. They are nourished by the vulnerability of obese, overweight, and even some normal-weight people who wish to shed their real or perceived excess pounds. Drugs, books, and new diets that "guarantee a 20-pound loss in 3 weeks" turn up each year at predictable times. In seeking ways to improve the likelihood of success for losing weight, maintaining weight loss, *and* achieving and maintaining fitness, I have sought commonalities among the circumstances of the men and women who have qualified for the National Weight Control Registry (NWCR). Founded by Wing and Hill in 1994 (see Wing & Hill, 2001 for review; Klem et al., 1997), the registry has been in effect for about 13 years as of this writing.

To qualify for the NWCR, people had to lose 13.6 kilograms (about 30 pounds) and keep this weight off for 1 year. In fact, they lost on average 30 kilograms, going from a BMI of 36.7 down to a BMI of 25.1—a remarkable achievement by any standard. They have pretty successfully guarded against regain for 5 years; the success of almost 15% of registry members has extended to 10 years. The elements shared by many of the registry's members are presented next, along with the recent report of Anderson and colleagues (2007):[8]

1. TRIGGERING STIMULUS   Fully 77% of the original NWCR list members initiated their lifestyle change after an event that shook them into action. Reasons were *medical* and *social*. Medical reasons may have arisen when a cardiologist warned that the patient's years, indeed months, were numbered absent substantial weight changes. Social reasons included actual or potential divorce because the spouse found the individual too fat, as well as the individual's being sufficiently upset by a look in the mirror. The potency of the triggering event must be appreciated because 46% of the participants had been obese from age 11 or younger, and an additional 25% had become overweight or obese between 12 and 18 years of age. That is, 71% of these 45-year-olds who achieved NWCR status had been obese for all of their adult lifetimes and had repeatedly tried dieting with limited success. Two issues concerning triggering events remain to be considered, however. First, how many unsuccessful dieters had had a triggering event of the same magnitude and intensity? Second, of the previous unsuccessful efforts by the registered NWCR members, how many had also been triggered by a particular event?

Ninety-one percent of the NWCR members had repeatedly dieted in the past. The total amount of weight previously lost through dieting averaged an astonishing 565 pounds per person—a figure considerable higher than the 200- to 400-pound lifetime weight losses that had been previously reported in the literature

---

[8]In this study, 66% of the patients (starting average weight of 383 and 317 pounds for males and females respectively) who had lost on the order of 100 pounds discontinued their medications, for an average savings of $100 a month.

on repeat dieters. Weight cycling (yo-yo dieting) is the common dietary pattern and reflects the inability of the majority of dieters to maintain the achieved weight level. *Losing weight is not the problem: keeping the lost weight off is.* Noncompliance, a major medical issue in general, is nowhere greater than in addiction and dieting. As indicated, the triggering event was a major motivational factor. Clearly a change had to have occurred in the individual's life to provide the motivational impetus to sustain at least a 5-year weight loss maintenance.

2. REDUCED FAT INTAKE   Average daily fat intake of NWCR members was about 24% of total food intake, a figure well below the 30% recommended by the National Institutes of Health. This was achieved by restricting intake of certain classes of foods (88% of participants), eating smaller portion sizes (44%), counting calories (44%), and substituting low-calorie milk shakes for regular meals. In the study conducted by Anderson and colleagues (2007), half of the participants ate liquid meal replacements (milk shakes), and the remainder ate low-fat meals under supervision.

Comment: Ledikwe and colleagues (2007) and Ello-Martin and colleagues (2007) recently demonstrated that reduced fat intake, alone or in combination with eating more fruits and vegetables, helped reduce body weight. Daily exercise was not recorded. The possibilities of long-term dieting through volume expansion and increased fruit and vegetable intake, especially in conjunction with high exercise levels (below) may be worth pursuing, especially because hunger ratings are diminished as volume intake remains high, but without a caloric cost (described by *Hetherington* and *Rolls* in Chapter 10).

3. HIGH EXERCISE LEVELS   The exercise levels of NWCR members—about 3000 kilocalories—exceeded the 1000-kilocalorie weekly minimum recommended by the American College of Sports Medicine. In the Anderson study, exercise levels were at 2000 kilocalories weekly. Different exercise strategies were followed: 55% of the NWCR members, mostly women, exercised in a group; the remaining 45%, mostly men, exercised "alone." The latter merits comment because at first blush it undercuts one of my central points: that enlisting a peer in the process is key to successful weight loss. Men's dominant exercise form was weight lifting during an era in which free weights were used. Weight lifting, especially free weights, is done with a partner who is integral to the process; it is an intense shared experience. Moreover, other solitary exercises, such as jogging, cycling, or walking are often group activities involving at least two people.

Comment: The importance of support groups, clinical support, and high exercise levels has been demonstrated experimentally in follow-up studies (Jeffery et al., 2003; Tate et al., 2007). Overweight participants (14–32 kilograms) were randomly assigned to a weekly exercise regimen of either 1000 or 2500 kilocalories per week for 18 months. All were on fat-restricted (≤20% total intake) diets of 1000 or 1500 kilocalories daily, depending on starting weight. Importantly, participants in the high-exercise group also worked out with one to three partners. All participants met weekly in small groups for the first 6 months of the study, biweekly during months 7 through 12, and monthly until the study was terminated at 18 months. Participants were seen once more at 30 months.

The findings are of considerable interest from a number of perspectives. First, the high-exercise group lost more weight than did the low-exercise group during the first 18 months. Second, group differences had disappeared by 30 months. Third, as in other reports, *weight loss reversed at the time that counseling sessions changed from weekly to biweekly, and this weight gain continued for the next 2 years.* Finally, 13 participants sustained their high levels of exercise beyond 18 months. Moreover, decreased caloric intake was integrated into their lifestyle change. At 30 months these 13 participants had lost a total of 12 kilograms. High exercise levels may increase fat oxidation; they have recently been shown to exert short-term effects (Hansen et al., 2007).

4. PERMANENT LIFESTYLE CHANGES   Achievements in the NWCR also came through permanent lifestyle changes. The *diets were not radical*; certain foods simply were no longer eaten, or portion sizes were reduced. Target weights were not necessarily set, and an average of 1 pound a week was lost. In other words, what occurred was not so much a clearly demarcated shift from weight loss to weight maintenance but more of a slide into the maintenance phase, which is compatible with the decision to become fit while losing weight. Weight change was achieved *without* weight loss drugs. Only 1% to 2% of the NWCR used any drugs at all, and those who did, used them for very brief periods of time.

One may ask—what can we take from this? Is there a recipe that will guarantee to make it work? Are these extraordinary people who are super motivated? As far as can be told, the successful dieters were ordinary people who had tried repeatedly to keep lost weight off. In Anderson's study, the 118 successful dieters constituted 18% of the 656-patient study group. No distinguishing features appeared to separate them from the unsuccessful dieters.

A confluence of four factors led to success in the NWCR participants (information on some of the points was not provided in Anderson et al., 2007). First, participants were very *highly motivated* to see their program through. Second, the primary mode of dieting was a *considerably reduced fat intake*. Third, weight maintenance featured *high daily caloric expenditure*. Fourth, successful dieters had *at least one person actively offering support*. This last point is obvious for individuals who are involved in group exercise or in weight loss programs, such as Weight Watchers, that provide a great deal of support through the process. Weight lifters also benefit from a partner who is vested in the process and supports and encourages the individual.

Reports of weight reversals abound in the literature when weekly meetings with the primary contact person are switched to biweekly or even monthly. Slowly surrendering what one has worked so hard to achieve is stressful, particularly for those who have tried repeatedly and failed. Knowing that the *maintenance phase of dieting has proven so difficult should alert the support person that his or her job is really just starting.* Clinicians supervising weight loss should *never start the disengagement* process when the client is first entering the weight maintenance phase of the program. In my view, the process of weight loss supervision should be treated as any other clinical process in which sensitivity and active support are extended to clients who are demoralized and have a low self-regard—in this instance, because of their appearance and lack of success in previous weight loss efforts. Clinical responsibilities extend well beyond the mechanics of tracking weight loss and giving useful suggestions. Struggles with weight loss parallel the difficulties experienced by people seeking to quit smoking, alcohol, or drugs. These parallels will be more fully developed in the next section.

A frame of reference

In conceptualizing the present and future status of obesity, I have been swayed by the arguments presented by *Wise* (see Chapter 4) and others thinking of overeating as an expression of addiction. This conceptualization can help guide means of prevention and reversal. Table E.1 draws parallels between obesity and addiction—parallels based on anatomy, function, and behavior, as well as the artificiality of the substances used.

ANATOMY   All investigated addictions, regardless of origin, share the common anatomical substrate that forms a dopaminergic arc along the medial forebrain

Table E.1
Commonalities between Overeating/Obesity and All Recognized Addictions

Characteristic	Overeating/obesity	Addiction
Neurology	Medial forebrain bundle	Medial forebrain bundle
Neurochemistry	Dopamine, O/C[a]	Dopamine, O/C[a]
"Addicting substances"	Manufactured	Manufactured
Cravings	Profound	Profound
Compliance	Poor	Poor
Reinstatement: cond. St.[b]	Yes	Yes
Reinstatement: drug/taste	Yes	Yes
Stress	Yes	Yes
Psychological dependence	Yes	Yes
Physiological dependence	No	Yes
Withdrawal	Delayed	Immediate

[a]O/C Opioid Cannabinoid
[b]Conditioned Stimuli

area rostral to the nucleus accumbens. Embedded in this matrix are opioid and cannabinoid elements that, when activated electrically or with the appropriate neurochemical agonists, elicit eating and self-stimulation in all animals studied, including humans. The anatomy and neurochemistry are remarkably conserved, as has been consistently demonstrated by track tracing, histochemistry, and functional MRI studies (documented by *Wise* in Chapter 4).

FUNCTION   Animals of different species are readily trained to work for electrical and neurochemical stimulation of these areas. Destruction of the lateral hypothalamic area, either electrolytically or through dopamine-selective neurotoxins, causes a dramatic syndrome, documented by Teitelbaum and Epstein (1962), that essentially eliminates all forms of motivated behavior and causes sensory indifference and severe motor dyskinesia, from which recovery is slow and tenuous. In humans, Parkinson's disease, also provoked by striatal dopamine depletion, most approximates this syndrome, reflecting motor compromise, very low affect, and sensory indifference.

Stimulating a number of the loci in the arc electrically or neurochemically elicits appetitive and appropriate consummatory behaviors with the objects in the environment, including eating, drinking, sex, attack, and infant retrieving. Studies of early genes with markers such as c-*fos* show that the crescent lights up during *any* of these behaviors along with the different sensory and motor systems that detect the proximal objects and the different neural systems involved in their consummation. Stated differently, mammalian motivated behaviors share an "hourglass" organization of diverse sensory and acquired sources funneling into a common motivational core. The efferents in parallel with representational systems allow an animal to locate the object that releases its consummatory act.

NEUROCHEMISTRY   From the perspective of reward and state maintenance, the major players in the circuit are dopamine, opioids, and cannabinoids. For present purposes, this is especially true for systems involved in energy conservation. My own studies and those of my colleagues examining rat and human infants have demonstrated that sweet taste and fat flavors cause endogenous opioid release that reduces crying and is analgesic in both human (Blass & Hoffmeyer, 1991) and rat (Blass et al., 1987; Shide & Blass, 1989) infants (Ren et al., 1997). Sugars and fats are rewarding to these infants (Shide & Blass, 1991). Newborn rats press a lever many times for infusions of milk into the mouth (Johanson & Hall, 1979), and human newborns are readily conditioned to tactile stimuli that predict sucrose delivery. It is reasonable to suggest that the conditioned stimulus induced a positive anticipatory change in affect because almost all of the infants in the study cried when sucrose no longer followed the predicting tactile stimulation (Blass et al., 1984).

Taste- and flavor-induced calming and analgesia are blocked by opioid, and to a somewhat lesser extent cannabinoid, antagonists. The fact that both systems are also found in the intestine and contribute to various digestive processes is of considerable interest from the perspective of energy conservation. Rao and colleagues (1997) investigated this question and, using direct calorimetry, reported a 13% reduction in energy expenditure in term and premature newborns when crying was arrested with a 1-milliliter taste of sucrose. Opioid determinants of ingestion are remarkably conserved; they are found even in mollusks (Kavaliers & Hirst, 1987).

The disruptive effects of dopamine depletion and blockade on a variety of behaviors have been extensively documented and reviewed (as noted by *Wise* in Chapter 4; Smith, 2004). In all animals studied, parallel effects of reduced behavior under dopamine blockade have been obtained. This has been verified through electrophysiology studies. Importantly, dopamine blockade appears to work on reinforcement systems so that the dose–response function relating, for example, deprivation to willingness to work for food is shifted to the right. There can be no doubt as to the centrality of these pathways in the organization of motivation and action.

CAPTURE OF ENDOGENOUS DOPAMINERGIC SYSTEMS DURING ADDICTION

These underlying mechanisms are at the core of every known addiction— whether behavioral or material. Accordingly, on functional MRI, core areas of the medial forebrain bundle dopaminergic systems all "light up" during administration of drugs such as amphetamine or cocaine *and* when sweet foods are eaten (Everitt & Robbins, 2005). The magnitude of the rise is greater for drugs, of course, reflecting the pharmacological action of an agent that is clearly beyond the physiological range. These findings are very important. They demonstrate that drugs of substance abuse utilize the pathways that normally function to sustain and be rewarded by motivational systems. Humans report sensations of pleasure when these areas are electrically stimulated, and all nonverbal animals work on incredibly demanding schedules to obtain electrical or chemical stimulation of the areas in the dopaminergic crescent.

Although one might shrug off demonstrations that animals will starve to death in the face of available food when working nonstop for electrical stimulation, the parallel in human drug and alcohol addictions characterized by unconquerable urges requires attention. This also is true, I maintain, for less dramatic addictive behaviors such as compulsive gambling, sexual addictions, and, to the point of the present essay, food addictions with the consequence of obesity. Reciprocally, we learn that the core pathways utilized by all drug addictions are the very ones that are engaged by motivated, vital behaviors such as feeding and sex.

Further parallels strengthen this position. All addictive drugs and alcohol are manufactured; that is, they are artificial. The same is true for energy-dense, superpalatable foods in the fat and sweet domains. In fact, in-house laboratories of food manufacturers have tasters on payroll who rate the appeal of the products, which are then tweaked appropriately to produce the most attractive tastes and flavors to best capture market share. There are other compelling parallels. As Wise argues (see Chapter 4)—as difficult as the first drink is to resist, the second drink is harder still. The same is true for overeating. Stress causes people to return to their addiction. Stressful situations likewise break down resolve, and dieters will again binge-eat large volumes of energy-dense food.

Engaging in other behaviors can also trigger the behavior in question. For example, smokers during the process of quitting make themselves exceedingly vulnerable if they have had too many drinks. The same holds for dieting. The list goes on. Eating an energy-dense food like a cheeseburger will trigger an overeating relapse in much the same way that snorting a row of cocaine will for a cocaine addict who has been clean for a period of time. All of these parallels have been documented again and again, giving credence to the idea that obesity through overeating in healthy individuals should be regarded as an addiction, just as smoking is. *The smoker is not necessarily ill at the moment, but the odds of morbidity and early mortality are substantial.* Smoking persistence and recruitment of new smokers despite common knowledge of smoking consequences underscore the challenges that are faced in reversing the obesity trend.

The bottom two rows of Table E.1 identify two important ways in which overeating differs from drug addiction. First, the crucial parallel of physiological dependence in obese individuals has not been established, despite efforts to do so. This is important. It predicts that compliance with drug abstinence should be more difficult than compliance with weight maintenance because the underlying physiological changes that are linked to the conditioned stimuli are far more profound. Accordingly, withdrawal triggered by the conditioned stimuli should come earlier and be more severe, and it is. I will return to this point.

Second, compliance is lost very early in the drug treatment period, generally in the first few weeks. In contrast, a much higher percentage of individuals succeed in losing weight but are generally not able to sustain the loss as weight creeps back after months of dieting. Lack of physiological withdrawal in overeaters and very severe withdrawal in people addicted to drugs predicts immediate, or very early, compliance difficulties. Passing the phase of severe withdrawal improves recovery chances considerably. Accordingly, a number of rehabilitation plans have specific subprograms dedicated to keeping the recovering addict in the program; the longer a person remains in a program and drug-free, the better are the odds of recovery. Such is also the case for adherence to diet and exercise programs.

Chronic overeating differs importantly from other forms of addictive behavior in that we must eat, thereby repeatedly performing the act that is at the core of overeating. We can avoid taking drugs or drinking alcohol or gambling; they all occur in assigned places that must be sought out. Moreover, the agents of abuse, drugs, and alcohol cannot be blatantly advertised, as can energy-rich foods. The public nature of the act, its biological imperative, and its cultural malleability, through advertising, form powerful vectors that align against successful weight loss or obesity prevention. This, of course, is exacerbated by a fiscally unlimited, highly motivated, and sophisticated mercantile establishment.

In short, I have argued that extensive overeating resulting in obesity should be considered an addiction, like smoking or compulsive gambling. As with all other addictions, overeating is acquired. *Overeating occurs in the absence of need.* In contemporary Western societies, overeating, like abuses of drugs or alcohol, is fueled by artificial, human-made, substances. Indeed, ingestive systems are vulnerable to a number of experiential classes of events. They are malleable even before birth (as *Lumeng* describes in Chapter 6). Social experiences have been specified that can broaden food acceptance and even overcome food aversions, as *Lumeng* and *Yeomans* discuss in Chapters 6 and 7). The effects are impressive, and the capacity of social factors to influence food intake, proximally and even at a distance, has independently appeared many times in this text. With rare exceptions, normal social interactions at table with family and friends increase eating [de Castro, 1994; Herman, et.al., 2003; *Hetherington* and *Rolls* (Chapter 10); *Harrison et al.* (Chapter 12)]. These powerful forces should be exploited to break addiction and maintain stable weight and fitness levels.

Nonetheless, viewing obesity as an addiction allows us to learn from the addiction literature by exploiting what works in facilitating abstinence. I will focus on this topic in the next section and integrate it with information from diet and exercise literatures and the chapters reported herein. I will then move to what can be achieved at a community level, on the basis of different literatures, and finally address possibilities on the national level based on strategies successfully used against exploitation by Big Tobacco, a first cousin of Big Ag.

Treatment and Prevention

The remainder of this epilogue is based on the *principle of fences*. The principle states that fences (barriers) should be erected to prevent contact with the source. It rests on the following assumptions:

1. Contact with an energy-dense source *cannot* be resisted.

2. The *farther* a barrier keeps the individual away from the source, the *weaker* the force to overeat.

3. Overeating is *not* in response to a physiological need.

4. Hunger and its consequent overeating are *elicited by stimuli that have previously been associated with eating.*

The *principle of fences* can be translated into pragmatic actions that are based on statistically reliable experimental reports and/or on proven weight loss and fitness approaches that have been documented in the clinical and exercise literatures.

Partnering

Ideally the partner should be a friend of long standing, with shared views on weight loss and like determination to do something about it. The vast majority of people in the NWCR partnered with other people, either through group membership or through activities such as weight lifting that cannot be solitary. The *social contract* has three vital features that can be exploited to facilitate weight loss and improve fitness. First, it offers mutual support when one partner wavers. The longer people are kept in addiction or weight loss programs, the better are the chances of success. Second, a partner provides a proximate model for agreed-upon resolutions, undertaken together. Third, the partnership can act distally; it is the *potential* converse of the phenomenon described by Christakis and Fowler (2007). With such an agreement, the standard set by the partner, in principle, can become the normative model that is followed.

Entering into a support alliance helps free members from being dependent on clinical approval and availability. As indicated earlier, after the frequency of visits to a therapist are shifted from weekly to monthly, patients start to put weight back on. Progress backslides in all psychotherapeutic settings when a therapist withdraws or is perceived to withdraw support for a client as therapy advances (Frank, 1971). If the obese dieter is perceived as going through addictive withdrawal and is vulnerable to relapse at times of stress, then the support that is in place at the start of the weight loss/fitness process should be actively maintained. Alliances help maintain that support.

Support networks work best for drug and alcohol addicts when firmly in place at the start of an abstinence program. The same social structures should also be in place when people embark on weight loss programs. Support networks, even for people losing weight independently, should include family and friends. This is especially true when children are making the effort. Praise goes a long way in reinforcing behavior. By the same token, gentle constraints are needed and appreciated when a child or adult starts to waver from the initiated path. Because dieting and maintaining a regular exercise schedule make for hard work, family and friends who enter the support nexus must remain alert to opportunities to reinforce even what may appear to be small achievements, and they must be prepared to offer support when needed. Primary partners should be actively monitoring themselves and each other.

Creating distal fences

Fences that put the greatest distance between the individual and available cheap foods are erected on the national level—a topic to which I will return. As individuals, alone or working with partner and family, the first outposts can be established at the market. The rule is simple: *if an energy-dense food is not in the house, then it cannot be eaten.*

Unsweetened, low-calorie cereals can be purchased rather than sweet, energy-dense ones. In fact, food manufacturers are producing low-calorie lines of cereal and investing considerable resources in advertising these items. A positive public reaction will sustain these changes. Individuals may have considerable difficulty resisting the purchase of energy-dense foods for themselves, especially when shopping with children who clamor for energy-dense foods seen on TV ads, that are placed at child eye level. Resistance is possible, however, if carefully prepared shopping lists that exclude or minimize energy-dense items are exchanged and partners shop for each other. Reciprocal food shopping is an effective first step because overweight people are drawn to food and not pushed by physiological need.

The second fence can be constructed at the level of food packaging and storage. *Wansink* and *Sobal* have shown repeatedly that considerably less is eaten when items—potato chips, for example—are provided in small packages. Although money can be saved on a per weight basis through bulk shopping, this is false economy when the direct and indirect costs of illness and missed work are taken into consideration. Accordingly, if purchasing energy-dense foods is truly necessary, purchases should be in small quantities and in small packages. When these foods are brought into the home, they should be stored remotely on the bottom shelf at the back of the cupboard. Likewise, foods that were stocked in larger quantities in people's homes by the experimenters were also eaten more frequently. Although clinical trials have not been conducted to address these issues, the experimental data are sufficiently robust to warrant instantiating these findings.

That said, although scaling issues are complex (as discussed by *Snyder* and *Bartoshuk* in Chapter 5), the qualitative space between the first and second fences is immediately appreciated when the temptation to snack strikes. In the first instance, food is not available and either a substitute (healthful) must be taken, or the pang left to wither. With the second, closer, fence in place, finding food might be a hassle, but it is doable. At the beginning especially, the support system in a household must be strong to get the family over this hump (see Ludwig, 2007, for instantiating diets in a household in which one or more children are obese).

The third barrier level is closer yet to the food and, on those grounds alone, will be less effective. This fence separates the already prepared food from the table. There are a number of posts in this fence, each of which has been empirically documented. One concerns serving manner. Rather than following the path of least resistance by placing the preparation pot itself on the table, or by transferring the food from pot to large serving bowl, one should serve food individually to each table member in appropriately modest portions. Likewise, seconds should also be prearranged in appropriately sized portions and not left piled in a serving bowl.

The oft-repeated comparison of portion size from the "good old days" to today is worth raising again. In Figure E.1, I compared a chocolate chip cookie, courtesy of Elizabeth Spelke, in a manner prepared, independently, by her mother and mine, with a cookie purchased at the Blue Colony Diner on Inter-

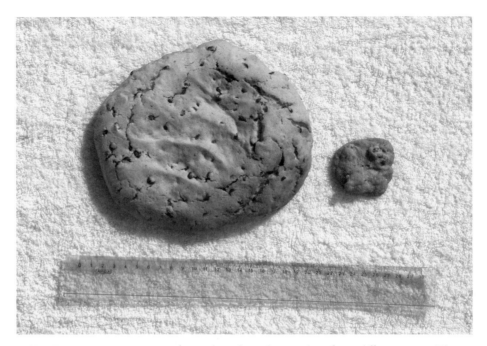

FIGURE E.1   A comparison of two chocolate chip cookies from different eras. (Photo by Elliott Blass.)

state 84 in Connecticut. The owners assured me that their cookie is a standard serving for one person—a fact that I have often observed. Differences in size do not misrepresent weight and calorie differences; the Blue Colony cookie weighs 322 grams and contains 1003 calories, according to the in-house baker (personal communication). Spelke's cookies of our youth, in contrast, average 11.6 grams and 30 calories each. One has to eat 33 of Spelke's cookies to come out calorically even with just one Blue Colony cookie. Generally savoring two or three of her cookies makes a tasty dessert or snack.

Another empirically validated fence post concerns distance from the table. As demonstrated by Painter, Wansink, and Hieggelke (2002), people who had a jar of chocolates placed on the adjacent desk in their office, and were therefore obliged to stand up and take a step or two to reach the chocolates, ate considerably fewer chocolates than when the jar was placed on their desk, necessitating only a reach. This scenario was brought into a laboratory meal setting in which considerably more macaroni and cheese was eaten with the serving bowl on the table than when it was a few steps away and the participants were obliged to get up for their additional helpings.

These suggestions gain empirical force when we recall the Rolls finding that satiety ratings at the end of a large meal were the same as after a more modest one. This is another instance in which the amount eaten is dictated by external factors. As discussed earlier, other factors include eating in a group of family and friends, and the distal determinant of considering as a normal standard the weight of a friend who has recently become obese. Thus, from the perspective of fences and their proximity to food, these efforts should succeed. Greater intensity is needed, however, so continued support from family and friends is especially important during maintenance. Again, the model of support for individuals who are in the process of quitting smoking is relevant.

Changing lifestyle

The need to alter lifestyle has been pretty standard fare since the demonstrations, about a decade ago, that lifestyle changes are as effective as planned exercise (see *Filiault*'s comments in Chapter 8). I emphasize just a few points. First, the change should be permanent, but it does not have to be major. It can be as simple as parking a distance from the workplace, thereby walking a few blocks to office or school, or walking the dog, or any other activity that is not currently practiced. Changes should be set up to be permanent, reversal coming only with considerable difficulty.[9] The changes are best exemplified by changes in the behavior of NWCR members who embarked on major exercise programs not to turn back, and in the 13 patients who retained their high levels of exercise in the report by Dunn and colleagues (2007).

From the perspective of eating, many pathways have led to weight reduction. These include simply cutting one calorie-dense food out of the diet, eating smaller portions, counting calories, and other forms of restriction. It is not for me to recommend one over the other. Permanent focused lifestyle change undertaken with a supportive friend considerably improves the likelihood of shedding pounds, keeping them off, and improving fitness.

Actions on a Community Level

As *Filiault* has documented (see Chapter 8), community exercise and fitness improve when opportunities to be outdoors in a safe and clean ambience are made available to neighborhood members and organizations. Unfortunately, such an initiative must take place at a grassroots level to overcome vested interests that often carry the political day. Fortunately, precedents provide guidance for how to make these organizational goals attainable. Community members have organized and approached local governments to volunteer to clean up park areas

---

[9]A good friend of mine, a world-class French patissier/boulangier, whose breadmaker left, took over that responsibility and turned pastry preparation over to others. As a result, he no longer got to taste the pies, tarts, and other delicacies during their preparation. He also started to play golf once a week, and has lost about 30 kilograms during the past 14 months. A perk for us and his other customers has been that as good as the breads had been, they are better yet under the magic of his touch.

and lay out public exercise/recreational venues. This is simply good politics. City councilmen and -women want to provide services that make them look good.

Once neighborhood residents have demonstrated a willingness to solve a problem, resources to create or improve local facilities become more readily available. They have ranged from providing cleanup materials and a city truck for trash removal, to leveling empty spaces, to providing benches, basketball courts, and open spaces for sitting, playing, walking, jogging, and so on. A crucial element is community safety. This, too, has been put into effect, through a combination of neighborhood groups working in conjunction with local law enforcement agencies. Again, proven strategies are available that allow people to clean up their neighborhoods, make them safe, and utilize local facilities for exercise and athletic and social activities. See *Filiault* (Chapter 8) for additional details, as in the Indianapolis project.

This approach reinforces individual behaviors at the level of mutual support and by providing the wherewithal for community gathering in a safer ambience. Success also empowers groups to take on other projects that reflect communal needs. To the point of the present efforts, boycotting local supermarkets has been successful in convincing market owners to offer affordable healthful foods and make less available energy-dense ones. The fundamental unit of leverage in making nutritionally viable foods available for consumption is the pocketbook.

Actions on a National Level

In Chapter 11, *Mullaly et al.* identify some of the theoretical and practical implications of proposing changes that have national implications, as in modifying programs that are already in place to improve fruit and vegetable availability and decreasing support for FLNV. Even without resistance from vested interests, the effects of change can be slow and can take unanticipated turns. To complicate matters, consumers face unified, entrenched mercantile and political forces, concentrated mainly in congressional agricultural committees and the USDA. Historically, the USDA protected the interests of agriculture and the consumer. This protection started as subsidies to *small farmers* during the Depression and during periods of food shortages to mitigate widespread hunger. Today, during times of energy surfeit, these subsidy policies have been turned on their ear. Eighty-five percent of USDA subsidies go to a very small number of very large agricultural businesses that produce mainly energy-dense products that can be marketed at low prices. Subsidies of fruits and vegetables are virtually nil.

These policies have direct consequences. Programs for increasing fruit and vegetable intake have not been systematically launched, nor have programs that make fresh fruits available in schools, despite the research report presented to Congress in 2003. To effect change on this and similar issues demands political leverage and will to change USDA policies and provide considerable subsidy support for fruits and vegetables. The choice of an inner-city mother to purchase *subsidized energy-rich, nutrition-poor* macaroni and cheese that enables her to feed her teenage family for $1 to $1.50 or to purchase *nutrition-rich, energy-poor unsub-sidized fruits and vegetables,* at present is a "no-brainer" that awaits correction through price supports and other changes in USDA distribution. Such changes will have immediate effects. A recent California study demonstrated that people who otherwise could not afford to purchase vegetables readily accepted and ate from a range of fruits and vegetables offered to them. Launching such a program has the potential of broadening inner-city children's food choices and nutritional quality. It should be initiated before children reach 4 years of age.

There is some hope, however, because the proposed Farm Bill is receiving Congressional and Media attention. In the political climate of February 2008, pressure to make the farm bill more equitable is coming from both bottom and top. Even President Bush recognizes the inequalities of cutting Food Stamp Programs while not decreasing subsidies to megafarms in seven states in the country's heartland. The current political climate may sustain consumer activism to make equitable changes in this farm bill that will benefit the ⅔s of the farmers who do not get any subsidies at all, will especially subsidize *produce* farms and will not pay taxpayer dollars to farms with annual takes of 2 million dollars.

A surreptitious video documenting vicious treatment of debilitated cattle in feedlots and slaughtering facilities gained instant, well-deserved national notoriety in February 2008. These animals, too debilitated to stand, that should not have been slaughtered for food, were pulled by their tails, kicked and moved by forklift to the slaughter area. The company spokesmen said that they were horrified by the treatment and immediately fired the perpetrators.

The USDA ordered the recall of 143 million pounds of beef[10] (not a typo) to guard against the possibility of mad cow disease and to reduce the likelihood the cattle had been contaminated by a particular virulent strain of *e. coli.* As of this writing, none were found among the remains of the 37 million pounds that had been distributed nationwide through federally subsidized school lunch programs. It is likely that about half of the meat had already been eaten. Ironically the company in question had received a USDA award for its performance in 2005–2006.

This event warrants its own chapter, if not book. But for now I want to make a few observations concerning USDA policies. There are about 7800 inspectors to cover an estimated 6200 plants that process cattle, hogs, chickens, and eggs. Some farm lots accommodate upwards of 100,000 head of cattle. How can the public expect even token supervision under these circumstances?

Second, cattle raised in feedlots are injected with growth hormone, for the obvious reasons, and with massive doses of antibiotics to stave off and hold at bay rumen infections that are caused by eating corn, a food that cattle had not evolved to eat or digest. Both the hormones and the antibiotics pass to us through eating.

Third, feedlots are incredibly densely populated. There is no grass, only concrete and earth that quickly becomes mud through rain- and snowfalls. The ani-

---

[10] At an estimate of 2,000 pounds a cow (generous) we are looking at a total of at least 71,500 cattle, assuming that everything was included in the poundage report, and not just edible meat.

mals live in their waste and take rest on slopes of concrete mounds so as to not to lie down in the mud. This is in conformity with USDA guidelines.

Fourth, the treatment that was filmed came as a shock to the company owners, who prided themselves on their past performance and transparency. Even if one grants that this was news to them, the cruel treatment must have been sufficiently widespread to be practiced publicly, without raising eyebrows. Was this business as usual? How could the USDA not have known about this practice?

Finally, it is reasonable to consider if the USDA has set an extremely high bar for declaring an animal unfit for human consumption. Must an animal be so debilitated as to not be able to stand to be eliminated from the food chain? Together, all of these situations should be taken very seriously because the number of major recalls out of concern for diseases that could be transmitted through beef has jumped from 5 in 2005 to 21 in 2007. The data are not yet in as to causality, but the literature on stress and decreased immune function is legion.

Addressing issues on a national level is beyond my expertise and the scope of this text. In Chapter 11, however, *Mullaly et al.* highlight some of the major issues that would be triggered by implementing what all would agree was an outstanding idea by Townsend (2006) to change the structure of the Food Stamp Program (FSP). These issues include the impact on poor people who are not in the FSP, and the agricultural changes that would have to be made to meet the demand surge for fruits and vegetables and the reduction in land used for grains. Because of weather and terrain constraints, crops are not interchangeable, as agriculturalists know. In short, the issues concerning food distribution and price supports must be addressed and changed as an integral part of correcting obesity spread at its source, but proposals to do so must be integrated and systematic. Changing people's consumption habits is far more difficult than changing their smoking habits. Although taxing FLNV is a fine idea (Brownell, 1994), it will not work unless alternative, healthful foods are available for poor people to purchase at a considerably reduced cost.

In the end, however, the obesity issue, if it changes at all, will change slowly. Diets have worked only to the extent that they have been followed through the maintenance period so that the individual can turn the overweight trend around. Absent the dedication to maintaining weight loss, a significant portion will be regained within a year, and all of it by 3 years following diet termination. In part failed goals reflect noncompliance; in part, exercise must be maintained at very high levels for the weight to be kept off.

Bergh et al. (Chapter 13) have provided a new approach that has been proven with anorexics and has had initial success with a population that had been very resistant to weight loss. This is a promising path to follow because the client is *actively engaged* with the computer screen that tracks eating rate and volume and adjusts her eating rate accordingly. Ideally this approach could be combined in the long term with the high-exercise programs that are integral to successful and sustained weight loss.

Concluding Remarks

This text has brought together experts in different areas that touch on obesity. The problem is one that we can attack from complementary fronts by focusing each salient on issues and institutions that range from individuals, alone and in small groups, to the community, to transportation systems, to state and federal political structures. Anything less than this broad effort will fail at the epidemiological level. Finally, even in the face of failure, the fact is that 40% of US adults are neither overweight nor obese, and over 70% of our children are of normal weight. Many of the programs identified herein, especially in the current chapter, can be brought to the service of overweight/obesity *prevention*. This is a good place to start.

Acknowledgments

I am obliged to David Blass, Joseph Blass, and Gerard Smith for time spent and suggestions made on an earlier draft of this chapter.

References Cited

Ammar, A. A., Sederholm, F., Saito, T. R., Scheurink, A. J., Johnson, A. E., & Södersten, P. (2000). NPY-leptin: opposing effects on appetitive and consummatory ingestive behavior and sexual behavior. *American Journal of Physiology – Regulatory, Integrative and Comparative Physiology, 278,* R1627–R1633.

Anderson, J. W., Conley, S. B., & Nicholas, A. S. (2007). One hundred-pound weight losses with an intensive behavioral program: changes in risk factors in 118 patients with long-term follow-up. *American Journal of Clinical Nutrition, 86,* 301–307.

Baker, J. L., Michaelsen, K. F., Sorensen, T. I. A., & Rasmussen, K. M. (2007). High prepregnant body mass index is associated with early termination of full and any breastfeeding in Danish women. *American Journal of Clinical Nutrition, 86,* 404–411.

Blass, E. M., Fitzgerald, E., & Kehoe, P. (1987). Interactions between sucrose, pain and isolation distress. *Pharmacology Biochemistry and Behavior, 26,* 483–489.

Blass, E. M., Ganchrow, J., & Steiner, J. (1984). Classical conditioning in newborn humans 2–48 hours of age. *Infant Behavior and Development, 7,* 223–235.

Blass, E. M., & Hoffmeyer, L. B. (1991). Sucrose as an analgesic in newborn humans. *Pediatrics, 87,* 215–218.

Brownell, K. D. (1994, December 15). Get slim with higher taxes [Editorial]. *New York Times,* p. A29.

Buzby, J. C., Guthrie, J. F., Kantor, L. S. (2003). *Evaluation of the USDA Fruit and Vegetable Pilot Program: Report to Congress.* Washington, DC: US Department of Agriculture. Retrieved August 2007 from http://www.ers.usda.gov/publications/efan03006/efan03006.pdf

Campos, P., Saguy, A., Ernsberger, P., Oliver, E., & Gaesser, G. (2006). Response: lifestyle, not weight should be the primary target. *International Journal of Epidemiology, 35,* 81–82.

Christakis, D. A., & Fowler, L. (2007). The spread of obesity in a large social network over 32 years. *New England Journal of Medicine, 357,* 370–379.

de Castro, J. M. (1994). Family and friends produce greater social facilitation of food intake than other companions. *Physiology & Behavior, 56,* 445–455.

Despere's, J.-P., Golay, A., Sjostrom, L., et al. (2005). Effects of Rimonabant on metabolic risk factors in overweight patients with dyslipidemia. *New England Journal of Medicine, 353,* 2121–2134.

Dunn, A. L., Marcus, B. H., Kampert, J. B., Garcia M. E., Kohl III, H. W., & Blair, S. N. (1999). Comparison of lifestyle and structured interventions to increase physical activity and cardiorespiratory fitness: a randomized trial. *Journal of the American Medical Association, 281,* 327–334.

Eckel, R. H. (2005). The dietary approach to obesity: is it the diet or the disorder? *Journal of the American Medical Association, 293,* 96–97.

Eckel, R. H., Kahn, R., Robertson, R. M., & Rizza, R. A. (2006). Preventing cardiovascular disease and diabetes: A call to action from the American Diabetes Association and the American Heart Association. *Diabetes Care, 29,* 1697–1699.

Ello-Martin, J. A., Roe, L. S., Ledikwe, J. H., Beach, A. M., & Rolls, B. J. (2007). Dietary energy density in the treatment of obesity: a year-long trial comparing two weight-loss diets. *American Journal of Clinical Nutrition, 85,* 1465–1477.

Everitt, B. J., & Robbins, T. W. (2005). Neural systems of reinforcement for drug addiction: from actions to habits to compulsion. *Nature Neuroscience, 8,* 1481–1489.

Frank, J. (1971). *Persuasion & Healing.* New York: Schocken Press.

Hansen, K. C., Zhang, Z., Gomez, T., Adams, A. K., & Schoeller, D. A. (2007). Exercise increases the proportion of fat utilization during short-term consumption of a high-fat diet. *American Journal of Clinical Nutrition, 85,* 109–116.

Hermann, C. P., Roth, D., & Polivy, J. (2003). Effects of the presence of others on food intake: a normative interpretation. *Psychological Bulletin, 129,* 873–886.

Hill, J. O., Hauptman, J., Anderson, J. W., Fujioka, K., O'Neil, P. M., Smith, D. K., Zavoral, J. H. & Aronne, L. J. (2000). Orlistat, a lipase inhibitor for weight maintenance after conventional dieting: a 1-y study. *American Journal of Clinical Nutrition, 69,* 1108–1116.

James, W. P. T., Astrup, A., Finer, N., Hilsted, J., Kopelman, P., Rossner, S., Saris, W. H. M., & Van Gaal L. F. (2000). Effects of Sibutramine on weight maintenance after weight loss: a randomized trial. *Lancet, 356,* 2119–2125.

Jeffery, R. W., Wing, R. R., Sherwood, N. E., & Tate, D. F. (2003). Physical activity and weight loss: does prescribing higher physical activity goals improve outcome? *American Journal of Clinical Nutrition, 78,* 684–689.

Johanson, I. B., & Hall, W. G. (1979). Appetitive learning in 1-day-old rat pups. *Science, 205,* 419–421.

Kavaliers, M., & Hirst, M. (1987). Slugs and snails and opiate tales: opioids and feeding behavior in invertebrates. *Federation Proceedings, 46,* 168–172.

Kirkham, T. C., & Tucci S. A. (2006). Endocannabinoids in appetite control and the treatment of obesity. *CNS & Neurological Disorders-Drug Targets, 5,* 275–292.

Klem, M. L., Wing, R. R., McGuire, M. T., Seagle, H. M., & Hill, J. O. (1997). A descriptive study of individuals successful at long-term maintenance of substantial weight loss. *American Journal of Clinical Nutrition, 66,* 239–246.

Ledikwe, J. H., Rolls, B. J., Smiciklas-Wright, H., Mitchell, D. C., et. al. (2007). Reductions in dietary energy are associated with weight loss in overweight and obese participants in the PREMIER trial. *American Journal of Clinical Nutrition, 85,* 1212–1221.

Leone, T., Pliner, P., & Hermann, C. P. (2007). Influence of clear versus ambiguous normative information on food intake. *Appetite, 49,* 58–65.

Ludwig, D. (2007). *Ending the Food Fight.* Boston: Houghton Mifflin.

McCarthy, W. J. (2000). Orlistat and weight loss. *American Journal of Clinical Nutrition, 71,* 846–847.

Mechoulam, R., Berry, E. M., Avraham, Y., Di Marzo, V., & Fride, E. (2006). Endocannabinoids, feeding and suckling – from our perspective. *International Journal of Obesity, 30,* S24–S28.

Mennella, J., & Beauchamp, G. (1999). Experience with a flavor in mother's milk modifies the infant's acceptance of flavored cereal. *Developmental Psychobiology, 35,* 197–203.

Nestle, M. (2002). *Food Politics.* Berkely, CA: University of California Press.

Painter, J. E., Wansink, B., & Hieggelke, J. (2002). How visibility and convenience influence candy consumption. *Appetite, 38,* 37–38.

Pedersen, P. E., & Blass, E. M. (1982). Prenatal and postnatal determinants of the first suckling episode in albino rats. *Developmental Psychobiology, 15,* 349–355.

Pratt, M. (1999). Benefits of lifestyle activity vs. structured exercise. *Journal of the American Medical Association, 281,* 375–376.

Rao, M., Blass, E. M., Brignol, M. M., Marino, L., & Glass, L. (1997). Reduced heat loss following sucrose ingestion in premature and normal human newborns. *Early Human Development, 48,* 109–116.

Ren, K., Blass, E. M., Zhou, Q-q., & Dubner, R. (1997). Suckling and sucrose ingestion suppress persistent hyperalgesia and spinal Fos expression after forepaw inflammation in infant rats. *Proceedings of the National Academy of Sciences, 104,* 1471–1475.

Rosenthal, R., & Fode, K. L. (1963). The effect of experimenter bias on the performance of the albino rat. *Behavioral Science, 8,* 183–189.

Rozin, P., & Kennel, K. (1983). Acquired preferences for piquant foods by chimpanzees. *Appetite, 4,* 69–77.

Rozin, P., & Schiller, D. (1980). The nature and preference for chili pepper by humans. *Motivation and Emotion, 4,* 77–101.

Schaal, B., Orgeur, P., & Arnould, C. (1995). Olfactory preferences in newborn lambs: possible influence of prenatal experience. *Behaviour, 132,* 351–365.

Seely, R., & Woods, S. W. (2003). Monitoring of stored and available fat by the CNSW: Implications for obesity. *Nature Reviews – Neuroscience, 4,* 901–909.

Shide, D. J., & Blass, E. M. (1989). Opioid-like effects of intraoral infusions of corn oil and polycose on stress reactions in 10-day-old rats. *Behavioral Neuroscience, 103,* 1168–1175.

Shide, D. J., & Blass, E. M. (1991). Opioid mediation of odor preferences induced by sugar and fat in 6-day-old rats. *Physiology & Behavior, 50,* 961–966.

Smith, G. P. (2004). Accumbens dopamine is a physiological correlate of the rewarding and motivating effects of food. In E. Stricker & S. C. Woods (Eds.), *Handbook of Behavioral Neurobiology, Neurobiology of Food and Fluid Intake* (pp. 15–42). New York: Plenum Press.

Smotherman, W., & Robinson, S. (1985). The rat fetus in its environment: Behavioral adjustments to novel, familiar, aversive, and conditioned stimuli presented in utero. *Behavioral Neuroscience, 99,* 521–530.

Speakman, J. R. (2004). Obesity: The integrated roles of environment and genetics. *Journal of Nutrition, 134,* 2090S-2105S.

Tate, D. F., Jeffery, R. W., Sherwood, N. E., & Wing, R. R. (2007). Long-term weight losses associated with prescription of higher physical activity goals. Are higher levels of physical activity protective against weight regain? *American Journal of Clinical Nutrition, 85,* 954–959.

Teitelbaum, P., & Epstein, A. N. (1962). The lateral hypothalamic syndrome: recovery of feeding and drinking after lateral hypothalamic lesions. *Psychological Review, 69,* 74–90.

Thornton-Jones, Z. D., Vickers, S. P., & Clifton, P. G. (2005). The cannabinoid CB1 receptor antagonist SR141716A reduces appetitive and consummatory responses for food. *Psychopharmacology, 179,* 452–460.

Townsend, M. S. (2006). Obesity in Low Income Communities: Prevalence, Effects, a Place to Begin. *Journal of the American Dietetic Association, 106,* 34–37.

US Department of Agriculture, Farm Service Agency (2005). Tobacco Transition Payment Program. Retrieved August 23, 2007 from http://www.fsa.usda.gov/Internet/FSA_File/ttppfinalrule.pdf

Wadden, T. A., Berkowitz, M. D., Womble, L. G., Sarwer, D. B., Phelan, S., Cato, R., Hesson, L. A., Osei, S. Y., Kaplan, R., Stunkard, A. J. (2005). Randomized trial of lifestyle modification and pharmacotherapy for obesity. *New England Journal of Medicine, 353,* 2111–2120.

Wing, R. R., & Hill, J. O. (2001). Successful weight loss maintenance. *Annual Review of Nutrition, 21,* 323–341.

INDEX